Routledge International Handbook of Food Studies

Over the past decade there has been a remarkable flowering of interest in food and nutrition, both within the popular media and in academia. Scholars are increasingly using foodways, food systems and eating habits as a new unit of analysis within their own disciplines, and students are rushing into classes and formal degree programs focused on food.

Introduced by the editor and including original articles by over 30 leading food scholars from around the world, *The Routledge International Handbook of Food Studies* offers students, scholars and all those interested in food-related research a one-stop, easy-to-use reference guide. Each article includes a brief history of food research within a discipline or on a particular topic, a discussion of research methodologies and ideological or theoretical positions, resources for research, including archives, grants and fellowship opportunities, as well as suggestions for further study. Each entry also explains the logistics of succeeding as a student and professional in food studies.

This clear, direct Handbook will appeal to those hoping to start a career in academic food studies as well as those hoping to shift their research to a food-related project. Strongly inter-disciplinary, this work will be of interest to students and scholars throughout the social sciences and humanities.

Ken Albala is Professor of History at the University of the Pacific in Stockton, California, where he teaches courses on the Renaissance and Reformation, Food History and the History of Medicine. He is the author of many books on food history including *Eating Right in the Renaissance* (University of California Press, 2002), *Food in Early Modern Europe* (Greenwood Press, 2003), *Cooking in Europe 1250–1650 (Greenwood Press, 2005), The Banquet: Dining in the Great Courts of Late Renaissance Europe* (University of Illinois Press, 2007), *Beans: A History* (Berg, 2007, winner of the 2008 International Association of Culinary Professionals Jane Grigson Award) and Pancake (Reaktion Press, 2008). He has coauthored two cookbooks: *The Lost Art of Real Cooking* (Penguin/Perigee, 2010) and *The Lost Arts of Hearth and Home* (Penguin, 2012). He has also edited the 4 volume *Food Cultures of the World Encyclopedia* (ABC-CLIO, 2010) and co-edits the journal *Food, Culture and Society*.

Routledge International Handbook of Food Studies

Edited by
Ken Albala

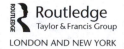

LONDON AND NEW YORK

First published in paperback 2014

First Published 2013
by Routledge
2 Park Square, Milton Park, Abingdon, Oxon OX14 4RN

and by Routledge
711 Third Avenue, New York, NY 10017

Routledge is an imprint of the Taylor & Francis Group, an informa business

British Library Cataloguing in Publication Data
A catalogue record for this book is available from the British Library

Library of Congress Cataloging-in-Publication Data
Routledge international handbook of food studies / edited by Ken Albala. – 1st ed.
    p. cm.
  Includes bibliographical references and index.
  1. Nutritional anthropology. 2. Food–Research. I. Albala, Ken, 1964–
  GN407.R88 2012
  394.1′2–dc23
              2012003797

ISBN: 978-0-415-78264-7 (hbk)
ISBN: 978-1-138-01949-2 (pbk)
ISBN: 978-0-203-81922-7 (ebk)

Typeset in Bembo by
Taylor & Francis Books

Printed and bound in the United States of America by
Edwards Brothers Malloy

Contents

Contents

Contributors

Julia Abramson teaches French and food studies at the University of Oklahoma. She is the author of the books *Learning from Lying: Paradoxes of the Literary Mystification* (2005) and *Food Culture in France* (2007), and she has published articles on topics including print representations of meat carving in Europe, the aesthetics and ethics of vegetable sculpture in contemporary society, vegetarianism in France, and the politics of French Empire gastronomic writing and the work of Grimod de la Reynière. Abramson is currently writing a new book, while also realizing, in cooperation with the Smithsonian Institution, the Oklahoma Humanities Council, and organizations throughout the state of Oklahoma, a project to engage public debate about food history and contemporary food culture.

Ken Albala is Professor of History at the University of the Pacific in Stockton, California, where he teaches courses on the Renaissance and Reformation, Food History and the History of Medicine. He is the author of many books on food history including *Eating Right in the Renaissance* (University of California Press, 2002), *Food in Early Modern Europe* (Greenwood Press, 2003), *Cooking in Europe 1250–1650* (Greenwood Press, 2005), *The Banquet: Dining in the Great Courts of Late Renaissance Europe* (University of Illinois Press, 2007), *Beans: A History* (Berg, 2007, winner of the 2008 International Association of Culinary Professionals Jane Grigson Award), and *Pancake* (Reaktion Press, 2008). He has coauthored two cookbooks: *The Lost Art of Real Cooking* (Penguin/Perigee, 2010) and *The Lost Arts of Hearth and Home* (2012). He has also edited the four-volume *Food Cultures of the World Encyclopedia* (ABC-CLIO, 2010) and co-edits the journal *Food, Culture and Society*.

Alison Hope Alkon is an assistant professor of sociology at the University of the Pacific. She is co-editor of *Cultivating Food Justice: Race, Class and Sustainability* (MIT Press, 2011). Her first monograph, *Black White and Green: Farmers Markets Race and the Green Economy* is due out from UGA Press in 2013.

Anne C. Bellows is University Professor, Chair in Gender and Nutrition, Institute for Social Sciences in Agriculture, University of Hohenheim, Germany. She is a geographer and focuses on issues of: Food and nutrition security, human rights – especially the right to adequate food and nutrition, food sovereignty and systems, urban agriculture; taking an approach characterized by a gender and justice perspective and carried out in the context of local and global relationships and analysis.

Rachel Black is Assistant Professor of Gastronomy and coordinator of the Gastronomy Program at Boston University. Black is the author of *Porta Palazzo: The Ethnography of an Italian* *market* (2012) and editor of *Alcohol in Popular Culture: An Encyclopedia* (2010). Black's current research focuses on wine, culture, and economics.

Anne Bower recently retired from teaching English at Ohio State University-Marion. She is the author of *African American Foodways: Explorations of History and Culture* (University of Illinois Press, 2007; paperback edition 2009); *Reel Food: Essays on Food and Film* (Routledge, 2004); and *Recipes for Reading: Community Cookbooks, Stories, Histories* (University of Massachusetts Press, 1997), and has also published food and culture articles in *Gastronomica* and the *Journal of Popular Culture*. She now lives in rural Vermont, teaching tai chi, gardening, and cooking, writing fiction and creative nonfiction, but retaining an interest in food studies.

Anthony F. Buccini holds a PhD in Germanic Linguistics from Cornell University and is an Associate in the Department of Linguistics, University of Chicago. He has published on a variety of topics in historical linguistics, language contact, and dialectology, especially on Dutch and other Germanic languages, and on Romance languages. His most recent linguistic article is "Between pre-German and pre-English: the origin of Dutch," *Journal of Germanic Linguistics* (Special issue on Dutch between English and German), 2010. In the field of food history he has been a regular contributor to the annual Oxford Symposium on Food and Cookery since 2005, when he was awarded the Sophie Coe Prize in Food History for "Western Mediterranean Vegetable Stews and the Integration of Culinary Exotica" (published 2006 in *Authenticity in the Kitchen. Proceedings of the Oxford Symposium on Food and Cookery 2005*). His work in food studies employs linguistic methodologies and models as part of his approach to topics in Mediterranean culinary history; see, for example, his 2010 paper "The Anatolian Origins of the Words 'Olive' and 'Oil' and the Early History of Oleïculture" in *Food and Language. Proceedings of the Oxford Symposium on Food and Cookery 2009*. He is currently preparing a monograph on the history of olive oil.

Kima Cargill is Associate Professor of Psychology in the Interdisciplinary Arts and Sciences Program at the University of Washington, Tacoma. Her work sits at the intersection of psychoanalysis and cultural anthropology and focuses on food and culture. Her research has been published in *The Psychoanalytic Review, Psychoanalysis, Culture, and Society,* and *Food, Culture, and Society*, among other publications. Dr Cargill teaches graduate and undergraduate courses focusing on psychoanalysis and culture. Her courses include Freud and His Critics, Mental Illness Across Cultures, and the Psychology of Food and Culture. She has taught in Latin America, Asia, and Africa.

Janet Chrzan holds a PhD in physical/nutritional anthropology from the University of Pennsylvania. Her research explores the connections between social activities, nutritional intakes, and mother and child health outcomes in pregnant teens. She teaches a variety of courses in the Anthropology Department and School of Nursing including food and culture, nutritional anthropology, world hunger, and topics in medical anthropology.

Jonathan Deutsch, PhD, is Associate Professor of Culinary Arts at Kingsborough Community College, City University of New York, and of Public Health at the CUNY Graduate Center.

Robert Dirks is an Emeritus Professor of Anthropology at Illinois State University. He has conducted research in areas of both food and nutrition. His publications include papers in *American Anthropologist, Annual Review of Nutrition, Current Anthropology, Journal of Nutrition,* and *World Cultures*. His most recent publication is *Come & Get It! McDonaldization and the Disappearance of Local Food from a Central Illinois Community*.

Margot Finn has a PhD in American culture and teaches courses on food studies, mass media, and the liberal arts at the University of Michigan. Her writing has been published in the journal *Folklore Forum* and several anthologies, and she is currently working on a book based on her dissertation, *Aspirational Eating: Class Anxiety and the Rise of Food in Popular Culture*.

Joan Fitzpatrick is the author of *Food in Shakespeare: Early Modern Dietaries and the Plays* (Ashgate, 2007) and a dictionary entitled *Shakespeare and the Language of Food* (Continuum, 2010). She has also edited a collection of essays entitled *Renaissance Food from Rabelais to Shakespeare: Culinary Readings and Culinary Histories* (Ashgate, 2010) and is currently preparing an edition of three early modern dietaries for the Revels Companion Library Series (Manchester University Press).

Beth M. Forrest is Assistant Professor of Liberal Arts in the bachelors program at the Culinary Institute of America. Her work has appeared in *Food and Foodways*, *Gastronomica*, and *Food and Culture and Society*, among other publications.

David Grumett is Research Associate in the Faculty of Divinity in the University of Cambridge, UK. He is (with Rachel Muers) author of *Theology on the Menu: Asceticism, Meat and Christian Diet* (Routledge, 2010) and editor of *Eating and Believing: Interdisciplinary Essays on Theology and Vegetarianism* (T&T Clark, 2008). He has also produced several articles, chapters, and contributions to reference works on topics in food and theology.

Lisa Heldke is Professor of Philosophy and Sponberg Chair in Ethics at Gustavus Adolphus College. The author of *Exotic Appetites: Ruminations of a Food Adventurer* (Routledge), she is also the editor or co-editor of several books, including *Cooking, Eating, Thinking: Transformative Philosophies of Food* (Indiana). She co-edits *Food, Culture and Society* with Ken Albala, and is on the editorial team for the forthcoming *Encyclopedia of Agriculture and Food Ethics* (Springer). She is currently at work with fellow philosopher Ray Boisvert, on a manuscript entitled *Philosophers at Table*.

Carol Helstosky is an associate professor of history at the University of Denver, where she has taught European history since 1997. She is the author of *Garlic and Oil: Food and Politics in Italy* (2004), *Pizza: A Global History* (2008), and *Food Culture of the Mediterranean* (2009), as well as many articles on the subject of food history and Italian cultural history. She is currently writing a book on the relationship between art forgery and the development of the art market in modern Italy. She is also the editor for the forthcoming *Routledge History of Food*.

Amanda Hesser, a co-founder of food52.com, was named one of the 50 most influential women in food by *Gourmet*. As a longtime staffer at *The New York Times*, Hesser wrote more than 750 stories and was the food editor at the *Times Magazine*. She has written the award-winning books *Cooking for Mr. Latte* and *The Cook and the Gardener*, and edited the essay collection, *Eat, Memory*. Her last book, a *New York Times* bestseller and the winner of a James Beard award, is *The Essential New York Times Cookbook*. Hesser is a trustee of Awesome Food.

Gina Hunter, a cultural anthropologist, is an associate professor of anthropology at Illinois State University. Her geographic specialization is Brazil and areas of scholarly interest are women's reproductive health; anthropology of the body, gender, and health; food systems; and pedagogy. Her research articles have appeared in *Medical Anthropology: Cross-Cultural Studies in*

Health and Illness, Women's Healthcare International, and *Pedagogy: Critical Approaches to Teaching Literature, Language, Composition, and Culture*.

Frederick L. Kirschenmann, a longtime national and international leader in sustainable agriculture, shares an appointment as Distinguished Fellow for the Leopold Center for Sustainable Agriculture at Iowa State University and as President of Stone Barns Center for Food and Agriculture in Pocantico Hills, New York. He also continues to manage his family's 2,600-acre certified organic farm in south central North Dakota. He is a professor in the ISU Department of Religion and Philosophy and holds a doctorate in philosophy from the University of Chicago.

Emily Broad Leib is a lawyer and senior clinical fellow in the Harvard Law School Health Law and Policy Clinic. Emily works with nonprofit organizations and government agencies to recommend food laws and policies aimed at increasing access to healthy foods and assisting small farmers and producers in participating in food markets. She supervises Harvard Law students engaged in these projects and co-teaches a course entitled "Food: A Health Law and Policy Seminar."

Stefanie Lemke is a senior researcher at the Department Gender and Nutrition, Institute for Social Sciences in Agriculture, University of Hohenheim, Germany. For her Masters she studied nutrition sciences and home economics, taught in a holistic and integrative manner. During her PhD studies, situated within rural sociology, anthropology, and nutrition sciences, and successive research projects, she experienced the challenges and advantages of working in multidisciplinary settings. Besides her academic engagement she was a nutrition consultant for various private and public institutions. The focus of her current work includes food and nutrition security; sustainable livelihoods; local food systems; gender; the right to adequate food; qualitative, mixed methods; and rights-based approaches.

Vivian Liberman, MLA, is Training Manager at Sofitel Cartagena Santa Clara in Colombia.

Baylen J. Linnekin is a lawyer and food writer and is the founding executive director of the Washington, DC-based grassroots nonprofit Keep Food Legal. He has presented his research on street food, agricultural law, food safety, food advocacy, social media, teaching food law, food rights and the US Constitution, and other topics at academic conferences around the country.

Arthur Lizie is Associate Professor of Media Studies and Communication Technologies and Chair of the Department of Communication Studies at Bridgewater State University. He has also taught at the University of Gastronomic Sciences in Italy. His first book, *Dreaming the World: U2 Fans, Online Community, and Intercultural Communication*, was released in 2009. He is currently conducting research on the food film genre and writing a global history of smoked food.

Lucy M. Long is the author of *Culinary Tourism* (2004), *Regional American Food Culture* (2009), and numerous articles on foodways. She has a PhD in folklore, an MA in ethnomusicology and taught folklore, American studies, popular culture, international studies, and tourism at Bowling Green State University, Ohio. She also founded and directs the non-profit Center for Food and Culture, based in Ohio, which serves as an international networking clearinghouse on all aspects of food in order to promote a deeper understanding of the ways in which food connects us all.

William Alex McIntosh is a professor in the Department of Sociology and on the Interdisciplinary Faculty of Nutrition. He teaches courses on the sociology of food and nutrition and research methods at both the graduate and undergraduate levels. Recent papers include "Writing the Food Studies Movement: A Commentary" in the journal *Food, Culture, and Society*, "Determinants of Time Children Spend Eating at Fast Food and Sit-Down Restaurants – Further Explorations" in the *Journal of Nutrition Education and Behavior* and "Mothers and Meals: The Effects of Mothers' Meal Planning and Shopping Motivations on Children's Participation in Family Meals" in the journal *Appetite*.

Alice McLean is the author of *Aesthetic Pleasure in Twentieth-Century Women's Food Writing: The Innovative Appetites of M.F.K. Fisher, Alice B. Toklas, and Elizabeth David and Cooking in America, 1840–1945*. A specialist in the literature of food and women's studies, she earned her PhD in English from the University of California, Davis and received an Honors Teaching Fellowship from Sweet Briar College (2004–9).

Katherine M. Moore is an archaeologist in the American Section of the University of Pennsylvania Museum of Archaeology and Anthropology. She received her PhD from the University of Michigan in 1989, and studies the origins of pastoralists and specialized hunters using animal bones from archaeological sites and stable isotopes. She has done fieldwork on the prehistoric cultural ecology of food production in North America, South America, and Central Asia.

Deirdre Murphy is Associate Professor of Liberal Arts in the bachelors program of the Culinary Institute of America. She earned her PhD from the Department of American Studies at the University of Minnesota.

Sarah Murray is a doctoral student in media and cultural studies in the Department of Communication Arts at the University of Wisconsin-Madison. Her research broadly encompasses taste cultures, niche media identities, feminist television studies, the relationship between television and new media, and food and media. She has most recently published on gender and reality television and has additional forthcoming work on modern food television.

Travis Nygard is Assistant Professor of Art History at Ripon College in Wisconsin. He received his PhD from the Department of the History of Art and Architecture at the University of Pittsburgh, where his dissertation research focused on the visual culture of American agribusiness during the nineteenth and twentieth centuries. He has published articles on the visual culture of agribusiness, murals made from corn, and ancient Mayan art. He is currently studying the social history of wheat in America, along with the gastronomist Kelly O'Leary.

Fabio Parasecoli is Associate Professor and Coordinator of Food Studies at the New School in New York City. His research focuses on the intersections among food, media, and politics. He is program advisor at Gustolab, a center for food and culture in Rome, and collaborates with other institutions such as the Universitat Oberta de Catalunya in Barcelona (Spain), the University of Gastronomic Sciences in Pollenzo (Italy), and ALMA Graduate School at the University of Bologna. Among his recent publications are *Food Culture in Italy* (2004), the introduction to *Culinary Cultures in Europe* (the Council of Europe, 2005) and *Bite me! Food in Popular Culture* (2008). He is general editor with Peter Scholliers of the six-volume *Cultural History of Food* (2012).

Thomas Piontek is Assistant Professor of English and Gender Studies at Shawnee State University in Portsmouth, Ohio. He is the author of *Queering Gay and Lesbian Studies* (Illinois University

Press, 2006) as well as articles, book chapters, reviews, and reference materials on film, popular culture, history, literature, and pedagogy.

Janet Poppendieck is Professor of Sociology at Hunter College, City University of New York. She is the author of *Free for All: Fixing School Food in America* (University of California Press, 2010), *Sweet Charity? Emergency Food and the End of Entitlement* (Penguin, 1999), and *Breadlines Knee Deep in Wheat: Food Assistance in the Great Depression* (Rutgers University Press, 1985).

Helen Rosner is an editor, writer, and occasional photographer. Currently the senior web editor at *Saveur*, she has formerly been an editor of *New York Magazine*'s restaurant blog *Grub Street*, a founding editor of the website EatMeDaily.com, and a cookbook editor.

Arlene Spark is Professor and Program Director of Public Health Nutrition at Hunter College and the Graduate Center at the City University of New York. She worked in pediatric preventive cardiology at the American Health Foundation and for more than 25 years has taught nutrition at the university level, including 12 years at New York Medical College. Since 1998, Dr Spark has been an associate professor at Hunter College and coordinator of the college's nutrition programs. She is also acting co-director of the Program in Urban Public Health. In 2007, CRC Press published her book – *Nutrition in Public Health: Principles, Policies, and Practice*.

Deborah Valenze is Professor of History at Barnard College, Columbia University, where she teaches courses on the history of food and early modern European history. She is the author of *Milk: A Local and Global History* (Yale University Press, 2011), and several books and articles on British social and cultural history. She is currently working on a project on food and the natural world in eighteenth-century Britain.

Jessica Walker is a first year PhD student in American studies. She received her BA from Bowdoin College in anthropology and gender and women's studies in 2009. Jessica's research interests focus on exploring the relationship between black women and their preparation, cooking, and consumption of "soul food." Other interests include material culture, black feminist anthropology, linguistic anthropology, and feminist theory.

Elizabeth Williams is a founder and President of the Southern Food and Beverage Museum in New Orleans, having always been fascinated by the way the lure of nutmeg and peppercorns motivated the exploration of the world. She is also a member of the adjunct faculty in the Food Studies Program at New York University. Much of her research and writing centers on the legal and policy issues related to food and foodways. Her book, *The A–Z Encyclopedia of Food Controversies and the Law* was published by Greenwood Publishing in January, 2011. She was for six years President and CEO of the University of New Orleans Foundation. Prior to the UNO Foundation, Williams was Director of the Arts Administration Program at the University of New Orleans. A graduate of Louisiana State University and Louisiana State University Law Center, she has served in the US Army as a Judge Advocate General (JAG). She has practiced law in Washington, DC and Louisiana. She is a member of the Folklife Commission, State of Louisiana.

Psyche Williams-Forson is Associate Professor of American Studies at the University of Maryland College Park and an affiliate faculty member of the women's studies and African

American studies departments and the Consortium on Race, Gender, and Ethnicity. She is co-editor of *Taking Food Public: Redefining Foodways in a Changing World and Building Houses Out of Chicken Legs: Black Women, Food, and Power* (2006). Her new research explores the role of the value store as an immediate site of food acquisition and the role of African-American women in underground economies in the late nineteenth and early twentieth centuries.

Introduction

Food studies is not exactly a new academic field. Scholars have been discussing food as long as there have been academic institutions of higher learning in the Western tradition, if not longer. However, it is only in the past 20 years or so that a critical mass of professional academics have devoted a signficant proportion of their energy to questions of food supply, patterns of eating, in fact, all aspects of food culture or foodways. The emergence of a field, if not perhaps a discipline, is signaled by regular conferences, academic journals, monograph series and encyclopedias as well as a permanent place in the curriculum, either within traditional disciplines or as proper food studies programs. By all these measures food studies is a thriving scholarly field, though defining it precisely is still a matter of lively debate.

Given the popularity of food courses and an ever-increasing number of scholars turning their attention to food, this Handbook is designed to offer some definition, to trace the many methodologies and theoretical positions that food scholars have employed and to provide sign-posts for the future. It is designed as a practical guide for students entering graduate programs as well as scholars in many disciplines hoping to jump on the food studies bandwagon. It is also for those still wondering what exactly is food studies, who does it and how. Leading scholars across a wide array of disciplines have written concise chapters outlining the most significant publications, prospects for future research as well as the meat and potatoes details, pardon the metaphor, of how to become a food scholar, such as resources, programs and job prospects.

Marshaling these chapters into a coherent whole has been a challenge, partly because there is not yet a comprehensive list of what disciplines belong in food studies. The chapters here consist primarily of those disciplines and interdisciplinary topics that have thus far garnered attention, but should by no means be considered exhaustive. For example anthropologists, sociologists and historians have been studying food for several generations. Newer fields such as communications as well as much older ones such as philosophy are now well represented among food scholarship, but not others, such as political science. In the end, most of the traditional humanities and social sciences boast numerous outstanding classics on food. These interact and borrow from other disciplines in ways that portend the emergence of a proper discipline of food studies, in much the same way gender studies or American studies have become academic departments in their own right. When job openings for food studies scholars proliferate, we will be certain that the discipline has arrived. For the moment, however, it is still most prudent for scholars to maintain a traditional disciplinary homebase to conduct research on food, hence the structure and scope of this Handbook, divided as it is, in ways that perhaps obscure the extremely interdisciplinary nature of this field.

The descision to omit most of the food sciences, with the exception of nutrition, was made simply because most biologists, food chemists and other scientists do not yet participate in the dialogue of critical food studies. Someday, we hope, that will change; humanists will address the discourse of science and scientists will better use the work of their colleagues in other disciplines. There are optimistic signs that this is beginning to happen, as the chapters here show.

Each chapter is written using the particular conventions of the discipline, especially in matters bibliographic. This seemed advisable, rather than force a single stylistic model onto the entire book. This way readers will see not only what each discipline says about food studies, but the format they use as well.

The unavoidable overlap among the chapters also points to a real strength in food studies. No food scholars work in a specialized niche cut off from colleagues in other disciplines. Taking account of work in other departments is absolutely necessary and it is often surprisingly refreshing to find colleagues working on similar questions stretched across several different disciplines. For many of us, food studies has become a welcoming home, one which we hope, especially after using this Handbook, you will join.

Ken Albala
University of the Pacific

Social sciences

The anthropology of food

Robert Dirks and Gina Hunter

In this chapter on the anthropology of food, the authors examine eating and drinking as social and cultural experiences. From the earliest anthropological considerations of food to major recent works, the chapter provides an overview of how anthropologists have approached the study of food and culture. Seminal works for major theoretical approaches are discussed and new areas of research are identified. Conveying the breadth of anthropology, the authors discuss the role of cooking in human evolution, archaeological investigations of feasting, historical studies of global commodity trade, and in-depth studies of the foodways of particular communities among other topics. The authors state that anthropological research on food is distinguished by a commitment to holistic perspectives, dedication to comparative methods, and an abiding concern for origins and primal causes. Each of these defining characteristics is described via recent examples from the literature. Although few programs or funding opportunities designated specifically for food anthropology exist, the authors present a number of valuable research tools, data sets, and internet resources available to interested scholars.

Anthropologists study food from different perspectives. Some look at eating and drinking in connection with other aspects of social life. Others are concerned with dietary matters and how food-related practices and beliefs affect physical well-being. These two points of view, referred to respectively as "the Anthropology of Food" and "Nutritional Anthropology," need to be considered together if one wants a truly complete picture of a food culture. However, for the purposes of this book we limit our concern in this chapter to eating and drinking as social and cultural experiences. Major topics explored within this tradition have included the foodways of particular peoples and regions; the dynamics of various food systems; the cultural effects of ancient foodways; the ethnohistory of specific commodities; food-habit formation and change; the sociocultural effects of food shortage; food-related beliefs, rituals, and symbols; eating habits and etiquettes; and systems of food classification and meal structure. Our review highlights common threads among these studies.

Historical background and major theoretical approaches

The anthropology of food has deep roots. E. B. Tylor (1865), the world's first professional anthropologist, planted the seeds when he worked to establish the fact (disputed at the time) that cooking qualified as a human universal. Colonel John Bourke (1885) wrote the anthropology of food's first dedicated paper, "The Urine Dance of the Zuni Indians of New Mexico" 20 years later. Inspired by his own ethnographic observations, the paper probed, as more recent anthropological studies have (e.g., MacClancy, Henry, and Macbeth, 2007), the very definition of edibility. Bourke invoked a historical explanation for the Zuni's ritualized ingestion of "vile aliment" by theorizing it was a cultural survival, a relic of what in the past must have been an occasionally necessary behavior for want of water. Robertson Smith, an Old Testament scholar and contemporary of Bourke, also wrote about food but without his penchant for speculative history. Regarding his own particular subject, Semitic sacrifice and sacrificial meals, Smith (1889) found meaning in their social functions.

Functionalist ideas dominated by the time a deliberate, programmatic anthropology of food debuted. Audrey Richards (1932, 1939), a student of theoretician Bronislaw Malinowski, led the way while working with nutritionists on a study of the Bemba of East Africa. Richards's observations focused on tribal social relationships and how they served nutritional needs. Her work and that of several like-minded investigators, including Raymond Firth (1934) and Meyer and Sonia Fortes (1936), produced robust accounts of food production, distribution, preparation, and consumption, including the many beliefs and rituals attached to each activity. Meanwhile, anthropologists in the United States turned to psychology for inspiration and began investigating the effects of child rearing, including feeding practices, on adult behavior (e.g., DuBois, 1941; Whiting and Child, 1953). Research took a decidedly practical turn and became more nutritionally oriented during the latter years of the Great Depression and throughout the Second World War. Still, there were theoretical benefits, including some understanding of how food habits changed (see Montgomery and Bennett, 1979).

Ecological thinking captivated general anthropology after the war. By the 1960s, this elevated food-related studies to a position of central importance within the field as a whole. Ethnographies about communities in virtually every corner of the world focused on the acquisition, sharing, and redistribution of food, exposing a generation of undergraduates to narratives about foodways in such faraway places as the Kalahari Desert (Lee, 1979) and the New Guinea Highlands (Rappaport, 1968). A number of investigators, most famously Marvin Harris (1966, 1977, 1985) and his collaborators (Harris and Ross, 1978, 1987), built their reputations on ecological explanations for the food preferences, taboos, and customary feasts of various peoples around the world.

Anthropologists more inclined to see culture as a manifestation of shared mentalities rather than as a reflection of practical necessities attracted substantial followings as well. Claude Levi-Strauss (1969, 1973, 1978) used ideas about food and cooking to develop his immensely influential structuralist theory, a set of ideas about the principles of cultural representation. Mary Douglas (1966), working independently but also seeking to understand representation, studied notions of purity, pollution, and taboo. Her analysis, based on a reading of Old Testament proscriptions, led to the conclusion that food taboos were all about categorical identities and symbolic boundaries.

A polemic developed – cultural ecologists and economic analysts (together referred to as materialists) on one side, structuralists on the other. Partisans engaged in fierce debates, but three books published in the 1980s quieted the controversy, in large part because of their eclecticism. The first two, Jack Goody's (1982) *Cooking, Cuisine and Class* and Sidney Mintz's (1985) *Sweetness and Power*, reintroduced food anthropologists to history and used it to show how both material conditions and symbolic representations changed over time. Goody's book revolved around the distinction between high and low cuisines. He explained why the difference exists in some societies and not in others by using comparative history as a framework for sociological and cultural analysis. Mintz's volume traced the history of sugar from luxury good to basic commodity. His narrative, focused on England, attended to changes in symbolic meanings, and sketched the nutritional functionalities behind the transformation. Ultimately, however, Mintz explained England's outsized commitment to sugar as a consequence of past economic and political events.

As food anthropologists were becoming more attentive to history, a decidedly less formalistic concern with food symbols that had been brewing for a decade or more crystallized in Mary Weismantel's (1988) *Food, Gender, and Poverty in the Ecuadorian Andes* and a number of other works (Kahn, 1986; Munn, 1986; Pollock, 1985). Weismantel focused on Zumbagua, a parish of mostly indigenous Ecuadorians. Through an exploration of their culture, her readers learned that diet, cuisine, talk about food, and kitchen routines all mattered. All contributed to a better understanding of Andean culinary history; current ecological and economic crises; changing cultural and political allegiances; categorical differences between men and women, old and young; and conflicts between traditional and modern ways.

Identity (national, ethnic, gender, generational) became a resounding theme within the anthropology of food. Clever variations abounded. Carol Counihan (2004), for example, recorded the life histories of the members of a single Florentine family, showing how extended family and gender relations became realized through food-related work and commensality. However, by the end of the millennium the food and identity theme had become well-worn and vulnerable to criticism. Jeremy MacClancy (2004: 63–64) suggested that too often anthropologists relied on vague, singular, and static notions of identity. Jon Holtzman (2009: 60) wondered if food itself harbors qualities that make it an especially cogent means of identification or whether Westerners simply nominated it as such. David Sutton (2001: 170) tried to move past the idea that food "symbolizes" identities. Examining the ways eating and drinking structure daily and ritual events on the Greek Island of Kalymnos, he found that food conveys memories and in so doing engenders and maintains historical consciousness. Holtzman (2009) came to a similar conclusion among the Samburu of Northern Kenya. There he documented dietary changes brought about by economic development, a decreasing commitment to a pastoral lifestyle, and an increasing dependence on "town food." The Samburu talked about these changes with contradiction and ambivalence, but it struck Holtzman that their foods had become important references for thinking about their predicament and key loci for historical consciousness.

Research methodologies

Anthropologists have studied food-related practices and beliefs from nearly every conceivable angle. This makes it difficult at times to tell what is distinctive about their discipline. However, certain ways of thinking pervade the enterprise and affect its methods. These traits include a commitment to holistic perspectives, dedication to comparative methods, and an abiding concern for origins and primal causes (cf., Anderson, 2005: 240–41).

Holistic perspectives

Anthropology's holism makes it a kind of synthetic discipline. Unlike analytic fields (e.g. economics) in the business of breaking phenomena down, anthropologists are more inclined to fit things together. Ecologists rely on essentially the same method: take disparate observations and ideas and show how they relate as components of a larger system. Previous generations of anthropologists who studied foodways in small-scale societies often came away with impressively comprehensive accounts that explicitly showed how eating and drinking were part of their subjects' domestic, economic, political, and spiritual lives. In addition to several of the works cited above, Rosemary

Firth's (1966) monograph about Malay peasants, Michael Young's (1971) work on the Goodenough Islands, L.C. Okere's (1983) and O.A. Anigbo's (1987) writings about the Nigerian Igbo, and Mick Johnsson's (1988) account of the Aymara of Bolivia immediately come to mind.

As anthropologists increasingly began to turn their attention to large-scale societies, food anthropologists followed suit. Investigators produced comprehensive accounts of foodways among minority groups (e.g., Goode, Theophano, and Curtis, 1984; Goode, Curtis, and Theophano, 1984; Gutierrez, 1984, 1992), residents of urban areas (e.g., Flynn, 2005a, 2005b), and members of local organizations (e.g., Curran, 1989). Theodore Bestor's *Tsukiji: The Fish Market at the Center of the World* (2004) tackled one of Japan's most famous alimentary institutions. Chapters on Tsukiji's place in Japanese history and the world economy set the stage. Descriptions of the role of fish in contemporary Japanese culture, the intricacies of Tsukiji's auctions, and the social relations among market participants come together to shed light on the otherwise dimly understood transactions that bring much of the world's fresh tuna to the consumers' table.

In addition to studying communities and organizations, food anthropologists have looked carefully at national and regional food systems. Colonel Bourke, shortly after his study of the Zuni, wrote anthropology's first regional study, "The Folk Foods of the Rio Grande Valley and of Northern Mexico" (1895). It offered a purely descriptive account of the traditional foods of the Mexican-American border region, which at that time was *terra incognita* as far as most Americans were concerned. Current works attend to systemic processes and institutions with widespread involvements. Edward Fischer and Peter Benson (2006), for instance, investigated Guatemalan broccoli imported into the United States. Broccoli epitomized middle-class American concerns with "eating right" but represented a new, export crop for Mayan farmers. Fischer and Benson described the networks binding American consumers to Mayan farmers and examined what compelled broccoli farming under extremely risky circumstances. Richard Wilk's (2006) work on Belizian foodways combined ethnographic, archaeological, and historical data to show how global processes produce local culinary traditions. Curiously, Wilk discovered that the most consistent local element in Belizean food culture is an appreciation of foods from other countries. At the national and regional levels, the foodways of extinct civilizations are also part of the Anthropology of Food's stock and trade. Assyriologist Jean Bottero's book, *The Oldest Cuisine in the World* (2004), recently attracted attention by combining archaeology with information gleaned from cuneiform inscriptions to describe the food culture of ancient Mesopotamia in considerable detail. Such comprehensive accounts usually require a cooperative approach. John Staller and Michael Carrasco, for example, collected papers about Mesoamerican foods from 25 regional experts, drawn from a variety of anthropological sub-fields and neighboring disciplines, including archaeology, ethnohistory, ethnography, ethnobotany, linguistics, ceramics, mythology, icono-graphy, and epigraphy. Published as *Pre-Columbian Foodways in Mesoamerica* (2010), a volume of nearly 700 pages, the collection surveyed production, distribution, redistribution, and consumption, projecting for the first time a truly big picture of Mesoamerica's ancient food system and key institutions. Overviews of modern national and regional foodways, though not nearly so inclusive as *Pre-Columbian Foodways*, have been compiled for the US (Brown and Mussell, 1984; Humphrey and Humphrey, 1988), the Middle East (Zubaida and Tapper, 1994), South Asia (Khare and Rao, 1986), and Oceania (Kahn and Sexton, 1988; Manderson, 1986; Pollock, 1992).

Comparative methods

Anthropology lays claim to global expertise based on its meticulous attention to the remains of the past coupled with its long-standing engagement with present-day populations from every corner of the earth, living in every kind of society imaginable. Data acquired worldwide, and even from the observations of non-human primates, pave the way for comparative studies as a means for testing ideas.

Case comparisons

Comparative studies range from simple to complex. Case comparisons, the simplest sort, are regularly used to support or debunk assertions based on the study of a single instance. Sidney Mintz (1985), for instance, sought to clinch his argument about the importance of political economy in promoting sugar in England by writing a final chapter comparing and contrasting its political and economic history with that of France, a nation never so committed to sugar as its neighbor across the channel. Using multiple case studies, Robert Dirks (1980) lent credence to Colin Turnbull's (1972) ethnographic account of the Ik, an African group ravaged by famine. Critics had found the depravities reported by Turnbull hard to believe (see *Current Anthropology*, Volume 15: 99–102; Volume 16: 343–58). Dirks marshaled more than a dozen accounts of food emergencies worldwide revealing similar responses to famine elsewhere in the world.

Controlled comparisons

In the controlled comparison, another anthropological standby, cases are selected based on the presence or absence of some particular trait. Jack Goody's (1982) aforementioned *Cooking, Cuisine and Class* relied on this approach. Goody lined up societies that distinguish between high and low cuisines on one side, societies that make no such distinction on the other, and asked: "Are there differences between the two sets that might explain their contrasting conceptions?" In a similar vein, Dietler and Hayden (2001) assembled numerous archaeological and ethnographic examples of ceremonial feasting from around the world and compared them to find consistencies. Their research revealed that institutionalized feasting has functioned worldwide to force surplus production. Feasting has contributed to the emergence of social inequity, has served to validate status, and has been associated with the production of prestige goods, including specialty foods (Hayden, 2001: 24).

Holocultural studies

Cross-cultural or so-called "holocultural" studies, the most complex of anthropology's comparative methodologies, depend on data from a large sample of societies to subject hypotheses to statistical tests. The first such study within the anthropology of food tested the theory that fluctuations in food supply helped explain annual rituals of conflict (Dirks, 1988) and looked at food supply in connection with the incidence of warfare (Ember and Ember, 1992) and the cultural value placed on social cooperation (Poggie, 1995). Subsequent research has examined food supply and storage in relation to the development of counting (Divale, 1999) and cultural attitudes toward salt (Parman, 2002).

Origins and primal causes

Anthropology's concern with human origins and the roots of social and cultural life sustains paleoanthropology, drives inquiries regarding animal and plant domestication, and inspires researchers' efforts to better understand human nature. In top-notch works like Bestor's *Tsukiji* (2004), the essential character of *Homo sapiens* is ultimately at issue. At one level, the book seems little more than a colorful tour of a curious institution. The author's deeper purpose, however, is to challenge conventional economic theory and formalistic conceptions about how markets work.

Addressing human nature from another angle, anthropological studies of food habits and dietary patterns have figured prominently in models of evolution. The "Man-the-Hunter" hypothesis, originated in the 1960s, maintained that the genus *Homo* evolved from a population of Australopithecines on account of greater reliance on tools, more aggressive predation, and increased meat consumption. More recently, Richard Wrangham (2009) proposed that while meat eating may have given impetus to the evolution of *Homo habilis* some 2.5 million years ago, the subsequent emergence of *Homo erectus* and the eventual development of *Homo sapiens* depended on the control of fire and the invention of cooking. Pre-digestion through the application of heat would explain observed reductions in chewing apparatus, increases in cranial capacity, and other anatomical changes. Socioculturally, it elucidates behavioral and organizational transformations inferred by comparing humans with other primates. Cooking, as Wrangham sees it, explains the emergence of relatively stable mating patterns and the sexual division of labor, particularly with regard to the universal predominance of females in the kitchen. His arguments cannot be substantiated by direct archaeological evidence because of the ephemeral nature of a camp fire, but by weaving together knowledge from a variety of fields, including biochemistry, nutrition, anatomy, physiology, zoology, primatology, evolutionary ecology, prehistory, history, ethnography, ethnology, economic anthropology, sociology, and time-motion studies, Wrangham constructs a plausible model.

Social and cultural anthropologists too have used multidisciplinary approaches to address some of the anthropology of food's bigger issues. Symposia organized by the International Commission on the Anthropology of Food and Nutrition (ICAF) periodically address such seminal topics as the dynamics of food sharing, the development of food preferences, and the relationship between food and status. In a resulting publication, *Food and the Status Quest* (Wiessner and Schiefenhovel, 1996), co-editor Polly Wiessner (1996) summarized what the various disciplines brought to the table. The primatologists indicated just how deep status seeking and rank formation is to the human phylogeny and laid down a baseline against which science can measure the effects of human culture. Archaeological papers put the status quest as expressed through food in a temporal perspective and underscored the influence of status-related food concerns on the production of food and drink and in driving social evolution. Ethnologists familiar with particular cultures in different parts of the world reported on a variety of food transactions and their effects on status. Taken together, their papers revealed a considerable measure of cultural pliability. Still, societies universally honor givers above receivers, and humans appear deeply and irrepressibly determined to affect status by alimentary means.

Avenues for future research

The anthropology of food will continue to explore a number of familiar areas in the years ahead. The social crises caused by migrants and the introduction of their foods has been a favorite topic in the past. Recent attention to the strengthening of old traditions in communities hosting newly arrived immigrants (Garine *et al.*, n.d.: 10) represents a new direction for research and suggests other viewpoints yet to be explored. Anthropologists still have much to contribute to the history of globalization from the perspective of local communities. In recent years, the challenge that industrial homogenization presents to the local specialty food and craft producers has engaged a number of anthropologists (e.g., Heath and Meneley, 2007; Terrio, 2000), but much remains to be done to better our understanding of the culture of niche foods. Studies of the role of food in marking ethnic, regional, and national identity remain popular, and signs of increasing theoretical sophistication bode well for their future.

The first steps have been taken in new directions. A quick review of recent doctoral dissertations shows few studies focused on the travels of particular food items and greater concern with how food preparation and consumption creates a sense of place and cultivates specific tastes. Investigations of taste may offer a rich avenue for exploring "food as food" (Holtzman, 2009), particularly if they include its physiological, emotional, aesthetic, class, and other socially relevant dimensions. The locavore movement and other reactions to globalization are fertile areas for future investigation, especially as energy and commodity prices increase to the point of altering the current economics of food trade. Anthropologists' grasp on food-related symbols and meanings and the structural aspects of food systems positions them well to consider the social consequences of economic change as well as issues of sustainability and food safety. Given the tremendous popularity in the US of cooking programming on television, celebrity chefs, and food-centered blogs, future investigators might also give more attention to culinary performance and the media as an arena of investigation.

The anthropology of food will become more quantitative in the future. Currently, the literature contains little numerical data and even less statistical analysis. This could hardly be otherwise in a field dominated by cultural anthropologists, many of whom dismiss quantitative research as narrowly conceived. Cultural anthropologists often maintain that a well-conceived qualitative study stands on its own. Ellen Messer (2004: 181–82) disputes this and indeed faults two otherwise well-regarded anthropologies of food, James Watson's (1997) study of McDonald's restaurants in the Far East and Richard Wilk's (2006) culinary history of Belize, as being too insular and disconnected from important themes in nutritional anthropology and other areas of food studies. Pressure on food anthropologists to broaden their methodological horizons and report such basics as how frequently foods are eaten is likely to increase in the future, particularly as standards of evidence and demands on accountability increase.

Practical considerations

Funding

The best way to secure support from funders is to investigate topics they see as socially relevant. MacBeth and MacClancy (2004: 4) refer to an environment of "hard-nosed pragmatism." It began in the UK during the 1990s, spread to the rest of Europe, and now prevails worldwide. Gone for the most part are the days of post-modernism when anthropologists had the luxury of contemplating the literary aspects of their work. In today's world, nutritional anthropology rates as more relevant than the anthropology of food. Nevertheless, studies of food ideologies, cultures of consumption, food disorders, agricultural organization, and McDonaldization remain in demand (MacBeth and MacClancy, 2004: 4).

No agency devotes itself exclusively to promoting the anthropology of food. However, the Wenner-Gren Foundation, which funds research in all branches of anthropology, has awarded dozens of food-related research grants over the past decade. Recently funded projects include studies of urban food markets and networks in Madrid; blood, food and sociality in Iran; longitudinal studies of health transition and culture change in Vanuatu; and the identities of millet versus rice consumers in Neolithic Northern China (www.wennergren.org/grantees).

The majority of food anthropologists hold teaching posts and conduct research on a part-time basis. The ordinary costs involved are absorbed primarily by the institutions that employ them. However, when it comes to big-ticket items, such as research trips far from home, investigators usually find it necessary to apply to various funding agencies for grants. Theodore Bestor's (2004: xix–xxi) support for *Tsukiji* appears typical. It materialized in bits and pieces, paying for research trips and teaching appointments over a period of 14 years. Bestor acknowledges the Japan Foundation, the US Department of Education Fulbright Program, the Joint Committee on Japanese Studies of the American Council of Learned Societies and the Social Science Research Council, the National Science Foundation, the New York Sea Grant Institute, and some ten other organizations.

Programs

Academic programs having to do primarily with the anthropology of food are few and far between. Indiana University offers the only PhD students select among anthropology's four major subfields (archaeology, biological anthropology, linguistics, and sociocultural anthropology) and take additional courses in food and nutrition. The School of Oriental and African Studies at the University of London has organized an MA program in the anthropology of food. Full-time students undertake a year of continuous study, using break periods to read and prepare coursework. The program focuses on the study of famine and the role of food aid in nutritionally insecure regions. At New Mexico State University, graduate students in anthropology can minor in food studies.

Research tools

One of the most important tools for anthropological research are the Human Relations Area Files. The files consists of full-text ethnographic and historical accounts of nearly 400 societies around the world, providing ready information about a great variety of cultures. A system of detailed, standardized indexing allows users to pull out facts about foods and other aspects of culture quickly and in its original context. Access to the Human Relations Area Files, either on microfiche or on the web (as the eHRAF Collection of Ethnography) is through member libraries. The more recently developed eHRAF Collection of Archaeology provides readily accessible information about prehistoric populations.

Robert Freedman's monumental, two-volume *Human Food Uses: A Cross-Cultural, Comprehensive Annotated Bibliography* (1981, 1983) constitutes another exceedingly valuable research tool. It lists and describes nearly every scholarly publication about food and every paper about food consumption presented at the annual meetings of the American Anthropological Association over a period of approximately 100 years. Other valuable bibliographies include Christine Wilson's (1979) *Food-Custom and Nurture: An Annotated Bibliography on Sociocultural and Biocultural Aspects of Nutrition* and Robert Dirks's *World Food Habits* (see below).

Data sets

Holocultural studies rely for the most part on a data set known as the Standard Cross–Cultural Sample (SCCS). Its development began in 1957 when Yale anthropologist George Murdock first published the World Ethnographic Sample, consisting of 565 cultures coded for 30 variables. Ten years later the sample contained 1,200 cultures coded for more than 100 variables. In 1969, Murdock and Douglas White developed the SCCS, consisting of 186 well-documented societies selected to represent a world sample of human experience and cultural expression. Currently, the SCCS is coded for more than 2,000 variables, including a large number having to do with subsistence, food supply, the division of labor, exchange and other forms of distribution, and child-rearing practices (see *World Cultures* [ISSN 1045-0564], a paper and internet journal).

Internet resources

The anthropology of food is represented on a handful of internet sites. For bibliographic references organized by region and topic, professionals and students alike turn to World Food Habits (www.foodhabits.info). Members of the American Anthropological Association's Society for Food and Nutrition have a blog site entitled Food Anthropology (foodanthro.wordpress.com) where members publicize their own research and comment on current issues. A network of European researchers maintain Anthropology of Food (aof.revues.org/index.html), an open-access web journal published in French and English since the early 1990s.

Scholarships and awards

The Society for the Anthropology of Food and Nutrition (SAFN) sponsors the annual Christine Wilson Award competition. Prizes are presented to the outstanding undergraduate and graduate research papers either in Nutritional Anthropology or the Anthropology of Foods.

Key reading

Anderson, E. N. (2005) *Everyone Eats: Understanding Food and Culture*. New York: New York University Press.

Anigbo, O. A. (1987) *Commensality and Human Relationship Among the Igbo*. Nsukka: University of Nigeria Press.

Bestor, T. C. (2004) *Tsukiji: The Fish Market at the Center of the World*. Berkeley: University of California Press.

Bottero, J. (2004) *The oldest cuisine in the world: Cooking in Mesopotamia*. Chicago, IL: University of Chicago Press.

Bourke, J. G. (1885) "The Urine Dance of the Zuni Indians of New Mexico." In *Annual Meeting of the American Association for the Advancement of Science*. Ann Arbor, MI.

——(1895) "The Folk Foods of the Rio Grande Valley and of Northern Mexico." *Journal of American Folklore* 8: 41–71.

Brown, L. K. and K. Mussell, eds. (1984) *Ethnic and Regional Foodways in the United States: the Performance of Group Identity*. Knoxville: University of Tennessee Press.

Counihan, C. M. (2004) *Around the Tuscan Table: Food, Family and Gender in Twentieth-Century Florence*. New York: Routledge Press.

Curran, P. (1989) *Grace Before Meals: Food Ritual and Body Discipline in Convent Culture*. Urbana: University of Illinois Press.

Dietler, M. and B. Hayden, eds. (2001) *Feasts: Archaeological and ethnographic perspectives on food, politics, and power*. Washington, DC: Smithsonian Institution Press.

Dirks, R. (1980) "Social Responses During Severe Food Shortage and Famine." *Current anthropology* 21: 21–44.

——(1988) "Annual rituals of conflict." *American Anthropologist* 90(4): 856–70.

——(n.d.) *World Food Habits Bibliography*. www.worldfoodhabits.info (accessed on April 18, 2012).

Divale, W. (1999) "Climatic instability, food storage, and the development of numerical counting: A cross-cultural study." *Cross-Cultural Research* 33(4): 341–68.

Douglas, M. (1966) *Purity and Danger: An Analysis of Concepts of Pollution and Taboo*. Baltimore, MD: Penguin Books.

DuBois, Cora (1941) "Food and Hunger in Alor." In *Language, Culture, and Personality: Essays in Memory of Edward Sapir*. L. L. Speir, A. I. Hallowell, and S. S. Newman, eds., pp. 272–81. Menasha: Sapir Memorial Publication Fund.

Ember, C. R. and M. Ember (1992) "Resource Unpredictability, Mistrust, and War: A Cross-Cultural Study." *Journal of Conflict Resolution* 36: 246–62.

Firth, R. (1934) "The sociological study of native diet." *Africa* 7(4): 401–14.

——(1966) *Housekeeping among Malay Peasants*. New York: Humanities Press.

Fischer, E. F. and P. Benson (2006) *Broccoli and Desire: Global Connections and Maya*. Stanford, CA: Stanford University Press.

Flynn, K. C. (2005a) *Food, Culture, and Survival in an African City*. New York: Palgrave Macmillan.

——(2005b) "Food, gender and survival among street adults in Mwanza, Tanzania." *Food and Foodways* 8(3): 175–201.

Fortes, M. and S. L. Fortes (1936) "Food in the domestic economy of the Talensi Africa". *Africa: Journal of the International African Institute* 9: 237–76.

Freedman, R. L. (1981) *Human Food Uses: A Cross-cultural, Comprehensive Annotated Bibliography*. Westport, CT: Greenwood.

——(1983) *Human Food Uses: A Cross-cultural, Comprehensive Annotated Bibliography: Supplement*. Westport, CT: Greenwood.

Garine, Igor de *et al.* (n.d.) *Nutrition and the Anthropology of Food*. IUAES Commission on the Anthropology of Food and Nutrition (ICAF).

Goode, J. G., K. Curtis, and J. Theophano (1984) "Meal Formats, Meal Cycles, and Menu Negotiations in the Maintenance of an Italian-American Community." In *Food in the Social Order*. M. Douglas, ed., pp. 143–218. New York: Russell Sage Foundation.

Goode, J. G., J. Theophano, and K. Curtis (1984) "A Framework for the Analysis of Continuity and Change in Shared Socio-Cultural Rules for Food Use: The Italian-American Pattern." In *Ethnic and Regional Foodways in the United States: The Performance of Group Identity*. L.K. Brown and K. Mussell, eds., pp. 66–88. Knoxville: University of Tennessee Press.

Goody, J. (1982) *Cooking, Cuisine and Class*. Cambridge: Cambridge University Press.

Gutierrez, C. P. (1984) "The Social and Symbolic Uses of Ethnic/Regional Foodways: Cajuns and Crawfish in South Louisiana." In *Ethnic and Regional Foodways in the United States: The Performance of Group Identity*. L.K. Brown and K. Mussell, eds., pp. 169–81. Knoxville: University of Tennessee Press.

——(1992) *Cajun Foodways*. Oxford: University of Mississippi Press.

Harris, M. (1966) "The cultural ecology of India's sacred cattle." *Current Anthropology* 7: 51–66.

——(1977) *Cannibals and Kings*. New York: Vintage.

——(1985) *The Sacred Cow and the Abominable Pig: Riddles of Food and Culture*. New York: Simon and Schuster.

Harris, M. and E. B. Ross (1978) "How Beef Became King." *Psychology Today* 12: 88–94.

——eds. (1987) *Food and Evolution: Toward a Theory of Human Food Habits*. Philadelphia, PA: Temple University Press.

Hayden, B. (2001) "Fabulous Feasts: A Prolegomenon to the Importance of Feasting." In *Feasts: Archaeological and Ethnographic Perspectives on Food Politics and Power*. M. Dietler and B. Hayden, eds., pp. 23–64. Washington, DC: Smithsonian Institution Press.

Heath, D. and A. Meneley (2007) "Techne, Technoscience, and the Circulation of Comestible Commodities: An Introduction." *American Anthropologist* 109(4): 593–602.

Holtzman, J. (2009) *Uncertain Tastes: Memory, Ambivalence and the Politics of Eating in Samburu, Northern Kenya*. Berkeley: University of California Press.

Humphrey, T. C. and L. T. Humphrey, eds. (1988) *"We Gather Together": Food and Festival in American Life*. Ann Arbor, MI: UMI.

Johnsson, M. (1988) *Food and Culture among the Bolivian Aymara*. Uppsala: Uppsala University Press.

Kahn, M. (1986) *Always Hungry, Never Greedy: Food and the Expression of Gender in a Melanesian Society*. Cambridge: Cambridge University Press.

Kahn, M. and L. Sexton (1988) "Continuity and Change in Pacific Foodways." In *Food and Foodways (special issue)* 3 (1–2).

Khare, R. S. and M. S. A. Rao, eds. (1986) *Aspects in South Asia Food Systems: Food, Society and Culture*. Durham, NC: Carolina Academy.

Lee, R. B. (1979) *The !Kung San: Men, Women and Work in a Foraging Society*. Cambridge and New York: Cambridge University Press.

Levi-Strauss, C. (1969) *The Raw and the Cooked*. New York: Harper & Row.

——(1973) *From Honey to Ashes*. New York: Harper & Row.

——(1978) *The Origin of Table Manners*. New York: Harper & Row.

Macbeth, H., ed. (1997) *Food Preferences and Tastes: Continuity and Change*. Oxford: Berghahn Books.

MacBeth, H. and J. MacClancy (2004) *Researching food habits*. Oxford: Berghahn Books.

MacClancy, J. (2004) "Food, identity, identification." In *Researching food habits*. H. Macbeth and J. MacClancy, eds., pp. 63–74. Oxford: Berghahn Books.

MacClancy, J., J. Henry, and H. Macbeth, eds. (2007) *Consuming the Inedible: Neglected Dimensions of Food Choice*. Oxford: Berghahn.

Manderson, L, ed. (1986) *Shared Wealth and Symbol: Food, Culture, and Society in Oceania and Southeast Asia.* New York: Cambridge University Press.

Messer, E. (2004) "Food, culture, political and economic identity: Revitalizing the food-systems perspective in the study of food-based identity." In *Researching food habits: Methods and problems.* H. Macbeth and J. MacClancy, eds., pp. 181–92. Oxford: Berghahn Books.

Mintz, S. (1985) *Sweetness and Power.* New York: Viking Penguin.

Mintz, S. and C. M. Du Bois (2002) "The Anthropology of Food and Eating." *Annual Review of Anthropology* 31: 99–119.

Montgomery, E. and J. Bennett (1979) "Anthropological studies of food and nutrition: The 1940s and the 1970s." In *The Uses of Anthropology.* W. Goldschmidt, ed. Special Publications of the American Anthropological Association, No. 11. Washington, DC: American Anthropological Association.

Munn, N. D. (1986) *The Fame of Gawa: A Symbolic Study of Value Transformation in a Massim (Papua New Guinea) Society.* Cambridge: Cambridge University Press.

Okere, L. C. (1983) *Food in Rural Igboland.* Washington, DC: University Press of America.

Parman, S. (2002) "Lot's wife and the old salt: Cross-cultural comparisons of attitudes toward salt in relation to diet." *Cross-Cultural Research* 36(2): 123–50.

Poggie, J. J. (1995) "Food Resource Periodicity and Cooperation Values: A Cross-Cultural Consideration." *Cross-Cultural Research* 29(3): 276–96.

Pollock, D. K. (1985) "Food and sexual identity among the Culina." *Food and Foodways* 1(1): 25–42.

Pollock, N. (1992) *These Roots Remain: Food Habits in Islands of the Central and Eastern Pacific.* Laie: Institute of Polynesian Studies.

Rappaport, R. (1968) *Pigs for the Ancestors.* New Haven, CT: Yale University Press.

Richards, A. (1932) *Hunger and work in a savage tribe: A functional study of nutrition among the Southern Bantu.* London: Routledge.

——(1939) *Land, labour and diet in Northern Rhodesia: An economic study of the Bemba tribe.* Oxford: Oxford University Press.

Smith, W. R. (1889) *Lectures on the Religion of the Semites.* New York: Appleton.

Staller, J. E. and M. Carrasco, eds. (2010) *Pre-Columbian foodways: Interdisciplinary approaches to food, culture, and markets in ancient Mesoamerica.* New York: Springer Publishing Company.

Sutton, D. E. (2001) *Remembrance of Repasts: An Anthropology of Food and Memory.* New York: Berg.

Terrio, S. J. (2000) *Crafting the Culture and History of French Chocolate.* Berkeley: University of California Press.

Turnbull, C. (1972) *The Mountain People.* New York: Simon and Schuster.

Tylor, E. B. (1865) *Researches into the Early History of Mankind and the Development of Civilization.* London: John Murray.

Watson, J., ed. (1997) *Golden arches east: McDonalds in East Asia.* Palo Alto, CA: Stanford University Press.

Weismantel, M. J. (1988) *Food, Gender, and Poverty in the Ecuadorian Andes.* Philadelphia: University of Pennsylvania Press.

Whiting, J. W. M. and I. L. Child (1953) *Child Training and Personality: A Cross Cultural Study.* New Haven, CT: Yale University Press.

Wiessner, P. (1996) "Introduction: Food, Status, Culture, and Nature." In *Food and the Status Quest.* P. Wiessner and W. Schiefenhovel, eds., pp. 1–18. Oxford: Berghahn Books.

Wiessner, P. and W. Schiefenhovel, eds. (1996) *Food and the Status Quest: An Interdisciplinary Perspective.* Oxford: Berghahn Books.

Wilk, R. (2006) *Home Cooking in the Global Village: Caribbean Food from Buccaners to Ecotourists.* Oxford: Berg.

Wilson, C. S. (1979) "Food – Custom and Nature: An Annotated Bibliography on Sociocultural and Biocultural Aspects of Nutrition." *Journal of Nutrition Education* 11(4): 211–64.

Wrangham, R. (2009) *Catching Fire: How Cooking Made Us Human.* New York: Basic Books.

Young, M. (1971) *Fighting with Food.* New York: Cambridge University Press.

Zubaida, S. and R. Tapper, eds. (1994) *Culinary Cultures of the Middle East.* London: Tauris.

2

The sociology of food

William Alex McIntosh

Sociologists study groups and food is produced, processed, and consumed by groups. Such groups include farms, food companies and families. Consumers vary regarding the degree of control they believe they have over their food choices. In addition individuals purposely establish relationships with others in order to achieve their goals. For those of low income, establishing reciprocal ties with others in order to obtain needed food in times of scarcity is a necessity. These others include relatives, friends, and store owners. Family meals are said to define families and creating family meals places a significant burden on adult females in families.

Despite this obvious connection between sociology and food, until recently sociologists were slow to address food as a legitimate subject matter for their discipline. After a slow start, sociological work on food has accelerated and I discuss here the progress sociologists have made since I published a book in 1996 that dealt with sociology and food and nutrition. This chapter picks up where that work left off but focuses more narrowly on food from recent rural sociological endeavors as well as food from a cultural perspective. Currently, the sociology of food is driven by rural sociologists, medical sociologists, and sociologists of culture among others.

History

With the exception of George Simmel's paper on the meal (1916) [see Symons 1994], the history of sociological involvement with food is very recent. The work of Ann Murcott (1983), who focused on culture and family conflict and Stephen Mennell (1996), whose efforts involved both developmentalism and culture, drew early sociological attention to food consumption. Alan Warde (1997) and Jukka Gronow (1997) have extended this work, but placed food consumption in a decidedly more general consumerism framework. If we consider food production, since the late nineteenth century, rural sociologists had the most consistent track record among sociologists with their studies of farmers and rural communities. Buttel *et al.* (1990) have done an excellent job of reviewing this work from then until the 1980s. This review noted that the most recent emphasis was on political, economic, and environmental forces that influence agriculture. Similar concerns drive current rural sociological studies. Notable contributors to this literature include Harriet Friedmann (1978), Phil McMichael (1994), Larry Busch and Bill Lacy (Busch *et al.*, 1992), Allessandro Bonanno and Doug Constance (2008) and many, many more.

Main sociological theories

Agency theory

Roots of contemporary agency theory can be found in Giddens (1984) structuration theory. The terminology used today is "agency," which is meant to emphasize actions individuals take in order to pursue goals. Parsons's (1937) social action theory involved actors who set goals that are based on societal values, using social norms as the means to accomplish them. At the same time, social actors must confront situational conditions (environments) that constrain action. Early versions of agency theory suggested cultural barriers to action; more recently, resource and power imbalances serve as barriers to action. Agency theory can be applied to food shoppers, eaters, gardeners, farmers, etc. Its use in the sociology of food thus far is limited, but it has great potential.

Wright and Middendorf (2008) have provided a recent example by describing a changing agrofood environment, using the battle over raw milk. States have prohibited the sale of raw milk, but raw milk consumers have found ways around such prohibition (i.e., the cowshare). Other consumer efforts have involved getting "food animals" better treatment. Such consumers participate as a part of an "alternative food system that attempts to operate outside the mainstream commodity-driven network" (Wright and Middendorf, 2008: 2).

DuPuis (2002) developed a cultural theory that builds on a theory of reflexive consumerism (a form of agency theory) and involves social constructionism (the view that issues and problems are defined by social groups; see the discussion below). She described this as a cultural approach and argues that "even when consumers are not part of a social movement they can still act politically if she or he takes into account various political claims and a product in the process of making a purchase" (DuPuis, 2002: 228). A reflexive consumer is "not a social activist and may not be 'committed to a particular ideology [and] in fact, may evince … false consciousness'" (DuPuis, 2002: 228). Such consumers may be influenced by activists, but are also influenced by the mainstream media and personal networks. Their goals are frequently more individualistic rather than communal: Not in My Body (NIMB) compared with Not in My Backyard (NIMBY).

Sociology of culture

While culture is frequently viewed as an environmental constraint in terms of the values, norms, beliefs and social sanctions it provides, it also provides legitimated means by which to carry out action. Swidler (1986) broadened the idea by arguing that culture is a toolkit that enables social action. Cultural capital represents both social environmental constraints but, in addition, is also a tool kit by which members of social classes know how to behave and to distinguish themselves from others. Studies of cultural capital frequently involve musical and artistic tastes, but Bourdieu (1984) devoted some of his work on cultural capital in France to food. Lamont (1994) unsuccessfully detected cultural capital differences among Americans; however, Johnstone and Baumann (2010) portrayed "foodie-ism" as a form of middle-class cultural capital. Parasecoli (2008: 132) observed that tourists often seek authentic foods in the cultures they visit and may attempt to learn how to replicate this to "impress their friends with their newly enhanced cultural capital." But others do not restrict food cultural capital to middle-class lifestyles. Bava *et al.* (2008) talked about the confluence of habitus, cultural capital, and constraints in everyday life for many people. Constraints call for compromises, which opens the door for convenience foods. Constraints not only include time but also lack of cooking skills. Without this form of cultural capital, cooks lack a willingness to experiment.

A sub-area of the sociology of culture is the sociology of consumption, which contains several perspectives. Much of this work can be characterized as what sociologists refer to as a social problems perspective, while others think of consumption as simply a set of cultural practices. Cultural sociologists who embrace a more social problems perspective include Thomas Cook, Juliet Shor, and others, who have taken on the advertising sector of the economy with regard to marketing to children, food ads in particular. Shor (2004: 10) referred to a cycle of work and spend in which luxuries become necessities: "a trip to Disneyworld becomes an expensive but urgent social norm." She argued that it is "children [who] had become the conduits from the consumer marketplace into the household, the link between advertisers and the family purse." She connected this to outcomes such as obesity, but this hypothesis needs further investigation. Cook's (2009) approach involved a greater degree of agency than Shor's in his examination of the "contentious negotiations" that take place between mothers and children over food and meals, observing that "the commercial aspects of food" inhere in these discussions. Ritzer (2011) coined the now-famous term "McDonaldization," drawing on Weber's notions of hyper-rationalization in the modern world. Ritzer saw this very rationalization as an attraction for consumers in terms of (1) rapid service, (2) consistent products, and (3) low costs due to efficiency measures. Most of the approaches just reviewed leave little leeway for agency. However, Warde (1997) develops a theory of consumption that has much in common with agency theory, drawing on Bauman for agency and Bourdieu for structural constraints. Both Warde and Gronow view consumption as a set of practices rather than as a social problem.

Others tend to see culture in terms of ethnicity and acculturation; sociologists have devoted a great deal of attention to this topic, but only a few have observed the importance of food in terms of ethnic identity, acculturation, or resistance to acculturation. Ray (2004) found, for example, that Bengalis acculturate when circumstances demand it – time and space constraints on breakfast and lunch – but maintain their cultural identity by consuming traditional foods at dinner. Dean *et al.* (2010) found similar compromises of traditional food practices driven in part by irregular work schedules but also exposure to new ideas regarding what constitutes a healthy meal, perhaps a reflection of acculturation. At the same time, those dietary changes are contextualized in terms of tradition or what Dean *et al.* (2010) referred to as the "reinvention of culture." Others who have experienced attempts at forced acculturation, particularly in regards to food, have employed agency as a means of resistance and achieving a degree of independence as Williams-Forson (2006) aptly demonstrated. During and after slavery in the US, Black women used chicken as a means of resistance and economic independence.

Social problems

From its inception, sociologists have concerned themselves with social problems. Sociological pioneers such as Durkheim raised concerns regarding potential anomie as a result of societal change. Marx is well known for his concerns regarding the exploitation of labor. Marx in particular was willing to do more than analyze these problems; he also spoke out against them. From the 1950s onward, thanks to C. Wright Mills (Horowitz, 1983), sociologists once again acted as societal critics. Mills focused on differential power and rewards in the US class system. Sociologists such as William Friedland (1981; Friedland and Barton, 1975) turned this critical light on agricultural production, particularly on the treatment of labor. *Food and Society* by Bill Whit (1995) served as social criticism of the consumption side of food. It is fair to say that both Friedland and Whit have taken a neo-Marxist view in their criticism.

The nature of social problems has always been contentious. While some sociologists have embraced particular problems as real (e.g., Mark Nord *et al.*, 2002 and food insecurity), others have argued such problems have been manufactured by interested parties (social constructionism). Perhaps the most contentious area of argument in sociology regarding food-related health issues is obesity. Sobal (1995) documented the medicalization of obesity, while Oliver (2006) and others have argued that in addition to physicians, bureaucrats and health researchers funded by the weight-loss industry and drug companies have turned a harmless difference in body size into a life-threatening epidemic. It is, of course, possible for weight issues to compromise health and still find that those with a vested interest in obesity have greatly exaggerated the problem. It is far from clear, however, that the majority of these researchers have received industry funding. Instead, many researchers have obtained support from the National Institutes of Health or the United States Department of Agriculture. A far more relevant point made by Guthman and DuPuis (2006) argues that capitalism not only produces obesity but also sells the proposed cures.

Prejudice and discrimination against "sized" individuals is well documented and few would dispute it. The feminist critique of obesity has tended to follow the same line as that of social constructionist critics, but has emphasized the fallibility of "masculine, material science" that ignores the experiences of women (Aphramor and Gingras, 2009). The eating disorder literature tends to treat eating disorders as a real problem, but blame it on the social construction of obesity and the slender body, examining how women are taught to view the experience of anorexia nervosa and obesity as two forms of deviant female bodies (Whitehead and Kurz, 2008). These are all legitimate issues for sociologists and others to continue to pursue. At the same time, too many sociologists have willingly contributed to the perception that body weight issues are mere social constructions.

A sociologist who avoids the pitfalls of social constructionism is Jan Poppendieck (2010), who has devoted her career to the study of food problems and the frequently unsuccessful efforts to solve them, including federal food assistance during the Great Depression, voluntary food assistance (i.e., food banks) in recent times, and failures in federally supported school breakfast and lunch programs.

Social capital

Multiple definitions of this concept exist; for Bourdieu (1986) it had to do with the deliberate creation of social relationships in order to obtain resources. This is similar to Nan Lin's (1999) definition, which puts social capital into a social network framework. Putnam (2000) and others viewed this as a community characteristic, where trust and reciprocity are required for the exchange of resources to take place.

Regarding social capital and food insecurity, Martin *et al.* (2004: 2645) found that both household (e.g., trust in neighbors; perceived social cohesion; willingness to help one another) and community-level social capital (neighborhood averages of household social capital) "decreases the odds of household food insecurity." Johnson *et al.* (2010: 306) argued that individual social capital ("if there is a problem in my community, people work to get it solved," etc.) was associated with higher levels of fruit and vegetable consumption, and Locher *et al.* (2005) found social capital was negatively associated with malnutrition among Black Americans. Dean and Sharkey (2011a) expanded on these ideas by adding inequality (perceived disparity). Such disparities are important because they are said to decrease both trust and social capital (Wilkinson, 1996). Some have viewed social capital as a part of collective social functioning (Garasky *et al.*, 2004, n.d.; Locher *et al.*, 2005), which refers to "the social, cultural, and historical commonalities of a particular community" (Dean and Sharkey, 2011a: 2). Dean *et al.* (2011b) found that collective social functioning reduced food insecurity among older adults.

Social capital also inheres in market relationships, particularly in neighborhoods and communities. Trust in relationships would be important for those lacking sufficient food resources; for example, a willingness to share food requires the sharer to feel reasonably confident that the recipient will reciprocate at some later time. Trust is a major issue when it comes to the food itself; people want to be able to trust the food they are about to ingest. In order to do so they must trust the source, but Giddens (1991) has argued that trust in authorities has declined with "reflexive late modernity." Consumers' trust of the food industry depends on the perception of industry member competence and willingness to act in the best interests of consumers (Sapp et al., 2009). Lack of such trust helps explain the attraction of local food for customers (Hinrichs, 2000) and some local food producers have pointedly strived for demonstrating trustworthy production methods (Bildtgard, 2008).

People implicitly trust their local grocery store not to sell them foods past the expiration date. Stores trust (sometimes) that customers' checks won't bounce. Deutsch (2002) described the trust and distrust that once characterized exchanges between neighborhood grocers and their customers, where issues of mistrust included quality, prices, and credit/repayment. At present such transactions would appear to be largely impersonal; customers deal with a different checker each time they make a purchase; they do not know either the manager or the owner. They trust perhaps because they have no alternative. However, Kaufman and Karpati (2007) mentioned shopping at bodegas as being attractive because those stores offered credit as money became short towards the end of the month. Communities with strong, local social capital are described as "civic" and Lyson (2004) argued that civic agriculture was found in such communities where, in addition, local agriculture was tightly woven into the communities' social and economic fabric; Flammang (2009) made a strong claim that the social capital needed for such communities begins with civic dinner tables. "Civic" dinner tables bear a close resemblance to family meal rituals (discussed below).

The family

Sociologists have a longstanding interest in family life ranging from the effects of parents, family structure, and socioeconomic status on child development; the effects of employment, particularly by wife-mothers on children and spouses, etc. More recently, an interest in the effects of fathers on children has grown as has attention to family meals and family meal rituals.

Sociologists have given much attention to gender roles and work outside the home and how this work affects family functioning and family members. Since the crude studies of the pre-1996 period in which children's nutrition was connected to mothers' employment, research has turned towards work hours, work schedules and work-to-family spillover issues. For example, Anderson et al. (2003) found that children were more likely to be overweight the more hours their mothers work over the children's life; furthermore this effect was stronger among mothers of higher SES. Miller and Han (2008) reported that non-standard work schedules are associated with overweight among adolescents. Employed women with children spend less time cooking than non-employed women (United States Bureau of Labor Statistics, 2011a, 2011b). Others, however, have reported few if any effects of mothers' work on children's eating. Recently, efforts to determine fathers' work-experience effects on children's eating have taken place; McIntosh et al. (2011) found that fathers' work schedules influence children's time spent in full-service restaurants. Qualitative work by interdisciplinary teams of nutritionists and sociologists has found that work stress, spillover, and work schedules make meal planning difficult for some and lead to less healthy food choices for dinner (Devine et al., 2006). Less planning means less frequent participation in dinner by children (McIntosh et al., 2010).

Turning to time use in families, economists have given the most attention to time spent cooking and eating; however, sociologists have come to see time as both an opportunity and a constraint on cooking and eating. The perceived value of cooking and eating with others is partially judged by the amount of time devoted to these activities. Thus the qualitative (Kaufmann, 2010) and quantitative data (Robinson and Godbey, 2007) that have suggested these time uses have shortened is met with concern. Less time cooking may produce less healthy or desirable meals; less time at the dinner table may lessen the impact of eating together. However, evidence here is mixed. Working women may spend less time cooking or eating (Gimenez-Nadal and Sevilla-Sanz, 2011), but work outside the home does not affect the amount of meal planning that occurs, the scheduling of family meals nor children's participation in those meals (McIntosh et al., 2010).

Time constraints generated by work hours and other demands lead to the purchase of convenience. It has been argued that with higher income, working women use market substitutions such as convenience foods to compensate for cooking time lost because of employment (Killewald, 2011). She reported weak evidence for this. Others found that women did most of the cooking in order to avoid family conflict (Began et al., 2008). According to Sayer (2005), men's time spent cooking has increased during the 1965 to 1998 time period and Tashiro (2009) reported that cooking time varies significantly by ethnicity. The study of time spent on household duties, particularly cooking, has clearly been neglected.

Cooking itself has only recently received attention from sociologists, who in the past lumped it into studies of the household division of labor. The purpose of the latter was to identify gender roles as well as inequalities that arose from such assignments, particularly when both husbands and wives were employed outside the household. More recently, DeVault (1991) and others have taken a 'work of caring' perspective, which has roots in definitions of gender distinction. DeVault's (1991) work provided evidence that women do most of the cooking in their homes as an act of love and caring. Famously, she describes that through constructing meals, families themselves are constructed. Bugge (2003) drew on similar notions about family meals and connects women's cooking to identity work. Resource and time constraints can make this a real challenge. However, Kaufmann (2010) noted that for some, given enough time, every day cooking as part of housework can be pleasurable. This can be tied to the weekend but not always. Overlooked in this literature are the skills that cooks need in order to prepare meals.

Sociologists have given sporadic attention to meals. Simmel (1916 [see Symons 1994]) in a mostly forgotten paper wrote about this, speaking of their contradictory nature: a social setting in which individuals ingest and enjoy foods as individuals. Later, family sociologists' research identified family dinner as an important family ritual (Bossard, 1948; Bossard and Boll, 1950). More recently, a debate has sprung up over the family meal's possible disappearance, which connects nicely with sociologists' ongoing debate over the disappearance of the family (Popenoe, 1993; Coontz, 1992) (both "disappearances" are greatly exaggerated). Others such as Murcott, (1983) and Lupton, (1996) have focused on the tensions that arise during meals among family members. Others have claimed its disappearance results from increased individualism abetted by technology, which encourages solitary eating; Lupton (1996) found that many adults did not participate in family meals because of highly unpleasant memories of family meals when growing up. Finally, the use of television and electronic communications media during family meals potentially destroys their social nature.

However, Zick and Stevens (2011) found that American adults spent more time eating than in the past and suggest this may contribute to the rise of obesity. They found that this increase was due to an increase in time eating as a secondary activity. In fact time spent eating as a primary activity declined slightly from 1975 to 2006–7, but time spent eating as a secondary activity doubled (from less than 20 minutes per day to over an hour). Women who earned more money spent more time eating as a secondary activity. Of interest, using the 2007 ATUS data,

Reifschneider *et al.* (2011) reported no association between time spent eating and drinking (either as a primary or a secondary activity) and obesity. Warde *et al.* (2007) treated time spent eating as an indicator of "household organization" and "social interdependence," finding that these vary across cultures regardless of globalization.

While the so-called decline of the family meal is mourned in many places including Japan, Europeans have used the family meal as a defense against the pressures of life on the family (Kaufmann, 2010). In addition while there is slippage from this model and the discipline and rules that maintain it, the family meal is valued by not only women but also men and children (Kaufmann, 2010; McIntosh *et al.*, 2009). Many consider it important, even when the atmosphere is unpleasant, and some see the possible disintegration of their own families should this meal disappear (Kaufmann, 2010). Research by DeVault (1991), Mestdag (2005), and McIntosh *et al.*, (2009) indicated family meals are still important to family members and occur with some frequency. At the same time it is fair to say that family meals are changing as more families eat watching TV or attending to their personal message delivery devices. Other adjustments to meals come through convenience foods and more easily prepared dishes.

Food social movements

Traditional social movements have political and/or economic goals (e.g., the civil rights movement, the labor movement), while new social movements tend to have non-political or economic goals, some of which are cultural (e.g., preserving local food – the Slow Food movement and *lardo di Colonnata*) (Leitch, 2003). Recent theorists have argued that social movement success depends not only on the movement organization but also the cultural context in which the movement operates. In this case, the anti-genetic engineering or anti-GMO movement was found to be successful in Britain but unsuccessful in the US. In Britain new discourse on GM food and technology described them as "unsafe, unnatural and associated with unknowable and uncontrollable public and environmental risks" (Schurman and Munro, 2009). The British discourse also argued Monsanto, the promoter of these foods, as an ugly American company, both arrogant and insensitive to European culture. According to these authors, such messages were less effective in the US, in part because American consumer culture includes greater trust in business than those found in Europe's. In addition the reaction of Europeans to such foods produced by US farmers and companies created a backlash among American consumers, because the anti-technology message seemed anti-American. But more importantly, the British grocery sector dealt with a more critical consumer culture while a more decentralized grocery sector in the US served a more trusting consumer culture. These conclusions regarding Americans' trust of business contradict Giddens's (1991) claims about late-modern reflexiveness and other findings regarding mistrustful American consumers mentioned earlier. Local food has also become a social movement (Starr, 2010), part of a broader healthy food movement described by Winson (2010). Proponents express concerns over energy use, pollution, sustainability, supporting local farmers, and local community building, and express alternative economics in which these issues are the basis of a bottom line rather than price (Jussaume and Kondoh, 2008).

Research methods

While there are many excellent qualitative studies in this growing field, it is clear that survey research dominated early research efforts. Qualitative methods have become more prevalent in the form of ethnographies and content analyses.

Quantitative methods involve survey research data (e.g., consumer perceptions of food, farming and buying local) (Weatherell *et al.*, 2003) as well as secondary data such as administrative records or economic consumption data (e.g., egg consumption per capita over time or the number of health clubs by country; health magazine circulation) (Maguire, 2008). Methods of analyzing such data range from ordinary least squares regression (e.g., Shaft *et al.*, 2009 on obesity in food deserts), log linear methods including logistic regression, principal components analysis, and Tobit models.

Fitzgerald (2001) used content analysis of English-language print media in the Reuters Business Briefing Database to confirm that while media sentiment towards GMO foods was very positive in 1995, since then, media coverage has moved to a neutral middle ground. Johnstone *et al.*, (2009) examined the interaction between the corporate world and the organic world, using content analysis, finding that corporations producing organic food have co-opted messages of local scale and support of family farming.

Qualitative methods include open-ended interviews and focus groups. Bugge (2011) utilized open-ended interviews to learn young Norwegians' perceptions of fast food, and Johnson *et al.* (2010) took advantage of the photo-elicitation method, using photos taken by women regarding their meal preparation and consumption. The women were then asked to describe why they took the pictures and what was special about the picture. The exercise generated a great deal of discussion about the influences of their mothers, grandmothers, and aunts on their food choices. Focus groups have examined the behavioral decisions involved in "producers' adoption of price management strategies" (Jackson *et al.*, 2009). Feminist scholars in sociology have relied on "the participatory and qualitative tradition," treating "women as subjects as well as producers of knowledge" (Trauger *et al.*, 2008: 434, 435), which can be used either in individual interviews or focus groups.

Unanswered questions

More work is needed on food as distinction; the research thus far has not dealt with the general population but rather a few subgroups within. The purpose is to determine where food cultural capital is restricted to certain segments of the upper-middle class or can be found in various forms among other groups. In addition, despite a great deal of qualitative work conducted by sociologists and others, we know only a little about the process by which meals are planned, prepared, and performed. Little is known about the actual act of cooking. Cooking is often an individual activity, but the preparer must take into account the potential eaters while drawing on skills and knowledge and struggling with constraint of both time and money. Where do these skills come from? From mothers? From experimentation and recipe reading? Investigations of time spent eating and where and with whom are in their infancy, but surely these investigations will provide us with greater insights into food choices, food behaviors, and food-related maladies. Studies of social capital consumers draw on when engaging grocers, restaurants, and other sources of food have received insufficient attention.

Programs in the sociology of food

One graduate program in food studies is overseen by a sociologist. The Food Studies Program at Chatham is directed by Dr Alice Julier and offers a Masters degree. The New School's Bachelors Program in Food Studies was recently established by Dr Fabio Parasecoli, also a sociologist. In addition several sociology graduate programs offer concentrations in food-related areas. Cornell University's Department of Developmental Sociology deals with issues in food production and distribution as well as community and civic organization. University of Wisconsin at Madison offers a specialty area in the sociology of agriculture and food systems; it emphasizes the structure of agriculture, issues surrounding the family farm, and industrialization of agriculture). Colorado State's Department of Sociology includes Agriculture and Food as an Area of Study, while graduate students in the Department of Sociology at the University of California at Santa Cruz have the opportunity to work on research projects in the Center for Agroecology and Sustainable Food Systems. The graduate program in sociology at Michigan State University includes food, environment, agriculture, science and technology as an area of study. This is described on the department's website as a program that studies "the relationship between cultural attitudes towards the production, exchange, and consumption of food and the evolving technology to alter agrifood processes." Penn State University's Rural Sociology Graduate Program includes agriculture and food systems as one of its "signature areas". "We examine social organization and change in agriculture and food systems in the U.S. and internationally. Our focus ranges from individual farmers and local farming communities to global institutions that intersect with agriculture and food systems. Recent work has addressed food system inequalities, the role of science and technology in agriculture, regional supply chains and agricultural clusters, global agrifood restructuring, knowledge systems, and multifunctionality."

Key reading

Allen, Patricia (2004) *Together at the Table*. College Park, PA: Penn State University Press.

Fine, Gary (1996) *Kitchens: The Culture of Restaurant Work*. Berkeley, CA: University of California Press.

Germov, John and Lauren Williams (2004) *Sociology of Food and Nutrition*. New York: Oxford University Press.

Hinrichs, C. Clare and Thomas A. Lyson, eds. (2007) *Remaking the North American Food System: Strategies for Sustainability*. Lincoln, NB: University of Nebraska Press.

Leider, Robin (1993) *Fast Food, Fast Talk: Service Work and the Routinization of Everyday Life*. Berkeley, CA: University of California Press.

Maurer, Donna and Jeffery Sobal (1995) *Eating Agendas: Food and Nutrition as Social Problems*. New York: Aldine De Gruyter.

McIntosh, Wm. Alex (1996) *Sociologies of Food and Nutrition*. New York: Plenum.

Mennell, Stephen, Anne Murcott, and Anneke H. van Otterloo. (1992) "The Sociology of Food: Eating, Dieting, and Food." *Current Sociology* 40: 1–148.

Sobal, Jeffery and Albert J. Stunkard (1989) "Socioeconomic Status and Obesity: A Review of the Literature." *Psychological Bulletin* 105: 260–75.

Sobal, Jeffery and Mary K. Nelson (2003) "Commensal Eating Patterns: A Community Study." *Appetite* 41: 181–90.

Sobal, Jeffery, L. K. Khan, and Carol A. Bisogni (1998) "A Conceptual Model of the Food and Nutrition System." *Social Science and Medicine* 47: 853–63.

Bibliography

Anderson, Patricia M., Kristen F. Butcher, and Phillip B. Levine. (2003) "Maternal Employment and Overweight Children." *Journal of Health Economics* 22: 477–504.

Aphramor, Lucy and Jacqui Gingras (2009) "That Remains to Be Said: Disappeared Feminist Discourse on Fat in Dietetic Theory and Practice." In *The Fat Studies Reader*. Esther Rothblum, Sondra Solovay, and Marilyn Wann eds. pp. 97–105, New York: New York University Press.

Bava, Christina M., Sara R. Jaeger, and Julie Park (2008) "Constraints upon Food Provisioning Practices in 'Busy' Women's Lives: Trade-offs which Demand Convenience." *Appetite* 50: 486–98.

Bildtgard, T. (2008) "Trust in Food in Modern and Late Modern Societies." *Social Science Information* 47: 99–128.

Bonanno, Alessandro and Douglas Constance (2008) *Stories of Globalization: Transnational Corporations, Resistance, and the State*. University Park, PA: Pennsylvania State University Press.

Bossard, James H. S. (1948) *The Sociology of Child Development*. New York: Harper.

Bossard, James H. S. and Eleanor Stoker Boll (1950) *Ritual in Family Life: A Contemporary Study*. Philadelphia, PA: University of Pennsylvania Press.

Bourdieu, Pierre (1984) *Distinction: A Social Critique of the Judgment of Taste*. Cambridge, MA: Harvard University Press.

——(1986) "The Forms of Capital." In *Handbook of Theory and Research for the Sociology of Education*, J. Richardson ed., pp. 241–58. Westfield, CT: Greenwood.

Bugge, Annechen Bahr (2003) "Cooking – As Identity Work." Presented at the 6th European Sociological Association Conference, September, Murcia, Spain.

——(2011) "Lovin' It? A Study of Youth and the Culture of Fast Food." *Food, Culture and Society* 14: 71–89.

Busch, Lawrence (2004) "Grades and Standards in the Social Construction of Safe Food." In *The Politics of Food*. Marianne Elisabeth Lien and Brigitte Nerlich eds., pp. 163–78, Oxford: Berg.

Busch, Lawrence, William B. Lacy, and Jeffrey Burkhardt (1992) *Plants, Power, and Profit: Social, Economic and Ethical Consequences of the New Biotechnologies*. New York: Blackwell.

Buttel, Frederick H., Olaf F. Larson, and Gilbert W. Gillespie, Jr (1990) *The Sociology of Agriculture*. Westfield, CT: Greenwood Press.

Center for Agroecology. (n.d.) casfs.ucsc.edu (accessed on July 17, 2011).

Chatham University Master of Arts in Food Studies. (n.d.) www.chatham.edu/academics/programs/graduate/mafs/curriculum.cfm (accessed on July 17, 2011).

Colorado State University. Graduate Program. (n.d.) sobek.colorado.edu/SOC/Graduate/info.html (accessed on July 17, 2011).

Cook, Daniel Thomas (2009) "Semantic Provisioning of Children's Food: Commerce, Care and Maternal Practice." *Childhood* 16: 317–34.

Coontz, Stephanie (1992) *The Way We Never Were*. New York: Basic Books.

Cornell University *Development Sociology* (n.d.) devsoc.cals.cornell.edu/cals/devsoc/about/index.cfm (accessed on July 17, 2011).

Dean, Wesley R. and Joseph R. Sharkey (2011a) "Food Insecurity, Social Capital and Perceived Personal Disparity in a Predominantly Rural Region of Texas: An Individual-Level Analysis." *Social Science and Medicine* 72: 1454–62.

Dean, Wesley R., Joseph R. Sharkey, and Cassandra M. Johnson (2011b) "Food Insecurity is Associated with Social Capital, Perceived Personal Disparity, and Partnership Status among Older and Senior Adults in a Largely Rural Area of Central Texas." *Journal of Nutrition in Gerontology and Geriatrics* 30: 169–86.

Dean, Wesley R., Joseph R. Sharkey, Kevin-Khristián Cosgriff-Hernández, Amanda R. Martinez, Julie Ribardo, and Carolina Diaz-Puentes (2010) "'I Can Say that We Were Healthy and Unhealthy': Food Choice and the Reinvention of Tradition." *Food, Culture, and Society* 13: 574–94.

Deutsch, Tracy (2002) "Untangling Alliances: Social Tensions Surrounding Independent Grocery Stores and the Rise of Mass Retailing." In *Food Nations: Selling Taste in Consumer Societies*. Warren Belasco and Philip Scranton eds., pp. 156–74, New York: Routledge.

DeVault, Marjorie (1991) *Feeding the Family: The Social Organization of Feeding Work*. Chicago, IL: University of Chicago Press.

Devine C. M., M. Jastran, J. Jabs, E. Wethington, T. Farrell, and C. Bisogni (2006) "'A Lot of Sacrifices:' Work-Family Spillover and the Food Choice Coping Strategies of Low Wage Employed Parents." *Social Science and Medicine* 63: 2591–603.

DuPuis, E. M. (2000) "Not My Body: BGH and the Rise of Organic Milk." *Agriculture and Human Values* 16: 151–60.

DuPuis, Melanie (2002) *Nature's Perfect Food: How Milk Became America's Drink*. New York: New York University Press.

Fitzgerald, Ruth (2001) "Content Analysis of Bias in International Print Media Coverage of Genetically Modified Food." *Rural Society* 11: 181–96.

Flammang, Janet A. (2009) *The Taste for Civilization: Food, Politics, and Civil Society*. Urbana: University of Illinois Press.

Friedland, William (1981) *Manufacturing Green Gold: Capital, Labor, and Technology in the Lettuce Industry*. Cambridge: Cambridge University Press.

Friedland, William H. and Amy Barton (1975) *Destalking the Wily Tomato: A Case Study in the Social Consequences in California Agricultural Research*. Davis: University of California, Department of Applied Behavioral Sciences.

Friedland, William H., Amy E. Barton, and R. J. Thomas (n.d.) *Manufacturing Green Gold: Capital, Labor, and Technology in the Lettuce Industry*. Cambridge: Cambridge University Press.

Friedmann, Harriet (1978) "World Market, State and Family Comparative Studies." *Society and History* 20: 399–416.

Garasky, S., Lois Wright Morton, and K. A. Greder (2004) "The Food Environment and Food Insecurity: Perceptions of Rural, Suburban, and Urban Food Pantry Clients in Iowa." *Family Economics and Food Review* 16: 41–48.

——(n.d.) "The effects of the Local Food Environment and Social Support on Rural Food Insecurity." *Journal of Hunger and Environmental Nutrition* 1: 83–103.

Giddens, Anthony (1984) *The Constitution of Society*. Berkeley, CA: University of California Press.

——(1991) *Modernity and Self-Identity: Self and Society in the Late Modern Age*. Stanford, CA: Stanford University Press.

Gimenez-Nadal, Jose Ignacio and Almudena Sevilla-Sanz (2011) "The Time-Crunch Paradox." *Social Indicators Research* 102: 181–96.

Gronow, Jukka (1997) *The Sociology of Taste*. New York: Routledge.

Guthman, Julie and Melanie DuPuis (2006) "Embodying Neoliberalism: Economy, Culture, and Politics of fat." *Environmental Planning D: Society and Space* 24: 427–48.

Hinrichs, C. Claire (2000) "Embeddedness and Local Food Systems: Notes on Two Types of Direct Agricultural Markets." *Journal of Rural Studies* 16: 295–303.

Horowitz, Irving Louis (1983) *C. Wright Mills An American Utopia*. New York: The Free Press.

Johnson, Cassie, Joseph R. Sharkey, Wesley R. Dean, and W. Alex McIntosh (2010) "'I'm the Momma' Using Photo-Elicitation to Understand Matrilineal Influence on Food Choice." *BMC Women's Health* 10: 21–34.

Johnson, C. M., J. R. Sharkey, and W. R. Dean (2010) "Eating Behaviors and Social Capital are Associated with Fruit and Vegetable Intake among Rural Adults." *Journal of Hunger and Environmental Nutrition* 5: 302–15.

Johnston, Hank and Bert Klandermans (1995) "The Cultural Analysis of Social Movements." In *Social Movements and Culture*, Hank Johnston and Bert Klandermans eds., pp. 3–24, Minneapolis, MN: University of Minnesota Press.

Johnston, Josée, Andrew Biro, and Nora MacKindrick (2009) "Lost in the Supermarket: The Corporate-Organic Foodscape and the Struggle for Food Democracy." *Antipode* 41: 509–32.

Johnston, Josée and Shyon Baumann (2010) *Foodies: Democracy and Distinction in the Gourmet Foodscape*. New York: Routledge.

Jussaume, Raymond A., Jr. and Kazumi Kondoh (2008) "Possibilities for revitalizing local agriculture: Evidence from four counties in Washington State." In *The Fight over Food: Producers, Consumers, and activists challenge the global food system*. Wynne Wright and Gerad Middendorf, eds., pp. 225–46, University Park, PA: Penn State University Press.

Kaufman, Leslie and Adam Karpati (2007) "Understanding Sociocultural Roots of Childhood Obesity: Food Practices among Latino Families of Brunswick, Brooklyn." *Social Science and Medicine* 64: 2177–88.

Kaufmann, Jean-Claude (2010) *The Meaning of Cooking*. Malden, MA: Polity.

Killewald, Alexandra (2011) "Opting Out and Buying Out: Wives' Earnings and Household Time." *Journal of Marriage and Family* 73: 459–71.

Lamont, Michele (1994) *Money, Morals, and Manners: The Culture of the French and the American Upper-Middle Classes*. Chicago, IL: University of Chicago Press.

Leitch, Alison (2003) "Slow Food and the Politics of Pork Fat: Italian Food and European Identity." *Ethnos* 68: 437–62.

Lin, Nan (1999) "Building a Network Theory of Social Capital." *Connections* 22: 28–51.

Locher, Julie L., Christine S. Richie, David L. Roth, Patricia Sawyer Baker, Eric V. Bodner, and Richard M. Allman (2005) "Social Isolation, Support and Capital and Nutritional Risk in an Older Sample: Ethnic and Gender Differences." *Social Science and Medicine* 60: 747–61.

Lupton, Deborah (1996) *Food, the Body, and the Self*. Thousand Oaks, CA: Sage.

Lyson, Tom (2004) *Civic Agriculture*. Lebanon, NH: Tufts University Press.

Martin, Katie S., Beatrice L. Rogers, John T. Cook, and Hugh M. Joseph (2004) "Social Capital is Associated with Decrease Risk of Hunger." *Social Science and Medicine* 58: 2645–54.

Maurer, Donna and Jeff Sobal (1995) *Eating Agendas: Food and Nutrition as Social Problems*. New York: Aldine De Gruyter.

McIntosh, W. A., W. Dean, C. C. Torres, J. Anding, K. S. Kubena, and R. Nayga (2009) "The American Family Meal." In *Meals in Science and Practice: Interdisciplinary Research and Business Applications*. Herbert L. Meiselman ed., pp.190–214, Boca Raton, FL: CRC Press.

McIntosh, Wm. Alex, Wesley Dean, Glen Tolle, Jie-sheng Jan, Jenna Anding, and Karen S Kubena (2010) "Mothers and Meals: The Effects of Mothers' Meal Planning and Shopping Motivations on Children's Participation in Family Meals." *Appetite* 55: 623–28.

McIntosh, Wm. Alex, Karen S. Kubena, Glen Tolle, Wesley Dean, and Jenna Anding (2011) "Determinants of Time Children Spend Eating at Fast Food and Sit-Down Restaurants – Further Explorations." *Journal of Nutrition Education and Behavior* 43: 142–49.

McMichael, Philip ed. (1994) *The Global Restructuring of Food Systems*. Ithaca, NY: Cornell University Press.

Mennell, Stephen (1996) *All Manners of Food*. Urbana: University of Illinois Press.

Mestdag, Inge (2005) "Disappearance of the Traditional Meal: Temporal, Social and Spatial Destructuration." *Appetite* 45: 45–62.

Michigan State University. (n.d.) www.sociology.msu.edu/overview_areas_sociology.php (accessed on July 17, 2011).

Miller, Daniel P. and Wen-Jui Han (2008) "Maternal Nonstandard Work Schedules and Adolescent Overweight." *American Journal of Public Health* 98: 1495–502.

Murcott, Anne (1983) *Sociology of Food and Eating*. Aldershot: Gower Press.

New School Food Studies Program. (n.d.) www.newschool.edu/bachelorsprogram/subpage.aspx?id=14304 (accessed on September 11, 2011).

Nord, Mark, Margaret Andrews, and Joshua Winicki (2002) "Frequency and Duration of Food Insecurity and Hunger in US Households." *Journal of Nutrition Education and Behavior* 34: 194–201.

Oliver, J. Eric 2006) *Fat Politics: The Real Story Behind America's Obesity Epidemic*. New York: Oxford University Press.

Parasecoli, Fabio (2008) *Bite Me: Food in Popular Culture*. Oxford: Berg.

Parsons, Talcott (1968 [1937]) *The Structure of Social Action: A study in Social Theory with Special Reference to European Writers*. Volume I. New York: Free Press.

Penn State. Graduate Program in Rural Sociology. (n.d) ruralsociology.aers.psu.edu/ (accessed on July 17, 2011).

Popenoe, David (1993) "American Family Decline, 1960–90: A Review and Appraisal." *Journal of Marriage and the Family* 55: 527–55.

Poppendieck, Janet (2010) *Free for All: Fixing School Food in America*. Berkeley: University of California Press.

Putnam, Robert (2000) *Bowling Alone: The Collapse and Revival of American Community*. New York: Simon and Schuster.

Ray, Krishnendu (2004) *The Migrant's Table: Meals and Memories in Bengali-American Households*. Philadelphia, PA: Temple University Press.

Reifschneider, Marianne J., Karen S. Hamrick, and Jill N. Lacey (2011) "Exercise, Eating Patterns, and Obesity: Evidence from the ATUS and Its Eating and Health Module." *Social Indicators Research* 101, 2: 215–19.

Ritzer, George (2011) *The McDonaldization of Society*. 6th edition. Thousand Oaks, CA: Sage.

Robinson, John and Geofrey Godbey (2007) *Time for Life: The Surprising Ways Americans Use Their Time*. Second edition. University Park, PA: Penn State University Press.

Sapp, Stephen G., Charlie Arnot, James Fallon, Terry Fleck, David Soorholtz, Matt Sutton-Vermeulen, and James J. H. Wilson (2009) "Consumer Trust in the U.S. Food System: An Examination of the Recreancy Theorem." *Rural Sociology* 74: 525–45.

Sayer, Liana C. (2005) "Gender, Time and Inequality: Trends in Women's and Men's Paid Work, Unpaid Work and Free Time." *Social Forces* 84: 285–303.

Schurman, Rachel and William Munro (2009) "Targeting Capital: A Cultural Economy Approach to Understanding the Efficacy of Two Anti-Genetic Engineering Movements." *American Journal of Sociology* 115: 155–202.

Shor, Juliet (2004) *Born to Buy: The Commercialized Child and the New Consumer Culture*. New York: Scribner.

Sobal, Jeffery (1995) "Medicalization and Demedicalization of Obesity." In *Eating Agendas: Food and Nutrition as Social Problems*. Donna Maurer and Jeffery Sobal eds., pp. 67–90, New York: Aldine de Gruyter.

Starr, Amory (2010) "Local Food: A Social Movement?" *Cultural Studies Critical Methodologies* 10: 479–90.

Swidler, Ann (1986) "Culture in Action: Symbols and Strategies." *American Sociological Review* 51: 273–86.

Symons, Michael (1994) "Simmel's Gastronomic Sociology: An Overlooked Essay." *Food and Foodways* 5: 333–51.

Tashiro, Sanae (2009) "Differences in Food Preparation by Race and Ethnicity: Evidence from the American Time Use Survey." *Review of Black Political Economy* 36: 161–80.

Trauger, Amy, Carolyn Sachs, Mary Barbercheck, Nancy Ellen Kiernan, Kathy Brasier, and Jill Findeis (2008) "Agricultural education: Gender identity and knowledge exchange." *Journal of Rural Studies* 24: 432–39.

United States Bureau of Labor Statistics (2011a) "American Time Use Survey. Eating and Drinking." data. bls.gov/cgi-bin/print/tus/current/eating.htm (accessed on June 22, 2011).

——(2011b) "Table 8. Time Spent in Primary Activities (1) for the Civilian Population 18 Years and over by Employment Status, Presence and Age of Youngest Children, and Sex, 2010 Annual Averages." www.bls.gov/news.release/atus.t08.htm (accessed on August 24, 2011).

University of California at Santa Cruz. (n.d.) Center for Agroecology and Sustainable Food Systems. http://casfs.ucsc.edu/about (accessed on July 17, 2011)

University of Wisconsin. (n.d.) ssc.wisc.edu/soc/grad/fac-interest.php (accessed on July 17, 2011).

Warde, Alan (1997) *Consumption, Food & Taste: Cultural Antimonies and Commodity Culture.* Thousand Oaks, CA: Sage.

Warde, Alan, ShuLi Cheng, Wendy Olsen, and Dale Southerton (2007) "Changes in the Practice of Eating: A Comparative Analysis of Time-Use." *Acta Sociologica* 50: 363–85.

Weatherell, Charlotte, Angela Tregear, and Johanne Allinson (2003) "In Search of the Concerned Consumer: UK Public Perceptions of Food, Farming, and Buying Local." *Journal of Rural Studies* 19: 233–44.

Whit, Bill (1995) *Food and Society: A Sociological Approach.* Dix Hills, NY: General Hall.

Whitehead, K. and T. Kurz (2008) "Saints, sinners and standards of femininity: Discursive constructions of anorexia nervosa and obesity in women's magazines." *Journal of Gender Studies* 17: 345–58.

Wilkinson, Richard G. (1996) *Unhealthy Societies: The Affliction of Inequality.* New York: Routledge.

Williams-Forson, Psyche A. (2006) *Building Houses out of Chicken Legs: Black Women, Food and Power.* Chapel Hill, NC: University of North Carolina Press.

Winson, Anthony (2010) "The Demand for Healthy Eating: Supporting a Transformative Food 'Movement'." *Rural Sociology* 75: 584–600.

Wright, Wynne and Gerad Middendorf (2008) *The Fight over Food: Producers, Consumers, and Activists Challenge the Global Food System.* University Park, PA: Penn State Press.

Zick, Cathleen D. and Robert B. Stevens (2011) "Time Spent Eating and Its Implications for American's Energy Balance." *Social Indicators Research* 101: 267–73.

3

Food and communication

Arthur Lizie

Two major themes arise from this review of literature. First, there is the idea that food is a central aspect of the ways in which we represent ourselves to ourselves and to others. Second, and more politically oriented, there is an understanding that public discourse around food is controlled by powerful interests within our society (typically corporations), and this has led to the promotion of unhealthy foods, and the misrepresentation and misappropriation of traditional foodways, all at the expense of the less powerful. The academic study of communication is concerned with understanding the ways in which humans share verbal and nonverbal symbols, the meanings of the shared symbols, and the consequences of the sharing. Broadly viewed, communication food scholarship looks at how, what, and to what effect meaning is created as message producers (typically, but not exclusively, corporations) create messages about food (advertisements, commercials, films) that circulate in culture and are interpreted by audiences. This chapter explores the theoretical and methodological approaches that communication scholars have used to investigate and explain how humans use food to create and share meaning, and then offers some ideas about future research and ways to get started in the field.

The academic study of communication is concerned with understanding the ways in which humans share verbal and nonverbal symbols, the meanings of the shared symbols, and the consequences of the sharing. Broadly viewed, communication food scholarship looks at how, what, and to what effect meaning is created as message producers (typically, but not exclusively, corporations) create messages about food (advertisements, commercials, films) that circulate in culture and are interpreted by audiences. This chapter explores the theoretical and methodological approaches that communication scholars have used to investigate and explain how humans use food to create and share meaning, and then offers some ideas about future research and ways to get started in the field.

Historical background of food scholarship in communication and major theoretical approaches in use

While this chapter is of interest to food studies scholars who want to know what's up in communication food research, it is designed primarily to offer a solid foundation in the current state of and opportunities in communication food scholarship for those in communication who are looking for guidance (or reassurance) in structuring their thinking about food or contemplating a foray into the field. As such, a principal assumption is that communication scholars conceptualize food studies from broad historical and intellectual traditions within communication rather than from singular theoretical approaches. So while the story here weaves in theoretical approaches, which are often unstated in the literature, it is designed so the reader can readily locate herself within the field of research.

The four intellectual fields that appear most often in the communication food studies literature are rhetoric, public relations, media effects and advertising, and cultural studies. Before looking at the history and current landscape of these four areas, it's important to mention what is and what is not being covered and why. The focus is on research that has appeared in communication books (mostly edited collections), in communication journals, and at communication conferences (the National Communication Association and International Communication Association conferences in particular). This methodological emphasis gives a strong indication of what the researchers and the communication discipline think of as counting as communication scholarship. However, within this wide look at communication food scholarship, some food-related communication scholarship and some communication-related food scholarship are not covered in depth for two reasons.

First, there are the research areas in which food-related communication scholarship is important but ultimately subsumed by larger disciplinary concerns. The two big areas here are health communication and marketing communication. While the communication aspects of health communication are salient and occasionally appear in the food-oriented literature, the concept of health (diet, nutrition, exercise, obesity, etc., but also, to a degree, food safety and food policy) is not reducible to concepts of food. In other words, health communication, which would cover everything from USDA information campaigns to doctor–patient communication, is its own field. While marketing uses communication techniques and there is a lot of research about the marketing of food, marketing is not reducible to communication and, further, one gets the sense that food in much of this research is simply an interchangeable commodity, no more or less relevant than if the subject were cars or watches or dishwashers.

Second, there is food scholarship that is essentially interdisciplinary and cross-disciplinary in nature to which communication scholars contribute. In these areas, this article is just the communication hand grasping the interdisciplinary trunk: for a better sense of the whole elephant, check out this book's section on food studies and popular media, especially the chapters on film, journalism, television, and cultural studies.

Rhetoric

Rhetorical analysis looks at how messages are constructed, by whom and the persuasive effectiveness of the messages. Rhetoric is historically linked to the analysis of public and political speech through Aristotle. Brummett (1981) followed this traditional political approach when he looked at how the 1980 US presidential candidates were rhetorically associated with gastronomic terms.

The earliest rhetorical food analysis pointed the way toward both linguistic and intercultural analysis of food discourse. Among these early studies, Penzl (1934) researched how different terms for poached eggs appeared throughout New England, Wagoner (1957) was bemused at the lack of culinary words in textbook French language instruction, and Teller (1969) looked at consistency in the use of French, Italian, German and Yiddish, Spanish, and "Oriental" culinary terms across 190 restaurant menus in Chicago. More recent rhetorical work has looked at health claims in food labeling/advertising (Welford, 1992) and tactics that American organizations use to frame obesity as an issue of personal responsibility (Thomson, 2009); the latter article mixes rhetorical analysis with a combination of Laclau and Mouffe's theory of articulation and

Foucault's spectacle of the scaffold. Also worth noting in this general realm are Janis, Kaye, and Kirschner's (1965) study, which found that food increases acceptance of persuasive information (but sadly felt the persuasion was sullied with "the extraneous gratifying activity of eating") and Lippincott's (2003) analysis of texts related to a gender-related controversy about how to present cooking information at the 1893 Chicago World's Fair.

Kenneth Burke's rhetorical theory of dramatism anchors both Meister's (2001) analysis of the commodified "Good Life" on the Food Network and Heinz and Lee's (1998) look at the rhetorical construction of beef as a discourse of tradition and masculinity in US culture. The latter research is augmented by a Marxist theoretical approach, which also serves as an intellectual backdrop to many cultural studies approaches to food and communication detailed below.

Rhetorical analysis at some point overlaps with discourse analysis, which looks at lived discourse (often interpersonal communication) and adopts a psychological approach to attempt to understand what is said and how it is said. Along this intellectual edge, Amberg and Hall (2010) used rhetorical theories of discourse analysis to look at the manner in which journalists present information about farmed salmon; Cook, Reed, and Twiner (2009) drew on discourse analysis to analyze how consumers think about organic food in the UK; and Sprain (2006) looked at internet discussion groups to establish two disparate sectors of organic-food audiences, tasteful consumers and political actors.

Public relations

Public relations is an applied field of communication concerned with the maintenance of a public image for a public entity (a corporation, a celebrity), or, more generously, with managing effective communication between an entity and its publics. In its analysis of effective communication strategies it shares ties with rhetorical communication studies and, in its focus on using those strategies to communicate information to consumers, it is closely related to marketing.

There are two major public relations areas of communication food studies research. The first cluster of research looks at marketing and branding strategies, such as Pendleton's (1999) examination of Procter & Gamble's introduction of Crisco, Blue's (2009) look at the branding of beef by the Alberta beef industry, and Ragas and Roberts' (2009) case study of how the Chipotle food chain builds brand loyalty through its corporate social responsibility program. The second cluster is associated with risk or crisis communication, designed to determine how best (for the entity) to communicate sensitive and/or controversial information to consumers. In this area, Qin and Brown (2006) tried to figure out how best to present information about genetically engineered salmon to the public, Rodriguez (2007) studied how people assess information about food safety (finding that ensuring trust rather than actually communicating information might be a better communication strategy), and Greenberg and Elliott (2009) analyzed the management of a 2008 Canadian food contamination outbreak.

Media effects and children's ads

Media effects research seeks to discover what mediated messages do to people. Research in this area is mainly quantitative and, within the communication field, is typically set against cultural studies, which uses qualitative methods to discover what people do with messages. The theoretical backbone for media effects research is cultivation theory. Cultivation theory was developed in the late 1960s by George Gerbner and his research team to study the effects that television viewing (programs and commercials – the television environment) has on its audience. Cultivation theory found television contributes to the shaping of an individual's social reality, and that heavy viewers tend to hold more mainstream opinions and to think of the world less optimistically than lighter viewers. Cultivation analysis is often buttressed by Bandura's social learning theory, which posits that attitudes and behavior are learned through observing modeled behavior. Cultivation analysis is closely linked with content analysis as a method.

Food cultivation analysis has been concerned with how food and eating have been portrayed in the media, what types of food have been portrayed, and how these portrayals impact attitudes and behaviors. This approach has historically converged on health issues, especially in the case of children, and now tends to focus on the role of mediated communication in the obesity crisis. While some studies focused on program content (Gerbner, Gross, Morgan, and Signorelli, 1981; Nucci and Kubey, 2007; Ochsenhirt and Kim, 2008; Greenberg and Elliott, 2009) – mostly finding that "bad" food choices are most often depicted – most studies look at the influence of commercials and advertising.

With a few exceptions (e.g., Aronovsky and Furnham, 2008), the advertising research breaks down into two major, overlapping areas, the effects of healthy/unhealthy food messages and the effects of messages on children (technically a subset of the first area). All forms of media come under scrutiny within this research, including television, newspapers, magazines, and the internet. The emphasis here is on research that focuses on how the advertising of food influences audience attitudes, beliefs, and behaviors about food, excluding most studies that focus more specifically on related but broader issues of health, nutrition, obesity, etc.

Due to the ease of data collection, magazines have been a prime artifact for media effects research. Lord, Eastlack, and Stanton (1987), Klassen, Wauer and Cassel (1991) and Parker (2003) all looked at the role of food and health messages in magazine ads. Fay (2003) looked at food advertising New Zealand in 50 years of magazines, finding that advertising increasingly depicted a world that diverged from real-world social trends in terms of convenience, tradition, and "naturalness." Mastin and Campo (2006) looked at *Essence*, *Ebony* and *Jet*, finding the ads filled with high calorie/low nutrient items while the articles preached balancing low calories with exercise; this study also used media advocacy theory, which states that since media help to shape public and individual perceptions, they have a responsibility to promote pro-social messages.

Research on the effects of food advertising on children has a history stretching back a half century, with much of the research coming in the areas of applied developmental and social psychology and, more recently, marketing and advertising (Livingstone, 2005). Even more recently, this research area has been the domain of public policy bodies, especially within the European Union. The current thinking on the effects of advertising on children is that it has a "modest" (but nevertheless important) direct effect on food attitudes and behavior, but that other environmental factors that aren't being measured probably have greater effects (Livingstone, 2005). Due to the interdisciplinary nature of this research, this article does not offer a full review of the literature on advertising to kids. Instead, for the most comprehensive meta-reviews of the area check out Livingstone (2005) and Livingstone and Helsper (2006), for the extension of the debate into the cyberworld, seek out Sanberg (2011), and, for a broader analysis, take a look at the other relevant chapters in this book (e.g., psychology, law, television).

Interesting advertising-to-children analysis that doesn't take a strictly content-analysis approach includes Gorn and Goldberg's (1982) experimental attempt to find a correlation between ads and children's food choices, Gram *et al.*'s (2010) look at how Danone combines health and entertainment ("nutria-tainment") messages in European television commercials, Elliott's (2009) study of how children make sense of and respond to "fun foods" marketed toward them, and Thomson's (2009) investigation of the dangers involved in the performative aspects of "advergaming" and online food marketing aimed at children.

Cultural studies

The study of food and communication from a cultural/ritual point of view has its deep roots specifically in the often-cited Barthes (2008/1961) work on the semiotics of food in everyday life, and more generally (but less frequently cited) in Foucault and Baudrillard's post-modern theories of power and culture, Bourdieu's work on class and distinction, various aspects of Marxist criticism, and the Frankfurt and Birmingham Schools' critical cultural analysis of culture. The cultural studies approach looks at how industries, texts, and audiences share symbols to create meanings. Beyond the act of explaining how these symbols circulate to construct culture, critical cultural inquiry also seeks to understand and illuminate cultural areas of contestation, especially ideology and all manner of individual and social identities. Arising from these varying influences, cultural studies is by nature an interdisciplinary field, one with many theoretical and methodological interests that map efficiently onto the interdisciplinary field of food studies. Cultural studies is also covered in the popular culture and media section of this book; this article focuses primarily on cultural studies approaches from communication points of view. For an introductory volume that incorporates many of the research concerns of communication/media food scholars through a cultural studies framework, see Parasecoli (2008), which begins to move disciplinary boundaries and simply tackles food studies issues.

There are a number of early communication-specific articles that tackle food from a cultural/ritual communication point of view. Among the earliest is Henderson's (1970) "Food as Communication in American Culture," which relies heavily on anthropological viewpoints, including the work of Margaret Mead, and ponders the development of a "special kind of scientist" who, in essence, is a food studies scholar. Goode (1989) takes a similar approach in the "food" entry of the *International Encyclopedia of Communications*. Goode bases her understanding on the work of Levi-Strauss; curiously, she fails to consider the relevance of mediated communication in the relationship between food and communication.

As with general academic interest in food, the years since the turn of the twenty-first century have seen a wealth of food-centric cultural studies research. In addition to the individual articles that appeared in numerous publications covered below, this scholarship explosion has included edited volumes on food and film (Bower, 2004), eating and culture (Rubin, 2008), the ideology of mediated food representations (LeBesco and Naccarato, 2008), and food as communication (Cramer, Greene and Walters, 2011). These volumes cover a wealth of communication and food cultural studies scholarship and include essential background for anyone interested in this area. As such, the individual articles within these volumes aren't covered here, but the reader is advised to consult these volumes as foundational material for future research.

Communication–food cultural studies research has primarily focused on the analysis of two related areas of social discourse, lifestyle construction and identity construction. Central to both areas is an interest in the ideological construction and normalization of the lived consumer-oriented environment. This research typically manifests itself in the analysis of texts that message producers – typically corporations – produce and how they are received by audiences (although there is not much communication food research in reception studies).

Lifestyle construction studies break off into two branches, corporate identity construction and consumer lifestyle construction. The corporate identity construction area shares a kinship with marketing and public relations scholarship, with all interested in issues of branding, corporate image and identity – it's really a matter of one side hoping to find out consumer preferences to exploit them and the other side hoping to find consumer preferences to protect, empower, and understand consumers/citizens. Among the more interesting articles in this area, Reynolds (2004) used an ethnographic approach to look at how Monsanto created identity through advertising, Beverland *et al.* (2008) used informant interviews to look at the construction of authenticity for Trappist and Abbey beer brands, finding that consumers have a difficult time judging authenticity through advertising, Girardelli (2004) used semiotic analysis to look at the Fazoli restaurant chain's mythical construction of Italian food, and Ketchum (2005) used close textual analysis to look how cooking shows on the Food Network constructed consumer fantasies.

The idea of constructing consumer fantasies ties in with the construction of consumer lifestyles. This area of research looks at how mediated texts normalize consumption and respond to/create market segments. Hanke's (1989) look at the production of a food lifestyle in Philadelphia publications in the 1980s is an early and instructive entry in the communication-oriented cultural analysis of food, but is rarely cited in the literature. Other important texts in this area include de Solier's (2005) look at how Australian TV cooking shows both educate consumers and create class distinctions (i.e., they produce cultural capital for viewers), Yang's (2005) look at how the US media supported food rationing efforts during the Second World War, and Schneider and Davis's (2010) look at the role of the magazine *Australian Women's Weekly* in societal taste arbitration around health foods. Dickinson *et al.*'s (2001) look at the relationship between mass media and food through a lens of consumption is also worth searching out.

Work that investigates the role of food in the creation and maintenance of group and individual identity clusters around intercultural and gender concerns. Intercultural research primarily focuses on how concepts about food translate from one culture to another (Gallagher, 2004; Ogan, 2007; Cheong, Kim, and Zheng, 2010), often focusing on the analysis of the use (often revulsion, then incorporation) of co-cultural and subcultural foodways by dominant national cultures (Fonseca, 2005; Pearson and Kothari, 2007; Chiaro, 2008; Lindenfeld, 2007; Han, 2007; Chand, 2007; Shugart, 2008; Hoecherl-Alden and Lindenfeld, 2010).

The social construction of gender roles is a primary area of research for cultural studies scholars. This area of communication food research has been conducted almost exclusively on mediated artifacts, such as Brownlie, Hewer and Horne's (2005) look at cookbooks as a site of gendered cultural construction, Swenson's (2009) look at how celebrity TV chefs both challenge and reify gender roles, and Cooks's (2009) look at the performance of food-as-social-act as a site of identity construction and resistance. Historically gender-oriented media analysis has been concerned with investigating how women are portrayed in the media, the imbalances of power in mediated presentations of women, especially in advertising images, and with celebrating empowering moments. Examples that continue this tradition in the communication food realm include Lindenfeld's (2005) look at how the film *Fried Green Tomatoes* at once empowers and undercuts its gender and race narratives, Shroff's (2005) analysis of the Indian film *Mirch Masala* (*Spices*), which discusses the use of the chili pepper as a symbolic device of female resistance, West's (2007) look at the construction of a politicized version of women and motherhood in a cookbook, and Nathanson's (2009) look at cooking shows and female temporality.

The past few decades have seen a greater interest in the study of the mediated construction of masculinity/ies. This look at food and masculinity has revealed that men are as constricted in their food-associated gender roles (e.g., TV chef) as women, but that constriction offers more privileges and tends to come at the expense of women. In terms of magazines, Hollows (2002) looked at the construction of cooking as a male practice in *Playboy* magazine in the late 1950s, while Parasecoli (2005) used a semiotic approach to discuss the discourse of the male body in men's fitness magazines. In terms of television, Brownlie and Hewer (2007) looked at masculine practices in the construction of celebrity chef Jamie Oliver, Smith and Wilson (2004) looked at how a local cooking show positioned the viewer and created a feminized contemporary southern male, and Buerkle (2009) looked at the production of masculinity against femininity and metrosexuality in beef advertisements from Burger King.

There are a few analytical approaches that don't fit neatly into the above categories, but are worth a mention. In terms of general communication studies, Reagan and Collins (1986) simply surveyed people about mediated sources for recipes, and Eaves and Leather (1991) looked at contextual communication in the relationship between McDonald's and Burger King restaurant design and consumer behavior. In media history, Collins (2009) looked at the evolution of televised cooking shows and Bonner (2009) looked at the early development of cross-promotion between television and cookbooks, focusing on the work of Graham Kerr. With globalization theories as a backdrop, Huey (2005) considered the most effective ways to transmit food information in the new media world.

Research methodologies

Communication food scholarship can broadly be broken down into three methodological approaches: rhetorical analysis, quantitative analysis, and qualitative analysis.

Not surprisingly, rhetorical studies tend to rely on rhetorical analysis (which, for our purposes, is a method). Straightforward rhetorical analysis investigates how texts create persuasive arguments (Brummett, 1981; Welford, 1992; Pendleton, 1999; Amberg and Hall, 2010). Other types of rhetorical analysis employed in the study of food include Burkean (Heinz and Lee, 1998; Meister, 2001), critical-rhetorical (Thomson, 2009), and historical-rhetorical (Lippincott, 2003).

Quantitative methodologies allow for hypothesis testing and the generation of statistical evidence to support claims, but they tend to lack real-world applicability. Media effects research is almost exclusively joined with content analysis as a methodology (e.g., Kaufman, 1980; Lord, Eastlack, and Stanton, 1987; Klassen, Wauer, and Cassel, 1991; Fay, 2003; Parker, 2003; Mastin and Campo, 2006; Harrison, 2006; Aronovsky and Furnham, 2008; Nucci and Kubey, 2007; Gram, Le Roux, and Rampnoux, 2010; Cheong, Kim, and Zheng, 2010). The content analysis method consists of identifying a sample, such as food commercials aired during the Super Bowl in 1990–2010, and then coding and counting what happens in the sample. This gives a strong indication of what happens in the commercials, but it's unclear how real people in the real world use or make sense of this information. The other quantitative methodology used on occasion is experimental research design (Janis, Kaye, and Kirschner, 1965; Gorn and Goldberg, 1982; Rodriguez, 2007).

Qualitative methods incorporate a wide range of analytical techniques. The most encompassing method is a cultural critique, which typically combines aspects of ethnographic participant–observation methods with critical textual analysis. To varying degrees, most of the cultural studies work cited here employs this technique (Hollows, 2002; Ketchum, 2005; Gallagher, 2004; Brownlie, Hewer, and Horne, 2005; Lindenfeld, 2007; Parasecoli, 2005, Pearson and Kothari, 2007; Han, 2007; West, 2007; Chiaro, 2008; Shugart, 2008; Cooks, 2009; Swenson, 2009; Buerkle, 2009; Hoecherl-Alden and Lindenfeld, 2010). Some studies also use a more straightforward ethnographic analysis (Eaves and Leathers, 1991; Reynolds, 2004; Huey, 2005, Fonseca, 2005).

Beyond this cluster of qualitative methods, there are numerous other qualitative methods that have been employed, including straightforward textual analysis (Teller, 1969; Wagoner, 1957), interviews (Reagan and Collins, 1986; Dickinson et al., 2011; Beverland, Lindgreen, and Vink, 2008), critical visual analysis (Brownlie and Hewer, 2007), semiotic analysis (Girardelli, 2004), history and cultural analysis (de Solier, 2005), focus groups (Qin and Brown, 2006; Elliott, 2009), historical research (Bonner, 2009; Yang, 2005), and survey research (Lazerson, 1980;

Knodell, 1976; Ochsenhirt and Kim, 2008). Discourse analysis (not the conversation-analysis type) also appears in the analysis of cultural and mediated discourses. Case studies or research projects have combined methods, such as viewer letters, textual analysis, and ethnographic research (Smith and Wilson, 2004), interviews, surveys, textual analysis (Ragas and Roberts, 2009), textual analysis and interviews (Ogan, Ciçek, and Kaptan, 2007), corpus analysis, interviews, and focus groups (Cook, Reed, and Twiner, 2009), and discourse analysis and interviews (Chrysochous, 2010).

Avenues for future research

Aside from any discussion that would deal with the cumbersome moniker communication food studies, there are two meta-questions that serve as a productive initial position from which to think about the future of communication food studies research. First, is communication food studies viable as an "area of concern" within communication, distinct from its divisional roots as outlined above? Put another way: do we need communication food studies, per se, or do we just need communication researchers to study food? The lack of common texts and an at-times willful ignorance of literature across the different sub-fields within communication food studies seem to make the establishment of a distinct field a difficult proposition. Perhaps a different thematic synthesis of the material outlined above would lead to the necessary foundation.

Second, if the answer to the first question is yes (or even maybe), will we be able to produce communication food theory that is distinct from a simple application of communication theory to food and food-related issues? From a review of the literature it is apparent that communication researchers find the study of food an apt, interesting, and productive application of intellectual propensities and skills, but is there anything intrinsically different about the ways in which we communicate about food as distinct from the ways in which we communicate about other areas of our lives? What would communication food theory look like?

Whether or not these larger questions get answered (or even discussed), there is still a great deal of work to be done expanding on the research here and exploring how food works in other communication divisions. Here are some possibilities.

For rhetoric, the big area of research is to establish a rhetoric of food. Food certainly has a large influence on how we live our lives: what are the rhetorical means by which we are persuaded about food and how does food qua food persuade us? In terms of rhetorical analysis, there are large swaths of public discourse that have gone unexplored from a communication point of view. Some avenues: How have public leaders (presidents, prime ministers) talked about food? How has food been used rhetorically (and visually) in election campaigns? What would a rhetorical analysis of the discourse surrounding the US Farm Bill reveal (and how has the discourse changed over time)? What rhetorical devices do message posters use in online discussion forums about food? Further, we lack an understanding of how ideas about food circulate within cultural arenas divorced from (or peripheral or parallel to) mediated areas. For example, what role does communication (persuasive or not) have in the CSA, farmers' market, and community gardens cultural arenas? Within the restaurant workers community?

For cultural studies, it's probably necessary to take a step back and ask the big question: What is the ideology of food? There have been discussions about the ideology of hunger, of food production, etc., but is there a bigger ideological landscape that needs to be mapped? Is it possible to answer this question in any meaningful way without falling into a trap of grand narratives, or is it simply a matter of asking about ideologies in relation to specific cultural iterations of nation, race, class, gender, sexual orientation, etc.? Beyond the "big" question, Parasecoli

(2008) points toward the multiplicity of mediated locations for the analysis of food in popular culture beyond those already discussed at length – animation, advertising flyers, popular music, etc. There is also a lack of audience-reception research on the social/cultural uses of food (and food media) and a lack of communication-oriented research on the role of pleasure in food and food-media consumption.

Practical considerations for getting started – funding, programs, archival sources, tools, data sets, internet resources, scholarships and awards, etc. (where and how?)

There are no undergraduate degree programs specifically dedicated to communication food studies, although food studies degree and certificate programs typically offer a smattering of communication courses, usually in media production and/or analysis. At the graduate level, there are two major programs conducted in English. Boston University has a communication concentration in its Master of Liberal Arts in Gastronomy program, and the University of Gastronomic Science (Italy) offers food and communication masters programs. In addition, aspects of the Open University of Catalonia's (Spain) Food Systems, Culture and Society Program are appealing to communication scholars.

Funding communication food studies projects is no more or less difficult than funding any project in the humanities and social sciences. In other words, it's hard. Lacking more reliable sources of funding found in the hard sciences, it's more a process of working the system. Wear out internal institutional sources (could your food project in the community be funded by your service learning office?). Scour NEH, USDA, and Fulbright grant opportunities. Piggyback research on conference or personal travel. Beg.

Fortunately, a good deal of communication food research can be done inexpensively. Most mediated sources for analysis are available for free online or through libraries. Surveys, interviews, focus groups, and other qualitative data collection methods are typically supported through academic institutions and require more time than money. The same often goes for the use of data analysis software, such as SPSS and NVivo.

Key reading

Barthes, R. (2008 [1961]) "Toward a Psychosociology of Contemporary Food Consumption." In *Food and Culture: A Reader*. C. Counihan and P. Van Esterik, eds., pp. 28–35, 2nd edition. New York: Routledge.

Bower, A. L. ed. (2004) *Reel Food: Essays on Food and Film*. New York: Routledge.

Cramer, J. M., C. P. Greene, and L. M. Walters, eds. (2011) *Food as Communication: Communication as Food*. New York: Peter Lang.

Dickinson, R., A. Murcott, J. Eldridge, and S. Leader, (2011) "Breakfast, time, and 'breakfast time': Television, food, and the household organization of consumption." *Television & New Media*, 2: 235–56.

Hanke, R. (1989) "Mass media and lifestyle differentiation: An analysis of the public discourse about food." *Communication* 11(3): 221–38.

LeBesco, K. and P. Naccarato, eds. (2008) *Edible Ideologies: Representing Food and Meaning*. Albany, NY: State University Press of New York.

Livingstone, S. (2005) "Assessing the research base for the policy debate over the effects of food advertising to children." *International Journal of Advertising* 24(3): 273–96.

Parasecoli, F. (2008) *Bite Me: Food in Popular Culture*. Oxford: Berg.

Rubin, L. C. ed. (2008) *Food for Thought: Essays on Eating and Culture*. Jefferson, NC: McFarland.

Shugart, H. A. (2008) "Sumptuous texts: Consuming 'otherness' in the food film genre." *Critical Studies in Media Communication* 25(1): 68–90.

Bibliography

Amberg, S. M. and T. E. Hall (2010) "Precision and rhetoric in media reporting about contamination in farmed salmon." *Science Communication* 32(4): 489–513.

Aronovsky, A. and A. Furnham, (2008) "Gender portrayals in food commercials at different times of the day: A content analytic study." *Communications: The European Journal of Communication Research* 33(2): 169–90.

Barthes, R. (2008 [1961]) "Toward a Psychosociology of Contemporary Food Consumption." In *Food and Culture: A Reader.* C. Counihan and P. Van Esterik, eds., pp. 28–35, 2nd edition. New York: Routledge.

Beverland, M. B., A. Lindgreen, and M. Vink (2008) "Projecting authenticity through advertising: Consumer judgments of advertisers' claims." *Journal of Advertising* 37(1): 5–15.

Blue, G. (2009) "Branding beef: Marketing, food safety, and the governance of risk." *Canadian Journal of Communication* 34(2): 229–44.

Bonner, F. (2009) "Early multi-platforming: Television food programmes, cookbooks and other print spin-offs." *Media History* 15(3): 345–58.

Bower, A. L. (Ed.). (2004) *Reel Food: Essays on Food and Film.* New York: Routledge.

Bradley, S. G., S. F. Rosaen, T. R. Worrell, C. T. Salmon, and J. E. Volkman (2009) "A portrait of food and drink in commercial TV series." *Health Communication* 24: 295–303.

Brownlie, D. and Hewer, P. (2007) "Prime beef cuts: Culinary images for thinking 'men'." *Consumption, Markets & Culture* 10(3): 229–50.

Brownlie, D., P. Hewer, and S. Horne (2005) "Culinary tourism: An exploratory reading of contemporary representations of cooking." *Consumption, Markets and Culture* 8(1): 7–26.

Brummett, B. (1981) "Gastronomic reference, synecdoche, and political images." *Quarterly Journal of Speech* 67(2): 138–45.

Buerkle, C. W. (2009) "Metrosexuality can stuff it: Beef consumption as (heteromasculine) fortification." *Text and Performance Quarterly* 29(1): 77–93.

Chand, A. (2007) "The Fiji Indian chutney generation: The cultural spread between Fiji and Australia." *International Journal of Media and Cultural Politics* 3(2): 131–48.

Cheong, Y., K. Kim, and L. Zheng (2010) "Advertising appeals as a reflection of culture: a cross-cultural analysis of food advertising appeals in China and the US." *Asian Journal of Communication* 20(1): 1–16.

Chiaro, D. (2008) "A taste of otherness eating and thinking globally." *European Journal of English Studies* 12(2): 195–209.

Chrysochou, P. (2010) "Food health branding: The role of marketing mix elements and public discourse in conveying a healthy brand image." *Journal of Marketing Communications* 16(1/2): 69–85.

Collins, K. (2009) *Watching what we eat: The evolution of television cooking shows.* New York: Continuum.

Cook, G., M. Reed, and A. Twiner (2009) "'But it's all true!': Commercialism and commitment in the discourse of organic food promotion." *Text & Talk* 29(2): 151–73.

Cooks, L. (2009) "You are what you (don't) eat? Food, identity, and resistance. *Text and Performance Quarterly,* 29(1): 94–110.

Cramer, J. M., C. P. Greene, and L. M. Walters, eds. (2011) *Food as Communication: Communication as Food.* New York: Peter Lang.

de Solier, I. (2005) "TV dinners: Culinary television, education and distinction." *Continuum: Journal of Media & Cultural Studies* 19(4): 465–81.

Dickinson, R., A. Murcott, J. Eldridge, and S. Leader (2001) "Breakfast, time, and "breakfast time": Television, food, and the household organization of consumption." *Television & New Media* 2: 235–56.

Eaves, M. H. and D. G. Leathers (1991) "Context as communication: McDonald's vs. Burger King." *Journal of Applied Communication Research* 19: 263–89.

Elliott, C. D. (2009) "Healthy food looks serious: How children interpret packaged food products." *Canadian Journal of Communication* 34: 359–80.

Fay, M. (2003) "A 50-year longitudinal study of changes in the content and form of food advertising in New Zealand magazines." *International Journal of Advertising* 22: 67–91.

Fonseca, V. (2005) "Nuevo Latino: Rebranding Latin American cuisine." *Consumption, Markets & Culture* 8(2): 95–130.

Gallagher, M. (2004) "What's so funny about Iron Chef? *Journal of Popular Film and Television* 31(4): 176–84.

Gerbner, G., L. Gross, M. Morgan, and N. Signorelli (1981) "Health and medicine on television." *New England Journal of Medicine* 305: 901–4.

Girardelli, D. (2004) "Commodified identities: The myth of Italian food in the United States." *Journal of Communication Inquiry* 28(4): 307–24.

Goode, J. (1989) "Food." In *International Encyclopedia of Communications*. Barnouw, E. ed., pp. 187–93. New York: Oxford University Press.

Gorn, G. J. and M. E. Goldberg, (1982) "Behavioral evidence of the effects of televised food messages on children. *Journal of Consumer Research* 9: 200–05.

Gram, M., V. de la Ville, A. Le Roux, N. Boireau, and O. Rampnoux (2010) "Communication on food, health and nutrition: A cross-cultural analysis of the Danonino brand and nutri-tainment." *Journal of Marketing Communications* 16(1–2): 87–103.

Greenberg, J. and C. Elliott, (2009) "A cold cut crisis: Listeriosis, Maple Leaf Foods, and the politics of apology." *Canadian Journal of Communication* 34: 189–204.

Han, A. (2007) "'Can I tell you what we have to put up with?': Stinky fish and offensive durian." *Continuum: Journal of Media & Cultural Studies* 21(3): 361–77.

Hanke, R. (1989) "Mass media and lifestyle differentiation: An analysis of the public discourse about food." *Communication* 11(3): 221–38.

Harrison, K. (2006) "Fast and sweet: Nutritional attributes of television food advertisements with and without black characters." *Howard Journal of Communications* 17(4): 249–64.

Heinz, B. and R. Lee (1998) "Getting down to the meat: The symbolic construction of meat consumption." *Communication Studies* 49: 86–99.

Henderson, M. C. (1970) "Food as communication in American culture." *Today's Speech* 18(3): 3–8.

Hoecherl-Alden, G. and L. Lindenfeld, (2010) "Thawing the forth: *Mostly Martha* as a German-Italian eatopia." *Journal of International and Intercultural Communication* 3(2): 114–35.

Hollows, J. (2002) "The bachelor dinner: Masculinity, class and cooking in *Playboy*, 1953–61." *Continuum: Journal of Media & Cultural Studies* 16(2): 143–55.

Huey, T. A. (2005) "Thinking globally, eating locally: Website linking and the performance of solidarity in global and local food movements." *Social Movement Studies* 4(2): 123–37.

Janis, I. L., D. Kaye, and P. Kirschner (1965) "Facilitating effects of "eating-while-reading" on responsiveness to persuasive communications." *Journal of Personality & Social Psychology* 1(2): 181–86.

Kaufman, L. (1980) "Prime-time nutrition." *Journal of Communication* 30(3): 37–46.

Ketchum, C. (2005) "The essence of cooking shows: How the Food Network constructs consumer fantasies." *Journal of Communication Inquiry* 29: 217–34.

Klassen, M. L., S. M. Wauer, and S. Cassel (1991) "Increases in Health and Weight Loss Claims in Food Advertising in the eighties." *Journal of Advertising Research* 30(6): 32–37.

Knodell, J. E. (1976) "Matching perceptions of food writers, editors, and readers." *Public Relations Review* 2(3): 37–56.

Lazerson, B. H. (1980) "Is a pizza a pie? *American Speech* 55(2): 146–49.

LeBesco, K. and P. Naccarato eds., (2008) *Edible Ideologies: Representing Food and Meaning*. Albany, NY: State University Press of New York.

Lindenfeld, L. (2005) "Women who eat too much: Femininity and food in *Fried Green Tomatoes*. In *From Betty Crocker to Feminist Food Studies: Critical Perspectives on Women and Food*. Avakian, A. V. and Haber, B. eds., pp. 221–45. Amherst and Boston: University of Massachusetts Press.

——(2007) "Visiting the Mexican American family: *Tortilla Soup* as culinary tourism." *Communication and Critical/Cultural Studies* 4(3): 303–20.

Lippincott, G. (2003) "'Something in motion and something to eat attract the crowd': Cooking with science at the 1893 world's fair." *Journal of Technical Writing and Communication* 33(2): 141–64.

Livingstone, S. and E. J. Helsper, (2006) "Does advertising literacy mediate the effects of advertising on children? A critical examination of two linked research literatures in relation to obesity and food choice." *Journal of Communication* 56(3): 560–84.

Livingstone, S. (2005) "Assessing the research base for the policy debate over the effects of food advertising to children." *International Journal of Advertising* 24(3): 273–96.

Lord, J. B., J. O. Eastlack Jr., and J. L. Stanton Jr., (1987) "Health Claims in Advertising: Is there a bandwagon effect? *Journal of Advertising Research* 27(2): 9–15.

Mastin, T. and S. Campo, (2006) "Conflicting messages: Overweight and obesity advertisements and articles in Black magazines." *Howard Journal of Communications* 17(4): 265–85.

Meister, M. (2001) "Cultural feeding, good life science, and the TV Food Network." *Mass Communication & Society* 4(2): 165–82.

Nathanson, E. (2009) "As easy as pie: Cooking shows, domestic efficiency, and postfeminist temporality." *Television & New Media* 10(4): 311–30.

Nucci, M. L. and Kubey, R. (2007) "'We begin tonight with fruits and vegetables': Genetically modified food in the evening news 1980–2003." *Science Communication* 29(2): 147–76.

Ochsenhirt, A. M. and Kim, S. (2008) "Influence of parental control of television viewing on children's attitudes and behaviors of food." *Journal of the Northwest Communication Association* 37: 10–35.

Ogan, C. L., Çiçek, F., and Kaptan, Y. (2007) "Reverse glocalization? Marketing a Turkish cola in the shadow of a giant." *Journal of Arab & Muslim Media Research* 1(1): 47–62.

Parasecoli, F. (2005) "Feeding hard bodies: Food and masculinities in men's fitness magazines." *Food & Foodways* 13: 17–37.

——(2008) *Bite Me: Food in Popular Culture*. Oxford: Berg.

Parker, B. J. (2003) "The use of nutrient content, health, and structure/function claims in food advertisements." *Journal of Advertising* 32(3): 47–55.

Pearson, S. and Kothari, S. (2007) "Menus for a multicultural New Zealand." *Continuum: Journal of Media & Cultural Studies* 21(1): 45–58.

Pendleton, S. C. (1999) "'Man's most important food is fat:' The use of persuasive techniques in Procter & Gamble's public relations campaign to introduce Crisco, 1911–13." *Public Relations Quarterly* Spring: 6–14.

Penzl, H. (1934) "New England terms for 'poached eggs'." *American Speech* 9(2): 90.

Qin, W. and Brown, J. L. (2006) "Consumer opinions about genetically engineered salmon and information effect on opinions: A qualitative approach." *Science Communication* 28(2): 243–72.

Ragas, M. W. and Roberts, M. S. (2009) "Communicating corporate social responsibility and brand sincerity: a case study of Chipotle Mexican Grill's "Food with Integrity" program." *International Journal of Strategic Communication* 3: 264–80.

Reagan, J. and Collins, J. (1986) "Sources for recipe information." *Journalism Quarterly* 63(2): 389–91.

Reynolds, M. (2004) "How does Monsanto do it? An ethnographic case study of an advertising campaign." *Text* 24(3): 329–52.

Rodriguez, L. (2007) "The impact of risk communication on the acceptance of irradiated food." *Science Communication* 28(4): 476–500.

Rubin, L. C. (Ed.). (2008) *Food for Thought: Essays on Eating and Culture*. Jefferson, NC: McFarland.

Sandberg, H. (2011) "Tiger talk and candy king: marketing of unhealthy food and beverages to Swedish children." *Communications: The European Journal of Communication Research* 36(2): 217–44.

Schneider, T. and Davis, T. (2010) "Advertising food in Australia: Between antinomies and gastro-anomy." *Consumption Markets & Culture* 13(1): 31–41.

Shroff, B. (2005) "Chili Peppers as Tools of Resistance: Ketan Mehta's Mirch Masala." In *From Betty Crocker to Feminist Food Studies: Critical Perspectives on Women and Food*. Avakian, A. V. and Haber, B. eds., pp. 246–56. Amherst and Boston: University of Massachusetts Press.

Shugart, H. A. (2008) "Sumptuous texts: Consuming "otherness" in the food film genre." *Critical Studies in Media Communication* 25(1): 68–90.

Smith, G. M. and Wilson, P. (2004) "Country cookin' and cross dressin': Television, southern white masculinities, and hierarchies of cultural taste." *Television & New Media* 5(3): 175–95.

Sprain, L. (2006) *Voices of Organic Consumption: An Ethnographic and Rhetorical Exploration of Organic Consumption as Political Consumption*. Unpublished paper presented at the International Communication Association, San Antonio.

Swenson, R. (2009) "Domestic divo? Televised treatments of masculinity, femininity and food." *Critical Studies in Media Communication* 26(1): 36–53.

Teller, J. W. (1969) "The treatment of foreign terms on Chicago restaurant menus." *American Speech* 44(2): 911–05.

Thomson, D. M. (2009) "Big food and the body politics of personal responsibility." *Southern Communication Journal* 74(1): 2–17.

Wagoner, R. A. (1957) "The French menu, a textbook blind spot." *Modern Language Journal* 57(41): 342–45.

Welford, W. (1992) "Supermarket semantics: The rhetoric of food labeling and advertising." *Et Cetera: A Review of General Semantics* 49(1): 3–17.

West, I. (2007) "Performing resistance in/from the kitchen: The practice of maternal pacifist politics and La WISP's cookbooks." *Women's Studies in Communication* 30(3): 358–83.

Yang, M. (2005) "Creating the kitchen patriot: Media promotion of food rationing and nutrition campaigns on the American home front during World War II." *American Journalism* 22(3): 55–75.

4

Historical background of food scholarship in psychology and major theoretical approaches in use

Kima Cargill

Psychology and food studies spans virtually every "sub-discipline" of the field. Methodologies vary and the utility of the scholarship spans from cultural and ethnic facets of food experiences to the neuronal level of how our brains respond to specific tastes, smells, and ingredients. Most of the scholarship has focused on a few circumscribed areas, namely eating disorders, obesity, and intake regulation, in addition to a smaller handful of scholarship which has championed the cultural and ethnic facets of the psychology of food. In recent years new work has emerged in clinical, cultural, cognitive, experimental, neuro, and evolutionary psychology.

Historically speaking, the discipline of psychology has paid surprisingly little attention to food and eating. Most of the scholarship has focused on a few circumscribed areas, namely eating disorders, obesity, and intake regulation, in addition to a smaller handful of scholarship that has championed the cultural and ethnic facets of the psychology of food. This body of work has begun to change more rapidly in recent years, with new work emerging in clinical, cultural, cognitive, experimental, neuro, and evolutionary psychology. Taken together, the discipline is arriving at a broader, though still nascent approach to food studies, with enormous possibility on the horizon.

Anna Freud began the study of food in its logical place: breastfeeding. In her essay "The Psychoanalytic Study of Infantile Feeding Disturbances" (1946), she was the first to argue that unhealthy eating behaviors in adulthood were rooted in early maladaptive family relationships. Anna Freud believed that ambivalence toward the mother may manifest itself as vacillating bingeing and purging behaviors, or that guilty feelings toward the mother would manifest themselves as an inability to enjoy food, or that jealousy of the mother's love for other children would manifest itself as greediness or insatiability. For decades after Anna Freud's work, most of the scholarship on the psychology of food continued in the psychoanalytic tradition, often using Sigmund Freud's oral stage of psychosexual development as the basis for understanding food-related pathologies. These ideas can't be put to experimental test, but as with much Freudian and psychoanalytic theory, the theory now seems dated to most and rests outside mainstream, contemporary psychology.

In contrast to the psychoanalytic tradition, experimental psychologists have been studying eating in humans and non-human animals for a shorter period, but with more scientific rigor. This research tends to be less about food per se, than about bodily functions and regulation. Largely regulated by the hypothalamus, hunger and thirst have been the subject of many decades of experimental research. Both brain anatomy and chemistry, specifically neurotransmitters such as dopamine and serotonin regulate meal size, thirst, and frequency. The best primer on experimental psychology and food is A.W. Logue's ambitious volume, *The Psychology of Eating and Drinking* (2004), which reviews the literature on thirst, hunger, satiety, taste preferences, disordered eating, and obesity. Written primarily to serve as a classroom textbook and with over a thousand references, it is an impressive review and synthesis of the extant scholarship on eating and drinking from experimental psychology. In addition to intake regulation and taste preference development, the book is also devoted to eating- and drinking-related pathologies, namely bulimia, anorexia, obesity, alcoholism, smoking, diabetes, and fetal alcohol syndrome. Logue reviews the etiology, course, and treatment of these disorders, as well as provides resources and referral information for those seeking treatment. Interestingly, there is a great deal of variation in how different people experience the taste of the same foods. What tastes bitter to some is undetectable to others. For example, researchers have determined that people can generally be classified into one of three groups: supertasters, tasters, and nontasters, based upon their gustatory sensitivity to phenylthiocarbamide, or the chemical that causes bitter tastes. Not only do each of us have different thresholds of phenylthiocarbamide sensitivity, but there are significant cross-cultural differences that may also serve to partially explain how certain components of cuisine have developed around the world. For example, about one-third of North Americans are non-tasters, meaning that beer, coffee, saccharin, and certain dark green vegetables are palatable, whereas about 10 percent of Chinese university students are non-tasters, meaning that the aforementioned food and drinks taste overwhelmingly bitter to them (Logue, 2004: 56).

Another excellent introductory volume to psychology and food studies is Elizabeth Capaldi's *Why We Eat What We Eat: The Psychology of Eating* (1996). This edited volume moves away from the strictly bodily cues of hunger and satiety, and instead examines eating patterns based on life experiences. The focus, then, is on how humans *learn* about eating, from conditioning experiences as well as from family and culture, rather than the purely physiological mechanisms involved in hunger, digestion, and eating. Partly written with practitioners in mind, this book advances the idea that healthful eating patterns can be learned. Comparisons of eating patterns are made between obese and non-obese individuals, as well as explorations of early factors in taste and flavor preferences, including the development of food preferences that begin prenatally. One contributor to this volume is Paul Rozin, often considered the most established "food psychologist." Outside of psychoanalysis and experimental psychology, other voices were mostly absent until Rozin, who had largely focused on laboratory work, began looking at cultural determinants of food, as well as influences of the ancestral diet (Rozin, 1996, 2007).

Additionally, Rozin has conducted research contrasting the French and American diets in order to better understand the "French Paradox" (Rozin et al., 2003). He argues that many factors account for the differences in diet and cultural relationships to food. First, the French focus more on the experience of food, rather than the consequences. They are also less concerned about variety, which is notable because psychologists have shown that increased variety is related to overweight and obesity. In one study, for example, French respondents stated that they preferred to have ten flavor choices for ice cream, rather than the 50 choices preferred by Americans. Food variety was crucial for our ancestors in order to avoid nutritional deficiencies, but in our contemporary world of overabundance (in many places in the world) variety does a disservice to the individual because it increases overall calorie consumption. Other factors identified by Rozin in explaining the French paradox are lifestyle: Homes and neighborhoods designed where walking and bicycling are easier than driving, small markets, bakeries, and butchers are easily accessible to many. Snacking between meals is not common, and a general attitude of moderation prevails over a drive toward abundance seen in the United States.

In *Desire, Ritual, and Cuisine* (Cargill, 2007) I write about the psychological experience of many food rituals, particularly those related to specific rites of passages that have been handed down over generations. I argue that many food rituals attempt to invoke the past, a group's history, or even the deceased. In the Mexican celebration *Día de los Muertos*, for example, altars are made for the dead and women spend all day preparing the favorite food of the deceased to place at the altar. Other food rituals invoke a temporal regression as a means of connecting with one's ancestors. In the highly ritualized Passover Seder, for example, the Seder plate contains important symbols of the holiday. Maror, the bitter herbs, are used as a symbol of the bitterness of slavery. Zeroa, a roasted shank bone, is a symbol of the Passover sacrifice. Salt water is also used to symbolize the tears of slavery. The Seder is a ritual meant to bridge the cultural space and emotional experience between generations, faraway places, and the rituals of one's ancestors. It is not only the telling of a story, but a reenactment. It is an important component of both religious identity and history in that it also tells the story of a people so that it is never forgotten. The Seder then is a mechanism by which psychological "genes" are handed down through generations and transmit political information through oral history (Volkan, 1997). The poignant role of food and food ritual in the intergenerational transmission of sociopolitical history can be seen in the humorous Jewish saying regarding religious holidays: "They tried to kill us, we won, let's eat."

In other recent research evolutionary psychologists have contributed to the knowledge base on food. Deirdre Barrett's book entitled *Waistland* (2007) examines how foraging behavior, adaptive in ancestral times, becomes maladaptive in our sedentary, prosperous society. Barrett's audience is those who want to lose weight and/or stop the cycle of dieting. In addition to explaining the evolutionary determinants for food preferences, she also covers the physiological responses to certain foods, particularly glucose. Using the concept of "supernormal stimuli" from ethology, she explains how artificial objects can appeal to our senses more than the natural stimuli for which those instincts were designed, leading us to crave high sugar, high fat, and high salt foods. Other researchers refer to these as "superfoods", referring to "hyperpalatable" foods that surpass the rewarding properties of traditional foods (Gearhardt *et al.*, 2011).

Although not a psychologist, primatologist Richard Wrangham (2009) argues that cooking food, which began probably about 500,000 years ago, is what originally separated humans from apes and from our non-human ancestors. Evolutionary psychologists would do well to build on Wrangham's work, particularly to understand behavior related to cooking and food acquisition. He argues that our ancestors discovered that the control of fire could be used to cook food, which offered crucial biological advantages, such as maximizing energy, impeding food spoilage, and improving overall food safety. Quite simply, the energy the body must expend to consume and digest raw food is significantly more than what it expends when the same food is cooked. The energy of the heat used for cooking effectively pre-digests food, allowing the body to preserve more of its energy, allowing for a net gain in calories – a crucial biological advantage when food was scarce. In other words, Wrangham argues that cooking food made digestion easier and so the human gut could grow smaller compared to other non-human primates. The enormous energy previously spent on digestion then allowed the human brain to grow larger. The advantages to cooking food were not just biological. The social changes to human life were revolutionary. Gathering around a fire required socializing, calmed the human temperament, and fostered cooperative living.

Not only did cooking food become biologically and culturally important some 500,000 years ago, but it seems that it also became psychologically important to our species. Taming fire and using it to cook food not only had profound evolutionary consequences, but profound psychological consequences as well. The act of finding food, gathering around the fire, cooking and consuming it, is a profoundly important experience, not just to the body, but to the self. It is around the fire, or the hearth, or the dinner table, that community happens (Cargill, 2012). "When fire and food combined … an almost irresistible focus was created for communal life … The enhanced value cooking imparts to food elevates it above nourishment and opens up new imaginative possibilities: meals can be sacrificial sharings, love-feasts, ritual acts, occasions for the magical transformations wrought by fire – one of which is the transformation of competitors into a community" (Fernández-Armesto, 2001: 13). In other words, cooking is what civilized the species.

Other recent work in food and psychology has been Brian Wansink's research at the Cornell Food and Brand Lab, extraordinary both in its findings, as well as in its implications for the obesity crisis. Wansink's *Mindless Eating* (2006) specifically focuses on consumer behavior and examines the myriad contextual cues, often very subtle, which prompt people to overeat. Wansink has ingeniously designed a lab that functions as a working restaurant, which allows him to conduct controlled experiments in a "real world" setting, where most diners presumably behave similarly to how they would in a real restaurant. For example, in his "bottomless soup bowl" experiment, Wansink rigs a device that allows a soup bowl to be discreetly and continuously refilled (as it's being eaten from). Diners who have the "bottomless bowl" continue to eat 73 percent more soup than diners with a regular bowl of soup without perceiving they are overeating.

In another series of experiments, Wansink found that when given a large free tub of popcorn, moviegoers ate more than those with the smaller container, even when the popcorn in both conditions was 14 days old. The implications for this research is simply enormous from a public policy perspective. For example, the USDA's Smarter Lunchroom Initiative, which does things like redesign school cafeterias and rename vegetable dishes, is based on these findings. Other findings include the discovery that children paying in cash in school lunch rooms purchase 30 percent more healthy food than when they pay with debit cards (Just and Wansink, 2009).

Also in the area of obesity, Adam Drewnowski has focused extensively on the relationship between poverty and obesity and the links between obesity and diabetes rates as moderated by access to healthy foods in vulnerable populations. This more recent epidemiological work has come on the heels of decades of his research on taste function and food preferences, including the perception of bitter and sweet, as well as the texture of fat. His work on the behavioral phenotype in human obesity examined how the development of obesity is influenced by family risk, but modified by dietary choice.

Yale psychologist Kelly Brownell, who directs the Rudd Center for Food Policy and Obesity, has done extensive research on food and public policy. Most recently he has examined the effect of taxing sugared soda and has lobbied extensively for states to implement such a tax in order to reduce consumption and generate revenue (Andreyeva, Chaloupka, and Brownell, 2011; Brownell and Ludwig, 2011). He has examined nutrition-related claims on breakfast cereals and how they influence parents' willingness to buy them (Schwartz, Vartanian, Wharton and Brownell, 2008), as well as the influence of licensed characters on packaged foods on children's snack preferences (Roberto, Baik, Harris and Brownell, 2010). Brownell has also been actively involved in the movement to provide nutritional information to consumers at chain restaurants and has conducted outcome research on its effects (Roberto, Schwartz and Brownell, 2009; Roberto, Larsen, Agnew, Balk and Brownell, 2010). Most recently Brownell and his associates have examined whether food can be addictive in the same ways as drugs and alcohol, specifically whether or not there are neural correlates between eating and drug use (Gearhardt, Grilo, DiLeone, Brownell, and Potenza 2011). Findings have shown that foods stimulate the same dopamine reward pathways as many drugs. In related research, the Rudd Center has developed and validated a Food Addiction Scale (Gearhardt, Corbin and Brownell, 2009) that can be used by clinicians and other researchers.

Neuropsychologists who study food and eating often focus on both smell and taste since they are tandem sensory processes. Much interesting research has been conducted on how the brain processes, encodes, and responds to odor and taste. For example, the "Proust Phenomenon" (Chu and Downes, 2000, 2002) refers to how odors, usually food odors, have the ability to cue very specific types of memories. Research on this phenomenon has found that food smells have an extraordinary capacity to trigger autobiographical memories. Not only do they trigger autobiographical memories, but old (in some studies 40-year-old memories), vivid, and emotional memories. Interestingly, Proustian type memories are associated with a specific stage of development, age six to ten years. Chu and Downes tested a hypothesis called "differential cue affordance value," which says that different sensory modalities carry different cue affordances – or the efficiency with which they access autobiographical memories. Olfaction was found to have a more powerful cue affordance and to retrieve memories that were much older than visual or verbal cues. One explanation is that the olfactory bulb projects to a number of structures involved in memory, hippocampus, amygdala, thalamus.

Research methodologies

Research methodologies in the psychology of food almost exclusively involve laboratory-based, experimental research. While it is not essential that a new researcher in this area use this approach, it is by far what dominates mainstream academic psychology publications. A.W. Logue, in the aforementioned classroom text on the psychology of eating and drinking, focuses almost entirely on controlled studies with rats. Brian Wansink, in his *Mindless Eating*, uses analogue studies in which participants are brought into his "restaurant," i.e. the lab that is part of his Cornell research facility. Drewnowski conducts quantitative research, sometimes in laboratory settings and sometimes using naturalistic observations in fast food restaurants or grocery stores. Reflecting dominant trends in psychology, the research that is quantitative and advances "psychology as a science" currently dominates the field.

Additionally, there remains theoretical scholarship and qualitative research that uses field-based and/or naturalistic modes of inquiry, more characteristic of anthropology. Paul Rozin's earlier research, for example on the acquisition of taste preferences for chili peppers in Mexico, falls into this category (Rozin *et al.*, 1982; Rozin, Mark, and Schiller, 1982). Wrangham's research on the socializing effect of cooking in early humans, i.e., how we were tamed by the use of fire, uses archeological data to support his theory.

As food studies research expands in psychology I expect also to see the expansion of multi-method studies, particularly those with both qualitative and quantitative methods. Many studies coming out in the journal *Food, Culture, and Society*, for example, are collaborative studies by scholars in different disciplines, such as social sciences and nutrition. These kinds of collaborations not only provide rich, cross-validating data sets, but also stand to serve students interested in food studies who can learn multiple theoretical and methodological perspectives by taking one class or by being involved in one research study. The central message though, to anyone looking at a future in food studies, is simply that in psychology there is room for *any* methodological approach, so long as it is rigorous and advances the current knowledge base.

Kima Cargill

Avenues for future research

Research on the psychology of food is ripe for innovation and growth, and given the wide berth of the discipline, there is room for inquiry in social, cultural, and biological fields of study. Interdisciplinary research is at the forefront of food scholarship, quite simply because of the myriad factors that influence food choice and eating.

Obesity and nutrition will continue to be two major areas of research. Where there will be a great need is in outcome research to assess the vast array of policy measures currently being implemented to curb obesity. Changes in school lunch programs, happy meals, and nutrition labels, to name a few, are all measures that will require widespread assessment. Additionally, conducting pilot and analogue research on such interventions in focus groups or lab settings is also crucial in designing such programs. Much of this research can also be informed by behavioral economics, which includes the very powerful determinant of one's economic situation on one's food choice. Drewnowski and Specter (2004), for example, demonstrate how previous food scarcity is correlated to obesity, because one's history of food uncertainty "teaches" one to consume as much as possible when food is abundant to stave off future starvation. The better we understand predictors and correlates of overeating, both at the individual and societal level, the better we can educate people and shape public policy to help curb this problem.

Advances in neuropsychology and the understanding of the human brain will also open many doors for food psychologists. Simply developing a better understanding of the complex relationship among all of the senses, but particularly taste and smell, has vast implications for the diagnosis and treatment of many psychiatric and medical disorders. Evaluating medicinal and/or preventive effects of certain foods on memory functions, for example, is another promising area of research. Some current correlational research, for example, has found a relationship between curry consumption, specifically yellow curry and its key ingredient turmeric, and a reduced likelihood of developing Alzheimer's or dementia in older adults (Ng et al., 2006). Also understanding the ways in which food, particularly sweet, salty, fatty foods, activate pleasure centers in the brain are essential in understanding obesity and overeating.

Continued work in evolutionary psychology will allow us to better understand our species' history of cooking and food. We need to continue to answer questions about how and why our dietary paths deviated from ancestral humans and other primates. Using fossils, archaeological evidence, and DNA to piece together longer evolution of adaptive eating behavior has tremendous implications.

Rapid globalization also opens up many research questions for food psychologists. How has culinary tradition historically contributed to the development of ethnic identity and how does that change with rapidly shifting migration patterns? Another place in which globalization (and overpopulation) converge with psychology is with the issue of sustainability, specifically the psychology of how Westerners, accustomed to prosperity and broad choices, will respond to dietary changes based on shifts in the food supply chain. For example, a recent New Yorker article chronicles entomaphagy (insect eating) and its rise in haute culinary circles, as well as its sustainability. While insect eating might be one of the most sustainable food practices, the biggest obstacle is convincing Westerners who aren't reality TV stars to do it. Here, work such as Paul Rozin's on disgust (Rozin, Haidt, and McCauley, 1993) has very practical implications for potential behavior modification.

In cognitive psychology and neuropsychology, the study of how certain foods and spices affect the brain and body is extremely promising. The aforementioned research on curry (turmeric) as a potential anti-Alzheimer's agent has enormous dietary and public health implications. Historically there has not been much empirical support for supplements or holistic medicine, but results from these recent studies suggest that there is tremendous potential in this area.

These are simply a few possible, and somewhat obvious trajectories in the psychology of food. There are so many exciting ideas, methodologies, and approaches that it's impossible to predict what innovation is around the corner.

Practical considerations for getting started

Ideally one might start focusing on food research beginning in graduate school, although in many cases that is challenging simply because there aren't a large number of programs with such foci. The University of Florida's Center for Smell and Taste offers courses in chemosensory clinical phenomenon to students in a variety of graduate programs, but does not currently offer its own graduate program of study. Students with an experimental focus might want to train with Brian Wansink at the Cornell Food and Brand Lab or Paul Rozin at University of Pennsylvania, two of the most established researchers in food psychology. Barring that, any quality training in rigorous qualitative or quantitative methodologies can be applied to food as a topic. One could theoretically become a food scholar in almost any area of psychology: social, cognitive, evolutionary, clinical, developmental, etc.

For those interested in clinical training in this area, Bastyr University offers a masters degree program in nutrition and clinical health psychology that integrates training in mental health counseling and nutritional counseling. Bastyr focuses on natural health arts and sciences, including naturopathic medicine and oriental medicine. Another applied area of note is clinical neuropsychology as it relates to smell and taste disorders. For example, in their recent book, *Navigating Smell and Taste Disorders* (2011), physician Ronald DeVere and food consultant Marjorie Calvert collaborate to develop treatments, recipes, and food preparation strategies for those with smell and taste disorders. Such intersections among nutrition, psychology, and medicine are only just being explored. Those with such applied clinical interests could pursue a variety of programs in nutrition, neuropsychology, or clinical health psychology for training.

At this time there are no programs, scholarships, or funding aimed specifically at studying the psychology of food. There are, however, many grants available for obesity and nutrition researchers.

In addition to the key readings listed below, some other good resources are the Cornell Food and Brand Lab website, which summarizes key findings, has a trove of teaching tools, and links to numerous YouTube videos that show the research in action. Another excellent resource is Dr Kelly Brownell's Open Yale course on the psychology, biology, and politics of food. This course has 23 sessions of 75 minutes each, which can be downloaded in either video or audio format. Also, the Rudd Center for Food Policy and Obesity contains full text articles of most of its research, along with policy recommendations, and current initiatives.

In sum, psychology and food studies spans virtually every "sub-discipline" of the field. Methodologies vary and the utility of the scholarship spans from cultural and ethnic facets of food experiences to the neuronal level of how our brains respond to specific tastes, smells, and ingredients. Attention to food is rapidly expanding, with implications for clinical treatment, public policy development, and policy evaluation.

Key reading

Brownell, K. D. (n.d.) *The psychology, biology, and politics of food (Yale Open Course)*. oyc.yale.edu/psychology/the-psychology-biology-and-politics-of-food (accessed on October 12, 2011).

Capaldi, E. D. (1996) *Why we eat what we eat: The psychology of eating* (1st ed.). Washington, DC: American Psychological Association.

Cornell University Food and Brand Labs. (n.d.) foodpsychology.cornell.edu/discoveries.html (accessed on October 11, 2011).

Freud, A. (1946) "The psychoanalytic study of infantile feeding disturbances." *Psychoanalytic Study of the Child* 2: 119–32.

Logue, A. W. (2004) *The Psychology of Eating and Drinking*. New York: Brunner-Routledge/Taylor & Francis Group.

Rozin, P. (2007) "Food and eating." In *Handbook of Cultural Psychology*. S. Kitayama and D. Cohen eds., pp. 391–416. New York: Guilford Press.

Rudd center for food policy and obesity (n.d.) oyc.yale.edu/psychology/the-psychology-biology-and-politics-of-food (accessed on October 12, 2011).

Wansink, B. (2006) *Mindless Eating: Why We Eat More than We Think*. New York: Bantam Books.

Bibliography

Andreyeva, T., F. J. Chaloupka, and K. D. Brownell, (2011) Estimating the potential of taxes on sugar-sweetened beverages to reduce consumption and generate revenue. *Preventive Medicine, 52*(6), 413–16.

Barrett, D. (2007) *Waistland: The (R)evolutionary Science Behind our Weight and Fitness Crisis* (1st ed.). New York: W.W. Norton & Co.

Brownell, K. D. (n.d.) *The psychology, biology, and politics of food (Yale Open Course)*. http://oyc.yale.edu/psychology/the-psychology-biology-and-politics-of-food, accessed on October 12, 2011.

Brownell, K. D. and D. S. Ludwig, (2011) The supplemental nutrition assistance program, soda, and USDA policy: Who benefits? *Journal of the American Medical Association 306*(12), 1370–71.

Capaldi, E. D. (1996) *Why We Eat What We Eat: The Psychology of Eating* (1st ed.). Washington, DC: American Psychological Association.

Cargill, K. (2007) Desire, ritual, and cuisine. *The Psychoanalytic Review 94*(2), 315–32.

——(2012) Food, consumption, and the psychology of cooking. In R. S. Stewart & S. Korol eds., *Food for Thought: A Multidisciplinary Look at Food in our World*. Sydney: Cape Breton University Press.

Chu, S. and J. J. Downes, (2000) Odour-evoked autobiographical memories: Psychological investigations of Proustian phenomena. *Chemical Senses 25*(1), 111–16.

——(2002) Proust nose best: Odors are better cues of autobiographical memory. *Memory & Cognition, 30*(4), 511–18.

Cornell university food and brand lab. (n.d.) http://foodpsychology.cornell.edu/discoveries.html, accessed on October 11, 2011.

DeVere, R. and M. Calvert (2011) *Navigating Smell and Taste Disorders*. New York: Demos Health.

Drewnowski, A. (1996) The behavioral phenotype in human obesity. In E. D. Capaldi (ed.), *Why we eat what we eat: The psychology of eating* (pp. 291–308). Washington, DC: American Psychological Association.

Drewnowski, A. and Specter, S. E. (2004) Poverty and obesity: The role of energy density and energy costs. *The American Journal of Clinical Nutrition 79*: 6–16.

Fernández-Armesto, F. (2001) *Food: A History*. London: Macmillan.

Freud, A. (1946) The psychoanalytic study of infantile feeding disturbances. *Psychoanalytic Study of the Child* 2: 119–32.

Gearhardt, A. N., W. R. Corbin, and K. D. Brownell (2009) Preliminary validation of the Yale food addiction scale. *Appetite 52*(2): 430–36.

Gearhardt, A. N., C. M. Grilo, R. J. DiLeone, K. D. Brownell, and M. N. Potenza (2011) Can food be addictive? Public health and policy implications. *Addiction 106*(7): 1208–12.

Goodyear, D. (2011) Grub. *New Yorker 87*(24): 38–46.

Haidt, J., P. Rozin, C. McCauley, and S. Imada (1997) Body, psyche, and culture: The relationship between disgust and morality. *Psychology and Developing Societies 9*: 107–31.

Just, D. R. and B. Wansink (2009) Better school meals on a budget: Using behavioral economics and food psychology to improve meal selection. *Choices 24*(3): 19–24.

Logue, A. W. (2004) *The Psychology of Eating and Drinking*. New York: Brunner-Routledge/Taylor & Francis Group.

Ng, T., P. Chiam, T. Lee, H. Chua, L. Lim, and E. Kua (2006) Curry consumption and cognitive function in the elderly. *American Journal of Epidemiology 164*(9): 898–906.

Roberto, C. A., J. Baik, J. L. Harris, and K. D. Brownell (2010) Influence of licensed characters on children's taste and snack preferences. *Pediatrics Pediatrics 126*(1): 88–93.

Roberto, C. A., M. B. Schwartz, and K. D. Brownell (2009) Rationale and evidence for menu-labeling legislation. *American Journal of Preventive Medicine 37*(6): 546–51.

Roberto, C. A., P. D. Larsen, H. Agnew, J. Baik, and K. D. Brownell (2010) Evaluating the impact of menu labeling on food choices and intake. *American Journal of Public Health 100*(2): 312.

Rozin, P. (1996) Sociocultural influences on human food selection. In E. D. Capaldi (Ed.), *Why we eat what we eat: The psychology of eating* (pp. 233–63). Washington, DC: American Psychological Association.

——(2007) Food and eating. In S. Kitayama and D. Cohen eds., *Handbook of Cultural Psychology*, pp. 391–416. New York: Guilford Press.

Rozin, P. and D. Schiller (1980) The nature and acquisition of a preference for chili pepper by humans. *Motivation and Emotion 4*(1): 77–101.

Rozin, P., L. Ebert, and J. Schull (1982) Some like it hot: A temporal analysis of hedonic responses to chili pepper. *Appetite 3*(1): 13–22.

Rozin, P., J. Haidt, and C. R. McCauley, (1993) Disgust. In *Handbook of Emotions*, M. Lewis and J. Haviland eds., pp. 575–94. New York: Guilford.

Rozin, P., K. Kabnick, E. Pete, C. Fischler, and C. Shields (2003) The ecology of eating smaller portion sizes in France than in the United States help explain the French paradox. *Psychological Science 14*(5): 450–54.

Rozin, P., M. Mark, and D. Schiller, (1980) The role of desensitization to capsaicin in chili pepper ingestion and preference. *Chemical Senses, 6*(1): 23–31.

Rudd center for food policy and obesity. (n.d.) http://oyc.yale.edu/psychology/the-psychology-biology-and-politics-of-food, accessed on October 12, 2011.

Schwartz, M. B., L. R. Vartanian, C.M. Wharton, and K. D. Brownell (2008) Examining the nutritional quality of breakfast cereals marketed to children. *Journal of the American Dietetic Association 108*(4): 702–5.

Volkan, V. D. (1997) *Bloodlines: From Ethnic Pride to Ethnic Terrorism*. New York: Farrar, Straus and Giroux.

Wansink, B. (2006) *Mindless Eating: Why we Eat More than we Think*. New York: Bantam Books.

Wrangham, R. W. (2009) *Catching Fire: How Cooking Made us Human*. New York: Basic Books.

5

Nutritional anthropology

Janet Chrzan

Nutritional anthropology uses a biocultural paradigm to examine how social structures and actions interact with ecological and biological systems to determine food availability, use, and nutritional health. Central questions of interest include how diet affected the evolutionary development of Homo sapiens, *cross-cultural food use, the relationship between environmental conditions and food procurement and nutriture, how human biological and cultural variation affects dietary practices and health, and how food use and nutrition interacts with parasitic, infectious and chronic disease. Doctorates in nutritional anthropology allow for primary research within academic and medical settings and applied work with health-related NGOs and governmental agencies.*

Nutritional anthropology traditionally has been defined as a combination of biological and cultural paradigms, which jointly are considered to determine food choice, consumption, and resulting nutriture. Biological nutritional anthropology, with theoretical roots in nutritional science, epidemiology and medicine, focuses on the health parameters and consequences of food acquisition, processing and physical incorporation on the conceptual levels of the individual, population, and species. It is concerned with the biological outcomes of overall nutriture and basic physiological health as a result of evolutionary processes, environmental conditions, agricultural practices, food processing techniques, culturally determined interactions with resources and health constraints, and individual capacities to absorb and utilize particular nutrients. Biological nutritional anthropology is generally fueled by either an evolutionary or health and epidemiology framework.

The anthropology of food or cuisine is embedded within the overall sociocultural anthropological continuum. Food is most often treated as a material marker for other cultural processes, such as gender (Counihan, 1999, 2004, 2009; de Certeau and Giard, 2008; Devault, 1991; Innes, 2001; Meigs, 1983; Weismantel, 1989), exchange relationships (Bestor, 2004; Flynn, 1999; Gewertz and Errington, 2010; Williams, 1984), age-related ritual practices (Von Gennep, 1907; Thompson, 1988) and class or ethnic parameters (Appadurai, 1988; Bourdieu, 1984; De Garine, 1996; Deitler, 1996; Goode *et al.*, 1984a; Goody, 1982; Ray, 2004; Roseberry, 1996). Food in this context becomes an item of significance within material culture serving to delineate wider cultural patterns and forces. Food is also treated as an element of meaning, either as a metaphor for cultural patterns (Douglas, 1974, 1984, 1987; Douglas and Nicod, 1974; Goode *et al.*, 1984b; Mintz, 1996; Sharman, 1991; Toomey, 1986) or as a part of a system of generalized culture-based perceptions of physical properties or internalized symbols (Fiddes, 1992; Levi-Strauss 1958, 1970, 1978; Lupton, 1996; Kahn, 1998; Meigs, 1983; Wilk, 2007). Food, the processes that create it from the raw plant and animal forms, as well as the social forces that determine usage, are also subject to political and historical analysis (Belasco, 1989; Chang, 1977; Ferguson, 2004; Levenstein, 1988, 1993; Mintz, 1985, 1996; Shapiro, 1986; Wilk, 2006). Food is also examined as a holistic system within cultural and historic parameters (Richards, 1932; Anderson, 1988; Mennell, 1996). In the sociocultural approach food is treated as a system of communication and praxis that provides organizing rituals of meanings and reveals patterns and structures of social action. The sociocultural anthropology of food is ably covered in this volume (by Dirks and Hunter) and will not be further addressed in this chapter. However, the parameters of that branch of food anthropology are mentioned here specifically because social processes affect how food is produced, acquired, distributed, prepared, and consumed and thus play an important role in nutriture.

Pelto, Goodman, and Dufour have neatly summarized what makes the human diet so compelling and so very different from that of other species (Pelto, Goodman, and Dufour, 2000: 4):

1. extreme omnivory;
2. cooking (boiling, roasting, frying, steaming) with flavor amendments (salt, etc.);
3. because of cooking humans spend more time preparing and altering food than do other animals;
4. elaborate systems of food distribution, sharing, and exchange;
5. systems of food preferences and prohibitions that are linked to systems of belief and social regulations through ideology and which affect dietary intakes.

Since every human society exhibits these food behaviors and since each is determined through learned cultural processes, anthropologists are provided with rich amounts of social material pertaining to food use and diet to study. This is equally true for the biological as well as the social aspects of commensality.

Historical background of food scholarship in nutritional anthropology and major theoretical approaches

In the near-dawn of anthropological theory Audrey Richards wrote "nutrition as a biological process is more fundamental than sex. In the life of the individual organism it is the more primary and recurrent want, while in the wider sphere of human society it determines, more largely than other physiological functions, the nature of social groupings, and the form their activities take" (Richards, 1932: 1). This quote highlights both the centrality of nutrition to everyday life (one that is, alas, too often ignored, especially in social systems of conceptual abundance) as well as the foci of nutritional anthropology. Nutritional anthropologists study how social processes that determine food intake affect health on the individual, population, and species levels. While some focus on the social processes and others on the health outcomes, the vast majority of nutritional anthropologists study the connection between the two using methods derived from nutritional sciences, medicine, and anthropology. The sub-discipline is inherently biocultural because it links the social and the biological, and almost all methods are designed to promote better measurement and analysis of these connections. Nutritional anthropology is theoretically grounded in biological and medical anthropology, nutrition, and studies of evolution and uses a system approach to model research queries. Nutritional anthropology is a vibrant area of medical research and many trained in the field work in health-related NGOs, bilateral, and governmental organizations in the developing and developed world.

Most published research in nutritional anthropology is found in journals and peer-reviewed books relating to nutrition, medicine, epidemiology, and food anthropology. Audrey Richards's pathbreaking work among the Bantu (Richards, 1932) was published at roughly the same time as several other foundational studies of the Maasai, Kikuyu, and Tallensi (Orr and Gilks, 1931; Fortes and Fortes, 1936). Early texts were usually driven by colonial needs to improve the health (and thus the labor potential) of "native" populations in colonial territories. After the Second World War a number of more anthropological studies were initiated and published, often with a broad interest in subsistence patterns in relation to health (see Ulijasek and Strickland, 1993: 1–3 for a review of these titles). Primary areas of interest were Oceania, Papua New Guinea, and Africa, with a good example of that research published in an edited volume in 1976 titled *Shared Wealth and Symbol: Food, Culture, and Society in Oceania and Southeast Asia* (Manderson, 1986). In 1974 the subfield came into its own with the establishment of the Council on Nutritional Anthropology, an interest group within the American Anthropology Association. That group has since become a full section within the AAA with – as of this writing – 290 members, and has been renamed the Society for the Anthropology of Food and Nutrition (SAFN). Comprehensive texts include *Nutrition and Anthropology in Action* (Fitzgerald, 1976), *Nutritional Anthropology: Contemporary Approaches to Diet and Culture* (Jerome, Kandel and Pelto, 1980), *Food and Evolution: Toward a Theory of Human Food Habits* (Harris and Ross, 1987), *Nutritional Anthropology* (Johnston, 1987), *Nutritional Anthropology: Prospects and Perspectives* (Ulijasek and Strickland, 1993), *Nutritional Anthropology: Biocultural Perspectives on Food and Nutrition* (Goodman, Dufour and Pelto, 2000) and *Nutritional Anthropology* (Jensen, 2008). Excellent review articles include "Nutritional Anthropology and Biological Adaptation" (Haas and Harrison, 1977), "The Anthropology of Food and Eating" (Mintz and Dubois, 2002), "You are what you eat and you eat what you are: the role of nutritional anthropology in public health nutrition and nutrition education" (Himmelgreen, 2002) and "Social Research in an Integrated Science of Nutrition: Future Directions" (Pelto and Freake, 2003). For a good overview of the subfield as a whole read the Goodman, Dufour, and Pelto volume; many of the edited readings are from anthropologists (and other nutrition-related scientists) whose work forms the backbone of the current study of nutritional anthropology.

To provide a quick overview of present efforts, nutritional anthropology uses methods, theory, and data from anthropology, public health, medicine, nutritional science, demography, human biology, plant and animal biology, agronomy and epidemiology to examine food acquisition, processing, consumption, and nutriture. Nutrition, broadly painted, looks at the effects of food on individual biochemical and behavioral equilibrium and is interested in clinical health and medical outcomes while respecting population-level (epidemiological) measures of health status. Anthropology seeks to understand the relationship of individuals to each other and to the cultures to which they belong in part to explain the processes that have evolved to satisfy basic physiological and psychological needs. Nutritional anthropology is methodologically both processual and scientific because it explores the processes by which humans use food to meet requirements of biological and behavioral functioning and a science that studies the chemical processing and biological use of food. Primary interests include food and culture connections, variation for optimal diets, disease variations and the social patterns, culture, and roles within food-getting and distribution behaviors (including gender issues, economic structures, and hunger outcomes) that determine access to food. Primary concepts studied include evolution, adaptation, variability, history, behaviors, beliefs, and the cultural paradigms that channel beliefs and behaviors. Core areas of research interest include comparative dietary adaptation to subsistence patterns (hunter-gatherers, pastoralists, agriculturalists, cash-croppers and industrial farmers) and ecological/environmental patterns (climate, altitude, stress, hunger, and malnutrition), dietary evolution (hominid evolution and paleobiological dietary programming of body size and metabolism), human biology (fertility, growth and development, lactation and senescence), demographics and life history theory (child feeding, weaning, food provisioning, and fertility) and applied nutritional anthropology (public advocacy, health assessment, early warning systems, stress and resiliency, food policy, economics of food production in relation to nutriture and program development). These topics cover the full range of most current food research and activism and since some of them are covered in other areas of this volume the theory discussed here will be limited to adaptation, evolution, life history theory and malnutrition.

Dietary and primate evolution

A number of anthropologists have examined nutrition as an adaptive agent contributing to the evolution of the species (Mann, 1972, 1981; Garn and Leonard, 1989; Gordon, 1987; Bogin, 1991; Johns, 1996; Wrangham et al., 1999; Unger et al., 2006; Unger, 2007; Wrangham, 2009). Evolution of diet refers both to the evolution of the human species as a result of particular types of food-getting behaviors as well as the evolution of the diet in response to adapted changes in Homo sapiens' physiology and culture. Recent research on food sharing has suggested that we are human because we share and cook our food and that our species proliferated in part due to provisioning behaviors (Aiello and Key, 2002; Aiello and Wells, 2002; O'Connell et al., 1999; Lovejoy, 2009). The human brain is enormously expensive to produce and maintain, which suggests our ancestors evolved to eat a more enriched diet than other hominines (Abrams, 1987; Leonard and Robertson, 1994; Aiello and Wheeler, 1995; Leonard et al., 2007). Eating more meat and fat increases nutrient density and cooking food aids absorption. Sharing food is the final key to ensuring species survivability because provisioning children and pregnant females increases fertility and health and can lead to population growth.

Other research acknowledges the co-evolution of human, pathogen, and food species, as witnessed by favism and lactose tolerance (Katz, 1987a, 1987b; Katz, Hediger and Valleroy, 1974; Katz and Voight, 1986; Kretchmer, 1972, 1978). Katz and colleagues describe this co-evolution as a biocultural lock and key mechanism that allows humans to unlock the nutritive potential of plant foods. Cuisine (food preparation and cooking) allows humans to release the nutrient potential of food items either by making them more palatable or by making necessary nutrients more available for absorption. The co-evolution in this model is learned (cultural) behavior that widens the range of potential dietary items and increases the diversity of diet choice and nutrient intakes. In this model, learned behavior is part of a suite of adaptive behaviors that have evolutionary consequences. For example, the need for greater nutrient densities to feed the growing brain directly affected GI tract development (Milton, 1993), choice of foods, and food-sharing behaviors while the larger brain allowed for increased learning about acceptable foods, social connections of greater complexity, and further reliance on learning and culture. Culture is used in place of somatic evolution, which allows for greater diversity of behavior specifically because it is not encoded in physical needs. For example, while most animals have relatively narrow diets determined by evolutionary development (the panda bear is a good example), humans exhibit extreme omnivory because they are able to utilize cooking to remove toxins, increase nutrient bioavailability and render foods more easily digested. In summation, our relationship with food has directly affected our evolution by allowing for the development of the large brain and omnivory, and has indirectly abetted micro-evolutionary processes to encourage adaptation and variability in response to disease vectors mediated by food intakes. Additionally, learned cultural behavior (cuisine) has modified our biotic environment through selective plant and animal breeding and food preparation techniques that can enhance health and physical development.

The idea that the human body evolved in response to the environment has led to the hypothesis that there may be an optimal diet for *Homo sapiens*. Specifically, many have recognized that our biology is still attuned to a different and "less modern" world because culture has altered the environment faster than we can adapt to the changes. Human societies have progressed from hunter-gathering to industrial agriculture within 10,000 years, a shift that has left our bodies, metaphorically, in the evolutionary dust and with a "Paleolithic body" in a post-modern world. Because until recently we were far more physically active, our need for high-density foods is still encoded in biological and cultural preferences, but our environment now makes high-density foods far more available, leading to what has been described as a mismatch between diet and biology that leads to obesity and other modern diseases (Lee, 1968; Eaton and Konner, 1985; Eaton, Konner and Shostak, 1988; Brown and Konner, 1987; Hockett and Haws, 2003; Gluckman and Hanson, 2006; Lieberman, 2006; Ulijasek and Lofink, 2006; Trevathan, 2007; Popkin, 2009; Konner and Eaton, 2010; Wiedman, 2010; Brewis, 2011). The popular press has embraced – with terrible enthusiasm – the idea of an ideal "Paleodiet" that fits the human genome perfectly, which has led to a number of texts of more-or-less decent quality purporting to provide the perfect diet for optimum fitness (probably the best-known author of this genre is Loren Cordain). The first and foundational text of this kind, *The Paleolithic Prescription* (Eaton, Konner and Shostak, 1988) was written by anthropologists using data derived from studies of ancient diets and those of modern hunter-gatherers. In that book they traced increased intakes of sodium, fat, and calories to some of the modern diseases of dietary affluence such as hypertension and heart disease. Other anthropologists have explored the different nutrient profiles of wild, gathered, or early agricultural foods in relation to the modern dietary (Speth and Spellman, 1983; Leiberman, 1987; Strickland, 1990; O'Dea, 1998; Gladwell, 1998; Milton, 2002). Without a doubt, the human diet has changed profoundly within the last 10,000 years. Exactly how those changes affect the health of modern humans is a primary field of enquiry in nutritional anthropology.

Variation, adaptation, malnutrition, and health outcomes

Concepts such as adaptation, natural selection, and adaptability are central to theory in nutritional anthropology, which relies heavily on the idea of adaptation to explain the physiological differences found in diverse populations (Ulijaszek and Strickland, 1993; Johnston, 1987; Ulijaszek, 1996, 1997; Goodman, Dufour, and Pelto, 2000; Trevathan, 2007). In this context, adaptation refers to biological and cultural change through natural selection, developmental processes, and through fitness-enhancing cultural actions. Because the human species is defined (in part) by the presence of culture, discriminating between specific adaptational mechanisms caused by biological and/or genetic change and adaptational changes due to cultural practices is nearly impossible (Thomas *et al.*, 1979). Given that all humans must consume nutrients to sustain and create life, it is reasonable to assume that human dietary practices have provided a template for the processes of adaptation on all levels including genetic, physiological, and cultural.

Genetic adaptation has been discussed above, but at the level of the species. Population-based differences are also important to understanding nutritional processes because some populations may have adapted to differences in the environment in ways that enhance nutrition and health. The ability to digest milk carbohydrates is one such population-level adaptation (Kretchmer, 1972; Simoons, 1979; Wiley, 2011). Another is the possibility that some human populations have a 'thrifty genotype' that allows for better utilization of calories – a benefit in an environment of scarcity but problematic when faced with widespread calorie availability (Neel, 1962; Hales and Barker, 2001; Benyshek and Watson, 2006). But genetic change is expensive and consequently it is more typical to find adaptation expressed in physiological changes such as growth stunting as a result of under-nutrition (Seckler, 1982; Martorell, 1989; Jenike, 2001; Dettwyler, 2008) or increased susceptibility to diet-related diseases (Barker, 2001). The easiest form of adaption is cultural, because it is almost instantaneous and requires no physical changes, most populations have relied upon adaptations that alter cuisine and food choice rather than human biology (Katz *et al.*, 1974; Katz and Voigt, 1986; Katz, 1987a; Dufour, 1993). In this light, agriculture must also be considered to be a form of cultural evolution (Boserup, 1965; Cohen, 1977; Larsen, 1995).

To better understand how nutrition can be a vehicle for adaption, it is examined as a stressor as well as a resource (Bailey, 1993; Stahl, 1984; Stinson, 1992) and as a modifier of other bio-logical processes affecting adaptation (Stini, 1975; Haas and Harrison, 1977; Haas and Pelletier, 1989; Ulijaszek, 1990; Ulijaszek and Strickland, 1993; Weiss, 1980). While the focus of most of these studies has been biological adaptation, especially in the form of specific nutrient needs and utilization, anthropologists have also explored the behavioral and cultural adaptations to food acquisition and avoidance of nutrient stress (Goodman *et al.*, 2000; Leatherman, 1998; Dewalt, 1998; Thomas, 1998; Godoy *et al.*, 2005). These biocultural approaches to nutritional adaptation provide a wider approach to the understanding of the development of adaptational systems in human biology and behavior, and provide one of the most robust modeling tools for understanding how food interacts with physical and cultural systems to contribute to health states.

Population variability is examined through analysis of variables that affect health, including protein and energy metabolism, micronutrient adequacy, fertility, pregnancy and lactation, child growth and development, seasonality and climatic determination of food-gathering and grow-ing capacities. Increasingly anthropologists are examining the economic structures of agriculture and food access to understand how food use is affected by employment categories, social class, ethnicity, and life stage (Ulijaszek and Strickland, 1993). Poverty and food security are the pri-mary foci of many nutritional anthropologists and form the bulk of current research, particularly in the study of changing economic patterns (Fitchen, 1997; Coen, 2005; Baro and Deubel, 2006; Crooks *et al.*, 2008; Himmelgreen and Kedia, 2009; Krishna, 2010). Within the last 50 years many of the physical and ecological constraints that determined the potential for food scarcity and malnutrition have been supplanted by social and economic factors that determine access to food. The shift from a planet with a vast peasant class to one with an even larger proletarian population has permanently altered food use patterns for almost every human. Much of the current work in this field examines the variables that contribute to malnutrition in rapidly changing (globalizing) populations.

The most vulnerable periods for malnutrition are those times when the body is undergoing rapid growth and development, primarily early childhood and pregnancy. For these reasons women and children are usually more likely to demonstrate the clinical signs of malnutrition and are more at risk for development of the disease states that are exacerbated by malnutrition. Health during pregnancy and childhood is determined by resource availability, risk avoidance and cultural models of appropriate feeding and care, making diet during those periods a perfect example of biocultural anthropology. The timing of supplemental feeding of children, the beliefs that determine appropriate pregnancy foods, even whom is expected to care for women and children (and how) all affect nutriture during these critical periods of life (Bogin, 1991; Rizvi, 1991; McDade and Worthman, 1998; O'Connell *et al.*, 1999; Van Esterik, 2002; Wilson *et al.*, 2006; Sellen, 2007; Trevathan, 2010). It is therefore not surprising that much of nutritional anthropology research has been directed at understanding how cultural and environmental varia-bility affect maternal and child health, a perspective that often leads to applied work in the AID and NGO world.

To understand the connections between food and environmental stressors scientists must be able to model the relationships. A first-level model is one that starts with the smallest unit of analysis (cellular contents? DNA?) and adds progressively until all possible fields of health action are included. From the cell, organ system, and organism arises the individual (the usual clinical focus) and from there, the family or household, the community, the state, nation, etc. Surrounding all, interpenetrating, are the natural and social worlds consisting of the physical environment and its resources as well as the political, economic and demographic social system that determine any given individual (or community) access to resources or exposure to risks. Each element or variable of these differing levels must be identified and tested to explore how it contributes to the outcome variable in question. While this model can be pictured as an onion, a more useful model breaks out the various elements to graphically map their relatedness and demonstrate relationships of correlation and causality. For instance, the classic 1990 model by UNICEF (available online at www.unicef.org/sowc98/sowc98.pdf, page 25, accessed March 25, 2012, and medanth.wikispaces.com/Food+Insecurity, accessed March 25, 2012) groups biotic and social variables into a homeostatic model that predicts child malnutrition and illness. Malnutrition is recognized as being a direct and indirect cause of illness and disease and a number of diseases (parasitism, infection, etc.) work synergistically with malnutrition to increase the effect of under-nutrition in the physical state (Scrimshaw, 2003). The UNICEF model is similar to the recent models developed by biocultural anthropologists to include the political and economic in modeling for disease and illness causation (Thomas, 1998). These models use homeostatic systems modeling to link outcomes to nutritional variables that play an important role in the etiology of malnutrition, but it must be emphasized they do not indicate that there is a positive relationship between malnutrition and functioning or that malnutrition can lead to adaptation that ensures health under conditions of scarcity. While the "small but healthy" (Seckler, 1982) hypothesis was popular in the 1980s, more recent research has demonstrated functional differences in those who are stunted due to food scarcity. These models are designed to map out relationships between risks and resources that contribute to malnutrition and ill health, and are very useful when doing applied work in food security, environment, and health.

Applied nutritional anthropology

Most nutritional anthropologists find themselves doing some form of applied work. Many are employed directly with NGOs, governmental and bilateral organizations that promote health and wellness, such as Save the Children, the WHO, and UNICEF. Many academic anthropologists are employed as consultants for specific projects in health and nutrition as well. There is a robust body of work in nutritional anthropology consisting of articles and books about doing applied work (Green, 1977, 1986; DeRose, Messer, and Millman, 1999; Pfeiffer and Nichter, 2008; Himmelgreen and Romero-Diaz, 2009). There is an even larger body of work realized from such endeavors published in academic journals as well as the 'grey press' or the papers issued by NGOs, government agencies, and think tanks (recent examples: Chaiken, 2010a, 2010b; Gerberg and Stansbury, 2010; Millard et al., 2011). Many of the methods used by nutritional anthropologists are of real use in assessing food security and famine, and are used to improve Famine Early Warning Systems (FEWS) (Torry, 1988; Brown, 2008; Hadley and Maes, 2009).

Research methods

Methods in nutritional anthropology are biocultural and run the gamut from sociocultural participant observation to clinical tests for blood chemicals, bone density, and genetic markers.

Most practitioners focus on specific methods but should be aware of and able to learn and use most methods and be able to understand lab reports. Designing research requires careful assessment of the best methods to test for specific outcomes given a known set of independent and dependant variables. Appropriate statistical methods must also be applied, and used initially to determine an optimal number of subjects for the study. Does this sound like medical research? It should, since many of the methods used are derived from the standard biological and medical anthropology toolbox. Just as medical anthropology spans sociocultural and biological methods and theory, so does nutritional anthropology. Nutritional anthropology studies tend to have smaller subject numbers than most studies in nutrition or medicine because it is still rooted in participant observation and getting to know the subjects and their cultures personally.

As might have been apparent in the section on variation and adaptation, much of the conceptual modeling for research arises from biological and ecological systems approaches. The UNICEF child health model and the biocultural synthesis models ably demonstrate how nutritional anthropologists 'think through' problems in their subfield. How they test the connections – measurement and analysis – is determined by the variables of interest. Another important consideration when designing research is the number of subjects, since a large number will mandate epidemiological methods while smaller groups are more amenable to qualitative and participant observation techniques. Most anthropologists use both qualitative and quantitative methods. Qualitative methods include participant observation, verbal and written questionnaires and interviews, focus groups and other metrics that can be sorted with the aid of text analysis methods such as NVivo (see Bernard, 2006 for a full analysis of anthropological methods). Quantitative and biological methods – ones that derive numbers or other similar metrics – include everything from various types of scaling of sociocultural data to clinical, nutritional, and epidemiological means to measure social and biological data. The SAFN, a section within the American Anthropology Association, will publish in 2013 a new and comprehensive methods manual. Until that manual is released the best books and articles to indicate how nutritional anthropology is "done" are the following:

- Axinn and Pearce: *Mixed Method Data Collection Strategies*, 2006.
- den Hartog, van Staveren and Brouwer: *Food Habits and Consumption in Developing Countries*, 2006.
- Gibson: *Principles of Nutritional Assessment*, second edition, 2005.
- Pelto, Pelto, and Messer: *Research Methods in Nutritional Anthropology*, 1989.
- Kedia and van Willigen: *Applied Anthropology: Domains of Application*, 2005.
- Macbeth, Helen and Jeremy MacClancey: *Researching Food Habits: Methods and Problems*, 2004.
- Margetts and Nelson: *Design Concepts in Nutritional Epidemiology*, second edition, 1997.
- Pellett: *Problems and Pitfalls in the Assessment of Human Nutritional Status*, 1987.
- Quandt (ed.): *Training Manual in Nutritional Anthropology*, 1986.
- Scrimshaw and Hurtado: *Rapid Assessment Procedures for Nutrition and Primary Health Care*, 1987.
- Tremblay and Bouchard: *Assessment of Energy Expenditure and Physical Activity Patterns*, 1987.
- Ulijaszek: *Human Energetics in Biological Anthropology*, 2005.
- Ulijaszek and Strickland: *Nutritional Anthropology: Biological Perspectives*, 1993.

Avenues for future research

The study of the relationships between humans, food, and health is a growing field. It is impossible to enter a bookstore, open an internet browser or pick up any magazine without being bombarded with information about what you should eat, how you should eat it, and what it will do to your body. Unfortunately, most of this information is generated by marketing firms or enthusiastic advocates of particular dietary ideologies. The ability to understand the science, translate it into language accessible to the layperson, and then explain clearly how food affects health is an ability that most nutritional anthropologists have, and it is currently in demand (and perhaps desperately needed).

Academic departments are often interested in employing degreed academics who can bridge multiple areas of a discipline, which nutritional anthropologists can because of their biocultural focus. Primary areas of academic research at this time include research in obesity etiology variables, diet variation and health, public health and preventative and palliative nutrition, and food/drug interactions. There is need for additional nutritional anthropologists to study how poverty affects diet and health, especially as the numbers of people receiving food stamps in the United States continues to climb. AID and other similar development agencies (health and economic) can use nutritional anthropologists, and there is much work to be done in food and agriculture interactions. For instance, agricultural practices have changed immensely within the last 50 years (post Green Revolution) and we are still learning about how those land-use and production changes are affecting dietary habits and health.

Another area of need is food, nutrition and health education on all levels including K–12, college, and public. Because nutritional anthropologists are able to speak about food, diet, nutrition and health they are uniquely qualified to design health and educational campaigns to encourage public knowledge and better food habits in all ages. Given the very large number of food endeavors of this sort (the White House's "Let's Move" campaign, for instance) there should be plenty of jobs available in the decade to come.

Finally, there is room for nutritional anthropologists in the food industry in food product development as well as research in sales and use. With the astonishingly high number of food products developed in the US alone each year (upwards of 20,000) food and nutrition anthropologists could create valuable – and well-paid – niches in the industry.

Practical considerations for getting started – funding, programs, archival sources, tools, data sets, internet resources, scholarships, and awards, etc. (where and how?)

To be a competent nutritional anthropologist the student will need to have a background both in science and social science, and to function as a professional will need a PhD. Ideally, a student will take biology, chemistry, biochemistry and nutrition as an undergrad in order to feel completely comfortable with scientific reasoning and to be able to understand publications in the health sciences. It is not a good idea to think that a graduate student can 'pick up' this information by taking a few courses in grad school in addition to anthropology because the level of understanding will be superficial. A thorough grounding in the biological sciences is required in addition to courses in anthropology, although in the long run an undergraduate degree in a scientific field may prove more useful than in anthropology with science on the side. Fortunately, most colleges now provide interdisciplinary programs that teach science with social science, often packaged as pre-med public health degrees or something similar. For instance at the University of Pennsylvania (where the author teaches) the primary undergraduate college offers interdisciplinary degrees labeled "Biological Basis of Behavior" and "Health and Societies." Many of the students in those majors take pre-med classes in addition to more specific courses in nutrition, psychology, medical sociology, or medical anthropology. All encourage good knowledge of scientific principles and the biological world. On the other hand, a pre-med focus with anthropology, sociology, or other social science major would also work, as would a science major such as nutrition, biology, or biochemistry. The important thing is to have enough training in human biology and nutritional science to understand how the body works and to be able to use that information to understand publications and design research.

For graduate school, a student should seek a program that offers biocultural frameworks and strong biological anthropology capacities rather than a department famous for food studies. Of course, to be able to combine food anthropology (or food studies) with biological anthropology would be ideal, and many departments include faculty with strengths in both those areas. Even better yet would be a school with a strong biological/biocultural anthropology program with faculty who do research on sociocultural aspects of food *and* that has a good nutrition science department and public health, medicine, or nursing programs. Nutritional anthropology research is usually conducted by teams of people from different health and social sciences. Schools with strong departments in those fields are more likely to have vibrant research programs that will provide opportunities for learning how to do nutritional anthropology, as well as a means to do a dissertation project without starting from scratch, which is not advised.

One way to find good programs is to become familiar with recent texts and journals and to find out what researchers and faculty are doing and where they are teaching. If you are looking to get a PhD it is important to go to a department where faculty members are doing active research. As much as aiming for the department with the famous 'silverback' professor who inspired you as an undergrad might seem like a good idea, the likelihood that the eminent one is either not doing active research or shortly to become emeritus is high, which could effectively make accomplishing the PhD much more difficult. A far better strategy is to see which young faculty (assistant or associate) is turning out regular articles of interest and aim for that department. You will walk into a situation with ongoing research, high enthusiasm, and faculty who wish to train graduates.

Most nutritional anthropology articles are published in the following journals:

- *Appetite*
- *Ecology of Food and Nutrition*
- *Food and Foodways*
- *Journal of Hunger and Environmental Nutrition*
- *Social Science and Medicine*
- *Journal of Nutrition Education and Behavior*
- *Human Biology*
- *Yearbook of Physical Anthropology*
- *American Journal of Human Biology*
- *American Journal of Physical Anthropology*
- *Food and Nutrition Bulletin*
- *Human Organization*
- *Annual Reviews of Anthropology, Nutrition, etc.*
- *Nutritional Anthropology* (currently not published)

Programs that currently (2011) have strong biocultural and/or nutritional anthropology offerings include (but are not limited to):

- The University of South Florida
- Emory University
- University of Indiana, Bloomington
- School of Oriental and African Studies (SOAS)
- University of California, Santa Barbara

- University of Kentucky
- New Mexico State University
- Johns Hopkins Bloomberg School of Public Health
- University of North Carolina, Chapel Hill

Funding in nutritional anthropology

As with all graduate programs, it is essential to secure full funding for the PhD. Loans are simply out of the question given the cost of a doctoral program in relation to the possible salary a doctorate in anthropology will command. Fortunately most departments are aware of this and now attempt to fund students fully, thereby making acceptance increasingly selective. You should not plan to go to graduate school on student loans. Seriously. Secondary sources of funding include NSF education grants as well as anything – and I do mean anything – you are able to scare up. Many schools offer smaller research grants, which should be pursued, and there are often grants available for specific types of research or research conducted in specific countries or regions. Your university should be able to help you locate these sources of research money. Perhaps the best option is to sign on with a faculty member who has ongoing research in order to accomplish doctoral data collection while drawing a salary as a research assistant or associate. This will accomplish several tasks at once: provide a willing advisor for research design and analysis, smooth over access to the country or site in which you will collect data, scaffold your work and data collection, guide your analysis and write-up, and provide an income while doing your doctorate.

There are no specific grants at this time for nutritional anthropology graduate work, so you will most likely apply to the NSF or one of the private foundations that fund health research (Ford, Gates, etc.). The only paper prize in nutritional anthropology is the Christine Wilson Award, which is given annually by the Society for the Anthropology of Food and Nutrition. You can find out more about the prize here: foodanthro.wordpress.com (accessed on March 25, 2012).

Finally, a word about scholarly organizations that have nutritional anthropologists as members ... and why you should plan to attend their meetings. The SAFN, the Society for Applied Anthropology and the Association for the Study of Food and Society all have annual meetings during which papers about current research are presented. As a graduate student it is very important to begin to socialize yourself into the culture of the profession, and the best way to do that is to attend these meetings to learn how established anthropologists frame their research, how they present it, and how they present themselves. Additionally, these meetings are superb places to meet other graduate students, learn what is happening in the field, become confident when you talk about your research, become known to other nutritional anthropologists, discuss research and research design, network, network, network, and drink a lot of beer. Before you know it, you will become familiar – and friendly – with most of the people in the field and you will start to think of yourself as a nutritional anthropologist.

Bibliography

Abrams, H. L. (1987) "The preference for animal protein and fat; a cross-cultural survey." In *Food and Evolution*, M. Harris and E. B. Ross, eds. Philadelphia, PA: Temple University Press.

Aiello, L. and C. Key (2002) "Energetic consequences of being a Homo Erectus Female." *American Journal of Human Biology* 14: 516–65.

Aiello, L. and J. Wells. (2002) "Energetics and the Evolution of the genus Homo." *Annual Reviews in Anthropology* 31: 323–38.

Aiello, L. and P. Wheeler (1995) "The Expensive-Tissue Hypothesis." *Current Anthropology* 36 (2): 199–221.

Anderson, E. N. (1988) *The Food of China*. New Haven, CT: Yale University Press.

Appadurai, A. (1990) "Introduction: commodities and the politics of value." In *The Social Life of Things: Commodities in Cultural Perspective*, A. Appadurai, ed. Cambridge: Cambridge Univeristy Press.

——(1988) "How to make a national cuisine: cookbooks in contemporary India." *Society for Comparative Study of Society and History* 30(1) (January): 3–24.

Axinn, W. G. and L. D. Pearce (2006) *Mixed Method Data Collection Strategies*. Cambridge: Cambridge University Press.

Bailey, R. C. (1993) "Seasonality of food production, nutritional status, ovarian function and fertility in Central Africa." In *Tropical Forests, People and Food*, C. M. Hladik, A. Hladik, O. F. Linares, H. Pagezy, A. Semple, and M. Hadley, eds. Man and the Biosphere Series Volume 13. UNESCO, and the Parthenon Publishing Group, Paris.

Barker, D. (2001) *Fetal Origins of Cardiovascular and Lung Disease*. London: Informa Healthcare.

Baro, M. and T. F. Deubel (2006) "Persistent Hunger: Perspectives on Vulnerability, Famine, and Food Security in Sub-Saharan Africa." *Annual Review of Anthropology* 35: 521–38.

Belasco, W. J. (1989) *Appetite for Change*. New York: Pantheon Books.

Benyshek, D. C. and Watson, J. T. (2006) "Exploring the thrifty genotype's food-shortage assumptions: A cross-cultural comparison of ethnographic accounts of food security among foraging and agricultural societies." *American Journal of Physical Anthropology* 131: 120–26.

Bernard, H. R., ed. (2006) *Research Methods in Anthropology: Qualitative and Quantitative Approaches*, 4th edition. Walnut Creek, CA: Altamira Press.

Bestor, T. (2004) *"Tokyo's Pantry": Tsukiji: The fish market at the center of the world*. Berkeley: University of California Press.

Bogin, B. (1991) "The evolution of human nutrition." In *The Anthropology of Medicine*, L. Romanucci-Ross, D. Moerman, and L.R. Tancredi, eds. New York: Bergin and Garvey.

——(1995) "Growth and development: recent evolutionary and biocultural research." In *Biological Anthropology: the State of the Science*, N. T. Boaz and L. D. Wolfe, eds. Bend, OR: International Institute for Uman Evolutionary Research.

Boserup, E. (1965) *The Economics of Agrarian Change Under Population Pressure*. New Brunswick, NJ: Transaction Publishers.

Bourdieu, P. (1984) *Distinction: A Social Critique of the Judgement of Taste*. Cambridge, MA: Harvard University Press.

Brewis, A. (2011) *Obesity: Cultural and Biocultural Perspectives*. New Brunswick, NJ: Rutgers University Press.

Brown, M. (2008) *Famine Early Warning Systems and Remote Sensing Data*. Berlin: Springer-Verlag.

Brown, P. and M. Konner (1987) "An Athropological Perspective on Obesity." *Annals of the New York Academy of Sciences* 499: 29–46.

Chaiken, M. (2010a) *Promoting Biofortified Vitamin A-rich Maize in Zambia: Nutritional and Gender Related Issues for Monitoring*. A Report Prepared for the International Center for Research on Women and the Bill and Melinda Gates Foundation.

——(2010b) *Promoting Biofortified High Iron Beans for Rwanda: Nutritional and Gender-Related Issues for Monitoring*. A Report Prepared for the International Center for Research on Women and the Bill and Melinda Gates Foundation.

Chang, K. C., ed. (1977) *Food in Chinese Culture*. New Haven, CT: Yale University Press.

Cohen, M. N. (1977) *The Food Crisis in Pre-history: Overpopulation and the origins of Agriculture*. New Haven, CT: Yale University Press.

Counihan, C. (1999) *The Anthropology of Food and the Body*. New York: Routledge.

——(2004) *Around the Tuscan Table: Food, Family, and Gender in Twentieth Century Florence*. New York: Routledge.

——(2009) *A Tortilla Is Like Life: Food and Culture in the San Luis Valley of Colorado*. Austin: University of Texas Press.

Crooks, D. L. (1998) "Poverty and nutrition in eastern Kentucky: The political-economy of childhood growth." In *Building a New Biocultural Synthesis: Political-Economic Perspectives on Human Biology*, Alan H. Goodman and Thomas L. Leatherman, eds. Ann Arbor: University of Michigan Press, 339–55.

Crooks, D. L., L. Cliggett, and R. Gillett-Netting (2008) "Migration following resettlement of the Gwembe Tonga of Zambia: The Consequences for Children's Growth." *Ecology of Food and Nutrition* 47: 363–81.

De Certeau, M. and L. Giard (2008) "The Nourishing Arts." In *Food and Culture: A Reader*, 2nd edition. Carole Counihan and Penny van Esteriks, eds. New York: Routledge.

De Garine, I. (1996) "Food and the status quest in five African societies." In *Food and the Status Quest*, P. Weissner and W. Schiefenhovel, eds. Providence, RI: Berghahn Books.

den Hartog, A., W. van Staveren, and I. Brouwer (2006) *Food Habits and Consumption in Developing Countries*. Wageningen, the Netherlands: Wageningen Academic Publishers.

DeRose, Laurie, Ellen Messer and Sara Millman, (1999) *Who's Hungry? And How Do We Know?* Tokyo: United Nations University Press.

Dettwyler, K. (2008) The biocultural approach in nutritional anthropology: case studies of malnutrition in Mali. In *Medical Anthropology*. Cecil G. Helman, ed. Farnham: Ashgate.

Devault, M. (1991) *Feeding the Family: the social organization of caring as gendered work*. Chicago, IL: University of Chicago Press.

Dewalt, B. R. (1998) "The Political Ecology of Population Increase and Malnurtition in Southern Honduras." In *Building a New Biocultural Synthesis: Political Economic Perpsectives on Human Biology*, Alan Goodman and Thomas Leatherman, eds. Ann Arbor: The University of Michigan Press.

Dietler, M. (1996) "Feasts and commensal politics in the political economy: food, power, and status in prehistoric Europe." In *Food and the Status Quest*, P. Weissner and W. Schiefenhovel, eds. Providence, RI: Berghahn Books.

Douglas, M. (1974) "Deciphering a meal." In *Myth, Symbol and Culture*, Clifford Geertz, ed. New York: W.W. Norton and Company.

——(1984) "Standard social uses of food." In *Food in the Social Order*, Mary Douglas, ed. New York: Russell Sage Foundation.

——(1987) *Constructive Drinking*. Cambridge: Cambridge University Press.

Douglas, M. and M. Nicod. (1974) "Taking the biscuit: the structure of British meals." *New Society* December: 744–47.

Dufour, D. (1993) "The bitter is sweet: a case study of bitter cassava (Manihot esculenta) use in Amazonia." In *Tropical Forests, People and Food*, C. M. Hladik, A. Hladik, O. F. Linares, H. Pagezy, A. Semple, and M. Hadley, eds. Man and the Biosphere Series Volume 13. UNESCO, and the Parthenon Publishing Group, Paris.

Eaton, S. B., and M. Konner (1985) "Paleolithic nutrition: a consideration of its nature and current implications." *New England Journal of Medicine* 312: 283–89.

Eaton, S. B., M. Konner and M. Shostak (1988) *The Paleolithic Prescription*. New York: Harper Collins.

Ferguson, P. P. (2004) *Accounting for Taste: The Triumph of French Cuisine*. Chicago, IL: The University of Chicago Press.

Fiddes, N. (1992) *Meat: A Natural Symbol*. London: Routledge.

Fitchen, J. M. (1997) "Hunger, Malnutrition and Poverty in the Contemporary United States." *In Food and Culture*, Carole Counihan and Penny Van Esterik, eds. New York: Routledge.

Fitzgerald, T. (1976) *Nutrition and Anthropology in Action*. Assen: Van Gorcum.

Flynn, K. C. (1999) "Food, gender and survival among street adults in Mwanza, Tanzania." *Food and Foodways* 8 (3): 175–202.

——(2005) *Food, Culture, and Survival in an African City*. New York: Palgrave Macmillan.

Fortes, M. and S. L. Fortes (1936) "Food in the domestic economy of the Tallensi." *Africa* 9: 237–76.

Garn, S. and W. Leonard (1989) "What Did Our Ancestors Eat? *Nutrition Reveiews* 47: 337–45.

Gerberg, L. and J. P. Stansbury (2010) *Food by Prescription in Kenya*. USAID/AIDSTAR-ONE PROJECT, Arlington, VA: Task Order 1.

Gewertz, D. and F. Errington (2010) *Cheap Meat: Flap Food Nations in the South Pacific*. Berkeley: University of California Press.

Gibson, R. (2005) *Principles of Nutritional Assessment*, 2nd edition. Oxford: Oxford University Press.

Gladwell, M. (1998) "The Pima Paradox." *The New Yorker*, February 2: 44–57.

Gluckman, P. and M. Hanson (2006) *Mismatch: The Lifestyle Diseases Timebomb*. Oxford: Oxford University Press.

Godoy, R., V. Reyes-Garcia, E. Byron, W. R. Leonard and V. Vadez (2005) "The Effect of Market Economies on the Well-Being of Indigenous Peoples and on their use of Renewable Natural Resources." *Annual Review of Anthropology* 34: 121–38.

Goode, J. G., K. Curtis and J. Theophano (1984a) "Meal formats, meal cycles, and negotiation in the maintenance of an Italian-American community." In *Food in the Social Order*, Mary Douglas, ed. New York: Russell Sage Foundation.

——(1984b) "A framework for the analysis of continuity and change in shared sociocultural rules for food use: the Italian-American pattern." In *Ethnic and Regional Foodways of the United States*, L. K. Brown and K. Mussell, eds. Knoxville: The University of Tennessee Press.

Goodman, A., D. Dufour, and G. Pelto (2000) *Nutritional Anthropology: Biocultural Perspectives on Food and Nutrition*. Mountain View, CA: Mayfield Publishing Company.

Goody, J. (1982) *Cooking, Cuisine and Class: A Study in Comparative Sociology*. Cambridge: Cambridge University Press.

Gordon, K. D. (1987) "Evolutionary perspectives on human diet." In *Nutritional Anthropology*, F. E. Johnston, ed. Alan R. Liss, New York.

Green, E. (1986) "A short-term consultancy in Bangladesh." *American Anthropologist* 88: 176–81.

——(1977) "Hyperendemic goiter, cretinism, and social organization in highland Ecuador." In *Malnutrition, Behavior, and Social Organization*, Edward Green ed. Maryland Heights: Academic Press.

Haas, J. D. and G. G. Harrison (1977) "Nutritional Anthropology and Biological Adaptation." *Annual Reviews of Anthropology* 6: 69–101.

Haas, J. D. and D. L. Pelletier (1989) "Nutrition and Human population biology." In *Human Population Biology*, M. A. Little, and J. D. Haas, eds. New York: Oxford University Press.

Hadley, C. and K. Maes (2009) "A New Global Monitoring System for Food Insecurity? *Lancet* 374(9697): 1223–24.

Hales, C. N. and Barker, D. J. P. (2001) "The thrifty phenotype hypothesis." *British Medical Bulletin* 60: 5–20.

Harris, M. and E. B. Ross (1987) *Food and Evolution: Toward a Theory of Human Food Habits*. Philadelphia: Temple University Press.

Himmelgreen, D. (2002) "You are what you eat and you eat what you are: the role of nutritional anthropology in public health nutrition and nutrition education." *Nutritional Anthropology* 25(1): 2–12.

Himmelgreen, D. and S. Kedia (2009) "The Global Food Crisis: New Insights into an Age-Old Problem." *National Association for the Practice of Anthropology Bulletin* 22: 193–200.

Himmelgreen, D. and N. Romero-Diaz (2009) "Anthropological Approaches to the Global Food Crisis: Understanding and Addressing the "Silent Tsunami"." In The Global Food Crisis: New Insights into an Age-Old Problem, David Himmelgreen and Satish Kedia, eds. *National Association for the Practice of Anthropology Bulletin* 22: 193–200.

Hockett, B. and J. Haws (2003) "Nutritional ecology and diachronic trends in Paleolithic diet and health." *Evolutionary Anthropology* 12(5): 211–16.

Innes, S., ed. (2001) *Kitchen Culture in America: Popular Representations of Food, Gender, and Race*. Philadelphia: University of Pennsylvania Press.

Jenike, M. (2001) "Nutritional Ecology: Diet, Physical Activity and Body Size." In *Hunter-Gatherers: An Interdisciplinary Perspective*, Catherine Panter-Brick, Robert Layton, and Peter Rowley-Conwy, eds. Cambridge: Cambridge University Press.

Jensen, B. (2008) *Nutritional Anthropology*. Global Vision Publishing House, Delhi.

Jerome, N., R. Kandel, and G. Pelto (1980) *Nutritional Anthropology: Contemporary Approaches to Diet and Culture*. London: Routledge.

Johns, T. (1996) *The Origins of Human Diet and Medicine*. The University of Arizona Press, Tucson.

Johnston, F. E. (1987) "*Nutritional Anthropology*. New York: Alan R. Liss, Inc.

Kahn, M. (1998) ""Men are taro" (they cannot be rice): Political aspects of food choices in Wamira, Papua New Guinea." In *Food and Gender: Identity and Power*, Carole M. Counihan and Steven L. Kaplan, eds. Amsteldijk: Harwood.

Katz, S. (1987a) "Food and biocultural evolution: a model for the investigation of modern nutritional problems." In *Nutritional Anthropology*, F. E. Johnston, ed. New York: R. Liss, Inc.

——(1987b) "Fava bean consumption: A case for the co-evolution of genes and culture." In *Food and Evolution: Towards a Theory of Human Food Habits*, Marvin Harris and Erica B. Ross, eds. Philadelphia: Temple University Press.

Katz, S. H. and M. M. Voight (1986) "Bread and Beer: the early use of cereals in the human diet." *Expedition* 28(2): 23–34.

Katz, S. H., M. L. Hediger, and L. A. Valleroy (1974) "Traditional maize processing techniques in the New World." *Science* 184: 765–73.

Kedia, S. and J. van Willigen (2005) *Applied Anthropology: Domains of Application*. Santa Barbara, CA: Praeger.

Konner, M. and Eaton, B. (2010) "Paleolithic Nutrition: Twenty-Five Years Later." *Nutrition in Clinical Practice* 25: 594–602.

Kretchmer, N.O. (1972) "Lactose and lactase." In *Human Physiology and the Environment in Health and Disease*, W.H. Freeman, San Francisco.

——(1978) "Genetic Variability and Lactose Intolerance." *Progress in Human Nutrition* 2: 197–205.

Krishna, A. (2010) *One Illness Away: Why People Become Poor and How They Escape Poverty*. Oxford: Oxford University Press.

Larsen, C. S. (1995) "Biological Changes in Human Populations with Agriculture." *Annual Review of Anthropology* 24: 185–213.

Leatherman, T. L., (1998) "Illness, Social Relations, and Household Production and Reproduction in the Andes of Southern Peru." In *Building a New Biocultural Synthesis: Political Economic Perpsectives on Human Biology*, Alan Goodman and Thomas Leatherman, eds. Ann Arbor: The University of Michigan Press.

Leonard, W. R. and Marcia L. Robertson (1994) "Evolutionary perspectives on human nutrition: the influence of brain and body size on diet and metabolism." *American Journal of Human Biology* 6: 77–88.

Leonard, W. R., J. J. Snodgrass, and M. L. Robertson (2007) "Effects of Brain Evolution on Human Nutrition and Metabolism." *Annual Review of Nutrition* 27: 311–27.

Levenstein, H. (1988) *Revolution at the Table: the Transformation of the American Diet*. New York: Oxford University Press.

——(1993) *Paradox of Plenty: A Social History of Eating in Modern America*. New York: Oxford University Press.

Levi-Strauss, C. (1958) *Structural Anthropology*. New York: Harper Colophon.

——(1970) *The Raw and the Cooked*, New York: Harper Colophon.

——(1978) *The Origins of Table Manners*. New York: Harper Colophon.

Lieberman, L. S. (1987) "Biocultural consequences of animals versus plants as sources of fats, proteins, and other nutrients." In *Food and Evolution*, M. Harris and E. B. Ross, eds. Philadelphia, PA: Temple University Press.

——(2006) "Evolutionary and anthropological perspectives on optimal foraging in obesogenic environments." *Appetite* 47: 3–9.

Lovejoy, C. O. (2009) "Reexamining Human Origins in Light of *Ardipithecus ramidus*. *Science* 326: 74a–e.

Lupton, D. (1996) *Food, the Body and the Self*. London and Thousand Oaks, CA: Sage Publications.

Macbeth, H. and J. MacClancey (2004) *Researching Food Habits: Methods and Problems*. New York: Berghahn Books.

Manderson, L. (1986) *Shared Wealth and Symbol: Food, Culture, and Society in Oceania and Southeast Asia*. Cambridge: Cambridge University Press.

Mann, A. (1972) "Hominid and Cultural Origins." *Man* 7: 379–86.

——(1981) "Diet and human evolution." In *Omnivorous Primates*, R. S. O. Harding and G. Teleki, eds. New York: Columbia University Press.

Margetts, B. M. and M. Nelson (1997) *Design Concepts in Nutritional Epidemiology*, 2nd edition. Oxford: Oxford University Press.

Martorell, R. (1989) "Body size, Adaptation and Function." *Human Organization* 48 (1): 15–20.

McDade, T. W. and Worthman, C. M. (1998) "The weanling's dilemma reconsidered: a biocultural analysis of breast feeding ecology." *Journal of Developmental and Behavioral Pediatrics* 19: 286–99.

Meigs, A. (1983) *Food, Sex and Pollution: a New Guinea Religion*. New Brunswick, NJ: Rutgers University Press.

Mennell, S. (1996) *All Manners of Food*, 2nd edition. Chicago, IL: University of Chicago Press.

Millard, A. V., Graham, M. A., Wang, X., Mier, N., Sanchez, E. R., and Flores, I. (2011) "Pilot of the Diabetes Education Empowerment Program in a high-obesity, low-income Hispanic community on the U.S.–Mexico Border." *Journal of Immigrant and Minority Health* 13(5): 906–13

Milton, K. (1993) "Diet and Primate Evolution." *Scientific American* August: 86–93.

——(2002) "Hunter-Gatherer Diets: Wild Foods Signal Relief from Diseases of Affluence." In *Human Diet: Its Origin and Evolution*, P. Unger and M. Teaford, eds. Westport, CT: Bergin and Garvey.

Mintz, S. (1985) *Sweetness and Power: The Place of Sugar in Modern History*. Penguin Books, New York.

——(1996) *Tasting Good, Tasting Freedom*. Boston, MA: Beacon Press.

Mintz, S. and C. Du Bois (2002) "The anthropology of food and eating." *Annual Review of Anthropology* 31 (1): 99–119.

Neel, J.V. (1962) "Diabetes mellitus: a "thrifty" genotype rendered detrimental by "progress"." *American Journal of Human Genetics* 14: 353–62.

O'Connell, J. F., K. Hawkes, and N. G. Blurton-Jones (1999) "Grandmothering and the evolution of *Homo erectus*. *Journal of Human Evolution* 36: 461–85.

O'Dea, K. (1998) "Affluence in developing countries and natural selection in man." In *Human Biology and Social Inequality*, S. S. Strickland and P. S. Shetty, eds. Cambridge: Cambridge University Press.

Orr, J. B. and J. L. Gilks (1931) *Studies of Nutrition: The Physique and Health of Two African Tribes*. Medical Research Council, Special Report Series no. 155, London.

Pellett, P. L. (1987) "Problems and Pitfalls in the Assessment of Human Nutritional Status." In *Food and Evolution: Toward a Theory of Human Food Habits*, M. Harris and E. B. Ross, eds. Philadelphia: Temple University Press.

Pelto, G. H. and H. C. Freake (2003) "Social Research in an Integrated Science of Nutrition: Future Directions." *Journal of Nutrition* 133(4): 1231–34.

Pelto, G., A. Goodman, and D. Dufour (2000) "The Biocultural Perspective in Nutritional Anthropology." In *Nutritional Anthropology: Biocultural Perspectives on Food and Nutrition*, A. Goodman, D. Dufour, and G. Pelto, eds. Mountain View, CA: Mayfield Publishing Company.

Pelto, G., P. Pelto, and E. Messer (1989) *Research Methods in Nutritional Anthropology*. New York: United Nations Publications.

Pfeiffer, J. and M. Nichter (2008) "What Can Critical Medical Anthropology Contribute to Global Health? A Health Systems Perspective." *Medical Anthropology Quarterly* 22 (4): 410–15.

Popkin, B. M. (2009) *The World is Fat: The Fads, Trends, Policies and Products that are Fattening the Human Race*. New York: Avery.

Quandt, S., ed. (1986) *Training Manual in Nutritional Anthropology*. Washington, DC: American Anthropology Association.

Ray, K. (2004) *The Migrant's Table: Meals and memories in Bengali-American Households*. Philadelphia, PA: Temple University Press.

Richards, A. (1932) *Hunger and work in a Savage Tribe*. London: George Routledge and Sons Ltd.

Rizvi, N. (1991) "Socioeconomic and cultural factors affecting interhousehold and intrahousehold food distribution in rural and urban Bangladesh." In *Diet and Domestic Life in Society*, Ann Sharman et al., eds. Philadelphia, PA: Temple University Press.

Roseberry, W. (1996) "The rise of yuppie coffees and the reimagination of class in the United States." *American Anthropologist* 98(4): 762–75.

Scrimshaw, N. S. (2003) "Historical concepts of interactions, synergism and antagonism between nutrition and infection." *Journal of Nutrition* 133: 316S–21.

Scrimshaw, S. and E. Hurtado (1987) *Rapid Assessment Procedures for Nutrition and Primary Health Care*. Berkeley: University of California Press.

Seckler, D. (1982) ""Small but healthy": a basic hypothesis in the theory, measurement and policy of malnutrition." In *Newer Concepts in Nutrition and Their Implications for Policy*, P. V. Sukhatme, ed. Puna: Maharashtra Association.

Sellen, D. (2007) "Evolution of Infant and Young Child Feeding: Implications for Contemporary Public Health." *Annual Review of Nutrition* 27: 123–48.

Shapiro, L. (1986) *Perfection Salad: Women and Cooking at the Turn of the Century*. New York: Farrar, Straus and Girous.

Sharman, A. (1991) "From generation to generation: resources, experience, and orientation in the dietary patterns of selected urban American households." In *Diet and Domestic Life in Society*, Ann Sharman et al., eds. Philadelphia, PA: Temple University Press.

Simoons, F. J. (1979) "Primary adult lactose intolerance and the milking habit: a problem in biologic and cultural interrelations. II. A culture historical hypothesis." *American Journal of Digestive Diseases* 15: 695–710.

Speth, J. D. and K. A. Spellman (1983) "Energy source, protein metabolism, and hunter-gatherer subsistence strategies." *Journal of Anthropological Archeology* 2: 1–31.

Stini, W. (1975) "Adaptive strategies of human populations under nutritional stress." In *Biosocial Interrelations in Population Adaptation*, E. S. Watts, F. E. Johnston, and G. W. Lasker, eds. the Hague: Mouton.

Stinson, S. (1992) "Nutritional Adaptation." *Annual Review of Anthropology* 21: 143–70.

Strickland, S. S. (1990) "Traditional economies and patterns of nutritional disease." In *Diet and Disease in Traditional and Developing Countries*, G. A. Harrison and J. C. Waterlow, eds. Cambridge: Cambridge University Press.

Thomas, R. B. (1998) "The Evolution of Human Adaptability Paradigms: Towards a Biology of Poverty." In *Building a New Biocultural Synthesis: Political Economic Perpsectives on Human Biology*, Alan Goodman and Thomas Leatherman, eds. Ann Arbor: The University of Michigan Press.

Thomas, R. B., B. Winterhalder, and S. D. McRae (1979) "An anthropological approach to human ecology and adaptive dynamics." *The Yearbook of Physical Anthropology* 22: 1–46.

Thompson, S. E. (1988) "Death, Food, and Fertility." In *Death Ritual in Late Imperial and Modern China*, J. L. Watson and E. S. Rawski, eds. Berkeley: University of California Press.

Toomey, P. M. (1986) "Food from the mouth of Krishna: socio-religious aspects of sacred food in two Krishnaite sects." In *Food Society and Culture*, R. S. Khare and M. S. A. Rao, eds. Durham, NC: Carolina Academic Press.

Torry, W. (1988) "Famine Early Warning Systems: The Need for an Anthropological Dimension." *Human Organization* 47(3): 273–81.

Tremblay, A. and C. Bouchard (1987) "Assessment of Energy Expenditure and Physical Activity Patterns In Population Studies." In *Nutritional Anthropology*, F. E. Johnston, ed. New York: A. R. Liss, Inc..

Trevathan, W. (2007) "Evolutionary Medicine." *Annual Reviews of Anthropology* 36: 139–54.

——(2010) *Ancient Bodies, Modern Lives: How Evolution Has Shaped Women's Health*. Oxford: Oxford University Press.

Ulijaszek, S. (1990) "Nutritional status and susceptibility to infectious disease." In *Diet and Disease in Traditional and Developing Countries*, G.A. Harrison and J. C. Waterlow, eds. Cambridge: Cambridge University Press.

——(1996) "Energetics, adaptatian, and adaptibility." *American Journal of Human Biology* 8: 169–82.

——(1997) "Human Adaptation and adaptability." In *Human Adaptablility: Past, Present and Future*, S. J. Ulijaszek and R. Huss-Ashmore, eds. Oxford University Press, Oxford.

——(2005) *Human Energetics in Biological Anthropology*. Cambridge University Press, Cambridge.

Ulijaszek, S. and H. Lofink (2006) "Obesity in Biocultural Perspective." *Annual Review of Anthropology* 35: 337–60.

Ulijaszek, S. and S. Strickland (1993) "*Nutritional Anthropology: Prospects and Perspectives*. London: Smith Gordon Company.

Unger, P. S. (2007) *Evolution of the Human Diet: the Known, the Unknown and the Unknowable*. Oxford University Press, Oxford.

Unger, P. and M. Teaford (2002) "*Human Diet: Its Origin and Evolution*. Westport, CT: Bergin and Garvey.

Unger, P. S., F. E. Grine, and M. F. Teaford (2006) "Diet in Early *Homo*: A Review of the Evidence and a New Model of Adaptive Versatility." *Annual Review of Anthropology* 35: 209–28.

UNICEF (1990) *Strategy for Improved Nutrition of Children and Women in Developing Countries*. Policy Review paper E/ICEF/1990/1.6, , New York: UNICEF.

Van Esterik, P. (2002) "Contemporary Trends in Infant Feeding Research." *Annual Review of Anthropology* 31: 257–78.

Weismantel, M. (1989) *Food, Gender, and Poverty in the Ecuadorian Andes*. Philadelphia: University of Pennsylvania Press.

Weiss, B. (1980) "Nutrition Adaptation and cultural maladaption." In *Nutritional Anthropology*, N. Jerome, R. Kandel, and G. Pelto, eds. Pleasantville, NY: Redgrave Publishing Company.

Wiedman, D. (2010) "Globalizing the Chronicities of Modernity: Diabetes and the Metabolic Syndrome." In *Chronic Conditions, Fluid States: Chronicity and the Anthropology of Illness*, L. Manderson and C. Smith-Morris, eds. New Brunswick, NJ: Rutgers University Press.

Wiley, A. (2011) *Re-imagining Milk*. New York: Routledge.

Wilk, R. (2007) "'Real Belizean Food': Building Local Identity in the Transnational Caribbean." In *Food and Culture: A Reader*, 2nd edition, C. Counihan and P. Van Esterik, eds. New York: Routledge.

——(2006) *Home Cooking in the Global Village: Caribbean Food from Buccaneers to Ecotourists*. London: Berg.

Williams, B. (1984) "Why migrant women feed their husbands tamales: foodways as a basis for a revisionist view of Tejano family life." In *Ethnic and Regional Foodways of the United States*, L. K. Brown and K. Mussell, eds. Knoxville: The University of Tennessee Press.

Wilson, W., J. Milner, J. Bulkan, and P. Ehlers (2006) "Weaning practices of the Makushi of Guyana and their relationship to infant and child mortality: A preliminary assessment of international recommendations." *American Journal of Human Biology* 18(3): 312–24.

Wrangham, R. (2009) *Catching Fire: How Cooking Made Us Human*. New York: Basic Books.

Wrangham, R., J. H. Jones, G. Laden, D. Pilbeam, and N. L. Conklin-Brittain (1999) The raw and the stolen: cooking and the ecology of human origins. *Current Anthropology* 40(5): 567–94.

6

Public health nutrition

Arlene Spark

This section opens with a historical perspective of public health nutrition from the 1800s to the present, and provides a list of the current goals of nutritionists working in the field of public health. The tools used by public health nutritionists vary, and may include geographic information systems (GIS); nutritional epidemiology; survey design, implementation and evaluation; and literature reviews known as meta-analyses. New areas of research in public health nutrition include examining the nutrition transition and learning how diet interacts with genes throughout life, affecting the expression of those genes and, consequently, tissue function and disease risk.

Historical background

The world faces both old and new public health challenges. The safety of our water and food from unintentional contamination has always challenged us. In fact, the founding event in the science of epidemiology was John Snow's use in 1854 of a spot map (the forerunner of geographic information systems, GIS) to make the connection between the quality of the source of water and cholera cases. Snow demonstrated an increased incidence of cholera in the households clustered around the Broad Street (London) water pump, which delivered sewage-polluted water. Currently, environmentalists are concerned with the effect on our water supply of hydraulic fracturing (fracking), which may result in water contamination near fracking sites.

Historically, we faced single nutrient deficiency diseases and protein and calorie malnutrition. The presence of severe malnutrition among the poor can render a population more susceptible to infection, as well as impeding their prospects of recovery. The health of the entire population, rich and poor, is undermined because malnutrition among the poor decreases their ability to ward off infectious diseases, which in turn leads to increases in infectious diseases in the population as a whole. Severe malnutrition now exists primarily in developing countries, but with international travel, its effects are seen globally, as infectious diseases are carried by travelers from the developing to the developed parts of the world.

The industrialized nations face the threat of agroterrorism, heart disease, cancer, the health of our increasingly elderly populations, and an obesity epidemic. Paradoxically, obesity is seen predominantly not only among the poor in developed countries but also among the more affluent in developing countries.

Mary C. Egan (a former associate director and chief nutritionist of the Bureau of Maternal and Child Health, Health Resources Administration, Department of Health and Human Services) provides a comprehensive overview of public health nutrition services from the mid-nineteenth through the mid-twentieth century, with special emphasis on mothers, children, and families.[1]

In the 1800s, efforts were focused on establishing state health departments and voluntary health agencies, initiating early nutrition investigations, and establishing milk stations and school lunch programs in large cities to supplement the diets of poor people and to combat the high rates of morbidity and mortality in infants and children. In 1867 the first state department of health was established in Massachusetts and by 1877 there were 14 state departments of health; in 1872 the American Public Health Association (APHA) was founded. The fields of community and public health nursing and of home economics, established in the 1850s and 1870s, respectively, served as precursors to public health nutrition, which narrowed the focus of both these fields.

Public health nutrition came of age in the early 1900s with the creation of the Children's Bureau (CB) in 1907, the pasteurization of milk in 1910, and the Massachusetts General Hospital's hiring in 1917 of its first nutritionist (called a "health instructor in foods"), the CB's launching of studies of the nutrition status of children, iodization of salt to prevent goiter, and the creation of an experimental food stamp program.

In the 1930s and 1940s, the economic depression, the Second World War and waves of immigration brought new milestones in the delivery of nutrition services to the public. The US government embarked on food and nutrition status surveys, which began focusing attention on groups at nutrition risk, such as infants, children, pregnant and lactating mothers, the elderly, children with developmental disabilities, and racial and ethnic minority groups, and there appeared the first qualifications for nutritionists in public health. These additional landmark events occurred during the maturing years of public health nutrition: the first conference on the role of State Health Departments in nutrition research (1961), passage for the Food Stamp Act (1965), the first White House Conference on Food, Nutrition and Health (1969), which ushered in the Head Start Program, and the first White House Conference on Aging (1971), which led to the establishment of the Nutrition Program for the Elderly.

The 1950s witnessed the founding of the Association of Faculties of Graduate Programs in Public Health Nutrition and the Association of State and Territorial Public Health Nutrition Directors. The War on Poverty in the 1960s called attention to income and health disparities, which resulted in the beginnings of programs in maternal and child health (MCH), migrant health, school lunch and breakfast, all of which employed public health nutrition personnel.

Key figures in the earliest days of public health nutrition include Ellen H. Richards, Lydia Roberts, Frances Stern, Marjorie G. Heseltine. Physicians whose work led to the identification of nutrients responsible for deficiency diseases are Lind (vitamin C and scurvy, 1753) and Goldberger (niacin and pellagra, 1914).

Our current food- and nutrition-related challenges make public health nutrition a multi-disciplinary field that requires expertise in the biological, quantitative, and social sciences. Because preventing disease is at the heart of public health, one must look towards the social sciences to understand health-related behaviors and their societal influences – critical elements in educating and empowering people to make healthier lifestyle choices. In addition to understanding nutrition and food science and the behavioral sciences, public health nutrition professionals are also required to have a background in biostatistics, epidemiology, environmental science, and health policy and management. Working in interdisciplinary teams, public health nutritionists provide evidence-based approaches to solving the population-based health problems, and develop programs and policies to prevent and ameliorate these conditions.

Thus, some of the goals of those working in public health nutrition are to: identify and assess diet-related health problems – of both undernutrition and overnutrition – among diverse population groups in developed and developing countries; identify the social, cultural, economic, environmental, and institutional factors that contribute to the risk of undernutrition and overnutrition among populations; demonstrate the linkages between agriculture, food, nutrition, and public health; develop educational, institutional, and other population-based intervention strategies to improve food security and reduce obesity; develop policies to reduce barriers to food insecurity and to improve the food and activity choices and nutritional status of diverse population groups; promote policies to ensure the safe production, distribution, and consumption of food; advocate for improved nutrition and physical activity opportunities for diverse population groups; apply population-based research findings to the development and implementation of nutrition policies and programs in the US and abroad; and investigate relationships between diet and disease by using the techniques of nutritional epidemiology.

Research methodologies

Because nutrition affects almost every public health challenge, public health nutrition draws on diverse, multidisciplinary teams to find solutions, and in doing so examines the continuum from the cell to the population. Currently, domestic and international research is addressing ways to define and stem the global obesity epidemic, decrease risks of cancer and diabetes through dietary means, supplement women's diets to improve maternal health, improve materno-fetal, infant, and child nutrition to protect survival and prevent adult onset chronic diseases, assess and prevent micronutrient deficiencies and their health consequences across the life stages, and develop and advocate food and nutrition policies to improve population.

Public health nutrition personnel in managerial and professional titles collect and analyze data to identify community needs prior to planning, implementing, monitoring, and evaluating programs designed to encourage healthy lifestyles, policies, and environments. Research conducted by public health nutrition professionals may also serve as a resource to assist individuals, other professionals, or the community, and may provide justification for the allocation of resources for health education programs. Personnel in public health nutrition conduct nutrition assessments, design programs, and evaluate nutrition interventions at the individual, community, and national levels. They collect data using dietary assessment tools, qualitative methods, and surveys using local, state, and national data, including surveillance data. They determine how population consumption patterns affect nutrition status, how to evaluate epidemiologic studies on nutrition and health and how to apply findings to practice. They design, implement, and evaluate evidence-based local, state, and national nutrition programs that address the needs of diverse and vulnerable populations.

In terms of obtaining information about an individual's diet, clinical nutritionists and dietitians use diet histories, 24-hour diet recalls and 72-hour foods records. However, for collection of comprehensive dietary data in large-scale epidemiologic studies, the most practical and economical method is the food frequency questionnaire (FFQ). Several have been developed for use with varying populations and for specific needs – the Willet FFQ (Harvard), and from the National Cancer Institute, the Block Health Habits and History Questionnaire and the Diet History Questionnaire. FFQs ask respondents to report their usual frequency of consumption of each food from a list of foods for a specific time period. Compared with other approaches, such as 24-hour dietary recalls and food records, the FFQ generally collects less detail regarding the foods consumed, cooking methods, and portion size. Therefore, the quantification of intake is not considered as accurate. However, unlike records or recalls, FFQs are designed to capture usual dietary intake. Most are completed independently by a respondent and are relatively inexpensive. Therefore, the FFQ is usually the method of choice in large-scale epidemiologic studies.

The research methodologies used by public health nutrition professionals include secondary analyses of food, nutrition, and health data from the National Center for Health Statistics (NCHS), a unit for the Centers for Disease Control and Health Promotion (CDC). The NCHS maintains literally hundreds of databases with information valuable to public health nutrition professionals. The major surveys used by public health nutrition professionals are: the National Health and Nutrition Examination Survey (NHANES), Behavioral Risk Factor Surveillance System (BRFSS), Youth Risk Behavior Surveillance System (YRBSS), National Health Interview Survey (NHIS). Public health nutrition professionals also contribute to the development and administration of local surveys, such as the New York City Health and Nutrition Examination Survey (NYC HANES). Countries around the world maintain their own health survey data, such as the Canadian Community Health Survey, which includes dietary data, is run by Statistics Canada and Health Canada www.hc-sc.gc.ca/fn-an/surveill/nutrition/commun/cchs_guide_escc-eng.php (accessed on March 26, 2012).

In addition to designing and analyzing surveys, public health nutrition professionals conduct research using the standard methodologies of epidemiology. Consider these research study examples, all of which deal with the health effects of consuming sugar-sweetened beverages (SSB): *Long-term, randomized, controlled trials* have examined the relationship between the consumption of SSB and body weight.[2] *Prospective, observational studies* have examined associations between the consumption of SSB and the risk of type 2 diabetes.[3] *Meta-analysis* demonstrated associations between the intake of SSB and body weight.[4] *Cross-sectional and longitudinal studies* have examined environmental risk factors for overweight children.[5]

A relatively new tool used in public health, the GIS, includes a set of hardware and software tools that help to visualize and to locate, rather than analyze, the patterns of a phenomenon. Mapping the nutritional terrain is one of the many areas of application of GIS methodologies. GIS presentations have made it easy to visualize where "food deserts" exist and where public health nutrition services should be targeted. A food desert is an urban area with little or no access to nutritious food. Residents living in food deserts are more likely to be overweight and have other diet-related health problems such as diabetes or hypertension. Almost any nutrition survey aiming to define the nutritional status in a certain area (at district, town, province, region, state, nation, or continent level) can be enhanced by a GIS presentation. Early warning systems mapping, poverty mapping, and vulnerability forecasts are examples of applications used by public health planners.

Public health nutrition policy scholars look for successful programs to address the nutritional problems of vulnerable populations, and in this way their work informs and directs policies and programs regarding food and nutrition. Researchers may synthesize existing information in the form of meta-analyses and systematic reviews to provide key information to policymakers on how to deal effectively with public health nutrition problems. They may also examine the impact of policies on important health outcomes, such as policies for obesity prevention and the promotion of physical activity.

Avenues for future research

Economics poverty and malnutrition are continued challenges in the developing world. The *nutrition transition* in industrialized nations from a scarcity of calories to a surfeit has led to the development of obesity and nutrition-related non-communicable diseases (NR-NCD), such as cardiovascular diseases, diabetes, and so on. At present, this transition is happening differently in Asia, Africa, the Middle East, Latin America, and Oceana compared to what occurred in the United States, Western Europe, and Japan at a similar stage in their economic development. Understanding the phenomenon of rapid onset of obesity and development of NR-NCDs is important for public health nutritionists and others who are challenged with planning strategies to prevent the continued increase in prevalence of obesity and its complications in the developing world.[6]

Cutting-edge areas that will be the focus of public health nutrition in the future include epigenetics. Environmental factors interact with genes throughout life, affecting the expression of those genes and, consequently, tissue function and disease risk. One such environmental factor is diet during critical periods of development, such as during prenatal life. Epigenetics, which refers to modifications to the DNA that regulate how much of a gene is produced, has been suggested to underlie these effects. Epigenetics explains why poor diet during pregnancy may compromise the long-term health of the offspring. For example, children born to mothers who consumed an unhealthy diet during pregnancy have an increased risk of type 2 diabetes, a significant contributing factor to heart disease and possibly also to cancer later in life. This knowledge presents new opportunities in cardiovascular and cancer risk reduction using dietary and lifestyle factors, which are goals of public health nutrition.

Getting started

Some public health nutritionists work in private-sector organizations. Many work at the community level. Those with at least the MPH degree and several years of experience and/or the registered dietitian (RD) credential are employed by public health agencies in government settings.

The functions, duties, and qualifications of public health nutrition personnel have been delineated in *Personnel in Public Health Nutrition for the 2000s*.[7] Those in managerial titles include public health nutrition directors, assistant public health nutrition directors, and public health nutrition supervisors. Those in professional titles include public health nutrition consultants, public health nutritionists, clinical nutritionists, nutritionists, community nutritionists, and nutrition educators. Those providing technical and support services include nutrition technicians (paraprofessionals) and community nutrition workers (who do not require academic preparation).

Personnel in public health nutrition are specialized nutrition professionals and paraprofessionals who provide and/or plan nutrition programs through organizations that reach people living in a designated community. Settings can include federal, state, city, or county government-operated public health departments and contracted services with public or private health centers, hospital ambulatory care clinics, health maintenance organizations, home health organizations, and specialized community health projects. Whether under governmental or non–governmental sponsorship, public/community health organizations generally operate under medical direction. They employ a multidisciplinary staff that includes nutritionists who work with physicians, nurses, social workers, health educators, dentists, epidemiologists, statisticians, health planners, community health workers, and environmental health specialists, among others.

The large number of different competency units identified as essential for effective public health nutrition practice reflects the breadth of skills, knowledge, and applications required to address the myriad problems encountered in public health nutrition practice. As it is unrealistic to expect an individual practitioner to have proficiency in all the competencies identified, this highlights the need for teamwork to ensure the competency mix required for effective work effort.[8]

One of the difficulties in identifying competencies relevant to public health nutrition relates to whether we are referring to the individual public health nutrition practitioner or the field as a whole. According to a study conducted in 2004,[9] many core competencies expected of public health nutritionists are similar to those of nutrition and dietetics, health education, and generic public health practice.[10] These competencies are described as analytical (nutrition monitoring and surveillance; assess the evidence and impact of health and health-care interventions, programs, and services and apply these assessments to practice; needs assessment – assessing population needs using various methods; applied research, research and development – appraise, plan, and manage research; interpret research findings and apply in practice; analyze the determinants of nutrition issues using a range of information sources; food monitoring and surveillance; scientific writing and dissemination of research; improve the quality of health and health-care services and interventions through audit and evaluation; and health economics and economic evaluation applications), sociocultural, and political (knowledge and understanding of the psychological, social, and cultural factors that influence food and dietary choices; and policy development); public health services (intervention management: Design, plan, implement, monitor, and evaluate nutrition strategies and programs for promoting health and well-being of the population, reduce inequalities; principles and practice of health education, health promotion theory, behavior change and health promotion policy and programs, public health methods; knowledge of food and nutrition systems and community food needs; provision of preventive nutrition programs; building capacity of the health workforce through training, up-skilling, and mentoring; service and prioritizing programs based on identified needs, their potential impact, as defined by objective measurable criteria; provide nutrition information to diverse audiences; health-care systems knowledge; provision of clinical nutrition services); communication (interpersonal communication and written); management and leadership (financial planning and management skills); and professional (ethics of public health nutrition practice; commitment to continual competency development and lifelong learning; values and participates in peer review; reflective practice to enhance performance).

Responsibilities, credentials, education, and training

A masters degree with graduate coursework in advanced nutrition and the core public health areas (biostatistics, epidemiology, health planning/administration, environmental health, health behavior and health education, and cross–cutting competencies) is recommended for managerial positions and public health nutritionist and public health nutrition consultant positions.

In addition to understanding the fundamentals of nutrition and food science, public health nutrition professionals have a background in the five core areas of public health: biostatistics, epidemiology, environmental science, health policy and management, and behavioral science.

Selected schools in the United States and the United Kingdom that offer the Masters of Public Health (MPH) degree, the Master of Science (MS) degree, or the doctorate (PhD, ScD, EdD, DPH) with a concentration in public health nutrition include the City University of New York, School of Public Health at Hunter College (www.cuny.edu/site/sph.html, accessed on March 26, 2012), Harvard University, School of Public Health (www.hsph.harvard.edu/departments/nutrition/prospective-students/public-health-nutrition/index.html, accessed on March 26, 2012), New York University, Steinhardt School of Culture, Education, and Human Development (mph.nyu.edu/academics/concentrations/public-health-nutrition.html, accessed on March 26, 2012), Tufts University, School of Medicine in cooperation with the Gerald J. and Dorothy J. Friedman School of Nutrition Science and Policy (www.tufts.edu/med/

education/phpd/mph/concentrations/nutrition/index.html, accessed on March 26, 2012), Johns Hopkins University Bloomberg School of Public Health (www.jhsph.edu/chn/academics accessed on March 26, 2012), University of Massachusetts—Amherst, Department of Nutrition (www.umass.edu/sphhs/nutrition/about/index.html, accessed on March 26, 2012), University of North Carolina, Gillings School of Global Health (www.sph.unc.edu/nutr/degrees, accessed on March 26, 2012), University of Tennessee at Knoxville, College of Education, Health and Human Sciences, Department of Nutrition (nutrition.utk.edu/phn/degree_offering_and_curriculum/dual_ms_mph/index.html, accessed March 26, 2012), and London School of Hygiene and Tropical Medicine (www.lshtm.ac.uk/study/masters/msphn.html, accessed on March 26, 2012).

Other advanced degree programs in nutrition (not all of which offer public health degrees) are listed on the Academy of Nutrition and Dietetics website (www.eatright.org/Becomean RDorDTR/content.aspx?id=8146, accessed on March 26, 2012).

An alternative qualification would be the RD credential with an undergraduate degree in community nutrition or dietetics, additional public health core coursework, plus three years of increasing or progressively responsible full-time work experience as a nutritionist in a public health organization.

The Academy of Nutrition and Dietetics recognizes programs that train entry-level practitioners in community nutrition. These programs are expected to provide students with the ability to:

- Supervise screening of the nutritional status of the population and/or community groups. Conduct assessment of the nutritional status of the population and/or community groups. Provide nutrition care for people of diverse cultures and religions across the lifespan, i.e., infants through geriatrics. Conduct community-based health promotion/disease prevention programs. Participate in development and evaluation of a community-based food and nutrition programs. Supervise community-based food and nutrition programs. Participate in coding and billing of dietetics/nutrition services to obtain reimbursement for services from public or private insurers.

- Manage nutrition care for diverse population groups across the lifespan. Conduct community-based food and nutrition program outcome assessment/evaluation. Develop community-based food and nutrition programs. Participate in nutrition surveillance and monitoring of communities. Participate in community-based research. Participate in food and nutrition policy development and evaluation based on community needs and resources. Consult with organizations regarding food access for target populations. Develop a health promotion/disease prevention intervention project. Participate in waived point-of-care testing, such as hematocrit and cholesterol levels. Conduct general health assessment, e.g., blood pressure, vital signs.

- For the managerial and professional titles, state licensure for nutritionists and managers who are responsible for policymaking, planning/evaluation/research, management, supervision, leadership, and resource development. For positions providing nutrition counseling to clients, registration from the Commission on Dietetic Registration as a dietitian (RD) is expected. Individuals with the RD credential have the professional training necessary to provide nutrition care to medically high–risk clients, and their local organizations would apply for participation in federal and other health-care cost reimbursement systems. Clinical nutritionists require a masters degree in advanced human and clinical nutrition, or the RD credential with additional coursework in advanced normal and clinical nutrition and/or completion of supervised training in dietetics plus three years of increasing or progressively responsible full-time work experience in clinical dietetics in a hospital, health-care facility, or community health organization.

Professional associations

In the United States, the major professional associations that represent professionals in public health nutrition include the Academy of Nutrition and Dietetics' practice groups: Hunger and Environmental Nutrition (www.hendpg.org, accessed on March 26, 2012) and Public Health/ Community Nutrition (www.phcnpg.org, accessed on March 26, 2012); the American Public Health Association's Food and Nutrition section (www.apha.org/membergroups/sections/ aphasections/food, accessed on March 26, 2012), and the Association of State and Territorial Public Health Nutrition Directors (ASTPHND) (www.astphnd.org, accessed on March 26, 2012). Globally, see: Nutrition Society (www.nutritionsociety.org, accessed on March 26, 2012) and World Public Health Nutrition Association (www.wphna.org/president_welcome.htm, accessed on March 26, 2012).

Notes

1 Egan, Mary C., "Public health nutrition: A historical perspective." *J Am Diet Assoc.* 1994, 94: 298–304.
2 James, J., P. Thomas, D. Cavan and D. Kerr, "Preventing childhood obesity by reducing consumption of carbonated drinks: cluster randomised controlled trial." *BMJ* 2004, 328: 1236; Sichieri, R., Paula Trotte, A., de Souza, R. A., and Veiga, G. V. "School randomised trial on prevention of excessive weight gain by discouraging students from drinking sodas." *Public Health Nutr* 2009, 12: 197–202; Ebbeling, C. B., Feldman, H. A., Osganian, S. K., Chomitz, V. R., Ellenbogen, S. J. and Ludwig, D. S. "Effects of decreasing sugar-sweetened beverage consumption on body weight in adolescents: a randomized, controlled pilot study." *Pediatrics* 2006, 117: 673–80; Albala, C., Ebbeling, C.B., Cifuentes, M., Lera, L., Bustos, N. and Ludwig, D. S. "Effects of replacing the habitual consumption of sugar-sweetened beverages with milk in Chilean children." *Am J Clin Nutr* 2008, 88: 605–11.
3 Matthias, B., Schulze, P. H., Manson, J. E., Ludwig, D. S., Colditz, G. A., Stampfer, M. J., Willett, W. C., and Hu, F. B. "Sugar-sweetened beverages, weight gain, and incidence of type 2 diabetes in young and middle-aged women." *JAMA* 2004, 292: 927–34; Montonen, J., Jarvinen, R., Knekt, P., Heliovaara, M. and Reunanen, A. "Consumption of sweetened beverages and intakes of fructose and glucose predict type 2 diabetes occurrence." *J Nutr.* 2007, 137: 1447–54; Palmer, J. R., Boggs, D. A., Krishnan, S., Hu, F. B., Singer, M. and Rosenberg, L. "Sugar-sweetened beverages and incidence of type 2 diabetes mellitus in African American women." *Arch Intern Med.* 2008, 168: 1487–92.
4 Vartanian, L. R., Schwartz, M. B. and Brownell, K.D. "Effects of soft drink consumption on nutrition and health: a systematic review and meta-analysis." *Am J Public Health* 2007, 97: 667–75.
5 Gillis, L. J. and Bar-Or, O. "Food away from home, sugar-sweetened drink consumption and juvenile obesity." *J Am Coll Nutr.* 2003, 22: 539–45; Ariza, A. J., Chen, E. H., Binns, H. J. and Christoffel, K. K. "Risk factors for overweight in five- to six-year-old Hispanic-American children: a pilot study." *J Urban Health.* 2004, 81: 150–61.
6 Popkin, B. M. "Part II. What is unique about the experience in lower- and middle-income less-industrialised countries compared with the very-high-income industrialised countries? The shift in stages of the nutrition transition in the developing world differs from past experiences!" *Publ Health Nutr.* 2002, 5: 205–14.
7 Dodds, J. M., ed. *Personnel in Public Health Nutrition for the 2000s.* ASTPHND, 2009. www.astphnd. org/resource_files/105/105_resource_file1.pdf (accessed on April 11, 2012).
8 Hughes, R. "Competencies for effective public health nutrition practice: a developing consensus." *Public Health Nutr.* 2004, 7: 683–91.
9 Hughes, R. "Competencies for effective public health nutrition practice: a developing consensus." *Public Health Nutr.* 2004, 7: 683–91.
10 Council on Linkages between Academia and Public Health Practice. *Core Competencies for Public Health Professionals.* Washington, DC: US Department of Health and Human Services, 2002.

Key reading

Books

Edelstein, Sari, ed. (2011) *Nutrition in Public Health: A handbook for developing programs and services*, 3rd edition. Washington, DC: American Public Health Association.

Frank, Gail C. (2008) *Community Nutrition: Applying Epidemiology to Contemporary Practice*, 2nd edition. Sudbury, MA: Jones and Bartlett Publishers.

Gibney, Michael J., Barrie M. Margetts, John M. Kearney, and Lenore Arab, eds. (2004) *Public Health Nutrition*. Hoboken, NJ: Wiley.

Spark, Arlene (2007) *Nutrition in Public Health: Principles, policies, and practice*. Boca Raton, FL: CRC Press.

Struble, Marie Boyle and David H. Holben (2006) *Community Nutrition in Action: An interdisciplinary approach*, 5th edition. Stamford, CT: Thomson/Wadsworth.

Vir, Sheila Chander, ed. (2010) *Public Health Nutrition in Developing Countries, Part I*. Cambridge: Woodhead Publishers.

Journals

Public Health Nutrition: published monthly on behalf of The Nutrition Society to disseminate research and scholarship aimed at understanding the causes of, and approaches and solutions to, nutrition-related public health achievements, situations, and problems around the world. Suitable for epidemiologists and health promotion specialists interested in the role of nutrition in disease prevention; academics and those involved in fieldwork and the application of research to identify practical solutions to important public health problems: www.nutritionsociety. org/publications/nutrition-society-journals/public-health-nutrition (accessed on March 26, 2012).

Occasional articles about public health nutrition in: *Journal of the Academy of Nutrition and Dietetics* (formerly *Journal of the American Dietetic Association*), *Journal of the American Public Health Association*, *Journal of Clinical Nutrition*, *Journal of Nutrition Education and Behavior*.

Newsletters

Hunger and Environmental Nutrition www.hendpg.org
Public Health/Community Nutrition www.phcnpg.org
Yale Rudd Center Newsletter www.yaleruddcenter.org/newsletter

Blogs

Appetite for Profit www.appetiteforprofit.com
Be Active Your Way Blog www.health.gov/paguidelines/blog
Bridging the Health Literacy Gap blogs.cdc.gov/healthliteracy
Food Politics www.foodpolitics.com
Genomics & Health Impact Blog blogs.cdc.gov/genomics
US Food Policy usfoodpolicy.blogspot.com
World Public Health Nutrition Association www.wphna.org/aboutthiswebsite.htm
Yale Rudd Center www.yaleruddcenter.org/blog
Young Public Health Nutrition Network sites.google.com/site/yphnutrition/yphn-blog

Centers

Center for Public Health Nutrition, University of Washington depts.washington.edu/uwcphn/about
Rudd Center for Food Policy & Obesity www.yaleruddcenter.org/blog

Other

Principles of Public Health Nutrition (web-based module) www.epi.umn.edu/let/nutri/principles/index.shtm

7

The archaeology of food

Katherine M. Moore

The archaeology of food combines laboratory methods to recover ancient foods, ancient food use, and ancient cuisine. Not all foods are likely to leave archaeological remains: animal bones are common and indicate the use of meat, but plant remains are unlikely to be found by archaeologists unless they have been accidentally charred. The study of cooking and serving has been approached through containers made of ceramic, stone, and wood. Interest in cooking equipment has expanded recently as techniques have been developed recently that recover faint residues of fats and other constituents of food from the insides of pots. Soil samples have yielded individual grains of food starch, greatly expanding our knowledge of the use of tubers, fruits, and grains. Linking these finds with artifacts and evidence from iconography, history, and human skeletal remains allows archaeologists to assess the connection between ancient food, ancient economies, and ancient social organization.

Historical background of food scholarship in archaeology and major theoretical approaches in use

Archaeology is the study of material remains to reveal past human behavior. The methods of archaeology are applied to the study of human evolution, anthropological research on the prehistoric societies and early civilizations of around the world, and research on the classical societies of the Mediterranean. Archaeologists study prehistoric or non-literate societies as well as historic and even present-day societies. Archaeologists have always acknowledged food as an important aspect of past cultures and economic systems, though few food remains were studied directly until recently. From the nineteenth to the twenty-first century the goals of understanding food in the archaeological record have expanded steadily, leading to an increase in the materials studied and the methods used (Samuel, 1996). Though the questions posed by each of these research communities vary, the research methods used to study ancient food around the world are shared between archaeologists and their collaborators in the natural and physical sciences. Two basic strands of research in food archaeology are the study of plant remains (paleoethnobotany or archaeobotany) and the study of animal remains (zooarchaeology). The specialists in these fields have distinct training and skills, but integrating these two strands has allowed rapid progress in studying ancient food (De France *et al.*, 1996; VanDerwarker and Peres, 2010). Since the 1990s, food archaeologists have sought a more complete record of hard-to-find foods, at the same time that they have sought a broader recognition of the influence of food production systems on political and social process.

Most archaeological food remains come from excavations at archaeological sites. Deposits with food remains are usually mixtures of foods and other materials discarded by households, and are not assumed to reflect individual food choice or consumption. Individual food intake may be reflected by traces on the human skeleton, or by discrete deposits such as funerary offerings. Some food remains are immediately recognized: bones and shells of ancient animals, for example. In contrast, most plant foods decompose after discard, leaving little for archaeologists to find. When plants are burned in processing, site cleanup, or as fuel, charred parts may preserve some tissue structure and survive burial. New methods allow recovery and identification of microscopic plant remains that were never charred.

Archaeological projects must commit to intensive recovery techniques to gather a representative sample of remains from all foods. Field archaeologists pass archaeological deposits through sieves to collect animal bone fragments (and many other kinds of artifacts).

A zooarchaeological specialist then studies the cleaned bone fragments to reconstruct the animals represented. A few uncharred plant remains are found intact because they have been preserved in a very dry or cold or acid setting, such as the stomach contents of the prehistoric human remains in Northern Europe known as "bog bodies" (Behre, 2008; Brothwell and Brothwell, 1988), or a dumpling found as a burial offering in a Bronze Age tomb in Xinjang, central Asia (Gong *et al.*, 2011). Otherwise, field archaeologists use fine sieves and water separation techniques (called flotation) to recover fragile traces of charred plant remains from archaeological deposits (Pearsall, 2000). An archaeobotanist then sorts and identifies the charred seeds, plant parts, and wood under low magnification. Microscopic remains, completely invisible to the naked eye during excavation, are collected in special soil samples to obtain ancient plant pollen, starch grains, phytoliths (silica bodies that form in plant cells), and raphides (particles of oxalates that form in leaves) (Torrence and Barton, 2006). At an even smaller scale, archaeologists collect samples to determine characteristic chemical signatures of ancient foods. This molecular level is a rapidly expanding area of research, leading to identification of such foods as milk, wine, and chocolate using gas chromatography, mass spectrometry, and infrared spectroscopy (Mukherjee *et al.*, 2005). Molecular traces come from charred lumps of burned food, from the residues that soaked into the clay of pottery vessels, and from the surfaces of ancient tools. In addition, the ability to study ancient food remains in terms of their DNA (Elbaum *et al.*, 2006; Li *et al.*, 2011) or their stable isotope ecologies (Brown and Brown, 2011; Schoeninger, 2009) has allowed precise reconstructions of the exact species being used and the region or ecology in which it was produced.

Food archaeology addresses fundamental questions about behavior millions of years old, a time period that captures the earliest traces of the archaeological record. Very basic questions arise in characterizing early human behavior: what foods were eaten by the first bipedal hominids (human ancestors and relatives) and their tool-using descendants? What impact did those foods have on the evolution of the human body or behavior (Jones, 2007)? Many insights come from the analysis of human fossil remains themselves. Methods in food archaeology have stretched to address material that is so remote in time and so faint in its imprint on the landscape. In the regions of Africa where the fossils of early human ancestors have been found, archaeologists seek evidence for the first deliberately flaked tool and the first bones marked by cuts from those tools. A key issue addressed by the zooarchaeology of these sites is whether the earliest humans hunted for themselves or scavenged from carcasses left by other animals, and if those early humans could control fire for cooking. These behaviors might be the baseline from which to infer that hominids tended to live in "family" groups of a male and female with offspring (Speth, 2010; Wrangham, 2009).

The interpretation of early hominid food remains has been continuously contested and modified. Study of faint traces of tools, tooth marks, and breakage on bones dating from three million years ago to two million years ago indicates that hominids scavenged carcasses, used tools to process meat, and were preyed upon by larger predators. Some bones may have been deliberately broken open to get the fatty marrow, even if the hominids never got the associated meat (Stanford and Bunn, 2001). No evidence has been preserved for plant use or for cooking for this period, but studies of hominid anatomy and the foods that would have been available suggest that they must have foraged for fruits, seeds, and underground root foods, and may have used fire to cook them (Stahl, 1984; Wrangham, 2008). Preliminary evidence has recently been offered for plant food intake for Neanderthal teeth from Iran and Belgium, approximately 40,000 years old. Evidence for grains and fruits comes from starch grains and phytoliths embedded in dental calculus, opening the possibility that such insights may provide substantive new data on the early importance of plants (Henry et al., 2011). Though these periods are remote in time, societies today are interested in such reconstructions of a "Paleolithic diet" and its possible lessons for a modern healthy diet (Kuipers et al., 2010).

One of the most profound transitions in the history of the human diet started in the period at the end of the last ice age (about 12,000 years ago) with the origins of the first farming societies. Agriculture, of course, is a completely new relationship between humans and food. We know that farming is associated with changing human settlement patterns, health status, work patterns, family and social life, and with new religious and legal systems. Recognizing these changes has driven the development of archaeological methods to pinpoint the first agriculture in time and to understand its spread to new areas (Pearsall, 2009; Price and Bar-Yosef, 2011).

Archaeologists searching for the origins of early crop plants such as wheat and barley have used water flotation to collect a sequence of charred ancient plant remains relating to the invention of farming (Cowan and Watson, 2006). The size and shape of ancient plant parts reflect human intervention in selecting, sowing, tending, and harvesting the first crops (Miller, 2006; Weiss and Zohary, 2011). Archaeologists note the rapid increase in implements for storing, grinding, and cooking grain (Willcox, 2002); later, the first ovens for bread are seen (Valamoti, 2002). The relationship between ancient farming and cooking is complicated. Cooking enhances the nutritional value of grains and other starchy foods and it initially appeared that ceramics had been developed around the same time farming arose. In this view, pots met the need to cook and store the new foods. It is now clear that while pottery is tightly associated with food processing and a less mobile lifestyle, in several cases (notably in east Asia and east Africa) pottery was invented to cook and store wild foods (Kuzmin, 2006). Some early cultivators did not use ceramics; and cooking has also been accomplished around the world using baskets, leather and stone containers, and even wooden boxes.

Grain agriculture became the most important source of plant food calories in the Near East and parts of East Asia and the Americas. In other regions, grain agriculture based on wheat, rice, or maize (corn) never developed. Many tropical regions had significant plant food sources in tubers and other underground storage organs (Torrence and Barton, 2006). Since these foods do not produce charred parts in cooking, archaeologists have used microscopic starch grains to study the origins of important crops like manioc (cassava) in Latin America, and taro in the Pacific. Such research attests to many independent locations of early agriculture, rather than a smaller number of centers of domestication known from research in the mid-twentieth century.

Zooarchaeologists study the origins of domesticated animals such as sheep, goats, and pigs by looking at proportions of different animal species in bones from early village sites; the sizes, proportions and ages of those animals; and the appearance of domestic species in places where they had not occurred as wild animals (Reitz and Wing, 2008). These clues suggest when and where animals had been domesticated. New research on the genetic diversity of wild and domestic herds has improved understanding of the specific wild ancestors of modern domesticated animals, and ancient DNA is now being collected from archaeological samples to link them to modern populations (Zeder, 2006).

It has been difficult to measure the immediate effect of animal domestication on human diet, since people had usually hunted the wild ancestors of the early herd animals in the first place. The need to provide domestic animals with food, water, and protection may have changed human lifeways more than having a supply of meat. The origins of milking and the preparation of dairy food relied on a particularly close human–animal relationship and resulted in completely new kinds of food and food preparation (Copley et al., 2005; Mukherjee et al., 2005). The analysis of fatty acid residues in ancient ceramic vessels from Turkey and the Near East has established the origin of ancient dairy use much earlier (6000 BCE) than had been suspected based on bone remains and other clues (Evershed et al., 2008). Storing and processing milk was a significant early use of pottery in this region. Dairying and using animals to pull plows or transport loads created a tightly integrated system of herding and farming, an enduring economic base for complex and expanding societies. The production of surplus food can be traced through the remains of substantial storage facilities. Such bins, pits, and silos indicate the importance of surplus in buffering against risk and amassing political influence (De Boer, 1988; Wesson, 1999).

Beyond the need for subsistence, humans have had a universal appetite for sweets and fatty foods, spicy foods, and intoxicating foods such as beer and wine. Fruits, the first sweet foods, can be traced from the charred remains of seeds and pits. The archaeology of honey is traced with using the remains of hive jars, pollen, and the lipids in beeswax (Crane, 1983). Archaeologists have less information about the archaeology of cane sugar and concentrated sweets such as dates (Nesbitt, 1993), agave (Flannery, 1986), and palm syrup.

The earliest concentrated fats used by humans would have been from marrow and the fatty parts of animal carcasses. The selection of skeletal parts and pattern of breakage on animal bones from archaeological sites reflects how important this source of energy must have been, especially in cold climates (Speth, 2010). Dairying also allowed the storage of the fats in butter and cheese, and did so without killing the animal (Copley et al., 2005; Berstan et al., 2004). The archaeological record of oil seeds and fruits has been most widely studied with charred olive pits (Foxhall, 2007) but olive oil residues in ceramics have also been recovered (Condamin et al., 1976).

Spices pose a particular problem for archaeologists because spices are used in small amounts and would rarely become charred and preserved. In the dry eastern desert of Egypt, spices such as pepper and coriander were identified inside Roman pots (Van der Veen, 2011). In tropical Latin America, intense sampling for the starches in the fruit case revealed the probable origin and spread of the chili pepper (Perry et al., 2007). The authors speculate that the geographic extent of maize (corn) overlaps so closely with that of chilis that the two foods appear to have been adopted as a culinary complex: a bland staple and an intensely flavored and nutritious condiment.

The origins of chocolate (in the form of spicy chocolate drinks in ancient Central America) illustrate how archaeologists have approached a rare food with special significance. Historical records show that cacao beans were important trade items and stores of wealth at the time of historic conquest in the sixteenth century (Coe and Coe, 2007). Epigraphers were able to identify a glyph associated with chocolate in Mayan script, and archaeologists working with chemists found chocolate residues in a pot bearing that glyph (Hall et al., 1990). Further glimpses of the role of chocolate came from a tomb offering of whole cacao beans (Prufer and Hurst, 2007). Chocolate residues from an even earlier period were determined to be from a beverage that had been prepared from the sweet pulp that surrounds the cacao bean in its pod, a different part of the plant than is famous today (Henderson et al., 2007). Recently, prehistoric chocolate residues were identified on distinctive ceramic jars in New Mexico, indicating the spread of a possibly ritually significant food from one broad region to another (Crown and Hurst, 2009).

Ancient wine and beer, all other issues aside, are another way that grain surpluses have been used and also another reason to make pottery containers. The association of fermented drinks with ceremonial and festive occasions is probably universal (Bray, 2002; McGovern, 1993). The containers for brewing, serving, and drinking liquids have allowed reconstruction of the scale and style of many prehistoric drinking events, even when the remains of the liquids served are faint (Mosely et al., 2005; Wright, 2004). The residues in such vessels indicate the sources of the fermented beverages, and in some cases, the flavoring and additives in them (McGovern et al., 2010).

Archaeologists posit that producing food surpluses for public feasts would have created significant pressure on hosts to intensify agricultural production. Evidence for substantial storage facilities, noted above, signals the accumulation of surplus. Participation in such large feasts strengthened the social relationships between group members and dramatized the hierarchy between host and guest (Dietler and Hayden, 2001; Hayden, 2009). In societies without money or military power, influence based on generosity would have been key political capital for early leaders. In many cases, drinking feasts are inferred in the archaeological record based on the containers involved and deposits of food remains in specific settings (Aranda et al., 2011; Bray, 2002; Wright, 2004). Archaeologists have also identified feasts centering on meat (Kelly, 2001; Ben-Schlmo et al., 2009). At the site of Durrington Walls, near Stonehenge, bone evidence for pig use was combined with data on the size and decoration of large pots (Albarella and Sergeantson, 2002) and the pork fats that had soaked into that pottery (Mukherjee et al., 2008), allowing archaeologists to reconstruct several aspects of the pork feasts. Such feasting events in the archaeological record must be distinguished from the dense remains of everyday food production and consumption. Evidence for very rapid deposition and special food items or vessels are some of the components of putative feasts. Archaeologists continue to model the economic impact of sponsoring periodic special events and compare those costs to the costs of food production for everyday consumption.

Since 2000, food archaeologists have attempted to address themes beyond those of the origins and abundance of particular foods. A new generation of research focuses on reconstruction of food production systems, cuisines, and the ecological impact of human subsistence. The huge diversity of contemporary cuisines raises the issue of discerning culturally based food choices in the archaeological record. Archaeologists can seek material markers of shared social identity from symbols or iconography on artifacts or from the organization of ritual space. Food can be approached in the same manner, as foods are produced in a social context using a complex body of scientific knowledge, technology, and belief. The flavors and aromas of the original foods are also considered as an indicator of social identity and as vehicles of memory. The coded messages in meal patterns, table manners, and food combinations are difficult to access in the archaeological record except in cases of spectacular preservation, as in the case where Mayan villagers fled from a volcanic eruption before they had washed the dishes (Sheets, 2003).

The search for social identity through the production and shared consumption of ancient foodstuffs has taken several approaches (Gremillion, 2011; Twiss, 2007). We assume that social experiences embedded in food production and consumption would have been powerful forces linking group members and ancestors, even when differences between two crops might seem mundane (Bush, 2004). When staple foods change over time or space, we assume that deep differences in daily life and in the social meaning of the foods are represented. At the most comprehensive scale, Smith (2006) sees entire agricultural landscapes in ancient India as the residue of culturally bounded food preference. Social boundaries have also been demonstrated in the archaeological record by noting the absence of an avoided or tabooed food. Careful archaeological research is required to separate a meaningful absence of a tabooed food from a case where a "missing" food was not recovered due to poor preservation or a sampling bias. A food can also decrease in prevalence when it becomes difficult or uneconomical to produce, even without changing symbolic content. In areas where pigs were taboo, the archaeological record presents a range of evidence for the efficacy and significance of the taboo (Hesse and Wapnish, 1997). Fine-grained case studies indicate cuisines that developed from application of Jewish dietary laws in fourteenth century Buda in Hungary (Daroczi-Szabo, 2004) and nineteenth century New York (Milne and Crabtree, 2001); both cases of social boundaries were maintained in tightly packed urban neighborhoods.

The archaeological record has captured the use of food to reinforce social memories where traditions of distant homelands were maintained at great cost. The perceived necessity to eat traditional foods has had a strong impact on economic decisions. In the expansion of Danish settlement to Greenland, food remains (and other artifactural remains) indicate that great effort was spent in trying to maintain a traditional European diet (Pierce, 2008). Food remains for the period following the Spanish colonization of North America and the Caribbean indicate that Spanish colonists had temporary success in bringing favored foods to the new lands, but that these supplies of imported foods could not be sustained locally. The eventual forced adoption of indigenous foods (maize, wild game) by European settlers would have been a material and symbolic break with the settler's remembered homelands (Scarry and Reitz, 1990). In sixteenth-century New Mexico, the food prepared in Spanish missions and indigenous villages reflected variable success in establishing new foods, cooking techniques, and agricultural methods. The Spanish residents in relatively elite compounds maintained their use of oven-baked wheat bread but accepted a number of local foods in addition to maize. Priests in the mission adopted more indigenous foods and relied more on maize foods cooked on a griddle (Trigg, 2004). Based on ethnographic and historical data, we assume the meanings of wheat bread for Catholic communion and maize as the representation of the indigenous maize goddess would have been important in this process.

Archaeological remains have the potential to reveal information about social practices (like eating) that may be seldom admitted or discussed. Archaeologists can measure the impact of differential access to food in societies where iconography and burial traditions suggest social status was marked. As noted, most food remains in the archaeological record represent household or community behavior, so differences in access to food based on age, gender, or status are blurred. Studies tracing the relationship between food access and social status have combined archaeological data with direct biological evidence. Rare data on individual food habits come from food items recovered in stomach contents, dental calculus, and fecal remains from latrines and privies (Reinhard and Bryant, 1992; Sobolik, 1994). Food archaeologists collaborate with biological anthropologists to estimate the food intake of individuals using the stable carbon and nitrogen isotope ecologies of food and human skeletal remains. Where preservation is favorable, the dietary intake of many individuals from one time period can be compared. Using isotope analysis, data have been gathered attesting to prehistoric differential dietary intake based on gender (Schulting and Richards, 2001), ethnic affiliation (Müldner and Richards, 2005), and elite social status (White et al., 2001). Information on the archaeology of food in early childhood comes from data on how babies were fed, based on stable isotope ratios of mother and infant skeletal remains. After the origins of agriculture and the introduction of new (to humans) foods like cow's milk and porridge, weaning was hastened, changing both social relations and the rate of population growth (Dupras et al., 2001; Schurr, 1998).

Avenues for future research

Techniques for identifying distinctive foodstuffs or constituents of foods on a molecular level have accelerated in the last ten years, and these advances are likely to continue as more samples are selected for analysis and as more baseline samples of traditional foods are obtained. Using microscopic identification of plant remains from starch grains, phytoliths, and pollen, food archaeologists will increasingly be able to identify previously under-represented or even unknown plant foods remains (Piperno, 2009). Archaeologists will be able to pick apart the stages of processing, storing, and preparing those foods in archaeological context. The study of physical wear traces on ceramics (Skibo, 1992) could also be fruitfully combined with the chemical study of food residues, but sampling has hampered this synergy so far. Microscopic and molecular techniques are in the early stages of wide application; so an important challenge is to establish standards for interpretation of cultural and dietary change based on limited samples. The most convincing reconstructions of past food use have been based on multiple samples from multiple sites (Perry *et al.*, 2007), and from combination studies where analysis of residues and microscopic remains are linked to a larger body of plant remains, animal bones, and artifacts (Evershed *et al.*, 2008; Zarillo *et al.*, 2008).

Archaeologists also seek to improve their understanding of cooking and other food processing techniques. More knowledge about food preparation would help us understand kitchen work and its physical stresses, the nutritional impact of food processing, and the sensory qualities of ancient foods. Grinding stones, ceramics, and other irregular kitchen surfaces can retain much detailed information about cooking practices (Pearsall *et al.*, 2004; Reber and Evershed, 2004). The importance of grinding has long been inferred from common finds of grinding stones and mortars (Curtis, 2001). The three material aspects of cooking (food, fuel, and the surface or container used) are all physically altered in predictable ways during cooking, but destruction from heating and the intensity of domestic activity have made cooking hard to study. Much of the burned bones archaeologists find were not burned in cooking; additionally, many of the charred plant parts recovered were not burned food but are instead the remains of burned brush or dung fuel. The smells of cooking food as well as burning fuels probably must have been important parts of the sensory environment of prehistoric settlements. The technology of controlling fermentation led to breads, beers, wines, fermented porridges, and many cultured dairy products, but archaeologists are just beginning to isolate the process in archaeological materials (Isaksson *et al.*, 2010).

Archaeologists have seldom managed to link evidence for individual foods or processing techniques to the study of cuisine in the sense that the word is used in historic and contemporary settings: the combinations of ingredients, flavours, and textures in meaningful combinations. Without this understanding, we offer only limited access to the shared social and symbolic values of those dishes. Intensive study of food remains in their archaeological context has begun to reveal food combinations such as maize and chili peppers (Perry *et al.*, 2007), or salty fermented fish sauce (Van Neer and Parker, 2007) to an early cuisine. Specific deposits such as funerary offerings have given archaeologists glimpses of special meals in almost pristine ancient contexts (Brothwell and Brothwell, 1988). New research combining molecular remains, serving vessels, and cooking facilities may be able to extend such insights to different kinds of meals and how culinary traditions changed over time. Ancient feasting and the role of feasting to maintain social bonds will continue to be a focus of study of food remains and of serving vessels in ceremonial sites. To interpret such research on direct food remains from the past, archaeologists will continue to study modern traditional food production and the traditional ecological knowledge stored in those techniques.

Practical considerations for getting started – funding, programs, archival sources, tools, data sets, internet resources, scholarships and awards, etc. (where and how?)

Food archaeology is a global initiative within the larger field of archaeology. In the US, it is linked to the discipline of anthropology and is also at home in classics and art history. Funding for all of these fields is limited and highly competitive. In some cases, researchers undertake their work as volunteers or rely on the availability of volunteer participants. In the US, funding for archaeological research in general comes from large governmental agencies such as the National Science Foundation and the National Endowment for the Humanities, from state and local governmental agencies charged with protecting cultural resources (the field of CRM or Cultural Resource Management), and from private foundations such as the Wenner-Gren Foundation and the National Geographic Society. The isotopic and molecular techniques used to complement traditional archaeology are expensive, but relatively small numbers of such samples are analyzed compared to the scope of zooarchaeology and archaeobotany in any one project. Archaeologists with samples of ancient food remains often need to go beyond their own departments and institutions to find the laboratories and instruments used for these molecular analyses. Most projects of this type are collaborations between archaeologists and chemists, botanists, geologists, and zoologists. In a few cases, food archaeologists have been funded by food trade groups and processors, notably in the support offered by the Hershey Foods Technical Center for research on early chocolate (Crown and Hurst, 2009; Hall *et al.*, 1990) and the support of vintners and brewers for work on wine and beer.

Archaeologists studying food work in museums or university departments and have advanced degrees in anthropology, archaeology, or classics. They collaborate with specialists in other fields, as noted, but within their field they also develop general backgrounds in archaeological fieldwork, the study of particular areas or regions, and the theoretical concerns of the larger fields in which they work. Research opportunities arise from new fieldwork, in collaborations with on-going research projects, and in work with museum collections. Some archaeological research on food is a standard part of archaeological analysis (e.g. the identification of animal bones from sites). Other research is the result of applying new techniques from outside archaeology, and some new collaborative methods have even changed the way that fieldwork is conducted (notably for the collection of ancient DNA). Food archaeologists also study modern and traditional food and cooking to better understand food production and the material remains that result from cooking, serving, and discard. Drawing on archival and epigraphic sources, food archaeologists connect texts about foods and even recipes to recreate ancient dishes. Here, archaeologists rely on the universal sensory qualities of foods and cooking techniques to recover some of the lost aspects of ancient menus.

The research base for the archaeology of food is huge but irreplaceably precious. The entire archaeological record contains the remains of food use and reflects food production in its structure. The act of doing archaeology by excavating sites destroys this record, so archaeologists plan field research deliberately. With each stroke of the shovel or pick, there is a single chance to make observations of the finds in place and collect appropriate samples. Archaeologists and their collaborators may need many years to study individual samples in detail. Museums, government storage facilities, and academic departments maintain critical archives of soil samples, bone samples, plant samples, and ceramics and other artifacts. Taking good care of those samples and the records associated with them has enabled recent decades of research on ancient food. Some ancient food remains are so well preserved that they are immediately recognized as they are discovered, the world's earliest noodles, for example (Lu *et al.*, 2005). Others, such as the red stains on pottery that were recognized as remains of very early wine (McGovern, 1993), were studied many years being first taken from the ground.

Decisions about sampling or destroying an item to find out more about it are carefully made. Access to samples for analysis may be restricted, since maintaining the physical integrity of artifacts is a cornerstone of museum practice. A single pottery fragment might be analyzed to determine the source for its raw materials, the techniques used to make it, the significance of its style and decoration, its use history and the foods with which it came into contact and why it was discarded. Tight coordination of specialists and their collaborators is essential in planning for such research.

Museums are physical libraries of potential new and renewed insights about food, cooking, and nutrition. Food archaeologists may maintain their own collections of modern plant and animal specimens to compare to ancient remains. They also consult herbaria collections and natural history museums to establish the biological baselines for ancient ecosystems. The starting place for information about artifacts and research records on them is the catalogs and databases maintained by most archaeology museums. Some large archaeological projects also maintain websites with detailed records about the excavations and artifacts from that location.

Neither individual museums nor individual projects can effectively link research conducted by many different teams, so several initiatives have created searchable databases of records from many different sites in one region or around the world. Two examples are the Digital Archaeological Repository, tDAR (www.tdar.org, accessed March 26, 2012) and the Alexandria Archives Open Source project (opencontext.org/projects, accessed March 26, 2012). There are also databases that organize information about food remains from many sites; see, for example, maps of plant remains in Western Asia (www.cuminum.de/archaeobotany/project.php#map, accessed on March 26, 2012), or the map of the spread of ancient maize (en.ancientmaize.com, accessed on March 26, 2012). It seems likely that information technology and the connectivity of the internet will continue changing this field before such databases fully achieve their goals. The archaeology of food has not yet become completely integrated into the traditional archaeology of soil layers and artifacts, so scholars searching for information about other sites and remains should use indexes of scientific research results in both the social sciences and the physical sciences.

Key reading

Bray, T. (2002) *The Archaeology and Politics of Food and Feasting in Early States and Empires*. New York: Kluwer Academic Publishers.

Brothwell, D. and P. Brothwell (1988) *Food in Antiquity*, expanded edition. Baltimore, MD: Johns Hopkins University Press.

Brown, T. and K. Brown (2011) *Biomolecular Archaeology*. Chicester: Wiley Blackwell.

Curtis, R. I. (2001) *Ancient Food Technology*. Leiden: Brill.

Deitler, M. and B. Hayden, eds. (2001) *Feasts: Archaeological and Ethnographic Perspectives on Food, Politics, and Power*. Washington, DC: Smithsonian Press.

Gremillion, K. J. (2011) *Ancestral Appetites: Food in Prehistory*. Cambridge: Cambridge University Press.

Pearsall, D. M. (2000) *Paleoethnobotany: A Handbook of Procedures*, 2nd edition. San Diego, CA: Academic Press.

Piperno, D. (2009) *Phytoliths: a comprehensive guide for archaeologists and paleoecologists*. Lanham, MD: Altamira Press.

Reitz, E. J. and E. Wing (2008) *Zooarchaeology*, 2nd edition. Cambridge Archaeology Manual. New York: Cambridge University Press.

Samuel, D. (1996) "Approaches to the Archaeology of Food." *Petits Propos Culinaires* 54: 12–21.

Torrence, R. and H. Barton, eds. (2006) *Ancient Starch Research*. Walnut Creek, CA: Left Coast Press.

VanderWarker, A. M. and T. M. Peres, eds. (2010) *Integrating Zooarchaeology and Paleoethnobotany: A Consideration of Issues, Methods, and Cases*. New York: Springer Verlag.

Bibliography

Albarella, U. and D. Sergeantson (2002) "A passion for pork; meat consumption at the British Late Neolithic site of Durrington Walls." In *Consuming Passions and Patterns of Consumption*. Preston Miracle and Nicky Milner eds., pp. 33–49. Cambridge: McDonald Institute for Archaeological Research.

Aranda, G. J., S. Montón-Subias, and M. Sánchez, eds. (2011) *Guess Who's Coming To Dinner: Feasting Rituals in the Prehistoric Societies of Europe and the Near East*. Oxford: Oxbow Books.

Behre, K.-E. (2008) "Collected seeds and fruits from herbs as prehistoric food." *Vegetation History and Archaeobotany* 17: 65–73.

Ben-Shlomo, D., A. C. Hill, and Y. Garfinkel (2009) *Feasting between the Revolutions: Evidence from Chalcolithic Tel Tsaf, Israel*. Journal of Mediterranian Archaeology 22: 139–50.

Berstan, R., S. N. Dudd, M. S. Copley, E. D. Morgan, A. Quye, and R. P. Evershed (2004) "Characterisation of 'bog butter' using a combination of molecular and isotopic techniques." *Analyst* 129: 270–75.

Bray, T., ed. (2002) *The Archaeology and Politics of Food and Feasting in Early States and Empires*. New York: Kluwer Academic Publishers.

Brothwell, D. and P. Brothwell (1988) *Food in Antiquity*, expanded edition. Baltimore, MD: Johns Hopkins University Press.

Brown, T. and K. Brown (2011) *Biomolecular Archaeology*. Chicester: Wiley Blackwell.

Bush, L. L. (2004) *Boundary Conditions: Macrobotanical Remains and the Oliver Phase of Central Indiana, A.D. 1200–1450*. Tuscaloosa: Alabama University Press.

Coe, S. and M. Coe (2007) *The True History of Chocolate*, 2nd edition. London: Thames and Hudson.

Condamin, J., F. Fromenti, M. O. Metais, M. Michel and P. Blond (1976) "The application of gas chromatography to the tracing of oil in ancient amphorae." *Archaeometry* 18: 195–201.

Copley, M. S., R. Berstan, S. N. Dudd, S. Aillaud, A. J. Mukherjee, V. Straker, S. Payne, and R. P. Evershed (2005) "Processing of milk products in pottery vessels through British prehistory." *Antiquity* 79: 895–908.

Cowan, C. W. and P. J. Watson (2006) *The Origins of Agriculture: An International Perspective*, 2nd edition. Tuscaloosa: University of Alabama Press.

Crane, E. (1983) *The Archaeology of Beekeeping*. Ithaca, NY: Cornell University Press.

Crown, P. and W. Jeffery Hurst (2009) "Evidence of cacao use in the Prehispanic American Southwest." *Proceedings of the National Academy of Sciences* 106: 2110–13.

Curtis, R. I. (2001) *Ancient Food Technology*. Leiden: Brill.

Daroczi-Szabo, L. (2004). "Állatcsontok a Teleki Palota törökkori gödréből [Animal remains from the Turkish Era Well of the Teleki Palace]. *Budapest Regisegei* XXXVIII: 159-160.

De Boer, W. R. (1988) "Subterranean storage and the organization of surplus: the view from eastern North America." *Southeastern Archaeology* 7: 1–20.

De France, S., W. F. Keegan, and L. A. Newsome (1996) "The archaeobotanical, bone isotope, and zooarchaeological records from Caribbean Sites in comparative perspective." In *Case Studies in Environmental Archaeology*. E. J. Reitz, L. A. Newsome, and S. J. Scudder eds., pp. 289–304. New York: Plenum.

Dupras, T., H. P. Schwarcz, and S. I. Fairgrieve (2001) "Infant feeding and weaning practices in Roman Egypt." *American Journal of Physical Anthropology* 115: 204–12.

Elbaum, R., C. Melamed-Bessudo, E. Boaretto, E. Galili, S. Lev-Yadun, A. A. Levy, and S. Weiner (2006) "Ancient olive DNA in pits: preservation, amplification and sequence analysis." *Journal of Archaeological Science* 33: 77–88.

Evershed, R., S. Payne, A. G. Sherratt, M. S. Copley, J. Coolidge, D. Urem-Kotsu, K. Kotsakis, M. Ozdogan, A. E. Ozdogan, O. Nieuwenhuyse, P. M. M. G. Akkermans, D. Bailey, R.-R. Andeescu, S. Campbell, S. Farid, I. Hodder, N. Yalman, M. Ozbasaran, E. Bıcakcı, Y. Garfinkel, T. Levy, and M. M. Burton (2008) "Earliest date for milk use in the Near East and southeastern Europe linked to cattle herding." *Nature* 455: 528–31.

Flannery, K. V. (1986) *Guilá Naquitz: Archaic Foraging and Early agriculture in Oaxaca, Mexico*. New York: Academic Press.

Foxhall, L. (2007) *Olive Cultivation in Ancient Greece: Seeking the Ancient Economy*. Oxford: Oxford University Press.

Gong, Y., Y. Yang, D. K. Ferguson, D. Tao, W. Li, C. Wang, E. Lü, and H. Jiang (2011) "Investigation of ancient noodles, cakes, and millet at the Subeixi Site, Xinjiang, China." *Journal of Archaeological Science* 38: 470–79.

Gremillion, K. J. (2011) *Ancestral Appetites: Food in Prehistory*. Cambridge: Cambridge University Press.

Hall, Grant D., S. M. Tarka, Jr., W. J. Hurst, D. Stuart, and R. E. W. Adams (1990) "Cacao residues in ancient Maya vessels from Rio Azul, Guatemala." *American Antiquity* 55: 138–43.

Hayden, B. (2009) "The proof is in the pudding: feasting and the origins of domestication." *Current Anthropology* 50: 597–601.

Henderson, J. S., R. A. Joyce, G. R. Hall, W. J. Hurst, and P. E. McGovern (2007) "Chemical and archaeological evidence for the earliest cacao beverages." *Proceedings of the National Academy of Sciences* 104: 18937–40.

Henry, A. G., A. S. Brooks, and D. R. Piperno (2011) "Microfossils in calculus demonstrate consumption of plants and cooked foods in Neanderthal diets (Shanidar III, Iraq; Spy I and II, Belgium)." *Proceedings of the National Academy of Science* 108: 486–91.

Hesse, B. and P. Wapnish (1997) "Can Pig Remains Be Used for Ethnic Diagnosis in the Ancient Near East?" In *Archaeology of Israel: Constructing the Past, Interpreting the Present*. N. Silberman and D. B. Small eds., pp. 238–70, Sheffield: Sheffield Academic Press.

Isaksson, S., C. Karlsson, and T. Eriksson (2010) "Ergosterol (5, 7, 22-ergostatrien-3β-ol) as a potential biomarker for alcohol fermentation in lipid residues from prehistoric pottery." *Journal of Archaeological Science* 37: 3263–68.

Jones, M. (2007) *Feast: Why Humans Share Food*. Oxford: Oxford University Press.

Kelly, L. (2001) "A case of ritual feasting at the Cahokia site." In *Feasts: Archaeological and Ethnographic Perspectives on Food, Politics, and Power*. M. Dietler and B. Hayden, eds., pp. 334–67. Washington, DC: Smithsonian Press.

Kuipers, R. S., M. F. Luxwolda, D.A. Dijck-Brouwer, S. B. Eaton, M. A. Crawford, L. Courdain, and F. A. Muskeit (2010) "Estimated macronutrient and fatty acid intakes from an East African Paleolithic diet." *British Journal of Nutrition* 104: 1666–87.

Kuzmin, Y. V. (2006) "Chronology of the earliest pottery in East Asia: progress and pitfalls." *Antiquity* 80: 362–71.

Li, X., D. L. Lister, H. Li, Y. Xua, Y. Cui, M. A. Bower, M. K. Jones, and H. Zhou (2011) "Ancient DNA analysis of desiccated wheat grains excavated from a Bronze Age cemetery in Xinjiang." *Journal of Archaeological Science* 38: 115–19.

Lu, H., X. Yang, M. Ye, K.-B. Liu, Z. Xia, X. Ren, L. Cai, N. Wu, T.-S. Liu (2005) "Millet noodles in Late Neolithic China." *Nature* 437: 467–68.

McGovern, P. (2003) *Ancient Wine: The Search for the Origins of Viniculture*. Princeton, NJ: Princeton University Press.

McGovern, P., M. Christofidou-Solomidou, W. Wang, F. Dukes, T. Davidson, and W. S. El-Deiry (2010) "Anticancer activity of botanical compounds in ancient fermented beverages." *International Journal of Oncology* 37: 5–21.

Miller, N. F. (2006) "Origins of plant cultivation in the Near East." In *The Origins of Agriculture, an International Perspective*, 2nd edition. C. W. Cowan and P. J. Watson, eds., pp. 39–58, Washington, DC: Smithsonian Institution.

Milne, C. and P. J. Crabtree (2001) "Prostitutes, a Rabbi, and a Carpenter—Dinner at the Five Points in the 1830s." *Historical Archaeology* 35: 31–48.

Mosely, M. E., D. J. Nash, P. R. Williams, S. D. deFrance, A. Miranda, and M. Ruales (2005) "Burning down the brewery: establishing and evacuating an ancient imperial colony at Cerro Baul, Peru." *Proceedings of the National Academy of Sciences* 102: 17264–71.

Mukherjee, A. J., M. S. Copley, R. Berstan, K. A. Clark and R. P. Evershed (2005) "Interpretation of $\delta^{13}C$ values of fatty acids in relation to animal husbandry, food processing and consumption in prehistory." In *The Zooarchaeology of Fats, Oils, Milk and Dairying*. J. Mulville and A. K. Outram eds., pp. 77–93, Oxford: Oxbow.

Mukherjee, A. J., A. M. Gibson, and R. P. Evershed (2008). "Trends in pig product processing at British Neolithic Grooved Ware sites traced through organic residues in potsherds." *Journal of Archaeological Science* 35: 2059–73.

Müldner, G. and M. P. Richards (2005) "Fast or feast: reconstructing diet in later medieval England by stable isotope analysis." *Journal of Archaeological Science* 32: 39–48.

Nesbitt, M. (1993) "Archaeobotanical evidence for early Dilmun diet at Saar, Bahrain." *Arabian Archaeology and Epigraphy* 1993 4: 20–47.

Pearsall, D. M. (2009) "Investigating the transition to agriculture." *Current Anthropology* 50(5): 609–13.

Pearsall, D. M., K. Chandler-Ezell, and J. A. Zeidler (2004) "Maize in ancient Ecuador: results of residue analysis of stone tools from the Real Alto site." *Journal of Archaeological Science* 31: 423–42.

Perry, L., R. Dickau, S. Zarrillo, I. Holst, D. M. Pearsall, D. R. Piperno, M. J. Berman, R. G. Cooke, K. Rademaker, A. J. Ranere, J. S. Raymond, D. H. Sandweiss, F. Scaramelli, K. Tarble, and J. A. Zeidler (2007) "Starch Fossils and the Domestication and Dispersal of Chili Peppers (*Capsicum spp.* L.) in the Americas." *Science* 315: 986–88.

Pierce, E. (2008) "Dinner at the edge of the world: Why the Greenland Norse tried to keep a European diet in an unforgiving landscape." In *Food and Drink in Archaeology I.* Sera Baker, Martyn Allen, Sarah Middle and Kristopher Poole, eds., Totnes: Prospect Books.

Piperno, D. R. (2009) "Identifying crop plants with phytoliths (and starch grains) in Central and South America: A review and an update of the evidence." *Quaternary International* 193: 146–59.

Price, T. D. and O. Bar-Yosef (2011) "The origins of agriculture: new data, new ideas." *Current Anthropology*, 52 (Supplement): S163–S174.

Prufer, K. and W. J. Hurst (2007) "Chocolate in the underworld space of death: Cacao seeds from an early Classic mortuary cave." *Ethnohistory* 54: 273–301.

Reber, E. A. and R.P. Evershed (2004) "How did Mississippians prepare maize? The application of compound specific carbon isotopic analysis to absorbed pottery residues from several Mississippi Valley sites." *Archaeometry* 46: 19–33.

Reinhard, K. J. and V. M. Bryant, Jr. (1992) "Coprolite Analysis: A Biological Perspective on Archaeology." *Papers in Natural Resources*, University of Nebraska. DigitalCommons@University of Nebraska – Lincoln: digitalcommons.unl.edu/natrespapers/46 (accessed on March 26, 2012).

Scarry, C. M. and E. J. Reitz (1990) "Herbs, Fish, Scum, and Vermin: Subsistence Strategies in Sixteenth Century Spanish Florida." In *Columbian Consequences. Volume II: Archaeological and Historical Perspectives on the Spanish Borderlands East.* D. H. Thomas ed., pp. 343–54. Washington, DC: Smithsonian.

Schoeninger, M. J. (2009) "Stable isotope evidence for the adoption of maize agriculture." *Current Anthropology* 50: 633–40.

Schulting, R. J. and M. P. Richards (2001) "Dating women and becoming farmers: new paleodietary and AMS dating evidence from the Breton Mesolithic cemeteries of Te'viec and Hoedic." *Journal of Anthropological Archaeology* 20: 314–44.

Schurr, M. R. (1998) "Using stable nitrogen-isotopes to study weaning behavior in past populations." *World Archaeology* 30: 327–42.

Sheets, P. (2003) "Uncommonly good food among commoners: growing and consuming food in ancient Ceren." *Expedition* 45: 17–21.

Skibo, J. (1992) *Pottery Function: A Use-Alteration Perspective.* New York: Plenum.

Smith, M. (2006) "The archaeology of food preference." *American Anthropologist* 108: 480–93.

Sobolik, K. D. (1994) "Paleonutrition of the Lower Pecos region of the Chihuahuan Desert." In *Paleonutrition: the Diet and Health of Prehistoric Americans.* K. D. Sobolik, ed., pp. 247–64, Carbondale, IL: Southern Illinois University Press.

Speth, J. D. (2010) *The Paleoanthropology and Archaeology of Big-game Hunting: Protein, Fat, or Politics?* New York: Springer.

Stahl, A. B. (1984) "Hominid dietary selection before fire." *Current Anthropology* 25: 151–68.

Stanford, C. B. and H. T. Bunn, eds. (2001) *Meat Eating and Human Evolution.* London: Oxford University Press.

Torrence, R. and H. Barton, eds. (2006) *Ancient Starch Research.* Walnut Creek, CA: Left Coast Press.

Trigg, H. (2004) "Food Choice and Social Identity in Early Colonial New Mexico." *Journal of the Southwest* 46: 223–52.

Twiss, K., ed. (2007) *The Archaeology of Food and Identity.* Carbondale, IL: Center for Archaeological Investigations, Southern Illinois University Carbondale, Occasional Paper no. 34.

Valamoti, S.-M. (2002) "Investigating the prehistoric bread of northern Greece: the archaeobotanical evidence for the Neolithic and the Bronze Age." *Civilisations* 49: 49–66.

Van der Veen, M. (2011) *Consumption, Trade, and Innovation: Exploring the Botanical Remains from the Roman and Islamic Ports at Quseir al-Qadim, Egypt.* Frankfurt: Africa Magna Verlag.

VanDerwarker, A. M. and T. M. Peres, eds. (2010) *Integrating Zooarchaeology and Paleoethnobotany: A Consideration of Issues, Methods, and Cases.* New York: Springer Verlag.

Van Neer, W. and S. T. Parker (2007) "First archaeozoological evidence for *haimation*, the 'invisible' *garum*." *Journal of Archaeological Science* 35: 1821–27.

Weiss, E. and Zohary, D. (2011) "The Neolithic Southwest Asian founder crops: their biology and archaeobotany." *Current Anthropology* 52 (suppl. 4): S237–54.

Wesson, C. B. (1999) "Chiefly Power and Food Storage in Southeastern North America." *World Archaeology* 31: 145–64.

White, C. D., D. M. Pendergast, F. J. Longstaffe, and K. R. Law (2001) "Social complexity and food systems at Altun Ha, Belize: the isotopic evidence." *Latin American Antiquity* 12: 371–93.

Willcox, G. (2002) "Charred plant remains from a 10th millenium B.P. kitchen at Jerf el Ahmar (Syria)." *Vegetation History and Archaeobotany* 11: 55–60.

Wrangham, R. (2009) *Catching Fire: How Cooking Made Us Human.* New York: Basic Books.

Wright, J. C., ed. (2004) *The Mycenaean Feast.* Athens: American School of Classical Studies.

Zarrillo, S., D. M. Pearsall, J. S. Raymond, M. A. Tisdale, and D. J. Quon (2008) "Directly dated starch residues document early formative maize (*Zea mays* L.) in tropical Ecuador." *Proceedings of the National Academy of Science* 105: 5006–11.

Zeder, M. (2006) "Central Questions in the Domestication of Plants and Animals." *Evolutionary Anthropology* 15: 107–17.

Humanities

8

Journalism

Helen Rosner and Amanda Hesser

Food journalism has gone through more changes in the past decade than it has in the past century. This chapter offers a brief history and evolution of journalism, as well as an exploration of the current forms, offline and online, of food journalism.

Introduction: What is food journalism?

For the most part, the phrase "food journalism" is interchangeable with "food writing." It's a tremendously diverse category of nonfiction that is only minimally defined by genre or format; instead, it applies to any sort of writing that deals with matters of food, cooking, food production, food culture, and the dozens of nooks and crannies in those categories. It can be historical, investigative, instructional, critical, inspirational, memoir driven, humorous, or all of the above. It's a running joke among food writers that any piece of journalism can be made into food writing simply by adding a sandwich. That's not far from the truth, particularly in contemporary food writing, where the food itself is often just a launching point for a broader story. Writes Eric LeMay in *Alimentum* (Winter 2011), good food writing "restores to food everything else, everything more, that food is about, which is just about everything."

Still, a large portion of the food writing canon is what old-schoolers refer to as "service journalism": stories with a clear, instructive takeaway, whether it's a recipe, a restaurant recommendation, or rules to keep in mind while you're grocery shopping or reheating left-overs. This sort of goal-oriented writing still makes up a large and important part of the category, as does the thoughtful recipe writing that makes up the core of most newspaper and magazine food sections. But the food has exploded into other areas of journalism in the last decades. Anthony Bourdain's scandalous back-of-the-house memoir *Kitchen Confidential* ushered us into the contemporary era of the rock-star chef, launching simultaneously both a hundred chefs' imitator book proposals, and a cottage industry of glossy, celebrity-style profiles of food industry types. With the publication of *The Omnivore's Dilemma* (2006) Michael Pollan almost single-handedly invented the category political food writing. Dining blogs like Grub Street (www.grubstreet.com) and Eater (www.eater.com) split their time between publishing food-related gossip, satire, and cultural criticism, and hard-news reportage about restaurants and chefs.

But even with the shifting boundaries of food journalism, some of the topic's defining elements remain the same. Journalism is not, by its very nature, an academic pursuit; it's writing that's done for a lay reader. As with conventional journalism, what all good food writing has in common is a combination of honest reporting, insightful analysis, and a commitment to the authenticity and integrity of the subject. But as a form of communication, food writing also has an obligation to entertain: we can't very well convey our message unless we can hang on to your attention until the point gets across. As Molly O'Neill says in her introduction to *American Food Writing* (2007), "A good piece of food writing is never just about the food; it is, among other things, about place and time, desire and satiety, the longing for home and the lure of the wide world." In other words, good food writing isn't something unique and special; it's merely good writing that just so happens to be about food.

Historical background of food scholarship in food journalism and major theoretical approaches in use

Before 1957, there was a lot of writing about food—crop levels, food transport and distribution—and plenty of recipe writing, but other than Brillat Savarin and a few gourmands with a pen, there was very little about the pleasures of eating and dining. In 1859, *The New York Times* published what is generally considered to be the paper's first restaurant review. Called "How We Dine" (read the full text at tinyurl.com/howwedine, accessed on April 11, 2012), and bylined to "The Strong-Minded Reporter of the Times," it's a witty and comprehensive rundown of the state of New York restaurants in the mid-nineteenth century, from Champagne at Delmonico's down through a lunch-counter sandwich.

New York was home to some of the first leading food writers and journalists, including Clementine Paddleford and James Beard, but for the first few decades of the twentieth century, most food writing was service journalism, led by an army of home economists, who did very little to improve how Americans ate.

In the late 1950s, *The New York Times* hired Craig Claiborne, a Southerner who'd studied cooking in Europe. Claiborne made cooking stylish and aspirational and soon New Yorkers—and home cooks around the country—were making goulash and crêpes for their dinner parties. In 1961, the same year *Mastering the Art of French Cooking* was published, Claiborne released *The New York Times Cookbook*. Both became bestsellers.

Then the internet happened

In the post-Craig Claiborne world, the tone and inquisitiveness of food journalism has stayed more or less the same, but the advent of the internet led to two drastic changes. First, with increased interest in blogs and websites dovetailing with the dawn of the golden age of food TV and cooking shows, "food" exploded as a topic worthy of popular interest. Suddenly the audience for writing about food, cooking, and eating was tremendous, and so the demand for writing on the subject became tremendous as well.

Second, much of that writing now found its home online. Blogs and online publications provided a seeming infinity of new outlets for food writing, amateur and professional alike, but the gradual shift in reader attention towards the internet led to something of a crisis for traditional print media. Declining print readership means fewer ad pages which means fewer editorial pages, and editorial staffs are increasingly assigning stories in-house to keep the budget down even more. (Magazine staffers generally don't get paid when they're writing for their own title.) As a result, a food writer selling a story to a print publication—already a tough enough task in boom times—has become even harder. But for every print magazine that slashes its well (or shutters entirely), a dozen new professional blogs open their doors to pitches and submissions, including online counterparts to print publications.

A partial taxonomy of food journalism

As we've mentioned, food journalism includes virtually every type of conventional nonfiction writing, as long as it concerns itself largely with a culinary matter. Any attempt to break down the entire canon into a comprehensive taxonomy is laughable; there's always something new coming up in the journalistic world, whether in style or subject, and that's a good thing. But the field can nevertheless be divided into some broad categories that, with a little wiggling, can fit most types of food writing. We've included examples for each—stories and books that define their genres, were particularly influential, or just happen to be our favorites.

Food memoir

My Life in France (2006) by Julia Child and Alex Prud'homme

Published posthumously, Julia Child's episodic account of her culinary awakening while living in Paris, Marseilles, and Provence is both the story behind *Mastering the Art of French Cooking* and a vivacious encapsulation of Julia's personality.

Gastronomical Me by M. F. K. Fisher

M. F. K. Fisher wrote one of the first books that ties together emotion and food. She recounts her marriages and her life in France and Switzerland, but it's really about how she ate through those years.

Kitchen Confidential (2001) by Anthony Bourdain

The first candid behind-the-scenes look at the life of a restaurant chef—the potheads, the aging leftovers, the misbehavior, and the dangers of cooking.

Blood, Bones, and Butter (2010) by Gabrielle Hamilton

It took nearly ten years for a culinary memoir to hit with remotely the same impact as *Kitchen Confidential*. Hamilton, a New York chef, writes honestly and poetically about the path that led her from an unconventional rural childhood to her New York City restaurant. It's as shocking and candid as Bourdain's book, but on a much more intimate, personal scale. It's not about blowing the lid off of a dark corner of the industry; instead, it's about humanizing the sort of chef who's usually written about only in hagiographic terms.

Investigative journalism and political activism

The Jungle (1906) by Upton Sinclair

Perhaps the most important piece of modern food activism, the book's depiction of the horrific working environments and squalid conditions of Chicago's meatpacking industry led to outrageous public response, and indirectly led to the establishment of the FDA. While a work of fiction, Sinclair's details were the result of two months' undercover investigation at meatpacking plants.

Fast Food Nation (2001) by Eric Schlosser

Arguably the instigator of the recent renaissance of investigative food journalism, Schlosser's indictment of the fast food industry attacks from all angles, from ingredient sourcing and processing to the social effects of marketing and advertising.

Supersize Me (film) (2004) by Morgan Spurlock

This documentary film has a simple premise: Spurlock eats nothing but McDonald's food for 30 days straight, and chronicles the disastrous health results. The film was so popular that it led to McDonald's retiring the "super-size" option from their value meal menus.

The Omnivore's Dilemma (2006) by Michael Pollan

Exactly a century after *The Jungle* came perhaps the second-most influential book about food politics in America. Pollan's magnum opus is structured as investigations of single meals in a variety of styles: Fast food, organic, and foraged.

Four Fish (2010) by Paul Greenberg

New York Times contributor Greenberg takes stock of the state of global fisheries through the lens of the four most popular varieties—tuna, salmon, cod, and bass—and makes the case that we should apply the same attitude of sustainability and ethics to seafood that we do to land animals.

Tomatoland (2011) by Barry Estabrook

Based on his story "The Price of Tomatoes," which ran in 2003 in *Gourmet* magazine, Estabrook traces the history of the tomato, from its Peruvian oranges to the current tasteless GMO spheres sold in midwinter, in the course revealing the plants' extraordinary pesticide load, and the tomato industry's reliance on exploitative immigrant labor.

Recipe and technique writing

"The Minimalist" series by Mark Bittman

Bittman's long-running column in *The New York Times* began in 1997 and concluded in 2011. Its simple, straightforward take on home cooking cemented Bittman as the expert on all things having to do with the home kitchen, and led to various book and television projects. Read the Minimalist archive at tinyurl.com/nytminimalist (accessed on April 11, 2012).

America's test kitchen

Christopher Kimball's perfection-driven approach to cooking aims to find flawless, perfectly repeatable recipes, and in doing so lets readers in on the copious testing that requires. With extended recipe headnotes detailing trial-and-error testing processes, detailed step-by-step instructions for even the simplest dishes, and a television, book, and magazine mini-empire, it's an essential voice in recipes.

Smitten Kitchen by Deb Perelman

In the pantheon of cooking blogs, Perelman's Smitten Kitchen (www.smittenkitchen.com) stands out as an exemplar of the form: Intimate but authoritative, peppered with personal anecdotes, lushly photographed, and beautifully designed. Smitten Kitchen largely features recipes from other sources, like cookbooks and magazines, but Perelman's detailed accounts of her cooking process and occasional recipe tweaks make the content wholly original.

Profile writing

"Don't Mention It" by Calvin Trillin, the *New Yorker*, April 15, 2001

Trillin's portrait of idiosyncratic New York chef/restauranteur Kenny Shopsin is intimate but universal, an endearing profile of a man who intentionally chooses to be anything but endearing. Trillin's long personal history with Shopsin is an essential part of the story.

Heat (2006) by Bill Buford

Buford's nonfiction book, which grew out of an article assignment for the *New Yorker*, models itself as a profile-cum-biography of celebrity chef Mario Batali: His childhood, his college years, and his peripatetic culinary training through New Jersey, London, Italy, and finally New York. But to fully understand what went into the making of the man, Buford follows in his footsteps, apprenticing with some of the same cooks and butchers Batali did, as well as working for a time at Batali's New York restaurant, Babbo.

Science

Cooking for Geeks (blog and book) by Jeff Potter

Potter celebrates the science of cooking in a wide-ranging blog (and now book), that explains how to cook a turkey faster, how to hack a sous vide machine, and how to cook with your office toaster.

On Food and Cooking (1997) by Harold McGee

A staple of uncountably many kitchens, McGee's famous red-jacketed book explains everything from why egg whites congeal to why salting meat changes its cooking process. With its encyclopedic organization and approachable tone, it's an indispensable food-science reference.

Modernist Cuisine (2011) by Nathan Myhrvold

At 2,438 pages and weighing over 38 pounds, Myhrvold (a former Microsoft CTO) has written a mega-cookbook that is quite possibly the largest ever published. The result of years of practical testing in a cooking laboratory decked out with tools ranging from a weapons-grade laser to a

50-G ultracentrifuge, the six-volume book covers scientific approaches to cooking and treating virtually all foods, along with recipes written in a scientific style.

History

Gastronomica and Alimentum

Academic quarterly *Gastronomica* (published by the University of California) and literary journal *Alimentum* take different approaches to food writing, but both distinguish themselves with top-notch historical writing, whether investigative or memoiristic.

The Food of a Younger Land (2009) by Mark Kurlansky

Kurlansky's research for a separate project led to his accidental discovery in the Library of Congress of a trove of American food writing from the 1920s and 1930s, essays by writers amateur and professional that were assigned as part of President Roosevelt's WPA project, with the goal of publishing a book called *America Eats*. That book never came to be, but Kurlansky curated and edited some of the strangest and most wonderful of its essays here, covering topics from sugaring in Vermont to rattlesnake cookery in Florida.

The Oxford Companion to Food (1999) by Alan Davidson

Alan Davidson spent 20 years researching and defining the major terms, ingredients, and people involved in the history of food. The book is arranged alphabetically with mostly short entries on topics from Isabella Beeton to vareniki.

The Oxford Encyclopedia of Food and Drink in America (2004) by Andrew F. Smith

Eight hundred brief capsules on the important people and events in American food history.

The Oxford Companion to American Food and Drink (2009) by Andrew F. Smith

A compendium, much like Davidson's, but focused on American foodstuffs, industry figures, and regional specialties—from Clarence Birdseye to whoopie pies.

Travel and cultural preservation

Gravy

The quarterly "foodletter" of the Southern Foodways Alliance is an ongoing journalistic arm of the alliance's goal of preserving and chronicling the food of the American South; it features stories from prominent names in contemporary food writing.

Saveur

This glossy food magazine covers the world of food through a lens of travel and culture; you're more likely to find a recipe for Emirati sweet potato halvah in its pages than a simple weeknight baked chicken.

Far Flung and Well Fed (2009) by R. W. Apple

New York Times writer Apple's decades-deep archive of food writing sets the standard for culinary travel journalism; whether eating street food in Bangkok or pies in the American southeast, his stories are equal part memoir and investigation. His later food essays are collected in this posthumously released anthology.

Criticism

"Le Cirque" by Ruth Reichl in *The New York Times* (1993)

Possibly the single most famous piece of contemporary restaurant criticism, then-*Times* critic Reichl offers a simultaneous critique of high-end New York restaurant Le Cirque and of the profession of food criticism itself: She visits the restaurant twice, once disguised as a clueless diner, and once as a regal (and un-anonymous) *Times* reporter. The first visit is atrocious, the later one, sublime, and a conversation about critical ethics was reignited that has not yet managed to die down. Find the review at www.nyu.edu/ipk/files/docs/events/Review_-_Le_Cirque_(Reichl).pdf (accessed May 1, 2012).

Jonathan Gold, *LA Weekly*

Longtime Los Angeles writer Jonathan Gold holds the distinction of being the only journalist ever to win the Pulitzer Prize for food journalism. His reviews and stories tend to focus more on LA's ethnic and hole-in-the-wall restaurants, rather than the city's glitzy high-end dining scene.

"Just a Quiet Dinner for Two in Paris: 31 Dishes, Nine Wines, a $4000 Check" by Craig Claiborne in *The New York Times* (1975)

When *Times* dining critic Craig Claiborne bid $300 for an all-expenses-paid dinner at any restaurant of his choosing anywhere in the world, he took it to the extreme, booking a trip to Paris with his friend Pierre Franey and eating (and subsequently writing about) the meal explained in the article's title. When the story was published, outrage and shock at Claiborne's excess was so widespread as to include condemnation from the Vatican.

The Art of Eating by Ed Behr

A 25-year-old newsletter out of Vermont, edited by Edward Behr. Behr reviews cookbooks, writes thoroughgoing articles on foodstuffs like dry-aged steaks and traditional goods like Provençal cheeses.

Gossip, ephemeral news, and metamedia

Off the Menu, in *The New York Times*

Florence Fabricant's regular column "charts restaurant news and dining trends," and has since its first appearance in the paper in January 1994. Running once or twice a week, it predated the restaurant-obsessed blog scene by over a decade; it remains an essential source for dining news.

Eater and Grub Street

Owned respectively by Curbed Media and *New York Magazine*, Eater and Grub Street cover similar territory—city-specific, hyper-detailed food news—and their shared territory has fueled a restaurant gossip arms race, developing and tearing down reality-based storylines as efficiently as any celebrity tabloid.

Lucky Peach

An "indie" food magazine created by chef David Chang, writer Peter Meehan, and the production company Zero Point Zero. A quarterly publication, it's published by McSweeney's.

Food blogs

The question of whether blogging counts as a type of formal journalism is a persistent one, though the ubiquity of the medium implies that the answer will soon be universally understood to be "yes." Still, the internet's ease of access—anyone with a wifi connection can start a blog and publish whatever she likes—means that the parameters of what counts as journalism are being questioned.

Traditionally, journalism has been defined as writing done for a publication, assigned and overseen by an editor whose job it was to incorporate a single piece of journalism together with other pieces to create a cohesive editorial whole: A newspaper, magazine, or journal. On the part of the reader, this process implied a degree of editorial oversight: Fact-checking, vetting of sources, and various additional codes of journalistic integrity. Many bloggers, both hobbyist and professional, maintain impeccable journalistic standards; however, the internet is a vast place and as of this writing, there aren't any official guidelines for independent online writers. (That's not to say efforts haven't been made: a Food Blogger's Code of Ethics exists at foodethics.wordpress. com, but it's not a formal association.)

In the early days of blogging, there was a widely held view that a person writing online wasn't to be taken as seriously as a journalist writing for print. This bias still exists today, though organizations like the James Beard Foundation have acknowledged the equality of online writing by, as of 2010, making their annual journalism awards medium-blind.

Some food blogs are hobbies, others are undertaken as full-time professional endeavors. For the most part online food writing can be broken down into several general categories:

- Online counterparts to print publications. Virtually every magazine and newspaper has a corresponding website; almost universally, these sites republish print content, and most of them contain additional blogs or verticals for web-exclusive stories and recipes.
- Online-only food publications. Multi-channeled online food magazines with full editorial mastheads have become an essential part of the online food-writing landscape. Sites like FOOD52 and Chow focus on recipes and techniques with great editorial depth; multi-city megasites like Eater and Grub Street provide hourly updates on restaurant news, as well as long-view assessments of the dining world.
- Professional personal blogs. Combining recipes with personal narratives and lifestyle inspiration, the most successful of these sites—often written by just one person, often begun as a hobby and becoming professional endeavors thanks to traffic-driven ad revenue (and not infrequently a book deal)—have a strong aesthetic point of view: The design, the style, and the typefaces on the page all combine with the writing and recipes to craft a complete and inviting world of which readers want to be a part.

Avenues for future research

Perhaps more than any other category of journalism, the engine of food writing is personal experience. But like any other form of journalism, it relies on an honest narrator. Even in criticism or opinion writing, there's an expectation of accuracy, and a prioritization of authenticity. This applies regardless of medium, and the future of food journalism will be the application of these principles to new media: The web and social media.

Individual food blogs

The self-contained, self-financing blog seems to be the wave of the future. The most succesful personal blogs are turning into fully fledged lifestyle brands: Ree Drummond, proprietor of Pioneer Woman, started as a food blog and has parlayed her avid readership into a TV deal, a bestselling memoir, and a children's book; many other food blogs seem poised to become full lifestyle brands supported by advertising revenue. Still, the internet is so young a medium with such a low barrier to entry that there's a large amount of content redundancy, and the types of sites that will sustain and thrive still remain to be seen.

Aggregation blogs

As with any category, websites dedicated to aggregation are flourishing, diverting traffic and revenue from sources of original content. The revenue model for original content online is still worrisome, but growing trends in social media usage point to declining importance of sites that curate others' content without providing their own unique stories or angles.

Print-counterpart blogs

The morphing form (and changing relevance) of the newspaper food section and of food magazines is the driving force behind the greatest amount of change. Print circulation might be going down, but the declining readership is more than made up for by an increase in online numbers. There's increasing demand at these outlets for web-specific content, as well as print content designed to translate well for the web.

Tablets and apps

Tablets, mobile devices, apps, and the media-inclusive nature of the internet are giving rise to tremendous demand for forms of journalism that go beyond the limitations of the written word: Videojournalism, photojournalism, audio journalism, and other interactive components are flourishing, as the reader comes to expect more interaction than the passive experience of simply reading. Just as cookbooks have been largely replaced by online recipes, multimedia recipes (with step-by-step photo or video components) seem poised to replace the static online recipe.

Social media

Facebook, Twitter, and other social media platforms have changed the way that we interact with information, whether we're on the creation side or the consumption side. Publications and journalists increasingly use social media as an equal partner to long-form writing in terms of disseminating ideas and stories both big and small; taken as a whole, a social media stream can be considered its own work. In 2010, the James Beard Foundation awarded their humor award to anonymous Twitter parodist Ruth Bourdain, based entirely on the whole of her tweets.

Practical considerations for getting started—funding, programs, archival sources, tools, data sets, internet resources, scholarships and awards, etc. (where and how?)

In an open Q&A session held on his Facebook page in March 2011, *LA Weekly* critic Jonathan Gold answered a reader's question about how to break into food writing:

> The best food writers I know have all gotten into it by accident. Ruth Reichl was studying to be an art historian. Colman Andrews edited a jazz magazine. Robert Sietsema played bass in a no-wave band. Jeff Steingarten was a lawyer. Alan Richman wrote about sports. I wrote about opera and new music. If you are meant to do this thing, this thing [kind] of finds you. That being said: read widely, eat widely, ask lots of questions, and be humble before the subject, because if you don't it will reach out and crush you like a bug. Also, it helps if you find a tiny corner of the food universe to call your own – become the go-to person on salsify, beefalo or Amish vegetable cookery.
>
> *(For the entire Q&A, which is largely about Los Angeles dining, visit tinyurl.com/jonathangold, accessed on April 11, 2012)*

There doesn't seem likely to be a better roadmap to becoming a successful food journalist than the one outlined in this paragraph: Be interested in the whole world, not just food. Read, eat, find stories, and tell them well. To this we would only add one thing: Learn how to cook, if you don't know already, and cook (and shop for groceries) regularly, whether or not you write about cooking. An intimate, practical understanding of the economics and science behind eating (which is what shopping and cooking amounts to) will serve you invaluably no matter what aspect of the world of food you choose to cover.

Academic degrees in food journalism

While a particular graduate or undergraduate degree is in no way a prerequisite for becoming a food writer, for some people it's a helpful stepping stone to their professional career. Virtually any academic program in journalism or creative writing will help establish a foundation of writerly skills and knowledge for the aspiring food writer; in seeking out a journalism program, pay particular attention to the depth of their criticism and cultural reporting curriculum, rather than hard news; in creative writing, look for courses in creative nonfiction, essay writing, and memoir. To go even deeper, pair writing and journalism courses with classes in sociology, anthropology, and history courses that are related to food, agriculture, gastronomy, and domesticity.

Food studies is such a young field that formal degrees in food writing are almost nonexistent; for the most part, food writing and communication is found as a sub-concentration within larger food studies programs, or as one-off courses within journalism or writing programs. Here are some of the very few programs that currently offer explicitly food-oriented degrees with a focus on writing.

PhD and terminal Masters programs

New York University Steinhardt School of Culture, Education, and Human Development: MA and PhD, Department of Nutrition, Food Studies, and Public Health

Established in 1996, the food studies program within NYU's nutrition department has the distinction of being the oldest Masters program in the United States exclusively devoted to food scholarship. The MA in Food Studies program includes two areas of concentration: Food Culture, and added in 2007, Food Systems, which focuses on issues related to food production. All students in either concentration must take a course in food writing, where they write reports, articles, pamphlets, and other informational materials related to their interest in food and nutrition. As an interdisciplinary department, students may take additional elective courses in journalism and writing.

Chatham University: Master of Arts in Food Studies

Chatham's Masters program focuses on global, environmental, and gender issues related to food. Students pick two concentrations from the three available: Food Politics, Food Markets and Marketing, and Communication and Writing; within the communication and writing concentration, students study food writing, food journalism, and other aspects of journalistic ethics and practice, advertising, recipe writing, and food criticism.

Boston University: Master of Liberal Arts in Gastronomy

Founded in 1993 by Julia Child and Jacques Pepin, BU's gastronomy program places an emphasis on hands-on learning. Students can choose from four concentrations within the program: Business, Communication, Food Policy, and History and Culture. As part of the communications concentration, students analyze food and culture in print, film, photography, television, the visual arts, and digital media.

Undergraduate programs

Very few undergraduate colleges offer true majors in food writing. If you're committed to that concentration, an independent major (or a degree at a school with self-designed majors, like NYU's Gallatin School) might be what you're looking for.

The New School: Food Studies Program

Food studies undergraduate courses can be taken as part of the New School's Bachelor's Program in the Liberal Arts. Areas of study within the program include Culinary History, Food Policy, The Food Business, Food and Health, and Food and Culture. Food politics is at the heart of the program, with particular emphasis on American farming structure, food production, distribution, quality, and nutrition; coursework may be done in conjunction with journalism and writing departments. A continuing education degree is also offered.

Champlain College: Professional writing major

This college's journalism major allows for a formal concentration on food writing.

Courses not affiliated with a university

Many culinary schools and non-academic professional writing programs offer one-off courses in food writing, food memoir, and food journalism. While these classes don't result in degrees or accreditation, they can be helpful for refining your skills, exploring the medium, and making connections with notable working food writers—in larger cities, you can count on meeting successful food writers as either teachers or guest lecturers in this sort of class.

Key reading

As with all forms of writing, the more you read in the world of food, the better your writing will be, and the more readily you'll find topics to write on and publications to write for. Read everything you can: Books, magazines, newspapers, journals, blogs, tweets, Facebook pages, Tumblr accounts. Read as many of the books and articles mentioned in this chapter as possible, as they're common touchstones within the industry.

Beyond the simple dictate to read everything, these are the key readings to be aware of if food writing is your goal:

- *Best Food Writing* annuals: Da Capo Press releases an annual anthology of what their editors consider to be the year's best food writing. Drawing from newspapers, magazines, blogs, and websites, it's an invaluable resource for getting a feel for current voices and topics in the food writing community.
- Essential magazines: *Bon Appetit, Saveur, Food & Wine, Cooks Illustrated, Gastronomica, The Art of Eating*. Many non-food-specific magazines also have strong food sections: *Esquire, Garden and Gun, Sunset*, the *Atlantic*, and most city rags like *Chicago, New York*, and *LA Magazines*.
- Newspaper food sections: Whether you live in these cities or not, stay on top of what's being written in *The New York Times*, the *Washington Post*, the *Guardian*, the *Times of London*, *SF Chronicle*, the *Boston Globe*, the *LA Times*, and more.

To truly ensure you don't miss anything (and to not become overwhelmed by the stream), curation/aggregation websites like Eater and Grub Street are useful content filters. But don't read just the stories that they pick up: Be investigative and curious in your own reading.

9

The cultural history of food

Deborah Valenze

The cultural history of food rests on a venerable foundation of classic works and methodologies in the historical literature. This essay traces the development of discussions of food by the Annales school of the 1920s, British Marxist historians, anthropological studies, and studies of consumption, including discussion of the notion of a "civilizing process." While earlier work concentrated on the role of producers and common people, more recent discussion has shifted attention to elites, personal taste, and aesthetics. Methodologies surveyed include the investigation of sensibilities of consumption, disciplinary practices related to the body, medicine and science, material history, agricultural history, and the history of luxury.

Anthropologists have usually claimed pride of place in the study of food, incorporating historical analysis as one of their most valuable tools. The cultural history of food proves how the relationship can be reversed by placing the study of food and cultural change at the center of a specifically historical analysis. While food studies is intrinsically multidisciplinary, this particular form of scholarship rests on a venerable foundation of classic works and methodologies in the historical literature. The following essay focuses selectively on works within the history of Western Europe and North America, and offers no pretensions to covering food history on a global scale. Its aim is to show how a shift in focus to historical analysis brings to the center of discussion the relationship between food and historical transformations, such as the rise of market society, the development of industrial modes of production, and state formation and the extension of bureaucratic regulations. Compared to anthropology, in which historical analysis is often diachronically linked to social practices or belief systems, the cultural historian will give priority to a narrative of change over time, contextualized within definitive historical developments. Political and economic structures, institutions, and social pressures are of primary interest to the cultural historian, even while narratives remain focused on food. Not all practitioners of cultural history have been historians; in fact, the field has developed in significant, new ways owing to the contributions of anthropologists, sociologists, and historical geographers, among others. A significant overlap exists between cultural history and culinary history. But it should be noted that the cultural history of food is distinct from the study of "food cultures," which are defined according to distinct regions or ethnic groups and more narrowly confined to subjects relating to the social formations around the preparation and consumption of food. The cultural history of food can be distinguished from culinary history by its tendency to fit its subject matter into frameworks related to historical change, rather than the other way around.

As early as the 1920s, innovative European scholars pointed the way toward recognition of the importance of food within a broad history of society. Drawing from the disciplines of anthropology and sociology, their work demonstrated the now familiar principle that the quest for food, along with the determination of what form it took, was situated at the center of social activity. Moreover, archeologists added the important point that the evolution of the human diet is inextricably intertwined with the origins of agriculture, a problem bearing directly on the formulation of culture as a concept (Anderson, 2005). As Massimo Montanari has suggested, the study of food "aspires to be something more, perhaps the entire history of our civilization" (Montanari, 1994: xi).

But what makes the historical study of food "cultural"? An inclusive definition of culture takes into account "[i]nherited artifacts, goods, technical processes, ideas, habits, and values" (Malinowski, 1931, cited in Burke, 2008: 29), and this agenda directs the food historian to reflect on defining issues of cultural formation. As Anna Meigs has pointed out, a full consideration of cultural dimensions demands that we look at "not just the physiological or nutritive aspects of food, but the social meanings and functions" that develop around its production and consumption (Meigs, 1997: 102). Historical data may be gleaned from a broad array of subject areas, including art, archeology, economic activity, prevailing philosophies, political organizations, religious beliefs and rituals, science, technology, and social groups, such as families, ethnic groups, or voluntary associations. In most cases, studies have focused on circumscribed regions or localities, though this particular methodological approach is changing and global linkages are of particular interest in current scholarship.

Historical background of studies in the cultural history of food

The *Annales* school, founded in the 1920s by Jacques Le Goff and Fernand Braudel, united the study of economies, societies, and the mental frameworks (*mentalités*) belonging to particular historical periods. Braudel's magisterial treatment of Mediterranean commerce included trade in food supplies and the pursuit of maritime occupations related to the procurement of food (Braudel, 1982, 1972). Other works examined provisions within modes of production that served as the organizational basis of economic and social life. The works of Marc Bloch and Jacques Le Goff offer some of the best foundational texts in the study of medieval European society, touching frequently on questions of food consumption, including hunger and its psychological impact (Bloch, 1961; Le Goff, 1988). Students of history later gained access to volumes of translated essays from the journal (e.g., Forster and Ranum, 1979). Emphasis on the embedded nature of food, especially in relation to food security, survival, and reproduction, enabled historians to envision wholly new ways of framing historical problems.

Humanitarian and nutritional interest in food during the Second World War inspired early scholarship on the subject. In Britain, scientists as well as historians produced wide-ranging accounts of the history of British food, valuable as much for their judgments on how to examine a nation's choices as they were for their interesting sources (see, for example, Drummond and Wilbraham, 1939). Redcliffe Salaman, a physician and geneticist by training, published a remarkable history of the potato, which described itself as a social rather than a cultural history, but its coverage of the different habitats, uses, and political implications of this globally essential food made it a much broader work of scholarship. Recent treatments have not supplanted its usefulness (Salaman, 1985; Smith, 2011; Reader, 2011; Zuckerman, 1999). Political developments in postwar Europe, particularly the emergence of the welfare state, created a setting favorable to the investigation of food as a social necessity. To a certain extent, the same was true in the United States, where a democratic awareness of dietary deficiencies across social classes and the rise of government assistance generated an interest in "food habits" and history (Cummings, 1940).

Socialism and communism in Europe and Britain had a considerable impact on historical scholarship, and this, in turn, led to increased interest in the subject of food. For the influential school of British Marxist historians, the subject served as a lightning rod of instances of class conflict in the history of capitalism. Though Marxist historians had been charged with economic determinism, scholarship of this era ultimately developed a more nuanced understanding of culture as a means of understanding historical change. Social historians broadened the framework of traditional history by focusing attention on common people and by raising new questions about ordinary life, including food consumption. In a controversial essay, Eric Hobsbawm brought historical analysis to the study of the impact of an uneven distribution of wealth in what became known as the "standard of living debate" during the classic phase of British industrialization (Hobsbawm, 1957). The ensuing discussion inspired scholars in other periods and fields to interrogate diverse issues surrounding the production, distribution, and consumption of food (Dyer, 1989). E. P. Thompson's discussion of the "moral economy of the crowd" (Thompson, 1971) included attention to the rituals and symbols of protest against changing marketing practices in the trade in grain and bread. Thompson brought to light the negotiation of popular political rights to affordable food that were inscribed in English law. The eventual abandonment of the Assize of Bread consigned English consumers to the vicissitudes of free trade in grain. By calling attention to the ethical component underlying laws governing necessities, Thompson showed how historians could discover conflict over issues of food justice in the past. The concept of a "moral economy" would, of course, migrate into anthropology and the study of non-Western cultures.

Social history in the following generation, grounded in issues of class conflict and economic change, generated important studies of food as an indicator of status and living standards. Of course, an enormous literature on the production of food grew within the history of agriculture and the rural world, not just Europe, but across every part of the globe and in all periods. In an environment favorable to "history from below," food histories were not seen as out of the ordinary, and several general works appeared, some of them with a cultural slant, and several of them authored from outside the academy. Reay Tannahill's *Food in History* (1973), for example, provided a cultural context for a narrative about changing diets through history. John Burnett's *Plenty and Want: A Social History of Diet from 1815 to the Present Day* (1979), an academic contribution, explored the striking contrasts in food consumption in different social classes in England. In a different vein, Waverly Root and Richard de Rochemont produced *Eating in America: A History* in 1976. Even from more conventional perspectives, particularly that of liberal reform, food as drink received attention (Harrison, 1971), though with less engagement of economic or social theory.

Anthropology was already exerting a definitive influence on the practice of social history by the 1980s, so it was not surprising that one outstanding example of food history should act as a focal point for further discussion. Probably the single most widely read book of food history in the Western world is anthropologist Sidney Mintz's *Sweetness and Power: The Place of Sugar in Modern History*, a historical study of political economy bound together with an anthropological investigation of work and food. In an original and provocative way, Mintz linked the worlds of production, especially slave labor, with that of consumption, probing the dietary adaptations generated by the adoption of sugar among different social classes in Europe and the Americas. The suggestive influences of his work proved to be innumerable: links between the fields of anthropology, history, and political economy forced historical discussion into further analysis of global trade and the "rise of the West." The fact of geographical separation between the realms of production and consumption, as just one example, set a model for future considerations of food in later studies of commodity chains and food regimes (Mintz, 1986).

Owing largely to the work of Massimo Montanari, the *Institut Européen d'Histoire et des Cultures de l'Alimentation* and the journal *Food and History* provide another approach to the cultural history of food. Montanari's many works of scholarship, including his survey of medieval and early modern European food history, *The Culture of Food* (1994), and most recently, his reflective collection of short essays, *Food is Culture* (2006), present every aspect of food history as thoroughly embedded in a broad set of cultural assumptions and practices. Quoting Hippocrates, he describes food itself as "a thing not of nature" and argues that human artifice – what we commonly refer to as culture – affects every step of food provisioning, from production to consumption. His attention to symbolic meanings surrounding food, coupled with attention to the history of ideas and belief systems, provide an interdisciplinary model of food writing unique to the academy.

From the 1980s, growing interest in cultures of consumption indicated a shifting center of gravity in the historical profession. While earlier interest had focused on economic and political change, the next generation of theoretical and empirical works now focused primarily on a more elaborated picture of the consumption patterns of commercial society. Cultural historians would find interpretative inspiration in the provocative work of Norbert Elias (1983, 2000) in order to theorize the impact of increasing wealth and changing practices of consumption. Focusing on increasing pressures in political life, Elias showed how competitive behavior resulted in an increase in sophistication and the rise of "civility" at court. Historians broadened his notion of the "civilizing process" to include matters of taste, as well as the extension of courtly manners, to an ever-widening circle of historical agents. Parallel shifts in scholarly interest occurred in the choice of agencies, from common people, working classes, and peasants to the emergent bourgeoisie and political and social elites. At the same time, studies came to focus on "identity-value conferred by commodities, the way they constitute the self and communicate it to others". As Alan Warde pointed out, the new wave of scholarship indicated that "personal taste and aesthetic judgment," as "critical assets in the project of self-development," replaced "use or exchange value as the central mechanism driving consumption decisions" (Warde, 1997: 2). Underlying assumptions of status hierarchies and practices of emulation offered a different paradigm, one that would differentiate the work of historians interested in culture from those who would continue to pursue issues grounded in political economy.

Research methodologies and theoretical approaches

Scholars interested in the cultural history of food would do well to examine the methodology used by Steven Mennell in Chapters 3 through 5 in his dazzling *All Manners of Food: Eating and Taste in England and France from the Middle Ages to the Present* (1985). As a historical sociologist, Mennell constructed a picture of prevailing and distinctive sensibilities in England and France, using Elias's theories of the civilizing process in order to elucidate the political and social bases of prescriptive behavior at French and English courts. For Mennell, the complex distribution of power and prestige becomes the framework for culinary choices at court. In England, he argued, little regard was given to distinguishing elite foods from those of commoners, and, in fact, such practices were decried as distinctly French. Mennell draws from contemporary accounts of food and behavior as well as cookery books in order to paint different pictures of refinement on either side of the Channel. In later chapters, he shows how "diminishing contrasts and increasing varieties" characterize twentieth-century consumption, reflecting the impact of new technologies of production and transport, along with the rise of a more modern attitude toward individualized consumption patterns.

Dietary regimes can also be seen as disciplinary practices working upon the body as a site of health and reproduction. The wide-ranging influence of Michel Foucault is an unmistakable influence in many works. Foregrounding religious beliefs and rituals, Caroline W. Bynum's *Holy Feast and Holy Fast: The Religious Significance of Food to Medieval Women* (1987) and Rudolph M. Bell's *Holy Anorexia* (1985) exerted important influence on scholars of women and gender. Ken Albala's *Eating Right in the Renaissance* (2002), an innovative study of understandings of food in Renaissance Europe, combined an interest in health and the body with a study of the changing adaptations of Galenic principles in the early modern period. The Renaissance table itself provided a stage for medical and bodily discourse; as Albala pointed out, physicians were often present to provide guests with on-site advice on the possible effects of the food items set before them.

As crucial agents in generating a knowledge base concerning food and the body, medicine and science provide important windows into questions of culture for food historians. Investigations into the history of medicine in Britain have traced the development of a field of human nutrition, showing how scientific concepts of dietetics and health have informed popular beliefs, public policy, and commercial strategies. Mark Finlay's essay on the medicinal uses of Liebig's extract of meat, for example, constructed the overlapping worlds of German laboratory science, capitalist investments in colonial Latin America, and the hunger for therapeutic foods in nineteenth-century Britain (Kamminga and Cunningham, 1995). Colonial involvements led to the European "discovery" of malnutrition in African populations, a subject that intersects with interdisciplinary work in the health sciences. Diseases commonly thought to be generated by microbes at the turn of the century required an entirely new paradigm when deficiencies in diet were finally understood (Worboys, 1988). Several works by David Smith on nutrition during the world wars have pointed the way to further research into the linkages between science, industry, and nutrition (Smith, 1995; Smith, 2000). Along parallel lines, yet from a social perspective, John Burnett and Derek Oddy's studies of food and nutrition place nutritional concerns at the center of a study of historical change and class difference (Burnett, 1999; Oddy, 1993; Geissler and Oddy, 2003).

The study of material history in Europe, meanwhile, continues to generate widespread interest in the history of provisioning, which has intermittently engaged with the role of culture defined more generally to mean broad consensus. Explorations of agriculture and other aspects of food production continue to inspire creative works of cultural history, such as Joan Thirsk's *Food in Early Modern England; Phases, Fads, Fashions, 1500–1760* (2006) and Steven L. Kaplan's *Good Bread is Back: A Contemporary History of French Bread* (2006). Following the inception of the International Commission for Research into European Food History in 1989, volumes of studies on selected topics, including health, material culture, food and the city, and eating out, have made available a wealth of research (Scharer and Fenton, 1998; Fenton, 2000; Atkins, Lummel and Oddy, 2007; Jacobs and Scholliers, 2003). The many essays on Germany and Europe by Hans Jurgen Teuteberg, for example, depend largely on a model of technological change (e.g., Teuteberg, 1992), while other European scholars interested in nutrition, such as Adel P. den Hartog (1995) and Ulrike Thoms (Fenton, 2000), or material culture, including Lydia Petránová (1985, 1997), Peter Scholliers (2001), and Martin Franc (Oddy and Petránová, 2005), have expanded the connections linking food to agriculture, labor, and changing styles of living.

Luxury products have attracted a great deal of interest in the cultural history of food. Inspired by Habermas's notion of a public sphere, a proliferation of studies of coffee and tea related those products to particular settings and styles of consumption (Cowan, 2007; Pendergrast, 2010; Kowaleski-Wallace, 1997). Schivelbusch's *Tastes of Paradise: A Social History of Spices, Stimulants, and Intoxicants* sketched a captivating picture of the European consumption of luxury imports, emphasizing the parallels between substances like tobacco and beer with more "tasteful" and conventionally accepted commodities like chocolate and coffee (Schivelbusch, 1992). Historians have traced the appearance of commercial establishments aimed at luxury consumption in the eighteenth century, particularly in Enlightenment Europe. Rebecca Spang's history of the restaurant is situated at the intersection of studies of consumption and sensibility during this definitive period of history. The changing meanings of a cup of restorative broth to a more generalized site for gourmandizing consumption makes the restaurant an ideal example of how elite clientele shaped new attitudes toward the body and pleasure (Spang, 2000).

Social historians working within the social sciences employ a more capacious notion of culture as something related to convention, somewhat theoretically aligned with a Marxist concept of cultural hegemony. Underlying much of this scholarship is a critique of capitalism, which is seen as creating its own "culture" of consensus and conformity. Harvey Levenstein's *Revolution at the Table: The Transformation of the American Diet* (1988) and *Paradox of Plenty: A Social History of Eating in Modern America* (1993) highlighted the role of giant, powerful corporations, a reverence for science within an influential middle class, and a diverse, diffuse working population in producing what became understood as a hegemonic construct of food culture. His critical treatments of the interplay between corporate power and middle-class reform laid the groundwork for further discussion of the role of capitalism in constructing modern food commodities. Warren Belasco's *Appetite for Change: How the Counterculture Took on the Food Industry, 1966–1988* (1989) developed this argument at greater length, demonstrating how food reformers and, in turn, the business of food responded to what were perceived as new cultural imperatives shunning the evils of modern society as they manifested themselves in food. Belasco's study was explicitly cultural in orientation: focusing on countercultural gurus and ecology movements, he illustrated how the rebellions of the 1960s expressed themselves through changes in eating orientations: "food was a medium for broader change" (Belasco, 1989: 28). On a more descriptive level, Margaret Visser's *Much Depends on Dinner: The Extraordinary History and Mythology, Allure and Obsession, Perils and Taboos, of an Ordinary Meal* (1986) extended an analysis of single items of food, such as salt and ice cream, to brief but incisive historical sketches of relevant changes in economic or political forces that made such items commonly available.

Cultural history offers the best means of understanding rejections of dietary norms in the past: as histories of vegetarianism have revealed, for example, reasons for avoidance of meat have differed greatly over time and according to region (Spencer, 1995; Preece, 2008; Stuart, 2006). The ethical dimensions of vegetarianism have demanded cultural histories based on religion and non-Western cultures (Adams, 1994). Other dietary reforms, such as Fletcherism and the popularity of health spas, have had a similar appeal to cultural historians (Merta in Oddy and Petráňová, 2005). Even more provocative is correlative interest in animals and society, intriguingly discussed in relation to food in Richard Bulliett's *Hunters, Herders, and Hamburgers: The Past and Future of Human–Animal Relationships* (2005).

Somewhat paradoxically, the post-modern breakdown of a notion of cultural consensus into myriad forms of identity has given rise to a proliferation of studies examining shared culinary traditions within ethnic groups or regional identities. Historians in this vein have tended to emphasize the interconnections among tastes and values associated with particular collectivities, presenting a framework of tradition in the face of forces of change. Hasia R. Diner's *Hungering for America: Italian, Irish, and Jewish Foodways in the Age of Migration* combined an examination of migration history and food practices to show how "women and men transformed food into the essence of identity and as the focal point of loyalty." Not simply an examination of food choices, Diner's work used data on occupational history, marketing, religious practices, and social and domestic spaces to create a variegated narrative of immigration history (Diner, 2001: 73). Other studies of particular regional cuisines, such as those by Jeffrey M. Pilcher, focus more specifically on historical forces impinging on food sources and thus more accurately belong to the social vein of culinary history (Pilcher, 1998).

Rebellion against normative cultural imperatives provides an entry into examining women, gender, and food in nineteenth- and twentieth-century history. As a field of its own, feminist food studies exists at the intersection of women's studies and numerous other disciplines. Early works included Dolores Hayden's *The Grand Domestic Revolution: A History of Feminist Designs for American Homes, Neighborhoods, and Cities* (1982), which revealed how thinking about women's crucial place in food preparation led to visionary designs of public kitchens at the Chicago World's Columbian Exposition in 1883. The career of Ellen Swallow Richards, the force behind the establishment of home economics as a division of academic study, appeared again in Laura Schapiro's *Perfection Salad: Women and Cooking at the Turn of the Century* (1986).

Academic studies of domesticity grappled with the more complicated tensions involved in women's experiences as caregivers and victims of oppression. Particularly in periods of conflict, women were called upon to ensure what Amy Bentley aptly termed "the icon of the ordered meal." In *Eating for Victory: Food Rationing and the Politics of Domesticity* (1998), Bentley blended anthropological and sociological theories with an investigation of American expectations of food during the Second World War. Using government documents, nutritional information disseminated during the war, and other sources of iconography, she shows how the numerous sources of prescriptive ideals of female domestic roles, including that of black servants, reinforced a sense of urgency around meal provision. Bentley's example became a model for the burgeoning area of feminist food studies (Avakian and Haber, 2005). Later works attempted to trace the meanings and impact of housekeeping literature, cookbooks, and advertisements on the population, particularly women. Mary McFeeley (2000) and Sherrie A. Inness (2001) reconstructed the ways in which a particular cultural model of female activity in the kitchen became normative in the twentieth-century United States.

European studies are more likely to investigate the relationship between gender, food provision, and social class. An early work of history that focused as much on power relations as food provision itself was Judith M. Bennett's *Ale, Beer, and Brewsters in England: Women's Work in a Changing World, 1300–1600* (1996), a fair reminder that cultural food history has been flourishing as a subset of women's history for some time. In examining motherhood in East London, Ellen Ross examined the particular ways that poor women managed household resources in order to feed children (Ross, 1993). Within European food studies circles of a later date, attempts to track the diffusion of distinctive food cultures, identified by time periods and regions, have inevitably revealed the central role of women (Oddy and Petráňová, 2005). The intersection of anthropology and history continues to enhance the analysis of issues of power invested in food production and consumption (Counihan and Kaplan, 1998).

The modern state has intervened in critical ways in matters relating to provisioning, whether owing to colonialism, war, or the welfare state. Cultural historians of food have found fertile material for analysis in the growth of state agencies and bureaucracies. The ideologies of capitalism, socialism, and communism provide contexts in which programs relating to food provision have flourished or foundered in the past two centuries. Studies of the Irish famine, which locate their origins in political economy, yet also extend the analysis to social and cultural contexts, remain an important part of the narrative of modern Western European history (Clarkson and Crawford, 2001). More recently, James Vernon has offered a bold analysis of the several ways in which hunger – whether defined as malnourishment or economic deprivation – intersected with humanitarian drives to mobilize against what were seen as detrimental features of modernity (Vernon, 2007). Wartime policies have offered historians and writers a plethora of opportunities to discuss how food distribution and shortages revealed the everyday workings of business and society (Davis, 2000; Zweiniger-Bargielowska, 2011; Collingham, 2011).

The power of modernity to construct food commodities with characteristics distinctly new and often alienated from their natural origins has created a flourishing subset of cultural histories. Distinct from popular commodity treatments, which often claim credit for changing the path of world history, cultural histories of food commodities aim to construct a context that is either deep (within one particular area of culture) or carefully delineated across space (usually according to a particular pathway of global trade). From a cultural perspective, commodity histories have revealed the ways in which consumers adopted products in ways that made them distinctly their own, according to time and place. The imaginative power of spices is at the heart of medieval historian Paul Freedman's recent study (Freedman, 2008). In the more modern case of canned food, cultural histories have shown how enlisted soldiers became accustomed to food that was of little interest to finicky consumer markets before the war, as in early twentieth-century France (Bruegel, 2002). Certainly the advertising industry joined in making certain products like milk more appealing to a broad public, as E. Melanie DuPuis has shown (DuPuis, 2002). The example of milk also reveals how cultural orientations, whether rooted in mythology, medicine, or science, can determine the power of a product to conjure up prevailing images of natural goodness and health (Valenze, 2011).

Most survey courses covering the cultural history of food necessarily find that certain key products demand attention: maize, meat, rice, milk, and beer reveal key transformations taking place in the provisioning of food on a large scale. Sydney Watts's recent treatment of meat in eighteenth-century Paris offers a fine example of cultural history built around one commodity (Watts, 2006). Thematic approaches like that of Susanne Freidberg's *Fresh: A Perishable History* (2009) can be illuminating. Accounts relying simply on technology tend to replicate models of modernization theory, but cultural history offers a way out of this trap by revealing the tensions and contradictions of modernizing trends.

Avenues for future research

Agriculture, the land, and the environment

Current interest in food sources is stimulating a renewed interest in the history of agriculture. Much more research needs to be done on the relationship between changes in food production and cultural factors impinging on agriculture, land usage, and the environment. Historians of science have opened up new areas of research in the history of weather and climate (Coen *et al.*, 2006). This area also may lead to investigation of cultural aspects of artisanal production, alternative farming, and animal liberation.

Health, the body, and the senses

Interdisciplinary work in the cultural history of the senses has made interesting new forays into subject areas relating to food and consumption (Ferguson, 2011). The cultural components of taste, for example, offer one such line of research (Korsmeyer, 2005). Sociobiology, the history of medicine, and economics have turned to new questions about the body and food raised by increasing obesity in recent years. Avner Offer's *Epidemics of Abundance: Overeating and Slimming in the USA and Britain since the 1950s* (1998) and the latest volume of essays from ICREF, *The Rise of Obesity in Europe: A Twentieth Century Food History* (Oddy, Atkins, and Amilien, 2009) sets out ideas for a research agenda for the future.

Migration of food and people

Long-distance trade networks transported food items across the globe from early times, and recent cultural histories of such exchanges demonstrate bold new strategies. Greatly influenced by the work of Alfred W. Crosby, the Columbian Exchange is now one of many paths of migration under study (Crosby, 1972, 1986). Judith A. Carney's exemplary study, *Black Rice: The African Origins of Rice Cultivation in the Americas* (2001), provides a model of transnational study of cultural transmission in an examination of systems of production in different settings. From a vantage point of political economy, Arturo Warman's global study of corn (or maize) is not so much a cultural history as a guide to the many forces shaping culture (Warman, 2003). James C. McCann looks more carefully at the interplay between science and agriculture in his investigation of corn through its encounter with Africa (McCann, 2005). Such studies have shown productive, new ways in which a single food can be approached through history.

How to get started

In order to locate a graduate program in history that can accommodate a cultural approach to food, prospective students may want to consider universities where food studies is already flourishing (New York University, Tufts University, School of Oriental and African Studies [SOAS], University of London) and expect to engage advisors from more than one department. But a research plan focused on food in cultural history can be done at many other institutions, as long as supervisors are open to having advisees involved in interdisciplinary work. Some universities may welcome students planning to combine history and anthropology (University of Michigan, Columbia University) or history and sociology. Many fields of interest can be pursued within environmental history (University of Wisconsin) or the history of science. New programs in Atlantic history (Johns Hopkins) or transnational histories involving Africa and Asia, by nature of their interdisciplinary foundations, will look favorably on interest in the history of food. Graduate programs expect students to demonstrate initiative and independence, so as long as research proposals reflect a foundational knowledge of history, a project focusing on food should fare well at a wide range of institutions.

The sources for cultural history are literally everywhere: big university libraries hold many early works, some still in the stacks, others housed in rare book libraries. Many important historical works on food commodities have been transcribed, reprinted, and/or translated into English. Volumes on health, diet, and illness will offer chapters on food choices. Handbooks on agriculture, animal husbandry, climate and weather, housewifery, motherhood, and childcare will mention food, too. Many old collections have been digitized (for British historians, Early English Books Online and Eighteenth-Century Collections Online are treasure troves); reference librarians can point to library subscriptions for many different regions. Google Books is now offering many works published before 1900 and crafty subject searching can turn up leads to volumes available in academic libraries. Newspapers, magazines, and other periodical literature, especially in particular fields of research (veterinarian journals, food testing research) should also be investigated. Students might consider centering a research topic on a particular individual involved in food research or activism in the past, or, in the case of the history of ideas, writers associated with particular philosophies (non–violence, humanitarianism, socialism). Certain fields of knowledge, such as organic chemistry, home economics, or nutrition, can prove rewarding as research areas. Sources for business history (trade journals for particular products, individual corporation histories, company papers) yield a great deal of information for cultural food historians. Archival research is necessary, once a topic has been narrowed down, so consider looking for particular collections: the papers of private individuals involved in reform, tax records of localities, accounts of institutions, such as military records and hospitals. Topics related to war, revolution, urban reform, government support for agriculture, and the welfare state will find state archives full of relevant data.

Key reading

Albala, Ken (2002) *Eating Right in the Renaissance*. Berkeley, CA: UC Press.
Bruegel, Martin (2002) "How the French Learned to Eat Canned Food." In *Food Nations*, W. Belasco and P. Scranton, eds., pp. 113–30. New York: Routledge.
Burke, Peter (2008) *What is Cultural History?* Second ed. Cambridge: Polity.
Flandrin, Jean-Louis and Massimo Montanari, eds. (1999) *Food: A Culinary History*. New York: Columbia Universtity Press.
Freedman, Paul (2005) "Spices and Late-Medieval Ideas of Scarcity and Value." *Speculum* 80, 4: 1209–27.
Freidberg, Suzanne (2009) *Fresh: A Perishable History*. Cambridge, MA: Harvard University Press.
Gabaccia, Donna R. (2002) "As American as Budweiser and Pickles? Nation-Building in American Food Industries." In *Food Nations*, W. Belasco and P. Scranton, eds., pp. 175–93. new york: Routledge.
Montanari, Massimo (2006) *Food is Culture*. Trans. Albert Sonnenfeld. New York: Columbia University Press.
——(1994) *The Culture of Food*. Trans. Carl Ipsen. Oxford: Blackwell.
Pilcher, Jeffrey (2002) "Industrial *Tortillas* and Folkloric Pepsi: The Nutritional Consequences of Hybrid Cuisines in Mexico." In *Food Nations*, W. Belasco and P. Scranton, eds., pp. 222–39. New York: Routledge.
Shaw, B. D. (1982–83) "'Eaters of Flesh, Drinkers of Milk': the Ancient Mediterranean Ideology of the Pastoral Nomad." *Ancient Society* 13/14: 5–31.
Trentmann, Frank (2001) "Bread, Milk, and Democracy: Consumption and Citizenship in Twentieth-Century Britain." In *The Politics of Consumption*, M. Daunton and M. Hilton, eds., pp. 129–63. Oxford: Berg.
Valenze, Deborah (2011) *Milk: A Local and Global History*. New Haven, CT: Yale University Press.
Worboys, Michael (1988) "The Discovery of Colonial Malnutrition between the Wars." In *Imperial Medicine and Indigenous Societies*. D. Arnold, ed., pp. 208–25. Manchester: Manchester University Press.

Bibliography

Adams, Carol J. (1994) *Neither Man Nor Beast: Feminism and the Defense of Animals*. New York: Continuum.
Albala, Ken (2007) *Beans: A History*. Oxford: Berg.
——(2002) *Eating Right in the Renaissance*. Berkeley, CA: University of California Press.
Anderson, E. N. (2005) *Everyone Eats: Understanding Food and Culture*. New York, New York University Press.
Arnold, David, ed. (1988) *Imperial Medicine and Indigenous Societies*. Manchester, Manchester University Press.
Ashley, Bob, Joanne Hollows, Steve Jones and Ben Taylor, eds. (2004) *Food and Cultural Studies*. London: Routledge.
Atkins, Peter J., Peter, Lummel, and Derek J. Oddy, (2007) *Food and the City in Europe Since 1800*. Aldershot: Ashgate.
Avakian, Arelen Voski and Barbara, Haber, eds. (2005) *From Betty Crocker to Feminist Food Studies: Critical Perspectives on Women and Food*. Amherst and Boston, MA. University of Massachusetts Press.
Belasco, Warren (1989) *Appetite for Change: How the Counterculture Took on the Food Industry, 1966–1988*. New York: Pantheon.
Belasco, Warren and Philip, Scranton, eds. (2002) *Food Nations: Selling Taste in Consumer Society*. New York: Routledge.
Bell, Rudolph A. (1985) *Holy Anorexia*. Chicago, IL: Chicago University Press.
Bennett, Judith M. (1996) *Ale, Beer, and Brewsters in England: Women's Work in a Changing World, 1300–1600*. New York and Oxford: Oxford University Press.

Bentley, Amy (1998) *Eating for Victory: Food Rationing and the Politics of Domesticity*. Urbana, IL: University of Illinois Press.

Bloch, Marc (1961) *Feudal Society*, trans. L. A. Manyon. Chicago, IL: University of Chicago Press.

Braudel, Fernand (1972) *Mediterranean and the Mediterranean World in the Age of Philip II*. Trans. Siân Reynolds. New York: Harper and Row.

——(1982) *Civilization and Capitalism, 15th to 18th Centuries*. Trans., rev. Siân Reynolds. New York: Harper and Row.

Bruegel, Martin (2002) "How the French Learned to Eat Canned Food," In *Food Nations: Selling Taste in Consumer Society*. W. Belasco and P. Scranton, eds., pp. 113–30. New York: Routledge.

Burke, Peter (2008) *What is Cultural History?* Second ed. Cambridge: Polity.

Burnett, John (1999) *Liquid Pleasures: A Social History of Drinks in Modern Britain*. London: Routledge.

——(1979 [1966]) *Plenty and Want: A Social History of Diet in England from 1815 to the Present Day*. London: Nelson.

Bynum, Caroline W. (1987) *Holy Feast and Holy Fast: The Religious Significance of Food to Medieval Women*. Berkeley, CA: University of California Press.

Cagle, W. R. and L. K. Stafford, (1999) *A Matter of Taste: A Bibliographic Catalogue of Inernational Books on Food and Drink in the Lilly Library*. New Castle, DE: Oak Knoll.

Carney, Judith A. (2001) *Black Rice: The African Origins of Rice Cultivation in the Americas*. Cambridge, MA: Harvard University Press.

Chang, K. C., ed. (1977) *Food in Chinese Culture: Anthropological and Historical Perspectives*. New Haven, CT: Yale University Press.

Clarkson, Leslie A. and E. Margaret, Crawford, *Feast and Famine: Food and Nutrition in Ireland, 1500–1920*. Oxford: Oxford University Press.

Coen, Deborah R., Fleming, James Rodger, and Jankovic, Vladimir, eds. (2006) *Intimate Universality: Local and Global Themes in the History of Weather and Climate*. Sagamore Beach, MA: Science History Publications.

Collingham, Lizzie M. (2011) *A Taste of War: World War Two and the Battle for Food*. London: Allen Lane.

Counihan, Carole M. and Kaplan, Steven L., eds. *Food and Gender: Identity and Power*. Amsterdam: Harwood Academic Publishers.

Cowan, Brian. (2007) *The Social Life of Coffee: The Emergence of the British Coffeehouse*. New Haven, CT: Yale.

Crosby, Alfred W. (1972) *The Columbian Exchange: Biological and Cultural Consequences of 1492*. Westport, CT: Greenwood.

——(1986) *Ecological Imperialism: The Biological Expansion of Europe, 900–1900*. Cambridge: Cambridge University Press.

Cummings, Richard Osborn (1940) *The American and His Food: A History of Food Habits in the United States*. Chicago, IL: Chicago University Press.

Daunton, Martin and Hilton, Matthew, eds. (2001) *The Politics of Consumption: Material Culture and Citizenship in Europe and America*. Oxford: Berg.

Davidson, Alan (1999) *The Oxford Companion to Food*. New York: Oxford University Press.

Davis, Belinda (2000) *Home Fires Burning: Food, Politics, and Everyday Life in World War I Berlin*. Chapel Hill: University of North Carolina Press.

Diner, Hasia R. (2001) *Hungering for America: Italian, Irish, and Jewish Foodways in the Age of Migration*. Cambridge, MA: Harvard University Press.

Drummond, J. C. and Anne Wilbraham (1939) *The Englishman's Food: A History of Five Centuries of English Diet*. London: J. Cape.

DuPuis, E. Melanie (2002) *Nature's Perfect Food: How Milk Became America's Drink*. New York: New York University Press.

Dyer, Christopher (1989) *Standards of Living in the Later Middle Ages: Social Change in England, c. 1200–1520*. Cambridge: Cambridge University Press.

Elias, Norbert (2000) *The Civilizing Process: Sociogenic and Psychogenic Investigations*. Trans. Edmund Jephcott. Oxford: Blackwell.

——(1983) *Court Society*. Trans. Edmund Jephcott. Oxford: Blackwell.

Ferguson, Priscilla Parkhurst (2011) "The Senses of Taste," *American Historical Review*, Vol. 116, No. 2, 371–84.

Flandrin, Jean-Louis and Montanari, Massimo (1999) *Food: A Culinary History*. Trans. Albert Sonnenfeld. New York: Columbia University Press.

Forster, Robert and Ranum, Orest, eds. (1979) *Food and Drink in History: Selections from the Annales, économies, sociétiés, civilizations*, Vol. 5, trans. Elborg Forster and Patricia Ranum. Baltimore, MD: Johns Hopkins University Press.

Freedman, Paul. (2008) *Out of the East: Spices and the Medieval Imagination*. New Haven, CT: Yale University Press.

Freidberg, Susanne (2009) *Fresh: A Perishable History*. Cambridge, MA: Harvard University Press.

Geissler, Catherine and Oddy, Derek J., eds. (1993) *Food, Diet, and Economic Change Past and Present*. Leicester: Leicester University Press.

Harrison, Brian (1971) *Drink and the Victorians: The Temperance Question in England, 1815–1872*. London: Faber.

Hartog, Adel P. den, ed. (1995) *Food Technology, Science, and Marketing: European Diet in the Twentieth Century*. East Linton: Tuckwell.

Hayden, Dolores (1982) *The Grand Domestic Revolution: A History of Feminist Designs for American Homes, Neighborhoods and Cities*. Boston, MA: MIT Press.

Hobsbawm, Eric J. (1957) "The British Standard of Living, 1790–1850," *Economic History Review*, N.S., 10, no. 1, 46–61.

Inness, Sherrie A. (2001) *Dinner Roles: American Women and Culinary Culture*. Iowa City: University of Iowa Press.

Kamminga, Harmke and Cunningham, Andrew, eds. (1995) *The Science and Culture of Nutrition, 1840–1940*. Amsterdam and Atlanta: Rodopi.

Kaplan, Steven L. (1996) *The Bakers of Paris and the Bread Question, 1700–1775*. Durham, NC: Duke University Press.

——(2006) *Good Bread is Back: A Contemporary History of French Bread*. Chapel Hill, NC: Duke University Press.

Katz, Solomon H. and Weaver, William Woys, eds. (2002) *Encyclopedia of Food and Culture*. New York: Scribners's Sons.

Kiple, Kenneth F. and Ornelas, Coneé Ornelas, eds. (2000) *The Cambridge World History of Food*. Cambridge: Cambridge University Press.

Korsmeyer, Carolyn, ed. (2005) *The Taste Culture Reader: Experiencing Food and Drink*. Oxford: Berg.

Kowaleski-Wallace, Elizabeth (1997) *Consuming Subjects: Women, Shopping and Business in the Eighteenth Century*. New York: Columbia University Press.

Le Goff, Jacques (1988) *Medieval Civilization*. Trans. Julia Barrow. Oxford: Blackwell.

Levenstein, Harvey A. (1993) *Paradox of Plenty: A Social History of Eating in Modern America*. New York: Oxford.

——(1988) *Revolution at the Table: The Transformation of the American Diet*. New York: Oxford.

McAvoy, Liz Herbert and Teresa Walters, eds. (2002) *Consuming Narratives: Gender and Monstrous Appetites in the Middle Ages and Renaissance*. Chicago, IL: Chicago University Press.

McFeeley, Mary (2001) *Can She Bake a Cherry Pie? American Women and the Kitchen in the Twentieth Century*. Amherst: University of Massachusetts Press.

Meigs, Anna (1997) "Food as a Cultural Construction" in Carole Counihan and Penny Van Esterik, eds. *Food and Culture: A Reader*. New York: Routledge.

Mennell, Stephen (1985) *All Manners of Food: Eating and Taste in England and France from the Middle Ages to the Present*. Oxford: Basil Blackwell.

Merta, Sabine (2005) "Karlsbad and Marienbad: The Spas and Their Cures in Nineteenth-Century Europe" in *The Diffusion of Food Culture in Europe from the Late Eighteenth Century to the Present Day*. D. Oddy and Petránová, eds., pp. 152–63, Prague: Academia,.

Mintz, Sidney W. (1986) *Sweetness and Power: The Place of Sugar in Modern History*. New York: Viking.

Mintz, Sidney W. and Christine M. DuBois (2002) "The Anthropology of Food and Eating." *Annual Review of Anthropology* 31: 99–119.

Montanari, Massimo (2006) *Food is Culture*. Trans. Albert Sonnenfeld. New York, Columbia University Press.

——(1994) *The Culture of Food*. Trans. Carl Ipsen. Oxford: Blackwell.

Oddy, Derek J. (2003) *From Plain Fare to Fusion Food: British Diet from the 1890s to the 1900s*. Woodbridge: Boydell.

Oddy, Derek J. and Petránová, eds. (2005) *The Diffusion of Food Culture in Europe from the Late Eighteenth Century to the Present Day*. Prague: Academia.

Oddy, Derek, Atkins, Peter, and Amilien, Virginie, eds. (2009) *The Rise of Obesity in Europe: A Twentieth century Food History*. Farnham: Ashgate.

Offer, Avner (1998) *Epidemics of Abundance: Overeating and Slimming in the USA and Britain since the 1950s*. Oxford: Oxford University Press.

Pilcher, Jeffrey M. (1998) *Que Vivan los Tamales! Food and the Making of Mexican Identity.* Albuquerque, NM: University of New Mexico Press.

Preece, Rod (2008) *Sins of the Flesh: A History of Ethical Vegetarian Thought.* Vancouver: University of British Columbia Press.

Reader, John (2009) *Potato: A History of the Propitious Esculent.* New Haven, CT: Yale University Press.

Root, Waverly and Rochemont, Richard (1976) *Eating in America: A History.* New York: Morrow.

Ross, Ellen (1993) *Love and Toil: Motherhood in Outcast London, 1870–1918.* New York: Oxford University Press.

Salaman, Redcliffe N. (1985 [1949]) *The History and Social Influence of the Potato.* Cambridge: Cambridge University Press.

Schivelbusch, Wolfgang (1992) *Tastes of Paradise: A Social History of Spices, Stimulants, and Intoxicants.* Trans. David Jacobson. New York: Pantheon.

Siegers, Yves, Bieleman, Jan, and Buyst, Erik, eds. (2009) *Exploring the Food Chain: Food Production and Food Processing in Western Europe, 1850–1990.* Turnhout: Brepols.

Simoons, Frederick J. (1991) *Food in China: A Cultural and Historical Inquiry.* Boca Raton, FL: CRC Press.

Smith, Andrew F. (2011) *Potato: A Global History.* London: Reaktion.

Smith, David F., ed. (1995) *Nutrition in Britain; Science, Scientists, and Politics in the Twentieth Century.* London: Routledge.

Smith, David F. and Phillips, Jim, eds. (2000) *Food, Science, Policy and Regulation in the Twentieth Century: International and Comparative Perspectives.* London: Routledge.

Spang, Rebecca (2000) *The Invention of the Restaurant: Paris and Modern Gastronomic Culture.* Cambridge, MA: Harvard University Press.

Spencer, Colin (1995) *The Heretic's Feast: A History of Vegetarianism.* Hanover, NH: University Press of New England.

Stuart, Tristram (2006) *The Bloodless Revolution: A Cultural History of Vegetarianism from 1600 to the Present.* New York: HarperPress.

Teuteberg, Hans Jürgen, ed. (1992) *European Food History: A Research Review.* Leicester: Leicester University Press.

Thirsk, Joan (2006) *Food in Early Modern England: Phases, Fads, Fashions, 1500–1760.* London: Hambledon Continuum.

Thompson, E. P. (1971) "The Moral Economy of the English Crowd in the Eighteenth Century," *Past and Present* 50: 76–136.

Trentmann, Frank (2001) "Bread, Milk, and Democracy: Consumption and Citizenship in Twentieth-Century Britain," in *The Politics of Consumption: Material Culture and Citizenship in Europe and America.* Daunton, Martin and Hilton, Matthew, eds., pp. 129–63, Oxford: Berg.

Turner, Bryan S. (1982a) "The Discourse of Diet," *Theory, Culture & Society* 1, 1: 23–32.

——(1982b) "The Government of the Body: Medical Regimens and the Rationalization of Diet," *British Journal of Sociology* 33, 2: 254–69.

Valenze, Deborah (2011) *Milk: A Local and Global History.* New Haven, CT: Yale University Press.

Vernon, James (2007) *Hunger: A Modern History.* Cambridge, MA: Harvard University Press.

Visser, Margaret (1986) *Much Depends on Dinner: The Extraordinary History and Mythology, Allure and Obsession, Perils and Taboos, of an Ordinary Meal.* New York: Grove.

Warde, Alan (1997) *Consumption, Food and Taste: Culinary Antinomies and Commodity Culture.* London: Sage.

Warman, Arturo (2003) *Corn and Capitalism: How A Botanical Bastard Grew to Global Dominance.* Trans. Nancy L. Westrate. Chapel Hill: University of North Carolina Press.

Watts, Sydney (2006) *Meat Matters: Butchers, Politics, and Market Culture in Eighteenth-Century Paris.* Rochester, NY: University of Rochester Press.

Worboys, Michael (1988) "The Discovery of Colonial Malnutrition Between the Wars," in *Imperial Medicine and Indigenous Societies.* D. Arnold, ed., pp. 208–25, Manchester: Manchester University Press.

Zuckerman, Larry (1999) *The Potato: How the Humble Spud Rescued the World.* New York: North Point Press.

Zweiniger-Bargielowska, Ina, Duffett, Rachel, and Drouard, Alain, eds. (2011) *Food and War in Twentieth-century Europe.* Farnham: Ashgate.

10

Culinary history

Ken Albala

Food history is a broad academic discipline encompassing many varied methodologies and theoretical positions, and employs practically any written document or artifact from the past as primary source material on which research is based. It employs both qualitative and quantitative approaches and borrows conceptual models freely from other disciplines. As a distinct subset of this larger field is culinary history, which is concerned foremost with what people in the past actually cooked, how and where food was served, and what particular dishes meant to the people who ate them. As such it focuses primarily on cookbooks, but also related gastronomic literature such as restaurant reviews, menus, guidebooks, and a wealth of related writings on diet, farming, herbal lore as well as historic cooking implements, paintings of kitchen scenes and historic sites related to food. The ultimate goal of culinary history is to engage with the past via food practices, largely from an aesthetic vantage point rather than as a means to discovering attitudes about class, gender, race, and other cultural values. The latter falls under the category of the social and cultural history of food.

Historical background

Culinary history is in fact among the oldest varieties of food history, stretching back to Athenaeus in third-century Naucratis, Egypt. His *Deipnosophistae*, recording banquets and eating habits of the ancient world, might be considered the first culinary history in the Western tradition. Within this work, for example, survive fragments of the oldest cookbook written by Athenaeus, who lived in Greek Sicily in the fourth century BCE. Comparable culinary histories exist outside the Western tradition as well, for example the "food canons" (*Shih ching*) by Meng Shen, written in the seventh century in T'ang Dynasty China, chronicles the origin and usage of every food consumed at court and grown in the imperial gardens. Renaissance humanists also commented upon the food customs and cooking methods of the ancients. Titles such as *Antiquitatum Convivialium* of J. Guglielmus Stuckius, Julius Caesar Bulengerus's *De conviviis libris quatuor* and Erycius Puteanus's *Reliquae convivii prisci* were all sophisticated culinary histories. These were professional scholars, and conducted research not essentially different from that done today. That is, they were not merely chronicling great feasts, but analyzing ancient food texts with a critical eye to understanding the gastronomic values and practices of the past.

Despite a few very early printed editions of historic cookbooks, such as that attributed to the Roman gourmand Apicius, or editions of medieval cookbooks printed in the late eighteenth and early nineteenth century, such as Richard Warner's *Antiquitates Culinariae*, it was not until the latter twentieth century that a concerted effort to make historic culinary texts available for research was made. Nor until then did archives consciously collect gastronomic works for the use of scholars.

Moreover, until recently the history of cooking was taken up more often by antiquarians and popular food writers rather than academic historians. William Carew Hazlitt's *Old Cookery Books and Ancient Cuisine* published in 1886 is characteristic of the first generation of this type of work. Similar popular titles continue to be published to this day. Academics have taken an interest only in the past few decades, though the field is still shared fairly equally with journalists and food writers. This has been to a great extent a boon, for while the scholars bring to the field rigorous methods of analysis and theoretical approaches to interpreting cooking texts, popular writers provide examples of lively engaging prose. Each influences the other in positive ways that few other food studies fields can boast.

Equally important is what has come to be called "living history" sites where historic cooking is presented to the public using authentic implements and fuel sources, often by people dressed in period costumes. Historic houses such as Hampton Court in the UK, Williamsburg and Plimoth Plantation in the US, Skanson outside Stockholm, which dates to the late nineteenth century, as well as working historic farms throughout Europe and the US, have reconstructed historic kitchens and cooked original recipes and were formerly even allowed to let visitors sample their work, before insurance companies and government safety regulations made this impossible. It is the synergy among these various practitioners of culinary history that has made it a dynamic and popular field.

Scholarly interest in culinary history may be said to have truly begun in the late nineteenth century, especially with the publication of the great bibliography of Georges Vicaire, which is still the standard reference work, though updated by the subsequent works of Bitting, Feret, and most recently Notaker. These simply collected for the first time bibliographic data on the full panoply of printed European cookbooks. Scholars began to notice the relationships among the printed cookbooks, those that borrowed from others, and in general how gastronomy progressed through the centuries.

Secondary works on food history with a largely gastronomic bent might look to the great chef Alexis Soyer's *Pantropheon* as the forerunner in the field, though it was also responsible for many of the misconceptions perpetuated well into the twentieth century. Much of the work of culinary historians has in fact been to dispel various recurrent myths about food in the past and objectively assess old cookbooks without modern bias or sensational gawking at the strange and seemingly disgusting things people once ate. They are hard pressed not to romanticize the past as well. Modern surveys of food history, although not necessarily with a culinary focus include Reay Tannahill's immensely popular *Food in History* first published in the 1970s, followed by the work of Maguelonne Toussaint-Samat, the landmark *Food: A Culinary History* edited by Jean-Louis Flandrin and Massimo Montanari, as well as the surveys of Felipé Fernandez-Armesto, Michael Symons, Linda Civitello, and more recently Paul Freedman.

Apart from the broader surveys two works in particular stand out as framing the dialogue and methodology of subsequent culinary histories: Stephen Mennell's *All Manners of Food*, which compares French and English culinary fashion in the early modern era, and Barbara Wheaton's *Savoring the Past*, which is about the development of French taste. Roughly contemporaneous with these was the work of literary scholars turning their attention to modern translations and editions of historic cookbooks; the work on medieval cookery by Constance Heiatt and Terence Scully is exemplary. Likewise a generation of historic cookery practitioners and commentators brought increased sophistication to the field, including Peter Brears, Charles Perry, Ivan Day, Karen Hess, Bruno Laurioux, and numerous others, including the cookbook authors Elizabeth David and Jane Grigson.

A number of food encyclopedias have also brought attention to cuisine as a legitimate field of study, again though not exclusively about cooking, they helped to popularize the topic. These include encyclopedias edited by Kenneth Kiple, Solomon Katz, Alan Davidson, and Andrew F. Smith. To these we should also add the numerous food series that are partly devoted to culinary history, such as those at the University of California Press, edited by Darra Goldstein, the University of Illinois, edited by Andrew F. Smith, Greenwood Press, edited by Ken Albala, as well as the food series at Routledge, Berg, Oxford, and Columbia Universities. A spate of single-subject food books starting with Redcliffe Salaman's work on the potato, through Betty Fussell's work on corn, Mark Kurlansky's on cod, has also spawned a minor industry of similar works, many of which are directly concerned with cuisines of the past.

Perhaps more important than all these secondary works has been the new editions of historic cookbooks issued most notably by Prospect Books, Arnaldo Forni in Italy, Applewood Books, as well as academic publishers on both sides of the Atlantic. That is, the most important primary source material for this field has been published and often translated only in the past two decades.

Journals that focus on culinary history include *Petits Propos Culinaires* (in English despite the title); *Food in History* and several others regularly feature relevant topics, in particular *Gastronomica*, and occasionally *Food Culture and Society* and *Food and Foodways*. There is also the Italian *Appunti di Gastronomia*. Edward Behr's *The Art of Eating* is also an excellent resource as are numerous newsletters (back issues of the now retired *Food History News* for example or the long defunct *Journal of Gastronomy* published the American Institute of Wine and Food). Slow Food also, not surprisingly, is often concerned with culinary history topics, reflected in its publications. Increasingly food blogs focusing on cuisine now proliferate, including websites like The Food Time Line.

The oldest continuing conference, which still remains the base for culinary historians, has been the Oxford Symposium on Food and Cookery founded by Alan Davidson and Theodore Zeldin. A congenial mix of academics, journalists, and enthusiasts, it continues to highlight some of the best work done in the field in its annual proceedings. Other conferences include the International Association of Culinary Professionals (IACP), who apart from the annual meeting also hold periodic conferences on food history, the International Ethnological Food Research Conference, which meets in a different European city every other year, the Institut Européen d'Histoire et des Cultures d'Alimentation (IEHCA) and the FOST Center in Brussels. The Association for the Study of Food and Society holds an annual conference and culinary history topics are certainly welcome there. Numerous cities in the US also boast active culinary history groups, the oldest of which are in Boston, New York, Southern California, Chicago, but also cities such as Austin, Ann Arbor, Washington, DC, and in Northern California also sponsor regular lecture series. Many of these groups organize regional conferences and offer scholarships and awards as well.

Food museums have also been an important part of the culinary history scene, such as the Southern Food and Beverage Museum in New Orleans and the Alimentarium in Vevey, Switzerland, or the now defunct Copia in Napa, California. Literally hundreds of small museums are connected to specific manufactured products or individual foods, such as the pasta museum in Rome or the Bad Reichenhaller Salt Museum in Germany. Larger museums such as the Smithsonian also regularly mount culinary exhibits; Julia Child's kitchen, for example, is one of the most popular exhibits in the Museum of American History.

How to get started

The mere use of cookbooks as a primary source does necessarily denote an interest in cookery per se. Cookbooks can be read for any number of reasons: to discern gender roles, to understand the social meaning of ingredients or cooking methods or modes of service, to trace food materials as they become available in markets through global trade. There are countless things gastronomic literature can reveal. The culinary historian is interested in the actual food, what was involved in its preparation and even how it tasted. To this end, culinary history is partly a species of archaeology and sometimes a recipe will only make sense after one has tried to cook it using original ingredients, historic implements and fuel sources and even period utensils.

Until recently culinary historians had to visit archives and rare book libraries to consult old cookbooks and culinary manuscripts. A good proportion of significant texts are still only found in such repositories. In the US the most important collections are found at the Schlesinger Library at Radcliffe, Harvard University, the Clements Library at the University of Michigan, the New York Public Library and New York Academy of Medicine, as well as the Szamarthy archives at the University of Iowa, the Lilly collections at Indiana University, the Aresty Collection at the University of Pennsylvania, the Sheilds Library at the University of California Davis, and the Fales Libary at New York University. Most rare book rooms in university libraries across the country hold a few important culinary texts, and one should not leave out the Library of Congress as well, especially the Pennell collection.

However, increasingly historic cookbooks and related gastronomic texts can be found online. Google Books is a remarkable resource, as are books on the Gutenberg site and the Feeding America site hosted by Michigan State, as well as Gallica at the Biblioteque Nationale and the Fons Grewe site at Barcelona. Independent groups also post electronic editions and translations, and many medieval cookbooks are easily found online, with mixed success. Thomas Gloning's site is a good place to start for these: www.uni-giessen.de/gloning/kobu.htm (accessed on March 28, 2012). The majority of early modern cookbooks can be found on EEBO (Early English Books Online), though you need to be at a library that subscribes to this very expensive electronic archive.

Research methodologies

The first and most important thing to remember when working with historic cookbooks and gastronomic literature is that very rarely are they accurate records of what people actually ate. Sometimes they do record menus of meals eaten, but more often they are prescriptive rather than descriptive. That means a researcher can be sure that a cookbook reflects the ideas and values of the author and perhaps by extension a set of readers who purchased the book, but this is almost never an indication of exactly how people cooked or what they ate. This is true of the earliest Mesopotamian recipes recorded on cuneiform tablets, to medieval manuscripts right down to modern cookbooks. They are all largely aspirational, meaning that readers may have mined them for ideas, or imagined cooking from them, but they are not evidence of actual practice.

Nonetheless, they do offer a wealth of information. The best way to read such texts is first to be clear about what you are interested in learning. One might simply identify ingredients to start. These can be tabulated, even quantified. Quite simply one can ascertain what kind of ingredients were available, how popular they were, and also what might be conspicuous by its absence. It is important not to jump to conclusions though, as recipe books might exclude simple dishes assuming everyone knew how to cook them, or vegetable recipes for similar reasons. Because cookbooks were often written for wealthy readers, sometimes common or lowly dishes were excluded. By this logic, one should not assume, for example, the dearth of vegetable dishes in a medieval cookbook means that wealthy people did not eat vegetables. It may be that the author simply didn't think they would be very impressive.

Next it is useful to identify fuel sources, cooking implements, and cooking methods. We are easily led astray by assumptions about modern cooking that seem to render directions confusing or inaccurate. Because old cookbooks often lack cooking times or temperatures or are written in short-hand form for professionals, modern redactors often guess at their meaning. As in all historic research, the context is especially important here. One absolutely must begin with the assurance that old cookbook authors knew what they were doing and achieved results that to them were worthy of recording. Of course there are sometimes mistakes and printers' errors, but if one assumes the recipe will not work, and consequently makes changes or substitutions, practically nothing will be learned about the past.

The context can be supplied by other gastronomic texts, images of cooking in old paintings, or even surviving implements in museums. For example, cooking in a suspended iron pot over a low flame will give very different results than in a modern stainless steel pot on a modern stove. Likewise roasting on a spit is nothing like baking in an oven or even using a modern rotisserie. While reading historic recipes, one must keep in mind a very different kind of kitchen.

Quite often a cookbook will also offer hints about who exactly is doing the cooking. It might be a professional for a large noble household. Quantities offer some clues, as does the source of ingredients. For example, if instructions include killing your animal first, this might point to a large estate or farm setting. If meat is bought already butchered and apportioned in small quantities, this might denote an urban setting. Sometimes the readership is directly addressed – it might be housewives, working-class mothers, bachelors, young inexperienced newlyweds. This will of course determine the cost and complexity of the recipes, the range of ingredients and equipment called for. Even when not directly addressed it is often possible to sleuth out exactly what kind of audience is targeted. Are the recipes meant to feed two people, or a small family; are they for everyday fare or special elaborate occasions? Is the book a small, cheap paperback or a large, expensive coffee table book or professional reference work? Cost alone is sometimes a good indication of the audience.

It is also useful to think about the ways ingredients are combined, the flavor combinations, condiments called for, and garnishes. These considerations will reveal an overall aesthetic sensibility that it might be possible to analyze in terms of historical progression. Art historians and music historians are accustomed to this kind of classification and categorization and they have a critical vocabulary for describing their subjects, often with precise periodization. In other words it is possible to describe cooking as being Baroque, Romantic, Modernist, much the same way other aspects of culture are described. Culinary history is only beginning to attain the sophistication of other disciplines in this regard.

One can also look for hints about presentation and service. Are there many courses, special utensils or serving dishes, table linens or napkins? Are there servants present to carve or apportion larger dishes, or ladle out soup? Is there a certain logic to the progression of the meal or is everything served at once? Does the author mention etiquette or seating arrangements or perhaps dining room decor? These are all ultimately relevant to gastronomy and changes in these aspects of dining may signal much broader cultural and social changes. A cookbook may also be explicitly connected to a restaurant, which offers an entirely different kind of information. Menus are naturally the best place to look for information about restaurant dining, but so too are advertisements, reviews, and culinary memoires. Advertisements in newspapers, magazines and in more recent media are also invaluable sources for research on manufactured goods, especially those that are marketed as convenience foods. Some manufacturers also issued small cookbooks to accompany their products, or even put recipes right on boxes and cans. For a complete picture of the entire gastronomic scene it is important not to neglect any possible resource, including cookware and utensils, ovens and other kitchen appliances. These are all directly relevant to reconstructing the culinary past.

Cookbooks may also have a particular angle. They might have been compiled by a certain community or group, or might reflect a specific ethnic tradition or region. They may cater to a certain dietary program for weight loss or physical training. They might be written specifically for people with dietary restrictions, vegetarians, diabetics, or those with allergies. Or a cookbook may appeal to a certain aesthethic niche – using farmer's market produce, using rare important ingredients, being sophisticated and authentic or homey and comforting. These are all important factors not only for discerning the values and preoccupations of the past, but also the gastronomic choices. Why, for example, do some cookbooks insist on fresh ingredients cooked from scratch while others use convenience foods and labor-saving devices? Why do some capitalize on the celebrity status of the author or advertise themselves as quick and convenient? For the culinary historian all these factors ultimately determine what ends up in the recipes.

Finally, the most important part of this research is actually cooking from historic texts. It is not of course requisite and many excellent studies in culinary history never take this final step. But in a certain sense it is like commenting on a painting without ever having seen it or on a piece of music without having heard it on period instruments. Tasting the past, coming to understand the embodied experience of cooks, and assessing the results aesthetically is only possible by getting a little messy. For the purposes of research rather than diverting entertainment, one must strictly adhere to the instructions offered. Substitutions will ruin the final affect. Modern cookware will tell you very little in the end. Original ingredients are a little harder since domesticated species of plants and animals have changed dramatically over time. A modern cut of pork, for example, might be quite different from what the author had in mind. Nonetheless, close approximation is possible. An onion is still essentially an onion. Assuming you have found all the ingredients and cookware and are using the proper fuel source, simply follow the instructions to the letter. The results are almost always astonishing.

For those foods that are not commonly described in detail, bread for example, fermented products such as pickles, cheese, or cured meats, the culinary historian must venture into less sure waters and delve into experimentation. Understanding that one can never replicate these exactly, especially since the ambient bacteria, weather conditions and myriad other factors will differ, it is still possible to reconstruct historic techniques, to at least gain a deeper understanding of these cooking and preservation methods by testing them. This type of work is akin to archaeological research that attempts to reconstruct foodways through interpreting replicas of physical remains in action. Authenticity is not really an issue here, it is more about understanding how an otherwise obscure object might have been used or how a technique was undertaken. The historian has the advantage of referring to surviving texts that offer clues about these processes, but again the extrapolation can only be an approximation.

Avenues for further research

Although many of the great classics in Western culinary history are now available in modern editions, the same can unfortunately not be said for the entire non-Western canon. The greatest single obstacle to the globalization of this field, to facilitate communication across language barriers, is the lack of translated sources. For speakers of English, there is practically nothing available as the basis for research. A few medieval sources from the Islamic world are now available, but almost nothing from Chinese or Indian culinary traditions, let alone from the rest of the world. Culinary history remains for the most part resolutely European and North American. There are no doubt people working on relevant topics elsewhere, but they are essentially cut off from the rest of the field.

Despite the coming of age of food studies in general, and the fact that food historians no longer have to explain what they do or struggle for respectability, the same cannot be said for culinary history. It does not have a firm foothold in academia and even among most professional food historians, it is an afterthought. There remains this lingering idea that somehow getting your hands dirty is not appropriate for detached scholarly inquiry. Perhaps for the same reason literary scholars don't write poetry, art historians generally don't paint and music historians don't perform. Perhaps they should. For food history, the aesthetic side of the story is one that deserves greater scrutiny, in tandem with these other arts. Until that happens, culinary history will remain the poorer, if sometimes more popular, relative to food history and food studies in general.

Key reading

Encyclopedias, reference works, and surveys

Albala, Ken (2011) *Food Cultures of the World Encyclopedia*. Santa Barbara, CA: ABC–CLIO.
Arndt, Alice (2006) *Culinary Biographies*. Austin, TX: Yes Press.
Civitello, Linda (2011) *Cuisine and Culture*. Hoboken, NJ: Wiley.
Davidson, Alan (1999) *The Oxford Companion to Food*. Oxford: Oxford University Press.
Fernández-Armesto, Felipe (2001) *Food: A History*. Oxford: Macmillan.
Flandrin, Jean-Louis and Massimo Montanari (1999) *Food: A Culinary History*. New York: Columbia University Press.
Katz, Solomon H. ed. (2003) *Encyclopedia of Food and Culture*. New York: Charles Scribner's Sons.
Kiple, Kenneth (2007) *A Moveable Feast: Ten Millenia of Food Globalization*. Cambridge: Cambridge University Press.
——ed. (2000) *The Cambridge World History of Food*. Cambridge: Cambridge University Press.
Pilcher, Jeffrey (2006) *Food in World History*. New York: Routledge.
Smith, Andrew F. (2004) *Oxford Encyclopedia of Food and Drink in America*. Oxford: Oxford University Press.
Strong, Roy (2002) *Feast: A History of Grand Eating*. London: Jonathan Cape.
Tannahill, Reay (1998) *Food in History*. New York: Crown Publishers.
Toussaint-Samat, Maguelonne (1992) *History of Food*. Oxford: Basil Blackwell.

Bibliography

Bitting, Katherine Golden, (2004 [1939]) *Gastronomic Bibliography*. Mansfield Centre, CT: Martino Publishing.
Feret, Barbara L. (1979) *Gastronomical and Culinary Literature: A Survey and Analysis of Historically-Oriented Collections in the U.S.A*. Metuchen, New York: Scarecrow Press.
Notaker, Henry (2010) *Printed Cookbooks in Europe, 1470–1700*. Newcastle, DE: Oak Knoll Press.
Vicaire, George (1890) *Bibliographie Gastronomique*. Paris: Roquette et fils.

Secondary sources

Achaya, K. T. (2002) *A Historical Dictionary of Indian Food*. New York: Oxford University Press.
Adamson, Melitta (2002) *Regional Cuisines of Medieval Europe*. New York: Routledge.
Albala, Ken (2007) *The Banquet: Dining in the Great Courts of Late Renaissance Europe*. Urbana and Chicago: University of Illinois Press.
Anderson, E. N. (1988) *The Food of China*. New Haven, CT and London: Yale University Press.
Beck, Leonard N. (1984) *Two Loaf Givers or A Tour through the Gastronomic Libraries of Katherine Golden Bitting and Elizabeth Robins Pennel*. Washington, DC: Library of Congress.
Belasco, Warren (1989) *Appetite for Change*. New York: Pantheon.
Bober, Phyllis Pray (1999) *Art, Culture and Cuisine*. Chicago, IL: University of Chicago Press.

Bower, Anne, ed. (1992) *Recipes for Reading: Community Cookbooks, Stories, Histories*. Amherst: University of Massachusetts Press.

Brears, Peter (2008) *Cooking and Dining in Medieval England*. Totnes: Prospect.

Cappatti, Alberto and Massimo Montanari (1999) *Italian Cuisine*. New York: Columbia University Press.

Carney, Judith (2001) *Black Rice*. Cambridge, MA: Harvard University Press.

Chang, K. C. (1977) *Food in Chinese Culture*. New Haven, CT: Yale University Press.

Coe, Sophie (1994) *America's First Cuisines*. Austin: University of Texas.

Cwiertka, Katarzyna (2006) *Modern Japanese Cuisine*. London: Reaktion.

Dalby, Andrew (1996) *Siren Feasts: A History of Food and Gastronomy in Greece*. London: Routledge.

Diner, Hasia (2001) *Hungering for America*. Cambridge, MA: Harvard University Press.

Eden, Trudy (2008) *The Early American Table*. DeKalb: Northern Illionois University Press.

Faas, Patrick (2003) *Around the Roman Table*. New York: Palgrave.

Fisher, Carol (2006) *The American Cookbook: A History*. Jefferson, NC: McFarland.

Flandrin, Jean-Louis (1997) *Arranging the Meal*. Berkeley: University of California Press.

Floyd, Janet and Laurel Forster (2003) *The Recipe Reader: Narratives, Contexts, Traditions*. Aldershot: Ashgate.

Gabbaccia, Donna R. (1998) *We Are What We Eat*. Cambridge, MA: Harvard University Press.

Gold, Carol (2007) *Danish Cookbooks*. Seattle: University of Washington Press.

Haber, Barbara (2002) *From Hardtack to Homefries: An Uncommon History of American Cooks and Meals*. New York: The Free Press.

Harris, Jessica B. (2011) *High on the Hog*. New York: Bloomsbury.

Henisch, Bridget Anne (1976) *Fast and Feast*. State College: Pennsylvania State College Press.

Higman, B. W. (2008) *Jamaican Food*. Kingston: University of the West Indies Press.

Humble, Nicola (2005) *Culinary Pleasures: Cookbooks and the transformation of British Food*. London: Faber and Faber.

Innes, Sherrie, ed. (2001) *Kitchen Culture in America*. Philadelphia: University of Pennsylvania Press.

Ishige, Naomichi (2001) *The History and Culture of Japanese Food*. New York: Kegan Paul.

Kamp, David (2006) *The United States of Arugula*. New York: Broadway Books.

Lehmann, Gilly (2002) *The British Housewife*. Totnes: Prospect Books.

Levenstein, Harvey (2003a) *Paradox of Plenty*. Berkeley: University of California Press.

——(2003b) *Revolution at the Table*. Berkeley: University of California Press.

Mendelson, Ann (1996) *Stand Facing the Stove: The Story of the Women Who Gave America The Joy of Cooking*. New York: Henry Holt.

Mennell, Stephen (1985) *All Manners of Food: Eating and Taste in England and France from the Middle Ages to the Present*. Oxford: Basil Blackwell.

Mintz, Sidney (1996) *Tasting Food Tasting Freedom*. Boston, MA: Beacon.

Montanari, Massimo (1994) *The Culture of Food*. Oxford: Blackwell.

Pettid, Michael J. (2008) *Korean Cuisine*. Reaktion.

Scully, Terence (1995) *The Art of Cookery in the Middle Ages*. Woodbridge: Boydell.

Shapiro, Laura (1986) *Perfection Salad: Women and Cooking at the Turn of the Century*. New York: Farrar, Straus and Girous.

Smith, Andrew F. (2009) *Eating History*. New York: Columbia University Press.

Spang, Rebecca L. (2000) *The Invention of the Restaurant*. Cambridge, MA: Harvard University Press.

Spencer, Colin (2002) *British Food*. London: Grub Street.

Theophano, Janet (2002) *Eat My Words: Reading Women's Lives through the Cookbooks They Wrote*. New York: Palgrave.

Trubeck, Amy (2000) *How the French Invented the Culinary Profession*. Philadelphia: University of Pennsylvania Press.

Wheaton, Barbara Ketchum (1983) *Savoring the Past: The French Kitchen and Table from 1300 to 1789*. New York: Simon and Schuster.

Willan, Anne (2000) *Great Cooks and their Recipes*. London: Pavilion.

Witt, Doris (1999) *Black Hunger*. Minneapolis: University of Minnesota Press.

11

Food and literature

An overview

Joan Fitzpatrick

Food has recently emerged as a topic for serious literary study. This chapter traces important developments in the field of literary criticism on food, considering the texts, authors, genres, and themes that have been the focus of attention, and the theoretical trajectory of such criticism. Since most critics tend to specialize in a particular historical period, the approach is broadly chronological but also considers those critical works tracing the development in literature across the centuries of food-related philosophical and psychological phenomena such as eating disorders. The chapter also considers where the study of food might take us in the future.

Until relatively recently the subject of food has been somewhat neglected by literary scholars, many of whom considered it rather too ordinary an area for investigation; it is notable, for example, that the first serious monograph on Shakespeare and food appeared only in 2007 (Fitzpatrick, 2007). Yet literary critics have begun to notice that much of what they research and teach involves food and the rituals surrounding its consumption. Literary critics who write about food understand that the use of food in novels, plays, poems, and other works of literature can help explain the complex relationship between the body, subjectivity, and social structures regulating consumption. When authors refer to food they are usually telling the reader something important about narrative, plot, characterization, motives, and so on. Many critics interested in food in literature are alert to the historical specificity of references to food, and this is especially true of literature written before the last century: explaining obscure foodstuffs and attitudes toward feeding that a modern reader might not grasp is an important part of the critic's job, and most literary critics have been influenced by food historians who have led the way in explicating esoteric foodstuffs and practices surrounding food. The literary canon is an important consideration here: critics writing about food in literature are conscious of ploughing new furrows and thus shaping what kinds of literary texts are worth exploring in terms of food. Food critics are making an important case for the serious study of food in respected literary texts: They are writing about food in nineteenth-century literature commonly studied in schools and universities, for example the work of Dickens (Hyman, 2009; Cozzi, 2010) and arguing for the centrality of food to phenomena hitherto thought beyond the remit of such analysis, for example the Romantic imagination (Morton, 2004; Gigante, 2005). Food critics are also drawing attention to literature currently at the edges of the canon, for example by exploring food and consumption in texts traditionally surveyed by historians: cookbooks, dietary literature, and so on, as well as literature by contemporary women writers (Sceats, 2000; Heller and Moran, 2003). They are thus making a strong statement about what deserves our attention and thus shaping future studies in this newly burgeoning area. The main aim of this chapter is to guide the reader toward some of the most important and original work done so far on literature and food, indicate the kinds of approaches critics tend to take, and consider which areas might well benefit from further exploration.

The historical background of literary criticism on food and major theoretical approaches in use

This section will trace important developments in the field of literary criticism on food; it will consider the texts, authors, genres, and themes that have been explored, as well as the theoretical trajectory of the criticism. Many literary critics specialize in a particular historical period, which means that those who are interested in food tend to write about food in the period they know best, and for this reason my approach is broadly period-based in scope. Although food has only recently emerged as a topic for serious literary study a lot has been written on the topic and so, although intended as a survey of key approaches to important literary texts and the issues they raise, this section should not be regarded as definitive.

Although Caroline Spurgeon did original work tracing conscious and unconscious images on food in Shakespeare's plays (Spurgeon, 1935: 83–84, 188–89), it is only relatively lately that early modernists have become interested in food in literature. An important monograph by Chris Meads, which traces the phenomenon of the banquet in non-Shakespearean drama, is typical of the debt to historical analysis in much of the work that has been produced by early modernists (Meads, 2002). Meads does not mention Ben Jonson at length but this dramatist's preoccupations with food and eating have been discussed in historically inflected criticism by others, although many works tend to focus more on the body, specifically Jonson's own large body, than food per se (Pearlman, 1979; Schoenfeldt, 1988; Boehrer, 1990). Other dramatists, and usually a specific play written by them, have been approached from the perspective of the symbolism of food whereby food stands for other things, for example nationalism and virtue (Williamson, 1979), sexual desire (Bryan, 1974; Anderson, 1962: 211; 1964), class difference, and social and religious observance (Cole, 1984: 86). Not much work has been done on non-dramatic literature, but some has focused on how certain texts have been described in terms of food, specifically sweet foods associated with excess (Hall, 1996; Craik, 2004) and explored the process of digestion and waste management in Spenser, Herbert, and Milton (Schoenfeldt, 1999). Robert Appelbaum (2006) invoked the work of the social historian Norbert Elias, specifically his reference to "the civilizing process," a phenomenon tied to (usually French) fashion. This eclectic study considers a range of genres from about 1450 to the early eighteenth century, from the first printed cookbook, dietary literature, and Shakespeare to John Milton's epic poem *Paradise Lost*, always with an eye to explaining what contemporary readers and audiences would have understood by references to food. Other critics have focused on food, especially eating, in Milton's poetry and prose (Gigante, 2000; Arvind, 2006); the significance of food, specifically bread and banquets in *Paradise Regained* (Cox, 1961; Franson, 1976); and books-as-food imagery in his *Areopagitica* (Smith, 1990; Cable, 1995; Schaeffer, 2000).

The first monograph on food in Shakespeare (Fitzpatrick, 2007) was especially interested in how the drama engaged with early modern dietary theories. Before this publication, influential articles on food in Shakespeare tended to consider individual plays (Charney, 1960; Candido, 1990) or unusual feeding, for example the animalistic, cannibalistic, or aggressive (Morse, 1983; Adelman, 1992); it is specifically medicinal cannibalism in Renaissance literature that is dealt with in Noble (2003; and further explored in Noble 2011) and the refusal of women to feed in Gutierrez 2003. That the subject of early modern food is gaining respectability amongst literary scholars, and increasingly discussed at academic conferences, is clear from the fact that in 2009 the journal *Shakespeare Jahrbuch* published a volume devoted to Shakespeare and food, containing essays on staging food in Shakespeare (Holland, 2009; Dobson, 2009), sugar in Shakespeare (Hall, 2009), and three representative foods (apricots, butter, and capons) in Shakespeare and early modern dietary literature (Fitzpatrick, 2009). Also published in 2009 was a special issue of the new journal *Early English Studies* with essays tracing early modern attitudes to vegetarianism (Borlik, 2009); food shortages (Knowles, 2009); the sexual dimension to food references (Lipscomb, 2009); gluttony and nationalistic foods (Fisher, 2009). A year later came a collection of international and interdisciplinary essays on food in the Renaissance, including Shakespeare, across drama, poetry, and prose from the late medieval period to the mid-seventeenth century (Fitzpatrick, 2010a), and a dictionary on Shakespeare and the language of food was published (Fitzpatrick, 2010b).

Although the early modern period has proved especially attractive to food critics, earlier and later periods have not been neglected. The collection of essays *Food and Eating in Medieval Europe* is typical of much of the scholarship that has emerged on food with its crossover between historical and literary analysis (Carlin and Rosenthal, 1998). As the editors of the volume point out: "The essays that can be categorized as falling within the realms of historical inquiry and historical methods go far beyond the 'what happened' menu of historical inquiry" (ix) while the essays on literature "serve to carry us from some of the hard realities of food production and consumption patterns into what we can think of as extra-nutritional aspects of this basic human endeavour" (x). The first essay in the volume, by Marjorie A. Brown, is a good example of historically inflected literary analysis since it offers a study of heroic poems from Old English literature, such as *Beowulf,* in an effort to illuminate further the evidence that has emerged from archeological excavations of feast halls (Brown, 1998). Another essay, by Elizabeth M. Biebel, considers what the food Chaucer's pilgrims eat can tell us about medieval attitudes to physical and spiritual nourishment (Biebel, 1998). The volume is alert throughout to the slippery nature of genre, and so texts that might traditionally have fallen under the category of historical document, for example English chronicles and the songs performed at feasts, are ripe for literary analysis (Marvin, 1998; Weiss, 1998). Another example of the interdisciplinary nature of much food writing is Caroline Walker Bynum's *Holy Feast and Holy Fast: The Religious Significance of Food to Medieval Women*, a study mainly historical in its trajectory but providing also a valuable discussion of food in the writings, including poetry, of women mystics (Bynum, 1987). Building upon Bynum's work primarily from the point of view of a literary critic, and focusing on writings by religious women on food from the medieval period to the nineteenth century, is Mazzoni (2005).

Collections of essays across periods have also emerged, for example *The Pleasures and Horrors of Eating*, which considers literature from the early modern period, through the eighteenth and nineteenth centuries, and right up to the twenty-first century (Gymnich and Lennartz, 2010). The focus here is on tracing an important shift in attitudes towards food and its consumption whereby we get "early modern ideas of the pleasures of eating, of the carnivalesque abundance of food changing into visions of horror, cannibalism and bulimia" (19) in eighteenth-century literature; later, in the nineteenth and twentieth centuries the literature reveals "a conjunction between eating and disease … or between eating and ontological pessimism which reveals that it is no longer the pleasure of food, but the horror of eating that provides modern culture with one of its prevalent semantic fields" (14).

The Romantics are the subject of an important collection of essays that, as the preface makes clear, presents studies that embrace phenomena from a variety of perspectives: literary, philosophical, and cultural (Morton, 2004). The more clearly "cultural" essays engage with eating in Hegel and what various foods tell us about the Romantic imagination but of particular interest to literary critics are essays that are "literary theoretical and cultural-historical" (xv) discussing milk and blood in Byron's poetry (Stabler, 2004); excessive consumption in late poetry by Keats and Shelley (Plotnitsky, 2004); the figure of disgust in Romantic literature, especially Keats (Gigante, 2004); the influence of views about digestion from John Locke onwards on writing by Mary Wollstonecraft (Youngquist, 2004). Gigante's later monograph explores the Romantic debt to Milton's *Paradise Lost* and *Paradise Regained*, specifically the notion that taste involves pleasure (Gigante, 2005).

The work of a number of female writers from the late eighteenth and early nineteenth centuries are explored in Moss 2009. This study of food in literature includes children's fiction by Maria Edgeworth, better known for her historical novel *Castle Rackrent*; novels by the Scottish author Susan Ferrier and Frances Burney and writings aimed at mothers by Mary Wollstonecraft. The focus throughout is on women's issues, specifically women's appetites and maternal feeding. Moss does not discuss Jane Austen at any length but Austen comes under book-length scrutiny in Lane 1995. Here we get a comprehensive analysis of Austen's own domestic arrangements, including the various times and types of meals with which she would be familiar and that appear in her letters and novels, before an exploration, in detail, of the role food, dining, and hospitality plays in the Austen *oeuvre*. Lane is interested in what Austen's use of food tells us about her characters, especially their moral status, for example pointing out that in Austen's novels "all the gluttons are men and all the (near-) anorexics women" (Lane, 1995: xiv). Important information is provided about the foods that were served in Georgian England and are mentioned by Austen, and explanations given of those dishes unfamiliar to a modern reader, for example white soup and route-cakes, as well as food-related words and phrases that have changed their meaning since Austen's time, for example that "mutton" could be a generic word for meat or dinner. Lane provides a fabulously useful index to all the foods mentioned in Austen's novels so that, for example, we can tell at a glance that coffee is mentioned lots of times, and olives only once, in *Sense and Sensibility*.

In 2008 a special section of the journal *Victorian Literature and Culture* devoted itself to the study of food and drink in the period. As its editors pointed out, although food studies has long been considered a legitimate field of enquiry amongst anthropologists, sociologists, historians, and psychologists, "in the camp of literary and cultural studies, it has remained – at least until recently – a devalued object of inquiry," which they suggest is due to food and cookery being associated with women and popular culture and thus raising "debates about the merits of feminist studies; the importance of maintaining the canon; and the value of the 'cultural turn' as a whole – as well as the field's broader lack of interest in the aesthetics of the quotidian" (Daly and Forman, 2008: 363). The editors tell us that their doubts about the validity of scholarship on Victorians and food disappeared when they saw the calibre of work submitted in response to their call for submissions to the journal.

A number of essays in *Victorian Literature* focus on the role of food and drink in nineteenth-century cultural history. Margaret Beetham applies the analysis of taste by the sociologist Pierre Bourdieu to Mrs Beeton's *Book of Household Management* (1861) specifically in relation to Beeton's argument that the way in which one dines indicates a person's rank (Beetham, 2008). Helen Day considers a complaints book from the archives of the Reform Club, a London dining establishment where Alexis Soyer, French chef and author of *The Modern Housewife* (1849) presided over the kitchen (Day, 2008). Day compares the complaints about cost, quality, and service that are detailed in the book with issues dealt with by Mrs Beeton in her advice to ladies on how best to run their household. Julie E. Fromer reveals what histories of tea can tell us about English national identity and the relationship between England and empire (Fromer, 2008); as Fromer notes, the tea history is "a slightly peculiar genre that blurs the boundaries between fiction and non-fiction, advertisement and travelogue, personal account and scientific treatise" (531). The same might be said of much of the writings that are of interest to food critics where the clear division between literary text and other categories can be unclear. For example, Thomas Prasch's essay on Alexis Soyer's new restaurant, the opening of which coincided with the Great Exhibition of 1851, engages with contemporary guide books, cookbooks, writings by Thackeray, and Henry Mayhew's novel *1851, or the Adventures of Mr. and Mrs. Sandboys and Family, Who Came Up to London to "Enjoy Themselves," and to See the Great Exhibition*; all these texts provide a way into exploring nineteenth-century English attitudes – specifically the attitudes of Londoners – towards foreign food (Prasch, 2008). The Great Exhibition itself is the focus of Paul Young's essay, which also mentions Mayhew's novel, and looks specifically at the role food and cooking played in the globalization that was central to the Exhibition (Young, 2008).

Those essays in *Victorian Literature* that are specifically literary in trajectory also tell us about nineteenth-century attitudes towards food and drink, and although they consider a range of texts from various perspectives a number of issues common to food critics recur including the political significance of eating certain types of food and instances of plenty and lack. Mrs Beeton provides the context for many nineteenth-century literary critics, evidence again of the crossover between what we traditionally regard as "literature" and other kinds of texts. Kate Thomas compares Beeton and Arthur Conan-Doyle, concluding that both are preoccupied with methods whereby, via ordinary routes, the middle class can acquire discernment (Thomas, 2008). Beeton also comes up in an essay by Heather A. Evans exploring the role of food in a children's tale by Beatrix Potter (Evans, 2008) and she is mentioned by Sharmila Sen on the national and ethnic significance of food in the little-known work *Curry & Rice (on Forty Plates); or, The Ingredients of Social Life at "Our" Station in India* by George Francklin Atkinson, a British captain in the Bengal Engineers (Sen, 2008). Potter is also one of many authors included in a collection of essays on food in children's literature from the nineteenth century to the modern day (Keeling and Pollard, 2009). *Victorian Literature* contains an essay on *Falk*, Joseph Conrad's short story featuring cannibalism, Paul Viltos explores Beeton's view on dining as an indicative of civility, revealing that Conrad problematizes simplistic notions regarding primitive savagery; in *Falk* joyless over-eating by the non-savage also indicates a lack of civility (Viltos, 2008). Cannibalism is a recurring feature of Conrad's writing and its significance in *Heart of Darkness* is considered in Collins (1998). Tara Moore shows that literature of all kinds (novels as well as periodicals) published around Christmas and featuring Christmas scenes, traditionally displays of plenty, are imbued with "national fears of famine" (Moore, 2008: 489); she argues that feminist critics who have focused mainly on female self-imposed starvation in Victorian literature have missed the rhetoric of social reform that many texts contain. Nineteenth-century literature was interested in the moral implications of eating the wrong thing or eating too much but also in other kinds of excess such as alcoholism, a condition that, like anorexia, was first recognized as a disease during the Victorian period. Yet, as Gwen Hymen points out in her discussion of alcohol abuse in Anne Brontë's novel *The Tenant of Wildfell Hall* it was not until the 1860s or 1870s that the addiction was considered anything other than a moral or social failing (Hyman, 2008). Noting that most critics of the novel have provided a feminist analysis of Helen Huntington, the wife of the drunkard Arthur, Hymen is more interested in what Arthur's drinking habits suggest about Brontë's political and moral views: Helen represents the views of the teetotal movement, Arthur the leisured class that is destroying itself and Gilbert, Helen's new love interest, the emerging and productive middle class that will destroy aristocratic entitlement.

Food and drink feature in a number of novels by the Brontë sisters and its cultural significance is also dealt with in Mergenthal 2010. Another work suggesting that food and drink is about more than simply sustenance is Deborah Mutch's essay, which explains the social significance of port, brandy, ale, and beer within the context of fiction serialized in socialist periodicals, which emphasized the social reasons for drunkenness amongst the working class whilst highlighting the hypocrisy of a heavy-drinking ruling class (Mutch, 2008).

More recently two monographs have made food the focus of their approach to nineteenth-century fiction (Hyman, 2009; Cozzi, 2010). Hyman continues her valuable work considering the neglected figure of the gentleman in Victorian literature, focusing on important male figures in a number of significant novels from the period including Jane Austen's *Emma*, Charles Dickens's *Little Dorrit* and Bram Stoker's *Dracula*. In her analysis of "class, gender, culture and the rhetorical construction of identity" (3) Hyman explores relevant socio-economic issues such as unhealthy consumptions, for example the commonplace adulteration of foodstuffs – a topic previously considered in the context of Dickens's novels and prose in Long 1988 – and the manner in which certain foods, for example gruel in *Emma* and the truffle in Wilkie Collins's *Law and the Lady*, signal the gentleman's status. Cozzi argues that food is "one of the most fundamental signifiers of national identity" (Cozzi, 2010: 5) and that novels reveal the construction of an English identity, one that emerges in the context of imperialism and industrialism and is created by and confirmed through food. Cozzi considers the significance of grain in the construction of England's rural past, especially in Hardy's *Mayor of Casterbridge*, the role of food in the construction of the middle-class gentleman in a number of novels by Dickens – a topic previously explored in relation to *David Copperfield* in Lewis 2009 – and how women and the foreigner figure in the construction of national identity in other important nineteenth-century novels. Monstrous appetites and what they indicate about Victorian attitudes to civility and savagery, specifically in the context of ethnicity, come up in the books by Hyman and Cozzi, both of whom engage with imperial anxieties about cannibalism in the work of Dickens, something also dealt with by James E. Marlow in an essay that explores Dickens's interest in ogres as evidence of a personal and professional anxiety not only of being eaten (re Freud) but of being present at the cannibalistic feast (Marlow, 1983). Eating to excess, and what that reveals, specifically in Dickens's *Martin Chuzzlewit* is dealt with in Paroissien (2010).

Amongst early twentieth-century fiction James Joyce, Virginia Woolf, and D. H. Lawrence have attracted the attention of food critics. Lindsey Tucker traces food and digestion in Joyce's great novel *Ulysses*, especially in relation to the movements of Leopold Bloom and Stephen Dedalus through the city of Dublin (Tucker, 1984) and Miriam O'Kane Mara takes the view that food refusal in a number of works by Joyce is worth exploring, not surprising perhaps given that famine is a recurring theme in Ireland's history (Mara, 2009). Virginia Woolf's difficult relationship with food, and what meals indicate about the process of existence, death, and mourning in her experimental novel *The Waves*, is explored in Utell (2008), whilst D. H. Lawrence, and other modernists including Woolf and Joyce, are discussed in the context of modernist food revulsion in Hollington (2010). Much of the literary criticism concerned with food in later twentieth-century women's fiction, written mainly by female, feminist critics, focuses on women's problematic relationships with food, for example not eating enough, eating too much, the preparation of food as a feminine endeavor, and the kitchen as a feminine space – criticism clearly influenced by Orbach (1978). In many of these studies the psychology of eating has taken the place of historical analysis, presumably because the reader is already familiar with the foods under discussion and so it is the manner in which they are consumed or avoided that is of most interest to these scholars. Typical of much feminist criticism of modern women's writing is

Sceats (2000), which considers the feeding mother and the starving female body. Sceats also considers what psychoanalytic theory can tell us about the cannibal motifs in Angela Carter's fiction and the wealth of food references in Margaret Atwood's fiction, writers who also come under close analysis respectively in Adolph (2009: 105–50) and Parker (1995). Although the collection of essays *Scenes of the Apple* deals with nineteenth- and twentieth-century women's writing, those essays on women's fiction, as opposed to their engagement in cultural politics, focus on the treatment of food in more recent material such as Toni Morrison's *Beloved* (Stanford, 2003) and the novels by Jeanette Winterson (Keen, 2003), the former emphasizing the interface between food and race, the latter between food and sexuality.

Research methodologies

Literary criticism on food has taken a variety of approaches, for example studies of food in the work of a particular author (Tucker, 1984; Lane, 1995; Fitzpatrick, 2007) and studies incorporating the work of a number of authors with critics taking a particular theoretical approach to their writing, for example feminism (Sceats, 2000; Adolph, 2009; Moss, 2009). Since most professional critics specialize in a particular historical period, most critical works also explore the workings of food in literature from a particular historical period but there are those that focus on the development in literature across the centuries of food-related philosophical and psychological phenomena such as eating disorders (Mazzoni, 2005; Gymnich and Lennartz, 2010). Not eating food, in the context of famine and food refusal, has also focused the attention of many critics (Gutierrez, 2003; Moore, 2008; Mara, 2009) as has unusual eating, specifically cannibalism (Marlow, 1983; Marvin, 1998; Noble, 2011). The interdisciplinary nature of much of the critical work done on literature that concerns itself with food is important: literary critics tend to focus not only on the usual suspects when it come to "lit crit" such as plays, novels, poems, but also other texts that have traditionally been beyond the remit of the literary scholar, such as dietary literature and cookery books (Appelbaum, 2006; Fitzpatrick, 2007; Thomas, 2008). The early modern period has witnessed a wealth of literary criticism on food in recent years, which reflects the empirical nature of much of the best literary criticism on food: explicating ingredients, dishes, and attitudes to feeding unfamiliar to a modern reader so as to facilitate their comprehension of the literary text in question. Historians have tended to lead the way and some of the best literary criticism takes a historical approach to writing about food, asking pertinent questions about the whys and wherefores of food consumption and how it relates to such issues as rank, gender, bodily health, national, and ethnic identity. Many of these works are keen to highlight the ways in which literature can inform us about the historical period in which it was written and vice versa.

Scholarship on Victorian literature has sought to interrogate nineteenth-century attitudes towards national identity, class, imperialism, and various problems surrounding food, including anxieties about food shortages, excess, and the adulteration of food (Cozzi, 2010; Hyman, 2009; Moore, 2008; Long, 1988) whilst critics on the Romantics have considered the role of the stomach in the context of the intellect (Morton, 2004; Gigante, 2005). Criticism on literature written in the twentieth century is more likely to be concerned with the psychology of eating (Tucker, 1984; Utell, 2008; Mara, 2009; Hollington, 2010), and female authors have attracted feminist critics concerned with body image and the gender politics of food and eating (Parker, 1995; Sceats, 2000; Adolph, 2009). In her essay on food in novels by the Brontë sisters Silvia Mergenthal notes that "food discourses revolve around a set of questions"; these questions are pertinent to all literary critics dealing with food across all periods and are worth repeating here:

What is considered edible?

How, and by whom, is food prepared and served?

When and how is food consumed?

How is the selection, preparation and consumption of food related to other discursive practices, for instance, to religious discourses which designate certain foodstuffs as sacred, others as profane, or to discourses of social distinction?

Finally, what, between the extremes of gluttony and self-starvation, is regarded as deviant with regard to consumption of food, and how should individuals who do not eat 'properly' be treated?

(Mergenthal, 2010: 206)

We might add more questions to the above, for example regarding gender, ethnicity, and so on, but this list works well as the basis for an interrogation by literary critics keen to probe what attitudes to food and diet might reveal about the literature itself, the historical period in which it was written, and human concerns about food.

Avenues for future research

There are no monographs devoted to Ben Jonson and food nor, aside from Meads's work on the banquet (2002), on the wealth of references to food and consumption in Jacobean drama generally; further work in these areas is needed. More work might also be done on early modern non-dramatic texts, specifically poetry and prose, which have received some attention (Hall, 1996; Schoenfeldt, 1999; Craik, 2004; Appelbaum, 2006) but require more; further study of Milton and Spenser would prove especially interesting. Although Shakespeare's plays have received some analysis in the first book-length study on the playwright and food (Fitzpatrick, 2007), much remains to be said and there is little critical material available on food in the sonnets and narrative poetry. Important inroads have been made in the study of the Romantics and the Victorians but there is little on eighteenth-century literature and it is surprising that, given the wealth of food references in Dickens, there is no monograph devoted to his engagement with food. Lane's monograph on Jane Austen is an important contribution to literary criticism and ought to provide the foundation for future work on Austen and food (Lane, 1995). Similarly, although fine work has been done so far on Margaret Atwood's detailed attention to food in her writing (Parker, 1995; Sceats, 2000: 94–124), a monograph could usefully broaden this body of knowledge.

Literary critics interested in food require good editions of literary and dietary texts, both canonical and marginal, so that the food references in these texts are made comprehensible to a wider readership, yet there is a clear gap in the market for editions upon which further research may be based. For example, dietary literature received some attention in the context of early modern literary culture in Appelbaum (2006) and Fitzpatrick (2007), but deserves fuller analysis in the context of early modern drama by Shakespeare and his contemporaries and other early modern writings. Most importantly, we need to be using modern critical editions based on the best early editions purged, where possible, of their errors. An edition of three important early modern dietaries is forthcoming (Fitzpatrick, 2013) but many more texts, dietaries, and other food-related books and pamphlets, languish unread because they are difficult to negotiate in their original editions. Another gap is the lack of reference works that might aid anyone interested in exploring literature and food. There are lots of good reference materials on the history of food, for example Davidson and Jaine 2006, but more works focusing specifically on literary references would facilitate research in this area. There is a dictionary on Shakespeare and the language of food (Fitzpatrick, 2010b) and similar works on the wealth of food reference by writers from other periods would be useful.

Critics tend to focus on one or two texts by an author where food most obviously features, for example Jonson's *Bartholomew Fair* or Austen's *Emma*, when more interrogation of references across an author's *oeuvre*, in the spirit of Lane (1995), might prove fruitful, as might more cross-period work on a particular theme or group of themes, such as Gymnich and Lennartz (2010). Additionally, work remains to be done on the relationship between gender and food; although much of the material on masculinity has constituted an original engagement with the literature under discussion, that on femininity, especially when focusing on the work of modern female authors, tends to focus specifically on what are perceived as female issues, such as problematic eating.

Ecocriticism might also prove a useful way into thinking about food for literary critics, illuminating how food consumption affects our fragile ecosystem, for example the destruction of rural landscapes and natural habitats in which plants and herbs thrive; the overproduction of beef to make fast food; the potential demise of bee colonies, and thus honey, which some experts claim is due to the use of pesticides. Victorian concerns about the adulteration of food speaks to our modern concerns about the dangerous substances regularly added to our food by the food industry and their genetic modification of natural foodstuffs. Eating disorders are not new – anorexia and gluttony have always been an issue – but obesity has become ubiquitous, at least in the developed world. Once the preserve of the rich gout-ridden gentleman, and thus, to some extent, a symbol of wealth, a fat body is no longer simply a feminist issue but has become undesirable for men and women and, along with alcohol abuse, constitutes a prominent concern for health professionals.

Practical considerations for getting started

There are a growing number of Masters programs in the US and UK offering courses on literature and food. The best way to locate which institutions have courses specializing in literature and food is to search the internet to find out where those scholars currently researching and publishing in this area are based, since many university departments encourage scholars to offer a course focusing on their specific area of specialism. The avenues for future research, noted above, might well take the form of PhD study under the supervision of a scholar who has published on food, and most will welcome informal queries regarding the viability of such a project. Many institutions offer funding in the form of bursaries or scholarships to pursue study in the humanities and it is worth consulting the websites of universities and research libraries to see what they have to offer, for example the Wellcome Trust in London will provide personal awards to undertake study in medical history and humanities (wellcome.ac.uk). External funding programs are also available to US and UK students who wish to study abroad (in the US or UK) and the Fulbright Commission offers valuable advice on opportunities available not only from Fulbright but other funding bodies, for example the British Council (fulbright.co.uk).

Keeping up to date on this growing area of scholarship will allow anyone interested in pursuing a career in food and literature to know what new publications they ought to be familiar with and what still remains relatively unexplored terrain. An important online resource for literary texts and criticism from all periods of English Literature is Chadwyck-Healey's

Literature Online (LION), access to which is via subscription. Other useful databases that require subscription include Early English Books Online (EEBO) and Eighteenth Century Collections Online (ECCO). The latest research on literary subjects including food is published in journal articles, and the definitive aid for discovering where articles on certain topics have been published is the Modern Language Association's International Bibliography (MLA-IB), sold by online subscription and included in LION, amongst other products. Online resources freely available on the web that are worth consulting for resources relating to literature and food include the following websites on culinary history:

www.historicfood.com
www.culinaryhistoriansboston.com/about.htm
www.culinaryhistoriansny.org

A good way to know who is working on what is to attend conferences where the cultural history of food comes up for discussion, for example the Oxford Symposium on Food and Cookery that takes place each year in England (www.oxfordsymposium.org.uk). Due to the burgeoning nature of interest in food and literature a number of large international meetings of scholars, for example the Renaissance Society of America, often include panel presentations and seminars especially devoted to the topic of food in literature; calls for papers for international conferences can be found at cfp.english.upenn.edu.

Key reading

Adelman, Janet (1992) *Suffocating Mothers: Fantasies of Maternal Origin in Shakespeare's Plays,* Hamlet *to* The Tempest. New York: Routledge.

Adolph, Andrea (2009) *Food and Femininity in Twentieth-century British Women's Fiction.* Farnham: Ashgate.

Anderson, Donald K., Jr. (1962) "The Heart and the Banquet: Imagery in Ford's *'Tis Pity* and *The Broken Heart.*" *Studies in English Literature, 1500–1900* 2: 209–17.

——(1964) "The Banquet of Love in English Drama (1595–1642)." *Journal of English and Germanic Philology* 63: 422–32.

Appelbaum, Robert (2006) *Aguecheek's Beef, Belch's Hiccup, and Other Gastronomic Interjections: Literature, Culture, and Food Among the Early Moderns.* Chicago, IL: University of Chicago Press.

Arvind, Thomas (2006) "Milton and Table Manners." *Milton Quarterly* 40.1, 37–47.

Beetham, Margaret (2008) "Good Taste and Sweet Ordering: Dining with Mrs Beeton." *Victorian literature and culture* 36: 391–406.

Biebel, Elizabeth M. (1998) "Pilgrims to Table: Food Consumption in Chaucer's *Canterbury Tales.*" In *Food and Eating in Medieval Europe.* Martha Carlin and Joel T. Rosenthal, eds. London: Hambledon, 15–26.

Boehrer, Bruce (1990) "Renaissance Overeating: The Sad Case of Ben Jonson." *Publications of the Modern Language Association of America* 105: 1071–82.

Borlik, Todd A. (2009) "'The Chameleon's Dish': Shakespeare and the Omnivore's Dilemma." *Early English Studies* 2: 1–23.

Brown, Marjorie (1998) "The Feast Hall in Anglo-Saxon Society." *Food and Eating in Medieval Europe.* Edited by Martha Carlin and Joel T. Rosenthal. London: Hambledon, 1–13.

Bryan, Margaret (1974) "Food Symbolism in *A Woman Killed With Kindness.*" *Renaissance Papers:* 9–17.

Bynum, Caroline Walker (1987) *Holy Feast and Holy Fast: The Religious Significance of Food to Medieval Women.* Berkeley: University of California Press.

Cable, Lana (1995) *Carnal Rhetoric: Milton's Iconoclasm and the Poetics of Desire.* Durham, NC: Duke University Press.

Candido, Joseph (1990) "Dining Out in Ephesus: Food in *The Comedy of Errors.*" *Studies in English Literature* 30: 217–41.

Carlin, Martha and Joel T. Rosenthal, eds. (1998) *Food and Eating in Medieval Europe.* London: Hambledon.

Charney, Maurice (1960) "The Imagery of Food and Eating in *Coriolanus*." In *Essays in Literary History Presented to J. Milton French*, Rudolf Kirk and C. F. Main, eds, pp. 37–55. New Brunswick, NJ: Rutgers University Press.

Cole, J. A. (1984) "Sunday Dinners and Thursday Suppers: Social and Moral Contexts of the Food Imagery in *Women Beware Women*." *Jacobean Miscellany*, vol. 4. James Hogg, ed., pp. 86–98. Salzburg Studies in English: Jacobean Drama Studies. Salzburg. Institut fur Anglistik und Amerikanistik, Universitat Salzburg.

Collins, Tracy J. R. (1998) "Eating, Food, and Starvation References in Conrad's *Heart of Darkness*." *Conradiana* 30.2: 152–60.

Cox, Lee Sheridan (1961) "Food-word Imagery in *Paradise Regained*." *English Literary History* 28: 225–43.

Cozzi, Annette. (2010) *The Discourses of Food in Nineteenth-century British Fiction*. Nineteenth-Century Major Lives and Letters. New York: Palgrave Macmillan.

Craik, Katharine A. (2004) "Reading Coryats Crudities (1611)." *Studies in English Literature, 1500–1900* 44: 77–96.

Daly, Suzanne and Ross G. Forman (2008) "Introduction: Cooking Culture: Situating Food and Drink in the Nineteenth Century." *Victorian Literature and Culture* 36: 363–73.

Davidson, Alan and Tom Jaine, eds. (2006) *The Oxford Companion to Food*. Oxford: Oxford University Press.

Day, Helen (2008) "A Common Complaint: Dining at The Reform Club." *Victorian Literature and Culture* 36: 507–30.

Dobson, Michael (2009) "'His Banquet is Prepared': Onstage Food and the Permeability of Time in Shakespearean Performance." *Shakespeare Jahrbuch* 145: 62–73.

Evans, Heather A. (2008) "Kittens and Kitchens: Food, Gender, and *The Tale of Samuel Whiskers*." *Victorian Literature and Culture* 36: 603–23.

Fisher, Joshua B. (2009) "Digesting Falstaff: Food and Nation in Shakespeare's *Henry IV* Plays." *Early English Studies* 2: 1–23.

Fitzpatrick, Joan (2007) *Food in Shakespeare: Early Modern Dietaries and the Plays*. Aldershot. Ashgate.

——(2009) "Apricots, Butter, and Capons: A Shakespearian Lexicon of Food." *Shakespeare Jahrbuch* 145: 74–90.

——ed. (2010a) *Renaissance Food from Rabelais to Shakespeare: Culinary Readings and Culinary Histories*. Aldershot: Ashgate.

——(2010b) *Shakespeare and the Language of Food: A Dictionary*. Student Shakespeare Library. London. Continuum.

——(2013) *Three Early Modern Dietaries: A Critical Edition*. The Revels Companion. Manchester: Manchester University Press.

Franson, John Karl (1976) "Bread and Banquet as Food for Thought: Experiential Learning in *Paradise Regained*." *Milton Reconsidered: Essays in Honor of Arthur E. Barker*. John Karl Franson, ed., pp. 154–92. Salzburg Studies in English: Elizabethan and Renaissance Studies. Salzburg. Institut fur Anglistik und Amerikanistik, Universitat Salzburg.

Fromer, Julie E. (2008) "'Deeply Indebted to the Tea Plant': Representations of English National Identity in Victorian Histories of Tea." *Victorian Literature and Culture* 36: 531–47.

Gigante, Denise (2000) "Milton's Aesthetics of Eating." *Diacritics* 30: 88–112.

——(2004) "The Endgame of Taste: Keats, Sartre, Beckett." *Cultures of Taste/Theories of Appetite: Eating Romanticism*. Timothy Morton, ed., pp. 183–201. New York: Palgrave Macmillan.

——(2005) *Taste: A Literary History*. New Haven, CT: Yale University Press.

Gutierrez, Nancy A. (2003) *Shall She Famish Then? Female Food Refusal in Early Modern England*. Women and Gender in the Early Modern World. Aldershot: Ashgate.

Gymnich, Marion and Norbert Lennartz, ed. (2010) *The Pleasures and Horrors of Eating: The Cultural History of Eating in Anglophone Literature*. Representations and Reflections. 1. Goettingen: V and R Unipress and Bonn University Press.

Hall, Kim F. (1996) "Culinary Spaces, Colonial Spaces: The Gendering of Sugar in the Seventeenth Century." *Feminist Readings of Early Modern Culture: Emerging Subjects*. Valerie Traub, M. Lindsay Kaplan, and Dympna Callaghan, eds., pp. 168–90. Cambridge: Cambridge University Press.

——(2009) "Sugar and Status in Shakespeare." *Shakespeare Jahrbuch* 145: 49–61.

Heller, Tamar and Patricia Moran, eds. (2003) *Scenes of the Apple: Food and the Female Body in Nineteenth- and Twentieth-century Women's Writing*. Albany: Albany State University of New York Press.

Holland, Peter (2009) "Feasting and Starving: Staging Food in Shakespeare." *Shakespeare Jahrbuch* 145: 11–28.

Hollington, Michael (2010) "Food, Modernity, Modernism: D. H. Lawrence and the Futurist Cookbook." *The Pleasures and Horrors of Eating: The Cultural History of Eating in Anglophone Literature*. Marion Gymnich and Norbert Lennartz, eds., pp. 305–21. Representations and Reflections. 1. Goettingen: V and R Unipress and Bonn University Press.

Hyman, Gwen (2008) "'An Infernal Fire in My Veins': Gentlemanly Drinking in *The Tenant of Wildfell Hall*." *Victorian Literature and Culture* 36: 451–69.

——(2009) *Making a Man: Gentlemanly Appetites in the Nineteenth-century British Novel*. Athens. Ohio University Press.

Keeling, Kara K. and Scott T. Pollard, eds. (2009) *Critical Approaches to Food in Children's Literature*. Children's Literature and Culture. New York: Routledge.

Keen, Suzanne (2003) "'I Cannot Eat My Words but I Do': Food, Body, and Word in the Novels of Jeanette Winterson." *Scenes of the Apple: Food and Female Body in Nineteenth- and Twentieth-century Women's Writing*. Edited by Tamar Heller and Patricia Moran. New York: State University of New York Press, 167–79.

Knowles, Katherine (2009) "Appetite and Ambition: The Influence of Hunger in *Macbeth*." *Early English Studies* 2: 1–20.

Lane, Maggie (1995) *Jane Austen and Food*. London: Hambledon.

Lewis, Daniel (2009) "The Middle-class Moderation of Food and Drink in *David Copperfield*." *Explicator* 67.2: 77–80.

Lipscomb, Robert (2009) "Caesar's Same-sex-food-sex Dilemma." *Early English Studies* 2: 1–13.

Long, William F. (1988) "Dickens and the Adulteration of Food." *The Dickensian* 84.3: 160–70.

Mara, Miriam O'Kane. (2009) "James Joyce and the Politics of Food." *New Hibernia Review* 13.4: 94–110.

Marlow, James E. (1983) "English Cannibalism: Dickens After 1859." *Studies in English Literature* 223.4: 647–66.

Marvin, Julia (1998) "Cannibalism as an Aspect of Famine in Two English Chronicles." *Food and Eating in Medieval Europe*. Martha Carlin and Joel T. Rosenthal, eds, pp. 73–86. London: Hambledon.

Mazzoni, Cristina (2005) *The Women in God's Kitchen: Cooking, Eating, and Spiritual Writing*. New York: Continuum.

Meads, Chris (2002) *Banquets Set Forth: Banqueting in English Renaissance Drama.* Manchester: Manchester University Press.

Mergenthal, Silvia (2010) "Dining with the Brontës: Food and Gender Roles in Mid-Victorian England." *The Pleasures and Horrors of Eating: The Cultural History of Eating in Anglophone Literature*. Marion Gymnich and Norbert Lennartz, eds, pp. 205–19. Representations and Reflections. 1. Goettingen: V and R Unipress and Bonn University Press.

Moore, Tara (2008) "Starvation in Victorian Christmas Fiction." *Victorian Literature and Culture* 36: 489–505.

Morse, Ruth (1983) "Unfit for Human Consumption: Shakespeare's Unnatural Food." *Jahrbuch der Deutschen Shakespeare-Gesellschaft West*, 125–49.

Morton, Timothy, ed. (2004) *Cultures of Taste/Theories of Appetite: Eating Romanticism*. New York: Palgrave Macmillan.

Moss, Sarah (2009) *Spilling the Beans: Eating, Cooking, Reading and Writing in British Women's Fiction, 1770–1830*. Manchester: Manchester University Press.

Mutch, Deborah (2008) "Intemperate Narratives: Tory Tipplers, Liberal Abstainers, and Victorian British Socialist Fiction." *Victorian Literature and Culture* 36: 471–87.

Noble, Louise (2003) "'And Make Two Pasties of Your Shameful Heads': Medicinal Cannibalism and Healing the Body Politic in *Titus Andronicus*." *English Literary History* 70: 677–708.

——(2011) *Medicinal Cannibalism in Early Modern English Literature and Culture*. Early Modern Cultural Studies. New York: Palgrave Macmillan.

Orbach, Susie (1978) *Fat is a Feminist Issue: The Anti-diet Guide to Permanent Weight Loss*. New York: Berkley Books.

Palma, Pina (2004) "Of Courtesans, Knights, Cooks and Writers: Food in the Renaissance." *Modern Language Notes* 119.1: 37–51.

Parker, Emma (1995) "You Are What You Eat: The Politics of Eating in the Novels of Margaret Atwood." *Twentieth-Century Literature* 41.3: 349–68.

Paroissien, David (2010) "Dyspepsia or Digestion: The Pleasures of the Board in *Martin Chuzzlewit*." *The Pleasures and Horrors of Eating: The Cultural History of Eating in Anglophone Literature*. Marion Gymnich and Norbert Lennartz, eds., pp. 221–35. Representations and Reflections. 1. Goettingen: V and R Unipress and Bonn University Press.

Pearlman, E. (1979) "Ben Jonson: An Anatomy." *English Literary Renaissance* 9: 364–94.

Plotnitsky, Arkady (2004) "Beyond the Inconsumable: The Catastrophic Sublime and the Destruction of Literature in Keats's *The Fall of Hyperion* and Shelley's *The Triumph of Life*." *Cultures of Taste/Theories of Appetite: Eating Romanticism*. Edited by Timothy Morton. New York: Palgrave Macmillan, 161–80.

Prasch, Thomas (2008) "Eating the World: London in 1851." *Victorian Literature and Culture* 36: 587–602.

Sceats, Sarah (2000) *Food, Consumption and the Body in Contemporary Women's Fiction*. Cambridge: Cambridge University Press.

Schaeffer, John D. (2000) "Metonymies we Read By: Rhetoric, Truth and the Eucharist in Milton's *Areopagitica*." *Milton Quarterly* 34.3: 84–92.

Schoenfeldt, Michael C. (1988) "'The Mysteries of Manners, Armes, and Arts': 'Inviting a Friend to Supper' and 'To Penshurst'." *"The Muses Common-Weale": Poetry and Politics in the Seventeenth Century*. Claude J. Summers and Ted-Larry Pebworth, eds., pp. 62–79. Essays in Seventeenth-Century Literature. 3. Columbia: University of Missouri Press.

——(1999) *Bodies and Selves in Early Modern England: Physiology and Inwardness in Spenser, Shakespeare, Herbert, and Milton*. Cambridge: Cambridge University Press.

Sen, Sharmila (2008) "The Saracen's Head." *Victorian Literature and Culture* 36: 407–31.

Smith, Nigel (1990) "*Areopagica* Voicing Contexts, 1643–45." *Politics, Poetics, and Hermeneutics in Milton's Prose*. Edited by David Loewenstein and James G. Turner. Cambridge: Cambridge University Press, 103–22.

Spurgeon, Caroline (1935) *Shakespeare's Imagery: And What it Tells Us*. Cambridge: Cambridge University Press.

Stabler, Jane (2004) "Byron's World of Zest." *Cultures of Taste/Theories of Appetite: Eating Romanticism*. Timothy Morton, ed., pp. 141–60. New York: Palgrave Macmillan.

Stanford, Ann Folwell (2003) "'Death is a Skipped Meal Compared to This': Food and Hunger in Toni Morrison's *Beloved*." *Scenes of the Apple: Food and Female Body in Nineteenth- and Twentieth-century Women's Writing*. Edited by Tamar Heller and Patricia Moran. New York: State University of New York Press, 129–47.

Thomas, Kate (2008) "Alimentary: Arthur Conan Doyle and Isabella Beeton." *Victorian Literature and Culture* 36: 375–90.

Tucker, Lindsey (1984) *Stephen and Bloom at Life's Feast: Alimentary Symbolism and the Creative Process in James Joyce's* Ulysses. Columbus: Ohio State University Press.

Utell, Janine (2008) "Meals and Mourning in Woolfe's *The Waves*." *College Literature* 35.2: 1–19.

Viltos, Paul (2008) "Conrad's Idea of Gastronomy: Dining in 'Falk'." *Victorian Literature and Culture* 36: 433–49.

Weiss, Susan F. (1998) "Medieval and Renaissance Wedding Banquets and Other Feasts." *Food and Eating in Medieval Europe*. Edited by Martha Carlin and Joel T. Rosenthal. London: Hambledon, 159–74.

Williamson, Cary Cecile (1979) "The Iconography of Food and the Motif of World Order in *Friar Bacon and Friar Bungay*." *Comparative Drama* 13: 150–63.

Young, Paul (2008) "The Cooking Animal: Economic Man at The Great Exhibition." *Victorian Literature and Culture* 36: 569–86.

Youngquist, Paul (2004) "Romantic Dietetics! Or, Eating Your Way to a New You." *Cultures of Taste/Theories of Appetite: Eating Romanticism*. Timothy Morton, ed., pp. 237–55. New York: Palgrave Macmillan.

12

Philosophy and food

Lisa Heldke

Philosophy has only recently begun the formal study of food, although philosophers have been discussing food since Plato. The philosophical study of food can be understood to take up four separate but related tasks ranging from least to most transformative. They are: (1) applying received philosophical categories to new or uncustomary topics in food; (2) reconceptualizing an existing philosophical discussion as a discussion in the philosophy of food; (3) reclaiming or recovering previous philosophical work relevant to the study of food; and (4) recasting familiar philosophical problems by way of analyses of food, thereby revealing new categories of philosophical understanding.

Philosophy has come to the food studies table rather more reluctantly than some other humanities disciplines. But while it has been slow to embrace the formal study of food, Western philosophy has always been concerned, in peripheral ways, with matters of eating and drinking. From Plato to Hume to Nietzsche, philosophers have reflected upon humans' relationships to food and drink, even if only to dismiss these concerns as inconsequential or base. As contemporary philosophers have begun to make food a topic of serious and concentrated study, they have also begun to revisit these earlier thinkers, in order to ask: how does our understanding of historic philosophers deepen when we consider their discussions of food as something more or other than casually chosen illustrations, examples and metaphors? Some contemporary philosophers of food believe that such work can fundamentally reshape the discipline; that beginning philosophy with questions about humans' relations to food not only will bring us to new understandings of historic figures, but also will invite us to reconsider the most fundamental, perennial problems of philosophy. What does it mean to be a person? What does it mean to know? What are our obligations to others? If we begin with the unavoidable fact of our being as *eaters,* and not just as *thinkers,* such fundamental rethinking inevitably follows.

Contemporary philosophers have come to study food for reasons both internal and external to the discipline. Internally, questions of humans' relations to food have arisen quite naturally, even necessarily, for theorists challenging a certain historical prejudice against the body, practice, ordinary everydayness, and temporality. It has come to seem odd, even unthinkable, that philosophy—the discipline that, more than any other, concerns itself with questions of meaning and value in human life—would be silent about food, a primary source of meaning and value. Philosophers working in this framework have, for instance, explored the aesthetic significance of food—showing how food reveals the impoverishment of the notion of "art," and the need for a more expansive definition of "the aesthetic" (see Korsmeyer, 1999). Others have used the model of the parasite (the "co-eater" or "table mate") to reconceptualize a fundamental onto-logical concept: substance (see Serres, 2007; Boisvert, *Parasite*). Still others have found in recipes an instance of theory making that resists arbitrary and invidious distinctions between reason and emotion, theory and practice (see, e.g., Heldke, "Recipes"). And others, acknowledging the presence of *culture* in *agriculture,* have looked to it as a way to revisit notions of community (see, e.g., Thompson 2010, 2007, 1994; Kirschenmann 2010).

One significant external reason for the rise in philosophical interest in food is the surge of public interest in, and attention to, food. Philosophers in the classroom have found in the subject an important lens through which to examine philosophical problems, particularly in ethics and environmental philosophy. Several anthologies have been created, partly in an effort to address the needs of such courses; examples include works by Fritz Allhoff and Dave Munroe; Ben Mepham; Gregory Pence; and David Kaplan.

Philosophers committed to public philosophy, and to expanding its role in public life, have found their insights valued in public debates about the safety of our food, the future of our food system, and the cultural meanings of our foods. However, while philosophy is welcomed into public conversations, it is the task of philosophers to push these conversations beyond formulaic moral dichotomies ("organic foods: yes or no?" "are genetically engineered seeds good or bad?"). Arguably, the chief contribution philosophy can make to discussions of food—in the public sphere *and* the academy—is to reveal underlying assumptions that bind and limit those discussions. Philosophy best contributes to public conversations about food not by solving or resolving ethical or aesthetic conundrums, but by problematizing the terms of those conundrums.

Historical background of food scholarship in philosophy and major theoretical approaches in use

One might argue, without irony, that Western philosophy began in considerations of food, and has never stopped. Plato, I noted, examines food with considerable regularity in his dialogues; in the *Republic,* the desire to consume meat and other luxuries leads the state to annex new territory—a move which necessitates war—and the *Timaeus* explains that the human digestive tract is long in order to enable us to think for long periods of time, uninterrupted by a growling stomach. (Plato is also one of those figures whose veneration of thinking led him to dismiss our stomachy nature as something that should be ignored whenever possible.) On the other end of that history, the contemporary French deconstructionist Jacques Derrida argues that the central ethical question is not "whether or not to eat but how to eat," a question that "comes back to determining the best, most respectful, most grateful, and also most giving way of relating to the other and of relating the other to the self" (quoted in Oliver, 2009: 105). And ethicists such as Peter Singer and Tom Regan answer that question by asserting what we ought *not* to eat: animals. Between these centuries, we find Michel de Montaigne's confession that he bites his fingers when he eats, so greedy is he; David Hume's discussions of literal tasting, in his essay "Of the Standard of Taste"; and Jean Anthelme Brillat-Savarin's famous proclamation "Tell me what you eat and I will tell you who you are," in his *Physiology of Taste.* (Indeed, philosophy seems particularly rich in food-related *aphorisms*; consider also Feuerbach's related assertion—much cleverer in the original German—that one is what one eats: "man ist was er isst"; and young Novalis's obser-vation—now flung by parents with painful frequency at offspring declaring their intention to major in the subject: "Philosophy bakes no bread.")

But is Brillat-Savarin really a philosopher? Or is Montaigne, for that matter? And would either Plato or Peter Singer call himself a philosopher of food? The answer to that last question is undoubtedly "no," and debates over the pedigrees of the first two figures are likely to go on forever. Part of the reason for the dispute over the philosophical credentials of Montaigne and Brillat-Savarin is, of course, precisely the fact that both figures take up subjects considered too menial, ordinary, or commonplace to be proper to so lofty a discipline as philosophy. Philosophy has, for the most part, displayed a neglect, even an abhorrence, of all things bodily; food, unavoidably, draws attention to our bodily being: we hunger, gobble, defecate, and eventually die, to be set upon by hungry worms. Who would wish to be reminded of these painful facts, when we could instead turn our attentions to the beauty of timeless truths?

Exceptions exist. Some food-related topics—the ethics of eating animals and the politics of famine—have been perennial staples of ethics and socio-political philosophy, and since the 1980s, eating disorders have been a topic of research for feminist philosophers. (Notably, all three of these topics concern themselves primarily with what one shouldn't, can't, or won't eat.) Much contemporary work on vegetarianism and animals pays homage to the work begun by Tom Regan and Peter Singer in the 1970s. In the 1980s, Amartya Sen, Susan George, Joseph Collins, and Frances Moore Lappe produced pathbreaking work (now considered to be the standard view) on the causes and consequences of hunger and of famine. And Susan Bordo's work on anorexia as a "crystallization of popular culture" opened new possibilities for feminist philosophical work on food, body, and personhood.

Work on philosophy of food that self-consciously identifies itself with the emerging discipline of food studies might be said to have begun in 1987, the year philosopher Richard Haynes founded the Agriculture, Food and Human Values Society. Five years later, Deane Curtin and Lisa Heldke published *Cooking, Eating, Thinking: Transformative Philosophies of Food,* which examined the question "how might fundamental philosophical problems be reshaped, were we to take seriously humans' relationships to food?" At about that time, Paul Thompson began to make agriculture a serious subject for environmental philosophers; his work *The Spirit of the Soil* was published in 1994. Five years after that, Carolyn Korsmeyer produced *Making Sense of Taste,* the first major work to treat food as a topic of aesthetic consideration.

Scholarly works in the philosophy of food produced since 1990 can be grouped according to a rough taxonomy that sorts them according to the kinds of philosophical tasks they undertake. I've identified four such tasks, arranged in order of "disruptiveness," from those that leave the philosophical terrain most undisturbed, to those that have the potential to effect the most profound changes to it.

- *Task 1: Applying received philosophical categories to new or uncustomary topics in food.* Works in this category undertake a somewhat conservative task, albeit one that also has radical potential: they add food-related topics to the list of problems and questions considered within the main subfields of philosophy. Aestheticians who debate the question "is cuisine an art, and if so, is it a high or low art?" are engaging in this first task. They are applying an established aesthetic concept—art—to an atypical topic—cuisine—and in so doing, are extending the legitimate domain of that concept. The entire field that goes by the name of "applied philosophy" might fall under this first task. Stated simply, applied philosophy considers how general theories—Aristotle's virtue ethics, Mill's utilitarianism—address specific concrete, everyday situations. For example, in their now-famous works on animals, Peter Singer and Tom Regan apply utilitarianism and virtue ethics, respectively, to argue against eating animals.
- *Task 2: Reconceptualizing an existing philosophical discussion as a discussion in the philosophy of food.* Work in this category shifts the camera angle to bring heretofore unnoticed food aspects

into focus. Consider: while vegetarianism has been a topic of philosophical discussion for centuries, it has generally been understood to be about *animals*. What happens if we think of vegetarianism as also being about *food and eating?* As philosophy of food becomes a more familiar field, I submit that a variety of existing philosophical topics can be understood to have connections to it. Hunger is another such topic, as is the notion of the commons. In the first case, it is not as if existing philosophical work on hunger denies that it is about food, but rather that placing the work in a context with other work explicitly addressing food exposes new features of the work and makes it resonate on new frequencies. In the case of the commons, discussing the concept in a food-focused context is indeed a relatively unexplored approach.

- *Task 3: Reclaiming or recovering previous philosophical work relevant to the study of food.* I've already suggested rereading Plato with an eye to his discussions of food; such a project is an example of this third task. Other Western philosophers are even more important to reclaim as proto food philosophers. Philosophers of agriculture working to create "new agrarianisms" are, for instance, recovering texts and concepts from theorists such as Virgil, Jefferson, and Emerson—texts that develop explicit theories about the roles of agriculture in culture. These new agrarians are further showing why and how the agrarian roots of other historical philosophers must be recovered and acknowledged. How have we covered over or forgotten the food and agriculture foci of our philosophical history?
- *Task 4: Recasting familiar philosophical problems by way of analyses of food, thereby revealing new categories of philosophical understanding.* How can the study of food disrupt or transform long-standing features of our philosophical map? How can it reveal unacknowledged philosophical presuppositions, thereby making the way for fundamentally new ways of philosophical thinking? I have already mentioned one significant example of this sort of recasting—namely, reconceiving humans as not simply thinkers, but eaters. How do the terms of the traditional mind/body problem shift if we take very seriously Plato's observation that we must eat in order to think? Similarly, how does the epistemological problem of how we can know the external world shift, if we notice (as John Dewey does), that "the problem of how a mind can know an external world ... is like the problem of how an animal eats things external to itself" (Dewey, 1988: 212)?

While these four tasks vary in their potential to affect philosophical thinking, even the least disruptive of them still disrupts; you can't ask whether cuisine is art without producing some boomerang effects upon future aesthetic discussions of the nature of painting or music, triggering a Task 4 discussion. Work of all four types plays important roles in developing philosophy of food and contributing to food studies. Here, I briefly discuss some of the significant works produced since 1990, using the taxonomy from above and grouping them by philosophical subdiscipline.

Ethics. Ethical questions are among the first and most likely questions to which philosophers have turned, as they have come to the study of food (just as they have been the questions philosophers in history have most often considered). Michiel Korthals's *Before Dinner* is a densely packed volume that undertakes both Tasks 1 and 3, to consider such issues as: Can we justify eating other animals? What are the responsibilities of consumers in a consumer society? How can we reconcile the promise and the peril of "high-tech" foods, such as those produced using sophisticated biotechnology? How does the just society adjudicate the matter of the nutrition of its citizens? In the spirit of Task 1, Korthals explicitly considers the concrete consequences of abstract ethical positions; in fact a central plank of his own ethical position is "applicationism," which acknowledges that "philosophical ethics has been overly concerned with the justification of principles … and far too little with the altogether different issue of their application" (Korthals, 2004: 51). This book—and a subsequent article, "The Birth of Philosophy and the Contempt for Food," also take up Task 3, cataloguing historical philosophers' observations about food production and consumption. In the latter work, he expresses hope that attention to the ethics of food "will change the philosophers' historical neglect" (p. 68).

Ethics and agriculture. Philosophers working on ethical issues in agriculture are perhaps the most active and prolific group of philosophers working on food, and have made the clearest marks on both philosophy and food studies. Agriculture in the twentieth century presents a host of pressing issues, including where and how our food will be grown, and even *what* will be grown. Among the most challenging issues are the nature of the present industrial agricultural system, and the promise and problems of the genetic engineering of our food supply. While they possess no specialized or unique body of *agricultural* knowledge, philosophers can and do bring to the debates on these issues an ability to excavate and interrogate the presuppositions on which they are founded.

Paul Thompson's *Food Biotechnology in Ethical Perspective* well exemplifies the contributions philosophy can make to this technical field. Thompson draws upon his sophisticated lay understanding of the science of biotechnology to consider ethical issues that arise for both animals and plants; consent, unintended consequences, trust, property. The work is an example of a Task 4 work, pressing, as it does, the limits of how we understand these philosophical concepts. It is also an instance of Task 2, insofar as Thompson is exploring issues that are often considered as philosophy of technology issues, but is framing them within a discussion that is explicitly about food.

Another, very different sort of project in ethics and agriculture situates itself in the tradition of agrarianism, and draws upon earlier agrarians, including Virgil, Jefferson, Emerson, and Thoreau. This is Task 3 work, reminding us of the role previous philosophers have assigned to agriculture, and rejuvenating that role for the present context. *The Agrarian Roots of Pragmatism,* a suggestively titled anthology edited by Paul Thompson and Thomas Hilde, makes explicit some of the ways pragmatism, the quintessentially American species of philosophy, emerged out of a context in which agriculture held a defining role in the culture.

At present, philosophy of agriculture often finds itself in conversation with philosophies of the environment—conversations that can minimize the degree to which agriculture is understood to involve growing *food.* Its conversations will certainly change and expand, as philosophy of agriculture comes to be more frequently cross-fertilized with philosophy of food. Such projects will likely be of the Task 2 variety.

Ethical vegetarianism. Feminist theorists have been particularly interested in the significance of meat eating for women; Carol Adams's work *The Sexual Politics of Meat* draws links between the oppression of women and the exploitation of animals to argue for vegetarianism, while *Animal, Vegetable or Woman,* by Kathryn Paxton George challenges arguments for vegetarianism from a feminist perspective. Deane Curtin works to develop what he calls a "contextual moral vegetarianism." His work slants toward Task 4, in that it upends received conceptions of personhood, putting in their place relational models that take seriously the adage "you are what you eat."

Social and political philosophy: hunger. Existing philosophical works that explore hunger often do so within the framework of distributive justice—by what means do we make decisions about how goods are distributed in a society or in the world? Significant bodies of work on hunger exist within both the literature of development ethics and the literature of environmental philosophy. In the former category is a collection of essays edited by William Aiken and Hugh LaFollette entitled *World Hunger and Morality*. Tom Regan's edited collection *Earthbound* couches issues of hunger in terms of environmental consequences. Regan suggests that all of environmental philosophy might be considered by way of the contents of one's dinner plate—a move that frames this work as a Task 2 kind of project.

Social and political philosophy: food, race/ethnicity and culture. Ethnic cuisines present an interesting terrain on which to explore questions about race, ethnicity, and culture. My own work *Exotic Appetites* explores "cultural colonialism," an attitude with which persons of racial privilege approach the food of the "ethnic" Other, and characterized by an obsession with novelty, a view of the Other as a resource for one's own use and adornment, and a passion for "authenticity." It is a kind of Task 1 work that shows the way to Task 4 projects.

Social and political philosophy: justice. Abby Wilkerson's work begins in Task 1, by extending the reach of the concept of justice to consider the matter of size and weight. It emerges into a Task 4 project of reconceptualizing justice in a way that renders the body an essential element of it. Situated in recent efforts in political philosophy to bring attention to the neglected significance of the body for the social contract, her forthcoming book demonstrates that the notion of obesity plays an extensive role in cultural politics, influencing social roles and relationships from the most intimate levels of personal identity to interactions between social groups and even nations.

Aesthetics. Elizabeth Telfer's *Food for Thought: Philosophy and Food* is a Task 1 work. It addresses the question "Is cuisine an art form?" Telfer concludes that it *is*, though a minor art form not capable of producing the highest, most profound sorts of aesthetic experiences. Telfer suggests that its pleasures are of a subordinate sort; a fine meal can enhance an evening at the symphony, resulting in an aggregate aesthetic experience more profound than attending the symphony alone. Carolyn Korsmeyer's *Making Sense of Taste,* on the other hand, is an example of a Task 4 work. In conducting her analysis of taste-the-sense alongside taste-the-aesthetic-sensibility, Korsmeyer asks why those forms of human creativity associated with sensory taste have been relegated to the aesthetic backwater, and, furthermore, why *aesthetic* taste has been defined in such a way as to marginalize or exclude them.

Value theory—aesthetics, ethics and social political philosophy—is, not surprisingly, the area of philosophy that has seen the most work on food. Ontology and epistemology, on the other hand, are relatively untapped to date. This is beginning to change. By exploring humans' relations to food on the most elemental levels (ingestion and elimination, for example), we cannot but come to question received Western notions of being and knowing that conceive of an absolute separation of knower from known, self from other. As Ray Boisvert observes: "Taking seriously our status as embodied and encultured … philosophers could actually begin to grasp philosophizing as a 'human' rather than as a 'mental' activity" (2001a). Work in these areas almost of necessity takes up Task 4, both transforming fundamental philosophical concepts transforming the fundamental relationships between and among philosophical categories.

Ontology: food and embodiment/body image. Feminist philosophers have often avoided the topic of food. Notable exceptions to this generalization are ecofeminist discussions of vegetarianism and of feminist development theorists' discussions of hunger. The other important exception involves the body and embodiment. The feminist philosophical literature on embodiment has, over the past two decades, presented a sustained, nuanced, and multi-faceted attack on received philosophical notions of human personhood, a central topic in ontology. According to the prevailing Cartesian model, humans are minds that are only accidentally attached to inferior bodies. Women, in Western thought, have been defined as more fully tied to our bodies and to all things bodily, because of our role in reproduction, our traditional tasks as caretakers of bodies, and our identification with sex and the sexual. As such, we have historically been regarded as incomplete or defective humans. Feminists have been at the forefront of challenging this ontological legacy, and explicating the ways in which it marginalizes and subordinates women.

Some feminists have examined these questions of embodiment specifically in terms of women's relations to food. The most well known and important of these theorists is Susan Bordo, whose work *Unbearable Weight* explores the construction of women's embodiment in contemporary culture, particularly through an examination of women's eating, both ordered and disordered. Her work "reads" in the bodies of the anorexic, the bulimic, and the "properly thin" woman manifestations of the historical Western disdain for, even hatred of, the body, extending all the way to Plato. Through her examination of contemporary women's relations to food, Bordo reveals ethical and social ramifications of our ontological commitments, and initiates a reconstitution of a fundamental Western ontological category.

Ontology: subject/object dualism. No philosophers of food have yet developed full-blown critiques of the fundamental ontological division between subject and object—between myself as a perceiver/possessor of the world and the items in the world that enter my vision. But eating profoundly violates this purportedly fundamental dichotomy. One piece that initiates such critique is Deane Curtin's "Food, Body, Person," in which he develops a relational model of the self that takes explicit account of the fact that, in eating, the "not-me" very literally becomes me.

Epistemology. In the twentieth century, scientific investigation (or an idealized version of it) has come to stand as *the* model of inquiry and knowing, in terms of which all other knowledge-producing activities are judged—and often found lacking. Science—or our idealized version of it—embodies the very qualities Descartes taught us to seek in our inquiry: Dispassion, disengagement, and an emphasis on abstract principles and timeless certainty. Foodmaking presents an interesting challenge to this model of knowing; my "Recipes for Theory Making," and "Foodmaking as a Thoughtful Practice" explore the suggestion.

Ray Boisvert presents a related proposal in his call for "convivial epistemology," which begins with the notion of humans as beings *living with* their surroundings—not subjects studying objects external to themselves. Such an understanding of knowing uproots a whole variety of received philosophical problems and preconditions, including, for instance, the problem of skepticism and the separation of fact and value. Boisvert's work—the essay "Convivial Epistemology" as well as other of his writings—stands as the clearest example of work that takes on the fourth task. His ways of examining food unearth the profound potential that it possesses to transform the very ways in which we ask the most basic questions of philosophy.

Research methodologies

Ray Boisvert notes: "At the intersection of food and philosophy, the key methodological consideration is flexibility. There must be a sensitivity to, and place for, empirical investigations, for hermeneutical strategies, for historical and sociological contextualization of positions … Philosophical texts cannot now be [approached as if] ideas exist independently of context … [The] history of ideas cannot be examined apart from history of social practices" (private correspondence). In addition to flexibility and contextuality, philosophy of food is motivated by a skepticism or curiosity about received categories, divisions, and hierarchies, and a willingness to rethink, reinvent, and restructure these in light of humans' profound, multifaceted relationships to food.

Whether or not there exist any such things as identifiable philosophical "methodologies" is a subject of considerable dispute among philosophers. It is more typical to sort philosophers according to schools or traditions of thought, which are characterized more by fealty to particular historical figures and questions than by particular methods of inquiry or analysis. It is, however, possible to make some meaningful methodological distinctions among these traditions, and to identify those that promise to be most useful and rewarding for philosophers.

Arguably, the school of philosophy that has been the most productive of, involved in, and influential upon, food studies is American pragmatism. The connection is unsurprising, given that pragmatist philosophy has traditionally rejected many of the traditional hierarchical dichotomies upon which other schools of philosophy have rested—dichotomies that have rendered the study of food unimportant, irrelevant, or impossible: mind versus body, theory versus practice and even reason versus emotion. Pragmatist philosophy begins from the understanding that philosophical questions begin in, and return to, the concerns of everyday human life. Thus, for example, the historical pragmatist John Dewey recognized the value of activities such as cooking and gardening for educating children in ways that do not reproduce the theory/practice dichotomy, while the contemporary pragmatist-inspired Ray Boisvert creatively draws upon bouillabaisse to conceive of a philosophy that replaces purity with complicated admixtures, and strict reasoning with "fuzzy logic;" and feminist pragmatist Heldke conceives of cooking as a "thoughtful practice" that resists the theory/practice division. Furthermore, pragmatist philosophy has significant connections to the tradition of agrarianism that has influenced the thinking of prominent philosophers of agriculture such as Paul Thompson and Fred Kirschenmann.

Continental philosophy has also shown a readiness to embrace some food-related themes. This, too is unsurprising; phenomenology, one influential strand of Continental thought, has concerned itself centrally with matters of bodily being, and existentialism, another important strand, has focused on conditions of human existence—both clearly approaches in which the matter of humans' relations to food bears considerable importance. The nineteenth-century Nietzsche devotes a considerable section of his work *Ecce Homo* to the matter of his own diet ("Why I Am So Clever), while in the twenty-first century, Kelly Oliver draws upon the work of deconstructionist Jacques Derrida to develop an "ethics of sustaining relationships" vis à vis other animals—an ethics that inevitably must address the matter of whether or not we eat them.

Avenues for future research

Philosophers interested in food might pursue one of two trajectories, one more focused on disciplinary interests and the other more directed toward participation in the multidisciplinary and interdisciplinary work of food studies. The opportunities to make meaningful contributions to both nascent projects are vast.

The most important disciplinary projects are Task 4 projects that use humans' profound, non-optional relationships to food to instigate rethinking of philosophical conceptions such as personhood, knowing, ethical agency, and aesthetic expression. A metaphilosophical question asks about the usual hierarchy that is presumed among philosophical subdisciplines: If we begin philosophy from humans' relations to food, do metaphysics and epistemology remain *the* foundational philosophical projects? Does aesthetics remain a secondary or even tertiary field? And do relations and dependencies among these subdisciplines remain unchanged?

Also intriguing are Task 2 projects that refocus existing conversations inside new contexts. I have mentioned revisiting vegetarianism as a philosophy of food, placing philosophy of agriculture in the context of philosophy of food, and reconsidering questions in philosophy of technology as questions about food. Many more such projects are possible.

Moving on to the second trajectory, there is important work for philosophers to do within food studies itself, by contributing to work on such crucial issues as: The perils and promises of genetically modified foods, and of organic foods; the future of the (alternative) food system(s); the "obesity epidemic"; food and authenticity; sustainability; food security and food sovereignty; food and identity; agrarianism; nationalism and cosmopolitanism; the food voice; food and disability; food and racial identity. While philosophy does not produce bodies of qualitative or quantitative data, nor is it the aggregator of historical knowledge, the discipline's capacities for drawing distinctions, teasing out assumptions, making conceptual connections, and posing critical questions are arguably important tools to include in the interdisciplinary research projects that the study of food, by its very nature, requires.

Practical considerations for getting started—funding, programs, archival sources, tools, data sets, internet resources, scholarships and awards, etc. (where and how?)

For philosophers, as for food scholars in many disciplines, the most important academic organizations are the Association for the Study of Food and Society (ASFS), and the aforementioned Agriculture, Food and Human Values Society (AFHV). Philosophers make up a small but significant percentage of members in both organizations. Philosophical organizations friendly to the study of food include the Society for the Advancement of American Philosophy (SAAP), the Society for Phenomenology and Existential Philosophy (SPEP), and the Society for the Philosophy of Creativity. Convivium: The Philosophy and Food Roundtable, a small organization, holds occasional sessions at meetings of the American Philosophical Association.

Food studies journals that publish significant numbers of philosophical articles include *Agriculture and Human Values* (the journal of the AFHV), *The Journal of Agricultural and Environmental Ethics,* and *Food, Culture and Society* (the journal of the ASFS).

The largest—indeed, perhaps the only—repository of food philosophy on the internet is housed at the University of North Texas, and is the work of David Kaplan. It can be found at www.food.unt.edu (accessed on April 2, 2012). The site is most valuable for its extensive and wide-ranging bibliography of food-related philosophy and philosophy-related food writing. It also features an introductory essay about philosophy of food. The ambitious site promises in the future to feature book reviews and arguments in significant food debates.

At the time of this writing, the publisher Springer is overseeing the production of a multi-volume encyclopedia, *The Encyclopedia of Food and Agricultural Ethics*, which will be available in both print and electronic forms. Edited by P. B. Thompson, R. Bawden, D. M. Kaplan, and K. Millar, it will serve as an invaluable resource, especially but not exclusively for persons interested in ethical, socio-political, and cultural aspects of food and agricultural production.

Students interested in graduate study in philosophy of food should consider whether they are primarily philosophers interested in the study of food, or food scholars who wish to take a philosophical perspective on their study. The latter would be best served by graduate programs in food studies that have a strong humanities focus, such as Boston University's Gastronomy Program. Students of philosophy who seek to write a dissertation on a food-related theme should consider philosophy programs strong in American pragmatism or Continental philosophy, or that describe themselves as pluralistic, since these departments are most likely to find the study of food legitimate, for reasons discussed above. It is wise to remember that the study of food is still relatively odd in philosophy departments, and will be genuinely unwelcome in some.

Key reading

Adams, Carol J. (1990) *The Sexual Politics of Meat: A Feminist Vegetarian Critical Theory*. New York: Continuum.
Aiken, William and Hugh LaFollette (1996) *World Hunger and Morality*. 2nd ed. Upper Saddle River, NJ: Prentice Hall.
Allhoff, Fritz and Dave Monroe (2007) *Food and Philosophy: Eat, Think and Be Merry*. Upper Saddle River, NJ: Wiley-Blackwell.

Boisvert, Raymond D. (2006) "Hungry Being: The Parasite." Unpublished manuscript.

——(2001a) "Food Transforms Philosophy." *The Maine Scholar* 14: 1–14.

——(2001b) "Philosophy Regains its Senses." *Food for Thought*. Special issue of *Philosophy Now* 31: www. pdcnet.org/collection/show?id=philnow_2001_0031_0000_0009_0011&file_type=pdf (accessed June 26, 2011).

Boisvert, Raymond D. and Lisa Heldke (forthcoming) *Philosophers at Table*. London: Reaktion.

Bordo, Susan (1995) *Unbearable Weight: Feminism, Western Culture and the Body*. Berkeley: University of California Press.

Brillat-Savarin, Jean Anthelme (2000) *The Physiology of Taste, Or Meditations on Transcendental Gastronomy*. Trans. M. F. K. Fisher. Berkeley, CA: Counterpoint.

Curtin, Deane (1992) "Food, Body, Person." In *Cooking, Eating, Thinking: Transformative Philosophies of Food*. Deane Curtin and Lisa Heldke, eds. Bloomington: Indiana University Press.

Curtin, Deane and Lisa Heldke (1992) *Cooking, Eating, Thinking: Transformative Philosophies of Food*. Bloomington: Indiana University Press.

Derrida, Jacques (2000) *Of Hospitality: Cultural Memory in the Present*. Stanford, CA: Stanford University Press.

——(1995) "Eating Well, Or the Calculation of the Subject" in *Points …: Interviews, 1974–1994*. Stanford, CA: Stanford University Press.

Dewey, John (1988) *Experience and Nature. 1925. The Later Works of John Dewey*. Volume 1. Carbondale: Southern Illinois University Press.

Garrison, Jim, and Bruce W. Watson (2005) "Food From Thought." *Journal of Speculative Philosophy* 19.4: 242–56.

George, Susan (1989) *How the Other Half Dies: The Real Reasons for World Hunger*. London: Penguin.

Heldke, Lisa (2003) *Exotic Appetites: Ruminations of a Food Adventurer*. New York: Routledge.

——(1988) "Recipes for Theory Making." *Hypatia: A Journal of Feminist Philosophy* 3.2: 15–30.

Heldke, Lisa, Kerri Mommer, and Cindy Pineo (2005) *The Atkins Diet and Philosophy*. Chicago, IL: Open Court.

Hume, David (1965) "Of the Standard of Taste." *Of the Standard of Taste and Other Essays*. Upper Saddle River, NJ: Prentice Hall.

Iggers, Jeremy, ed. (2001) *Philosophy Now* Special issue *Food for Thought* 31: www.pdcnet.org/collection/show?id=philnow_2001_0031_0000_0009_0011&file_type=pdf (accessed on 25 June, 2011).

——(1996) *The Garden of Eating: Food, Sex and the Hunger of Meaning*. New York: Basic Books.

Jager, Ronald (2004) *The Fate of the Family Farm*. Lebanon, NH: University Press of New England.

Kaplan, David, ed. (forthcoming) *The Philosophy of Food*. Berkeley: University of California Press.

——*The Philosophy of Food Project*. University of North Texas, food.unt.edu (accessed on 24 June, 2011).

Kass, Leon R. (1994) *The Hungry Soul: Eating and the Perfecting of Our Nature*. Chicago, IL: University of Chicago Press.

Kirschenmann, Fred (2010) *Cultivating an Ecological Conscience: Essays from a Farmer Philosopher*. Lexington: University Press of Kentucky.

Korsmeyer, Carolyn (2011) *Savoring Disgust: The Foul and the Fair in Aesthetics*. Oxford: Oxford University Press.

——(1999) *Making Sense of Taste: Food and Philosophy*. Ithaca, NY: Cornell University Press.

Korthals, Michiel (2008) "The Birth of Philosophy and the Contempt for Food." *Gastronomica: The Journal of Food and Culture* 8.3: 62–69.

——(2004) *Before Dinner: Philosophy and Ethics of Food*. Dordrecht: Springer.

Kuehn, Glenn (2005) "How Can Food Be Art?" In The Aesthetics of Everyday Life. Andrew Light and Jonathan Smith, eds., New York: Columbia University Press.

Light, Andrew (1999) "Dining on Fido: The Aesthetic Dilemma of Eating Animals." In *Animal Pragmatism: Rethinking Human–Nonhuman Relationships*. Andrew Light and Erin McKenna, eds., Bloomington: Indiana University Press.

Light, Andrew and Erin McKenna (1999) *Animal Pragmatism: Rethinking Human–Nonhuman Relationships*. Bloomington: Indiana University Press.

Mepham, Ben T., ed. (1996) *Food Ethics (Professional Ethics)*. New York: Routledge.

Montmarquet, James (1989) *The Idea of Agrarianism: From Hunter-Gatherer to Agrarian Radical in Western Culture*. Boise: University of Idaho Press.

Nietzsche, Friedrich (2009) *Ecce Homo: How One Becomes What One Is*. Oxford; Oxford University Press.

Oliver, Kelly (2009) *Animal Lessons: How They Teach Us to Be Human*. New York: Columbia University Press.

Pence, Gregory E. (2002) *The Ethics of Food: A Reader for the Twenty-First Century*. Lanham, NJ: Rowman & Littlefield.

Plato (1992) *Republic*. Trans. G. M. A. Grube. 2nd ed. Cambridge: Hackett.

——(1952) *Timaeus*. Trans. F. M. Cornford. New York: Humanities.

Probyn, Elspeth (2000) *Carnal Appetites: Foodsexidentities*. London and New York: Routledge.

Regan, Tom, ed. (1984) *Earthbound: New Introductory Essays in Environmental Ethics*. Philadelphia, PA: Temple University Press.

——(2004) *The Case for Animal Rights: Updated with a New Preface*. Berkeley: University of California.

Sen, Amartya (1982) *Poverty and Famines: An Essay on Entitlements and Deprivation*. Oxford: Clarendon.

Serres, Michel (2009) *The Five Senses: A Philosophy of Mingled Bodies*. Trans. Margaret Sankey and Peter Cowley. New York: Continuum.

——(2007) *The Parasite*. Trans. Lawrence Schehr. Minneapolis: University of Minnesota.

Singer, Peter (1975) *Animal Liberation: A New Ethics for Our Treatment of Animals*. New York: Random House.

Singer, Peter and Jim Mason (2006) *The Way We Eat: Why Our Food Choices Matter*. New York: Rodale Inc.

Telfer, Elizabeth (1996) *Food for Thought: Philosophy and Food*. London: Routledge.

Thompson, Paul B. (2010) *The Agrarian Vision: Sustainability and Environmental Ethics*. Lexington: University Press of Kentucky.

——(2007) *Food Biotechnology in Ethical Perspective*, 2nd edn. Dordrecht: Springer.

——(1994) *The Spirit of the Soil: Agriculture and Environmental Ethics*. New York: Routledge.

Thompson, Paul B. and Thomas Hilde, eds. (2000) *The Agrarian Roots of Pragmatism*. Nashville, TN: Vanderbilt University Press.

Thompson, Paul B., R. Bawden, D. M. Kaplan, and K. Millar, ed. (forthcoming) *Encyclopedia of Food and Agricultural Ethics*. Dordrecht: Springer.

Walters, Kerry S. and Lisa Portmess (1999) *Ethical Vegetarianism: From Pythagoras to Peter Singer*. Albany: State University of New York Press.

Watson, Richard (1999) *The Philosopher's Diet: How to Lose Weight and Change the World*. Rev. ed. Boston, MA: David R. Godine.

Wilkerson, Abby (forthcoming) *The Thin Contract: Social Justice and the Political Rhetoric of Obesity*. Chicago, IL: Open Court.

——(2011) "Food and Disability Studies: Vulnerable Bodies, Eating or 'Not Eating.'" *Food, Culture & Society* 14.1: 17–28.

——"'Obesity,' the Transnational Plate, and the Thin Contract." *Radical Philosophy Review* 13.1 (2010): 43–67.

13

Linguistics and food studies

Structural and historical connections

Anthony F. Buccini

The chapter illustrates ways in which food studies intersect with linguistics, the study of language structured as a system, including variation and change over time and space. Work in the allied fields of anthropology, semiotics, and discourse analysis is briefly touched upon, followed by a survey of lexical semantic analyses of taste terms, verbs of ingestion, and cooking methods. Especially relevant for food history are etymologies and other historical linguistic research that can shed light on cultural history not documented in written texts. A critical methodological appraisal is included, to guide non-specialists in judging the validity of purported etymologies.

Introduction

Language is the fundamental tool and communal institution of human societies and so it is in countless ways tied to the production, preparation, and consumption of food; linguistics, as the study of how language is structured and functions as a system – synchronic or structural linguistics – and how language varies and changes across time and space – diachronic or historical linguistics – is therefore naturally concerned with virtually all social activities related to food, albeit generally in an indirect way. Some aspects of the relationship between food and language are typically regarded today as falling more within the purview of academic disciplines other than linguistics in the narrow sense, namely, anthropology, semiotics, discourse analysis. For example, analysis of cross-cultural variation in the offering of food may naturally involve a linguistic component but itself concerns primarily the anthropologist (e.g. Brown and Levinson, 1987: 45ff. Chen, 1990/91). Similarly, the broader meaning of foodstuffs with iconic value in society, such as "wine" or "steak" (e.g. Barthes, 1972), falls largely outside linguistics in the narrow sense and within the field of semiotics. Looking at the language of recipes or menus or restaurant critiques stands likewise outside the boundaries of the traditional concerns of linguists and within those of students of discourse analysis (e.g. Zwicky and Zwicky, 1980; Strauss, 2005; Bonazzi, 2009; Carroll, 2010).

In this chapter I focus on the structural and historical approaches to language study and thus on linguistics in the narrow sense as an auxiliary field to food studies. Though the two broad subfields of structural linguistics and historical linguistics are interrelated in myriad ways, it makes sense to draw a line between how the two can be related to food studies. In the first case, structural linguistics can shed light on how cuisine is constructed as a semiotic or symbolic system and how such a system changes over time. In the second case, historical linguistics serves as a practical tool in the study of the history of specific foodstuffs, composed dishes, cooking utensils, etc., and thus of the social location and historical development of specific cuisines.

Historical background of food scholarship in linguistics and major theoretical approaches in use

There is no established or well-defined field that brings together linguistics, in the narrow sense defined above, and food studies. Given that, research that brings the fields together in a sustained fashion has largely been wanting with but a few exceptions. Consequently, the bulk of work that addresses shared concerns has been carried out either from the perspective of the food scholar or from that of the linguist, and while much of this work has been invaluable in the development of our understanding of food and cookery, in many cases the one-sidedness of the two approaches has had a deleterious effect on the progress of the field.

Focusing on work done by linguists, we note that the primary point of intersection between food studies and synchronic linguistics is in the field of lexical semantics, the study of meaning at the level of the word. This work generally entails the analysis of terms within a more or less broad semantic domain – e.g. kinship terms, color terms, terms for cooking methods – and an investigation of the semantic relations between those terms, asking questions such as which concepts are given a name, what oppositions hold among such names, what connotations or metaphorical extensions are associated with their use, etc. A fundamental detailed study of a food-related lexical field in English is Lehrer's (1969) article, "Semantic Cuisine," which explores the terminology of cooking within the theoretical framework of structuralist semantics. Also noteworthy is Lehrer's (1983) subsequent monograph on the language of "wine talk" in English, which analyzes the use of hundreds of words related to wine description and further includes the results of a series of experiments that demonstrate the semantic variability among speakers. A different sort of a work on food by a linguist who defies simple categorization is McCawley's (1984) *The Eater's Guide to Chinese Characters*. Its primary goal is to help non-readers of Chinese decipher the writing they encounter in restaurants but the book additionally contains numerous insights into the Chinese culinary lexicon.

Lexical semantic analyses can serve as a springboard for further investigations in either of two directions. On the one hand, one can attempt to find reflections of the structures discovered in one semantic field elsewhere in the language and more generally in the cultural institutions of the society that uses the language in question, as has been done most famously by the anthropologist, Lévi-Strauss (1978: 495) using precisely the intersection of food and language as his focal point: "Thus we can hope to discover how, in any particular society, cooking is a language through which that society unconsciously reveals its structure … " On the other hand, one can look at semantic domains from a comparative, cross-linguistic perspective with an eye toward elucidating the linguistic and cultural differences that exist between two speech communities. Comparative studies focusing on color terms (e.g. Berlin and Kay, 1969) can inform and, to a degree, have informed subsequent semantic studies relating to food, such as Backhouse (1994), which is first and foremost a detailed analysis of taste terms within Japanese but which then considers future paths of research along cross-linguistic/cross-cultural lines (164ff.). Kuipers (1984) in an important study of gustatory words in Weyéwa (Eastern Indonesia) also comments on the limitations of applicability of color term research to investigations of the semantics of taste.

Another very basic semantic domain related to food and cookery that has garnered sustained interest among linguists from a cross-linguistic perspective is that of the terms (and underlying conceptualizations) of the ingestion of food and drink. Indeed, an entire volume, *The Linguistics of Eating and Drinking* (Newman, 2009), has recently been dedicated to this topic and while the orientation of the various authors' contributions is very much linguistic in nature, they present a wealth of data and observations drawn from a wide variety of languages that are of interest to food scholars. Related to the work of the scholars whose pieces appear in the Newman volume is Ye (2010), which supplements cross-linguistic analysis focusing on Mandarin and Shanghainese with further brief consideration of the diachronic aspect of the terms of ingestion in Sinitic.

A further area of cross-linguistic lexical semantics relating to food studies involves the comparative analysis of cooking terminology, addressing in the first place questions of how the terms in one language correspond to those in another (e.g., the differing semantic ranges of German *braten* vs. English *to fry* vs. Dutch *bakken*, or how – if at all – the distinctions between Italian *friggere/soffriggere/saltare* can be rendered in other languages), but then conceivably progressing to address further questions: With a more linguistic orientation, regarding lexical organization, or with a more anthropological orientation, regarding other loci or levels of cultural structure, or finally, with a more purely culinary orientation, regarding, for example, a focus on the deeper conceptual and structural differences between specific cuisines. Again, Lehrer (1972) is to be cited here for the range of the cross-linguistic analysis of cooking terminology (with data from nine languages from around the world) in her paper critiquing Lévi-Strauss's (1965, 1978: 490ff.) culinary triangle; from a partially different perspective, see also Harrison (1983) in this regard.

In addition to cross-linguistic comparisons of the sort just described, one can of course also make comparisons between different stages within the history of one and the same language and with that one enters into the field of diachronic lexical semantics. The degree to which this line of inquiry with a specific focus on the culinary has been followed by linguists is limited but an exemplary piece, albeit with a very narrow focus, is Sihler (1973), which features a detailed analysis of the relationship between the terms *to bake* and *to roast* in modern English but also a consideration of how that relationship has changed over time.

The sort of semantic study presented in Sihler (1973) represents the lynchpin, as it were, that connects the three traditional language-related fields that have had the most sustained impact on food studies, namely, philology, lexicography and etymology: the semantic analysis, both synchronic and diachronic in nature, informs the broader understanding of historical texts, contributes directly to the compilation of lexicographical material, and in turn fleshes out the history of the individual word. Though these fields of study are regarded today by some linguists of a narrow theoretical perspective as at best marginal to their view of language study, the three represent core activities in the rise of linguistics as a scientific field in the course of the nineteenth century, and the kinds of investigations they entail continue to have relevance to less narrow approaches to linguistic theory, as well as to virtually all academic disciplines of a historical nature in both the humanities and the social sciences.

Of the three fields just mentioned – philology, lexicography, and etymology – the last named is in a very real sense the most basic. Indeed, the beginnings of the modern field of linguistics as a scientific discipline revolved to a considerable degree around etymological research, and specifically coincided with a relatively sharp break from a long-standing tradition of what the purpose of etymology was and how it had previously been done in the Western world. Traditionally, etymology was viewed as a scholarly tool to serve the more fundamental intellectual endeavors of philosophy and rhetoric, whereby the "original" or "true" meaning of a word could be ascertained and, for many philosophers and rhetoricians, a word's relationship to the natural world could thus be discovered (see, e.g., Liberman, 2009: 8ff., 239ff.; Geeraerts, 2010: 2ff.). The stock in trade of etymology was drawing connections between words not closely or not obviously related to one another, be they words in the same language, from different stages of a language, from different dialects or languages, or some combination thereof. In drawing such connections, some measure of phonetic or orthographic similarity between the words was required, but there existed no accepted guidelines for what entailed a legitimate kind or degree of phonetic/orthographic resemblance to justify the proposed etymological relation and so no objective means whatsoever to judge their relative worth. The fact of the matter is that any such phonetic or orthographic resemblances were very much secondary to the semantic relationship seen by the etymologist between allegedly related words, rendering etymology in general very much a semantic word game, albeit one with a learnèd and especially philosophical and/or poetic orientation that was essentially unfettered by any actual issues of linguistic history; as Liberman (2009: 240) puts it:

> For a long time, the main method of etymology was dissecting a word and adding, subtracting, and transporting letters. Socrates already used it. (We [linguists] do the same, but according to rules guided by the facts of history!) Those methods are easy to mock, for they are indeed silly.

The most notable bit of mockery in this regard is the oft-cited (but possibly apocryphal) comment attributed to Voltaire by Max Müller (1864: 238): "L'étymologie est une science où les voyelles ne font rien, et les consonnes fort peu de choses" – etymology is a science where vowels count for nothing and consonants for little.

The transition from this sort of semantically driven "speculative etymology" of the philosopher and rhetorician to the modern "scientific etymology" of the linguist involved a number of steps, of which the fundamental one was the development of the concept of the regular sound correspondence (see, e.g., Campbell, 2004: Ch. 5; Hock and Joseph, 2009: Ch. 4). With the establishment of this principle, there came in place a means by which the phonetic relationship between allegedly related words could begin to be judged in an essentially objective way and in turn there also came an inversion of the primacy of semantics over form (phonetic or orthographic) that characterized the spirit of speculative etymology; semantic connections henceforth became subordinate to and restrained or channelled by the requirements of what was known from the study of linguistic data about phonological form and how it changes. And once some rules were introduced, the possibility arose for dialogue and adjustment between what was learned generally both about semantic change and about formal – to wit, phonological and morphological – change; in other words, the sophistication of the semantic analyses themselves grew within the context of the broader concern with linguistic reality.

The discovery of the principle of regular sound correspondences, the subsequent elaboration of the comparative method and language reconstruction, and the gradual development of closely related subfields of linguistic investigation such as dialectology, language contact studies and sociolinguistics all have indirect but very important implications for the study of food history. In the first place, an accurate account of a given language's history builds on but also contributes to a more general understanding of the social and cultural dynamics at work within the community in which the language was spoken. Since the theoretical and methodological tools of historical linguistics allow us, moreover, to go to a certain degree beyond what extant historical records directly show us, we can thereby gain insights into cultural and culinary matters that are in nature pre-historical or what one might call "para-historical" or "sub-historical," by which I mean matters occurring in historical periods but outside the contemporary historical record.

A particularly interesting example of the use of the comparative method extending beyond purely linguistic ends is Watkins's (1995) study of Indo-European poetics (on the methodology, see especially 3ff.) and though that work has only indirect connections to food studies (e.g., through agriculture in chapter 17), there is a strong tradition of using the comparative method and linguistic reconstruction with an eye toward identifying cultural items, institutions, and notions reflected in the proto-language. With direct bearing on food studies is some of the research involving long-range linguistic reconstruction and especially studies attempting to identify likely homelands of peoples in the period when a given reconstructed proto-language is believed to have been spoken; in such discussions, flora and fauna and thus also food sources are particularly important pieces of evidence, as are any terms relating to agricultural practices that can be reconstructed. Probably the first language family to be studied in this manner was Indo-European and the field has produced an extensive literature; for recent works of interest here, see for example Gamkrelidze and Ivanov (1995: especially part II), Mallory and Adams (2006: especially Chapters 9, 10, 15, 16). Linguistic/cultural reconstructions related to questions of homelands of proto-populations for many other language families of interest to food scholars now exist; for example, in North America there is the comparative research done on the Algonquian (Siebert, 1967) and Iroquoian (Mithun, 1984) languages. As a further example, one notes the recent research on the Bantu language family of Africa, which, building on earlier discussions of Proto-Bantu foodways (Polomé, 1982), goes much further in attempting to reconstruct as detailed a picture as possible of the earliest culinary culture of the Bantuphone community (see Schoenbrun, 1993; Ricquier and Bostoen, 2010).

Another line of research involving long-range reconstruction with a bearing on food studies addresses the question of the degree to which the spread of agriculture was related to the spread of languages. The view that the link was very strong – the farming/language dispersal hypothesis – is associated particularly with the work of the archaeologists Renfrew and Bellwood, but brings together not only the various disciplines concerned with the domestication of plants and animals and the development of farming methods, but also the work of students of human genetics and, of course, historical linguists; for a broad overview of this research and criticism thereof, see the contributions in Bellwood and Renfrew (2002).

On account of the nature of the evidence available in the study of prehistory and historically remote periods, it is generally possible to reconstruct to a reasonable degree what basic foodstuffs a given language community consumed. On occasion, the lexical evidence allows us to ascertain further information, such as basic cooking methods, basic utensils related to food preparation or consumption, and on occasion also secondary alimentary products, such as "butter" or "dough" or "mead," and with that one begins to get glimpses into the nature of an ancient cuisine. As we proceed into historical periods in which there is direct and indirect textual evidence of culinary culture, it would seem perhaps that linguistic reconstruction would be otiose but such is not the case. Given the general relationship in many societies between literary sources and the social groups that produce them, the picture of the culinary culture of a given society we get from those sources may be very skewed and incomplete, with the foodways of the less affluent sectors of the population being largely or wholly ignored – such is the case in Europe from classical times on through the Middle Ages and well beyond, and a similar situation long obtained in the Islamic world as well. The limited or absent direct textual evidence for the culinary culture of whole sections of a society can be supplemented to a degree with indirect historical evidence, but the same tools required for the study of prehistoric foodways must also be brought to bear, namely archaeological and linguistic evidence, and in this way historical linguistics in the broadest sense can here play a role similar to its role in the field of ethnohistory (cf. Trigger, 1975: 53). With a certain degree of historical contextualization, the linguistic contribution to uncovering past cultural complexes, including the culinary, can transcend reconstruction or explication of individual lexical items and extend to broader analyses of sociolinguistic dynamics and the dynamics of language (and dialect) contact, which in turn can provide new perspectives on and fuller contextualization of social and cultural developments generally. A study along these lines is Buccini's (2006) account of the development and distribution of summer vegetable stews (*ratatouille, cianfotta, samfaina*, etc.) around the Western Mediterranean, in which an analysis of the various names for this type of stew, with extensive reference to dialectal material, is used in conjunction with known historical contacts and population movements within the region during the early modern period. This not only sheds light on the history of this family of dishes but beyond that offers evidence for earlier adoption of the New World vegetables (peppers, tomatoes, etc.) than scholars have generally believed, on account of the direct evidence we have for resistance to their use in botanical and culinary texts from the period – the dialectal evidence is a crucial element in getting past the limitations of those texts and getting a view of the foodways of the poor, which differed markedly from those of the more affluent and literate.

Such investigations, which are firmly within the field of food studies but carried out by a linguist who draws heavily upon linguistic evidence in the course of the argument, are not numerous but in this regard the work of Perry stands out in particular. His discussions of families of dishes found across a wide array of culinary cultures are notable for the combination of extensive philological work with culinary insights and linguistic analyses of lexical material from multiple languages, especially Arabic, Persian, and Turkish; see e.g., Perry (2001) on *būrān* or Perry (2010) on *korma*, etc. (other examples of Perry's work appear in the same volume as Perry, 2001).

Historical linguists, in the ordinary course of conducting their research, have in passing contributed much to the field of food studies by producing etymologies that serve a key role in the writing of food and culinary history and the fruits of this labour are most easily encountered in the many etymological dictionaries that have been compiled in a linguistically rigorous fashion. In many cases, however, etymologies relating to culinary matters proposed by linguists with little or no especial interest in or knowledge of that particular cultural domain are inadequate, either through missed connections of one form to another or through unconvincing semantic analyses of the material. Application of sophisticated linguistic analyses to culinary questions in a sustained fashion is something that only in recent times has come to the fore, as in some of the works just mentioned above, and with this further possibilities for significant advances in our knowledge and understanding of food history are possible, as a genuine dialogue between food historians and linguists develops. What I have in mind here is the sort of work in which an old and seemingly intractable linguistic problem, such as the etymology of the words "olive" and "oil," is approached with as much of a concern for the relevant historical data as for the linguistic data, as in Buccini (2010), where I argue that the Greek word from which "olive" and "oil" derive is itself a borrowing from Anatolian, a possibility that, if correct, forces us to revise received notions about the early history of oleïculture and in turn contributes more broadly to our understanding of the history of arboriculture.

Building on both the semantic studies and the historical research discussed above, linguists can also make significant contributions to the field of food studies in the areas of food-related lexicography and philology and in recent decades this has been increasingly the case. A considerable body of food-related research by linguists with a particular focus on lexicography is brought together in the three-volume proceedings of a conference held in Naples (Silvestri *et al.*, 2002). The conference and proceedings grew out of an ongoing major international scholarly project, namely, the *Atlante Generale dell'Alimentazione Mediterranea*, which promises to be an indispensable resource for the study of culinary culture in the Mediterranean region; for samples of the detailed lexical entries – with etymological information, related idioms, etc. – to appear there, see in particular the articles in the first volume. The second and third volumes are devoted to related research on specific topics in lexical semantics of culinary terms from various regions of Italy and other Mediterranean countries, a portion of it in the venerable tradition of the *cose e parole/Sachen und Wörter* approach (a notable early illustration of which is Schuchardt, 1912). Other recent work in food-related lexical semantics with ties to the *Sachen und Wörter* approach are Buccini (2009) on Greek and Italian names for *muscari comosum*, and Buccini (2007) on *spaghetti alla carbonara* and related dishes; the latter emphasizes the need to distinguish between the invention of a dish and the invention of a particular name for a dish. In the field of lexicography, another recent contribution to culinary studies from Italy is Pinnavaia's (2010) study of food and drink idioms in English. Relating more to food history is Dalby's (2003) reference work on food in the ancient world, which features semantic and etymological discussions for many of the entries.

Dalby, a linguist with an especially strong background in classical philology, has edited and translated important historical source works for food studies, such as Cato's *On Farming* (1998) and more recently the *Geoponika* (2011). The aforementioned scholar of Near Eastern languages, C. Perry, has also edited and translated historical works of significance, such as Arabic cookbooks *The Description of Familiar Foods* (2001) and *The Book of Dishes* (2005), bringing to bear both linguistic and philological expertise.

Research methodologies

In the previous section, I focused on work by linguists with bearing on the field of food studies and their work naturally follows the theoretical and methodological frameworks of their subfields in linguistics. In this section, I consider some aspects of the use of linguistic argumentation in the work of food historians and call attention to some methodological pitfalls that commonly arise there.

As mentioned above, the area where linguistic research most often is of direct concern to food scholars is etymology. Many food scholars are extremely careful in their use of linguistic and especially etymological evidence in their discussions of culinary matters, relying whenever possible on contributions established by linguists. In instances where no such appeal can be made, the prudent path to take is to suggest with caution and not base further arguments too much on an uncertain or unsound etymological base. The simple fact of the matter is that while it is obviously quite possible for a non-linguist to propose a (non-trivial) etymology that is convincing and correct, it is in practice something that does not occur especially often. First off, the basic etymologies regarding the core culinary vocabulary in the major and also many minor languages with which food scholars are generally concerned in their research have by and large already been done in the course of general historical or lexicographical work on those languages by linguists. Of course, there are undoubtedly many partially or wholly wrong etymologies that have been published by linguists as well, but where these errors occur it is typically the case that the error has been in a sense caused by the difficulty of the problem at hand; such is likewise the case with the many words for which historical linguists have felt it necessary to declare that their origins remain "uncertain", "unknown", or "obscure".

The difficulties in discovering a non-trivial etymology are often both numerous and complex, for ideally a good etymology accomplishes all of the following: (a) it accounts completely for the relationship of the sounds in the word in question and its proposed etymon(s) and does so in accord with known sound laws, patterns of phonological adaptation in borrowing, etc., which pertain to the language(s) involved; (b) it similarly accounts for the morphology of the word in question where required; (c) it provides a convincing account of any and all semantic changes that the word has undergone. All of these accounts of form and meaning need also to be matched appropriately with what is known concerning the historical use of the word, e.g. the details regarding attestation. In the case of a proposed etymology that invokes borrowing from one language to another, the complexities can increase considerably, insofar as one must then deal with the analysis of data from two (or conceivably more) languages and additionally give a reasonable account of the proposed socio-historical setting in which the borrowing was made. Questions of relative and absolute chronology must always be taken into consideration. Furthermore, care must be taken to avoid the common pitfall of anachronistically projecting the central status of the modern standard variety of a given language back in time – wherever possible one must identify the specific dialect(s) of relevance to the matter at hand. For example, in considering colonial-era European loanwords in Native American languages, one looks not to the modern standard varieties as the possible sources but rather to the dialects of French, Dutch, Spanish, etc. as spoken in the actual time of contact (i.e. the seventeenth or eighteenth centuries). But this then entails knowledge of the demographics of the colonial situation, as well as a solid grounding in historical dialectology. In short, what starts as a seemingly small problem concerning an individual word can in fact require a surprisingly large and time-consuming research project.

Enthusiasm and conviction are not substitutes for a deep understanding of the principles of language variation and change, as one can see from the work on cultural influences from Egypt and the Near East in early Greece by M. Bernal; in his three volumes of *Black Athena* historical linguistics and etymological arguments feature most prominently, but the lack of rigour in Bernal's approach to these and his inclination to generate in forced fashion linguistic evidence in support of his overarching claims have with justification been sharply criticized by linguists (e.g. Jasanoff and Nussbaum, 1996) and others. One finds partially analogous uses of linguistic argumentation in the literature on cookery and food history, albeit on a smaller scale. For example, in the extensive writings of C. Wright on Mediterranean food, there is an unmistakable tendency on his part to attribute culinary items and practices first and foremost to Arab influence (e.g., Wright, 1992, 1999). Of course, the Arab influence in matters culinary around the Mediterranean has indeed been extremely important, and a research agenda of trying to discover hitherto unseen instances of that influence is a very reasonable one. What is less reasonable is the tendency to include in historical arguments only etymologies that serve the overarching agenda even when those etymologies are flawed or highly speculative and are presented in lieu of more reasonable ones that do not fit the agenda. If the goal is to present an accurate appreciation of the role of Arab influence throughout Mediterranean cookery, flimsily argued etymologies do not serve the purpose, especially in those instances when etymological evidence is potentially of central importance to shedding light on a difficult problem, as with the early history of pasta (see, e.g., the suggested etymology of *maccheroni* in Wright, 1996–97; cf. Wright, 1999: 618ff.).

Even in instances where a given etymology is not crucial for understanding the broader issue at hand, some food historians feel compelled to supply one but do so more to the detriment of their own main point than to its benefit. Such is the case with Hess's (1992: 89–100) proposed etymology of the name of the dish "Hoppin John," which she offers in her generally sound, culinary oriented elaboration of Littlefield's (1981) work on the importance of African slaves in the development of rice cultivation in colonial South Carolina. This particular etymology (deriving "Hoppin John" from a posited phrase of very mixed linguistic parentage, *bahatta kachāng*, the first element being from Hindi via Persian and Arabic, the second Malay "perhaps by way of Malagasy") is noteworthy for the degree of mismatch between the manner of presentation, which suggests that the etymology had been carefully researched using sound linguistic and historical reasoning, and the actual argumentation offered, which harkens directly back to the sort of speculative etymologizing that Voltaire disparaged where seemingly anything goes: "Keeping in mind the historical consonant shift and the predilection for metathesis and elision … " (100). For example, Hess asserts that in the first word of the phrase, *b* becomes *p* and switches places with the *h*; *aṭṭa* is deleted and *in* is inserted, but this without any reference to established sound laws in any actual language.

Such etymological flights of fancy are unfortunately still not rare in the literature on food history and while it is understandable that they occur frequently in popular writing about food, they need to be eliminated from work that otherwise looks to provide us with a real understanding of the culinary past. Good etymologies can be very entertaining and they can of course be crucial bits of evidence in a historical argument, but as Liberman (2009: 166) says: "A bad etymology is not better (in fact, it is much worse) than no etymology at all … "

For a recent and detailed discussion of the methodologies used currently by etymologists, one can consult Durkin (2009), which can be supplemented with basic works on historical linguistics (e.g., Campbell, 2004; Hock and Joseph, 2009). Another recent contribution specifically concerned with etymology is Liberman (2009), which is an entertaining work but also one that contains many valuable insights and much information; of particular interest here is his chapter on methodology (158ff.), which includes a list summarizing important principles. Given the importance of cultural contacts and exchanges in food history, an understanding of the current state of the study of language contact, both with regard to the social dynamics that affect linguistic transfer and to the structural aspects of language contact, would be worth having. In this regard, the topic of loan phonology should be of especial interest to food scholars. Recent important general works on language contact are Van Coetsem (1988), Thomason and Kaufman (1988) and Van Coetsem (2000).

While it may well be (and should be) daunting for non-linguists to tackle difficult etymological problems, it is important that all food historians have a reasonable sense of what makes an etymology good or bad, more likely or less likely correct, in order to be able to judge better the relative merits of those proposed by others. And in many cases, there are etymologies that have been proposed by linguists with little interest in or understanding of culinary matters that can only be properly revised or rejected by those who have a deep knowledge of those culinary matters.

Avenues for future research

Interdisciplinary research which genuinely brings together linguistics and food studies has hitherto been relatively quite limited. Consequently there remain many topics on which such collaboration is a real desideratum. Hand in hand with ongoing research in culinary history should go a concerted effort to reject or revise etymologies that are wanting with respect either to their linguistic underpinnings or their connection to culinary culture.

Given the advances in recent decades by linguists in understanding how language contact works and the degree to which food studies are concerned with instances of cultural/culinary contact, it seems natural that interdisciplinary work focus on contact. From a practical standpoint, there is once again much to be gained for food studies through more sophisticated analyses of food-related word borrowings but linguistics has another, more general way of contributing to food studies here: by observing patterns of transfer, one gains insight into the inner structure of language and an understanding of what linguistic domains are more or less stable, more or less open, more or less susceptible to change in different situations. Looking at cuisine – which, like language, is itself a semiotic system – from this linguistically informed perspective, one begins to see more clearly what can reasonably be called "culinary grammar" (Buccini, 2008: 67; Buccini, 2011: 74; n.b. this conception of culinary grammar is rather different from that of Montanari, 2006: 99–103).

Many lines of inquiry bringing together lexical semantic research and food studies are yet to have been explored, particularly with regard to cross-linguistic topics.

For a list of suggestions by a culinary historian of what culinary historians can learn from linguists, see Laudan (2010).

Practical considerations for getting started

There are as yet no academic programs specializing in linguistics and food history. Students interested in applying linguistic methodology to food studies should seek a linguistics program that includes training in historical linguistics and/or lexical semantics; those interested in pursuing historical linguistics would benefit greatly from exposure to the related subfields of dialectology, socio-linguistics and language contact. For investigating food-related semantic fields in languages other than one's own native language, a course in field methods is highly recommended. Students at institutions without a program in linguistics may be interested in the courses offered through the Linguistic Society of America's Summer Institutes in odd-numbered years; see lsadc.org for more information.

Etymological dictionaries are increasingly available in online versions; note, however, that in many cases an affiliation with a university library may be needed in order to access the database.

With regard to grants and fellowships, there is no funding source specifically devoted to the intersection of linguistics and food studies. A possibility worth considering might be support from the American Council of Learned Societies, which funds humanistic research in a number of fields, including linguistics and history, and which accepts applications from independent scholars as well as from those with an academic affiliation.

Key reading

General linguistics

Bloomfield, Leonard (1984 [1933]) *Language*. Chicago, IL: University of Chicago Press.
(Classic work, still an excellent introductory text for the non-linguist, despite its age.)

Lexical semantics

Geeraerts, Dirk (2010) *Theories of Lexical Semantics*. Oxford: Oxford University Press.
Lehrer, Adrienne (1969) "Semantic Cuisine." *Journal of Linguistics* 5: 39–55.

Historical linguistics

Campbell, Lyle (2004) *Historical Linguistics. An Introduction*. Cambridge, MA: MIT Press.
Hock, Hans Heinrich and Brian D. Joseph. (2009) *Language History, Language Change, and Language Relationship. An Introduction to Historical and Comparative Linguistics*. New York: Mouton De Gruyter.

Language contact

Thomason, Sarah Grey and Terrence Kaufman (1988) *Language Contact, Creolization and Genetic Linguistics*. Berkeley: University of California Press.

Van Coetsem, Frans (1988) *Loan Phonology and the Two Transfer Types in Language Contact*. Dordrecht: Foris.
——(2000) *A General and Unified Theory of the Transmission Process in Language Contact*. Heidelberg: Carl Winter.

Etymology

Durkin, Philip (2009) *The Oxford Guide to Etymology*. Oxford: Oxford University Press.
Liberman, Anatoly (2009) *Word Origins ... and How We Know Them. Etymology for Everyone*. Oxford: Oxford University Press.

Food studies and language

Hosking, Richard, ed. (2010) *Food and Language. Proceedings of the Oxford Symposium on Food and Cookery 2009*. Totnes: Prospect.

Bibliography

Backhouse, A. E. (1994) *The Lexical Field of Taste. A Semantic Study of Japanese Taste Terms*. Cambridge: Cambridge University Press.
Barthes, Roland (1972) *Mythologies*, trans. Annette Lavers. New York: Hill & Wang.
Bellwood, Peter and Colin Renfrew, eds. (2002) *Examining the Farming/Language Dispersal Hypothesis*. Cambridge: McDonald Institute for Archaeological Research.
Berlin, Brent and Paul Kay. (1969) *Basic Color Terms: Their Universality and Evolution*. Berkeley: University of California Press.
Bernal, Martin (1987–2006) *Black Athena*. (3 Volumes). New Brunswick, NJ: Rutgers University Press.
Bonazzi, Andrea (2009) "Per uno studio della lingua dei menu." In *Linguisti in contatto. Ricerche di linguistica italiana in Svizzera*. Atti del Convegno, Bellinzona, B. Moretti, E. Pandolfi, M. Casoni, pp. 16–17 November 2007. Bellinzona, pp. 59–70. (Postprint available at: www.zora.uzh.ch, accessed on March 29, 2012.)
Brown, Penelope and Stephen C. Levinson (1987) *Politeness. Some Universals in Language Usage*. Cambridge: Cambridge University Press.
Buccini, Anthony F. (2006) "Western Mediterranean Vegetable Stews and the Integration of Culinary Exotica." In *Authenticity in the Kitchen. Proceedings of the Oxford Symposium on Food and Cookery 2005*, Richard Hosking ed., pp. 132–45. Totnes: Prospect.
——(2007) "On *Spaghetti alla Carbonara* and Related Dishes of Central and Southern Italy." In *Eggs in Cookery. Proceedings of the Oxford Symposium on Food and Cookery 2006*, Richard Hosking, ed., pp. 36–47. Totnes: Prospect.
——(2008) "From Necessity to Virtue: The Secondary Uses of Bread in Italian Cookery." In *Food and Morality. Proceedings of the Oxford Symposium on Food and Cookery 2007*, Susan Friedland, ed., pp. 57–69. Totnes: Prospect.
——(2009) "The Bitter – and Flatulent – Aphrodisiac: Synchrony and Diachrony of the Culinary Use of *Muscari Comosum* in Greece and Italy." In *Vegetables. Proceedings of the Oxford Symposium on Food and Cookery 2008*, Susan R. Friedland, ed., pp. 46–55. Totnes: Prospect.
——(2010) "The Anatolian Origins of the Words 'Olive' and 'Oil' and the Early History of Oleïculture." In *Food and Language. Proceedings of the Oxford Symposium on Food and Cookery 2009*, Richard Hosking, ed., pp. 52–61. Totnes: Prospect.
——(2011) "Continuity in Culinary Aesthetics in the Western Mediterranean: Roman *Garum* and *Liquamen* in the Light of the Local Survival of Fermented Fish Seasonings in Japan and the Western Mediterranean." In *Cured, Fermented and Smoked Foods. Proceedings of the Oxford Symposium on Food and Cookery 2010*, Helen Saberi, ed., pp. 66–75. Totnes: Prospect.
Campbell, Lyle (2004) *Historical Linguistics. An Introduction*. Cambridge, MA: MIT Press.
Carroll, Ruth (2010) "The Visual Language of the Recipe: A Brief Historical Survey." In *Food and Language. Proceedings of the Oxford Symposium on Food and Cookery 2009*, Richard Hosking, ed., pp. 62–72. Totnes: Prospect.

Chen, Victoria (1990/91) "*Mien Tze* at the Chinese Dinner Table: A Study of the Interactional Accomplishment of Face." *Research on Language and Social Interaction* 24: 109–40.

Dalby, Andrew (ed. and trans.) (1998) *Cato. On Farming (De Agricultura). A modern translation with commentary.* Totnes: Prospect.

——(2003) *Food in the Ancient Word A to Z.* London and New York: Routledge.

——(ed. and trans.) (2011) *Geoponika (Farm Work). A Modern Translation of the Roman and Byzantine Farming Handbook.* Totnes: Prospect.

Durkin, Philip (2009) *The Oxford Guide to Etymology.* Oxford: Oxford University Press.

Gamkrelidze, Thomas V. and Vjačeslav V. Ivanov (1995) *Indo-European and the Indo-Europeans* (two vols). Berlin and New York: Mouton De Gruyter.

Geeraerts, Dirk (2010) *Theories of Lexical Semantics.* Oxford: Oxford University Press.

Harrison, Alan F. (1983) "Making Sense of Cuisine: From Culinary Triangle to Pyramid Using Lehrer's Tetrahedron as a Stepping Stone." *Anthropological Linguistics* 25: 189–210.

Hess, Karen (1992) *The Carolina Rice Kitchen: The African Connection.* Columbia, SC: University of South Carolina Press.

Hock, Hans Heinrich and Brian D. Joseph (2009) *Language History, Language Change, and Language Relationship. An Introduction to Historical and Comparative Linguistics.* New York: Mouton De Gruyter.

Jasanoff, Jay H. and Alan Nussbaum (1996) "Word Games: The Linguistic Evidence in *Black Athena*." In *Black Athena Revisited*, Mary R. Lefkowitz and Guy MacLean Rogers, eds., pp. 177–205. Chapel Hill and London: University of North Carolina Press.

Kuipers, Joel C. (1984) "Matters of Taste in Weyéwa." *Anthropological Linguistics* 26: 84–101.

Laudan, Rachel (2010) "What can the Culinary Historian Learn from the Linguist? Ten Suggestions." In *Food and Language. Proceedings of the Oxford Symposium on Food and Cookery 2009*, Richard Hosking, ed., pp. 209–16. Totnes: Prospect.

Lehrer, Adrienne (1969) "Semantic Cuisine." *Journal of Linguistics* 5: 39–55.

——(1972) "Cooking Vocabularies and the Culinary Triangle of Lévi-Strauss." *Anthropological Linguistics* 14: 155–71.

——(1983) *Wine and Conversation.* Bloomington: Indiana University Press.

Lévi-Strauss, Claude (1965) "Le triangle culinaire." *L'Arc* 26: 19–29.

——(1978) *The Origin of Table Manners. Introduction to a Science of Mythology: 3.* (John & Doreen Weightman trans.) New York: Harper & Row.

Liberman, Anatoly (2009) *Word Origins … and How We Know Them. Etymology for Everyone.* Oxford: Oxford University Press.

Littlefield, Daniel C. (1981) *Rice and Slaves: Ethnicity and the Slave Trade in Colonial South Carolina.* Urbana and Chicago: University of Illinois Press.

Mallory, J.P. and D.Q. Adams (2006) *The Oxford Introduction to Proto-Indo-European and the Proto-Indo-European World.* Oxford: Oxford University Press.

McCawley, James D. (1984) *The Eater's Guide to Chinese Characters.* Chicago, IL: University of Chicago Press.

Mithun, Marianne (1984) "The Proto-Iroquoians: Cultural Reconstruction from Lexical Materials." In *Extending the Rafters. Interdisciplinary Approaches to Iroquoian Studies,* Michael K. Foster, Jack Campisi, Marianne Mithun, eds., pp. 259–81. Albany: State University of New York Press.

Montanari, Massimo (2006) *Food is Culture.* (Trans. Albert Sonenfeld.) New York: Columbia University Press.

Müller, Max (1864) *Lectures on the Science of Language* (Second Series). London: Longman, Gren, Longman, Roberts, & Green.

Newman, John, ed. (2009) *The Linguistics of Eating and Drinking.* Amsterdam and Philadelphia, PA: John Benjamins.

Perry, Charles (2001) "*Būrān*: Eleven Hundred Years in the History of a Dish." In *Medieval Arab Cookery,* Maxime Rodinson, A. J. Arberry, & Charles Perry, pp. 239–50. Totnes: Prospect.

——(2001) "The Description of Familiar Foods." In *Medieval Arab Cookery,* Maxime Rodinson, A. J. Arberry, and Charles Perry, pp. 272–465. Totnes, Prospect.

——(2005) *A Baghdad Cookery Book.* Petits Propos Culinaires 79. Totnes: Prospect.

——(2010) "*Korma, Kavurma, Ghormeh*: A Family or Not So Much?" In *Food and Language. Proceedings of the Oxford Symposium on Food and Cookery 2009,* Richard Hosking, ed., pp. 254–57. Totnes: Prospect.

Pinnavaia, Laura (2010) *Sugar and Spice … Exploring Food and Drink Idioms in English.* Monza: Polimetrica.

Polomé, Edgar (1982) "The Reconstruction of Proto-Bantu Culture from the Lexicon." In *Language, Society, and Paleoculture,* Anwar S. Dil, ed., pp. 316–28. Stanford, CA: Stanford University Press.

Ricquier, Birgit and Koen Bostoen (2010) "Retrieving Food History through Linguistics: Culinary Traditions in Early Bantuphone Communities." In *Food and Language: Proceedings of the Oxford Symposium on Food and Cookery 2009,* Richard Hosking, ed., pp. 258–69. Totnes: Prospect.

Schoenbrun, David (1993) "We Are What We Eat: Ancient Agriculture between the Great Lakes." *The Journal of African History* 34: 1–31.

Schuchardt, Hugo (1912) "Sachen und Wörter." *Anthropos* 7: 827–39.

Siebert, Frank T. (1967) "The original home of the Proto-Algonquian people." In *Contributions to Anthropology: Linguistics I (Algonquian),* A. D. DeBlois, ed., pp. 13–47. Ottawa: National Museum of Canada.

Sihler, Andrew (1973) "Baking and Roasting." *American Anthropologist* 75: 1721–25.

Silvestri, Domenico, Antonietta Marra, and Immacolata Pinto, eds. (2002) *Saperi e sapori mediterranei. La cultura dell'alimentazione e i suoi riflessi linguistici* (3 vols). Naples: Università degli Studi di Napoli "L'Orientale."

Strauss, Susan (2005) "The linguistic aestheticization of food: a cross-cultural look at food commercials in Japan, Korea, and the United States." *Journal of Pragmatics* 37: 1427–55.

Thomason, Sarah Grey and Terrence Kaufman (1988) *Language Contact, Creolization and Genetic Linguistics.* Berkeley: University of California Press.

Trigger, Bruce (1975) "Brecht and Ethnohistory." *Ethnohistory* 22: 51–56.

Van Coetsem, Frans (1988) *Loan Phonology and the Two Transfer Types in Language Contact.* Dordrecht: Foris.

——(2000) *A General and Unified Theory of the Transmission Process in Language Contact.* Heidelberg: Carl Winter.

Watkins, Calvert (1995) *How to Kill a Dragon. Aspects of Indo-European Poetry.* Oxford: Oxford University Press.

Wright, Clifford A. (1992) *Cucina Paradiso. The Heavenly Food of Sicily.* New York: Simon & Schuster.

——(1996–97) "Cucina Arabo-Sicula and Maccharuni." *Al-Masāq* 9: 151–77.

——(1999) *A Mediterranean Feast.* New York: William Morrow.

Ye, Zhengdao (2010) "Eating and Drinking in Mandarin and Shanghainese: A Lexical-Conceptual Analysis." In *ASCS09: Proceedings of the 9th Conference of the Australasian Society for Cognitive Science,* W. Christensen, E. Schier, and J. Sutton, eds., pp. 375–83. Sydney: Macquarie Centre for Cognitive Science. www.maccs.mq.edu.au/news/conferences/2009/ASCS2009/html/ye.html (accessed on April 12, 2012).

Zwicky, Ann D. and Arnold M. Zwicky (1980) "America's National Dish: the Style of Restaurant Menus." *American Speech* 55: 83–92.

14

Food and theology

David Grumett

Current work on food and theology is indebted to prior developments in religious studies, social anthropology, and sociology. Patristics and church history have provided foundations, notably critiques by feminist scholars in these disciplines of medieval fasting. Biblical studies has also produced valuable findings, as have theological engagements with culture, ritual, and liturgy. Scholars of food and theology now need to appraise further their inherited tradition, engage non-theological interest in food, shape church practice and witness, and consider the wider implications of practice-focused theology. As well as extending theological understanding of food, this will renew the discipline of theology.

The current expanding multidisciplinary interest in food, and the emergence of the discipline of food studies, provide theologians with both a challenge and opportunities. The challenge lies in connecting often abstract theological concepts to the material reality of people's daily lives. The opportunities offered are to recover rich traditions of theological reasoning that have in fact been shaped by material life, and to understand how theory and practice might be reconnected in the present day.

Food might be assumed to be of greater interest to religious studies scholars than to theologians, and with good reason. Religious studies is centrally concerned with the customs, rituals, narratives, and myths that structure the daily lives of people of faith and their communities, and food is likely to be part of each of these. Theologians certainly have much to learn from the close engagement with empirical life that religious studies at its best achieves. But religious studies does not usually interrogate the texts, theories, and doctrines that motivate and sustain empirical practices. That is the task of the theologian, and how he or she might pursue this task with regard to food is the subject of this chapter.

The task is complicated because the way in which theology functions varies between religions. Understood as a coherent body of rational reflection about God and divine revelation, theology has been central to Christianity since early in its history. Judaism and Islam, the other great monotheistic faiths with discrete historic identities, possess similar traditions of reasoning about God, although the place of food in daily life is better understood in these than in Christianity. This is due to food's clearer ritual significance in them. In some other religions, in contrast, it is debatable whether theology is even possible. Many scholars of Buddhism, for example, have viewed it as non-theistic and not amenable to rational investigation. Hinduism is often regarded as more susceptible to theological enquiry, not least because of its scriptural basis, yet it is a more diffuse tradition than either Christianity, Judaism, or Islam.

Because food is less well understood in Christian theology than in the theologies of these other religions, this chapter will take Christian theology as its main focus. Some important theological ideas about food in Jewish and Muslim theology will also be identified, however, not least because they confront similar food issues. Moreover, because religions address common fields of human experience, the theories and practices of one religion may usefully inform understanding of another. Furthermore, because food often serves as a boundary marker between different religions, the food practices of one religion sometimes arise in explicit reaction against those of another religion.

Historical background of food scholarship in theology and major theoretical approaches in use

Food has classically been viewed as a more important topic in religious studies than in theology. This is due partly to the greater engagement of religious studies with social anthropology and other empirically focused disciplines, in which food is identified as a basic need and signifier in human life. Work done in religious studies therefore forms an important part of the recent background to new work in food and theology. In his pioneering comparative study of taboos against consuming various kinds of flesh, Frederick J. Simoons (1961) surveyed various motives against such consumption, including religious motives, and showed that meat is a uniquely significant and problematic food across many cultures. Nonetheless, Simoons extended his project in a much later study (1998) to encompass taboos against a range of plants. These seminal works demonstrate that food avoidances and disciplines are cross-cultural aspects of human life, and challenge theologians to recognize and comprehend their continued existence today.

In Britain, pioneering sociological perspectives on vegetarianism were developed by Julia Twigg (1983, 1979). These remain key starting points for understanding a range of religiously motivated dietary abstentions, and address issues that include: Food status and hierarchy; attitudes to life, death, and corruption; and the discourses and representational systems surrounding food choices. Twigg also produced (1981) the first scholarly history of vegetarianism in Britain, from where it was exported to the United States, giving special attention to the theological and other belief factors that contributed to its rise. More recent research (Gregory, 2008) has deepened understanding of this historical context.

Food issues were brought into closer proximity with biblical theology by the renowned social anthropologist Mary Douglas. In order to account for the food taboos in Leviticus and Deuteronomy, Douglas (1966: 51–71) employed the concepts of pollution and taboo, for which she became widely known. She argued that those animals that failed to fit into a clear set of categories were deemed "abominable" and therefore unfit for human consumption. For example, in order to be counted clean, fish needed to possess scales and fins; those that did not were unclean. In other words, food choices were shaped more by avoidance than by positive acceptance. The best example is the pig, which has a cloven hoof but does not chew the cud. On this account, pork avoidance can be traced to beliefs about the cosmological structuring of the world by God, but is in practice motivated and perpetuated by a visceral, irrational sense that pork is unclean and inconsumable. While Douglas continued her work, Jean Soler (1979) published a compelling argument that, in the Mosaic law, predatory animals were just as much to be avoided as the uncategorizable, liminal animals on which Douglas focused. Gillian Feeley-Harnik (1981) has convincingly argued for the continuing importance of food rules and wider issues surrounding dining and diet in the New Testament. These contributions have been usefully assessed by Seth Kunin (2004: 29–98) and Walter Houston (1993). Douglas, in her later work (2001: 134–75), embraced an explanation of food avoidances based on the categories of creation, covenant, and fertility. She explicitly refuted her earlier concept of abomination, for which she nevertheless remains better known, regarding the consumption of unclean foods not as the contravention of purity but as the infringement of holiness.

The other important theological antecedent to new interest in food and theology is found in studies in Patristics and church history that reveal food's major significance in the religious and social life of earlier eras (Bazell, 1997; Henisch, 1976). Attention has rightly been directed as far back as the desert fathers (Leyerle, 2004), who were famed for their prodigious dietary abstinence, even if their biographers might have exaggerated the literal details of this abstinence. The principal role model for these hermits was John the Baptist, whom many early interpreters believed ate not locusts and honey, which they regarded as incompatible with his ascetic life, but plant roots (Kelhoffer, 2005; see Matthew 3.4, Mark 1.6). In this strictly ascetic tradition the most serious sin was not lust, as commonly supposed, but gluttony (Miller, 1990). Yet despite the prominence of dietary issues in accounts of these hermits' lives, studies usually devote more attention to issues surrounding virginity and sexuality. Strict fasting is now uncommon even in monasteries, although its reinstitution has been advocated by the French Benedictine Adalbert de Vogüé (1989).

Within Patristics and church history, a more recent theological approach to food has been via critical retrievals of traditions of abstinence and fasting. These have tended to synthesize a wide historical period, arguing that early writers such as Jerome continued to influence the practice of later centuries. In particular, feminist medieval historians have debated at length whether medieval women mystics such as Catherine of Siena should be classified as anorectic. Following the pioneering study of Rudolph Bell (1985), several have argued that such a classification is in fact valid and, moreover, that such fasting was a means by which celibate male clerics were able to gain indirect power over women's bodies (Rousselle, 1998; Shaw, 1998; Grimm, 1996; also Vandereycken and Van Deth, 1994). But it has also been argued that the reality was somewhat more complex. By fasting, women were able to gain a degree of autonomy from the structures of male priestly mediation and social control, within the boundaries imposed on them (Walker Bynum, 1987). Because the social and belief matrices within which medieval fasting took place were so different from those within which modern anorexia is situated, comparisons of the two must be made with care.

Research methodologies

Biblical studies

As shown earlier in this chapter, a good part of the development of theological interest in food has been inspired by biblical studies. This is because so much of scripture, at least in the Jewish and Christian traditions, is concerned in different ways with everyday material life and its theological and spiritual significance. But much of this earlier work in biblical studies was focused on a small selection of texts (although see Sharon, 2002) and has not probed sufficiently deeply their historical contexts. With regard to the Hebrew Bible/Old Testament, Nathan MacDonald has addressed both these problems, producing two studies. One is textually focused, considering the role of food in constructing Israelite identity (2008a). The other draws primarily on archaeology in order to reconstruct actual dietary practice and compare this evidence with textual claims (2008b), finding much corroborating evidence.

In New Testament studies, social scientific approaches have provoked fresh interest in aspects of material life such as food. David Horrell (2005) takes food as the key test case in his examination of the construction of Christian identity in Paul's letters. Horrell shows how the different food practices that existed among the early Jewish Christians and Gentile Christians produced issues that needed to be negotiated by an approach to rules and boundaries that introduced a measure of flexibility into an important field of social interaction. Mission was essential if nascent churches were to continue to grow, and hospitality was part of this. Such hospitality included commensality, in which people of differing traditions shared common food around a common table.

In assessing the impact of biblical texts on food practices, varying reception contexts must also be considered. For example, in monastically governed Christian communities in Celtic Ireland the Mosaic food laws were partly reinstituted in order to differentiate Christians from pagans (Grumett, 2008). Such a reappropriation would have been improbable in a region in which Jews were numerous, such as southern France. In that context, Christians would likely have defined themselves polemically against these laws in order to secure the same objective of enacting their distinctiveness (Fabre-Vassas, 1999).

Theological engagements with culture

To attend to food is to attend to everyday, material life. That life is patterned by traditions of practice, which exhibit forms of implicit rationality that are important theological sources. As such, traditions of practice both possess normative value and inform theologians working in the present day. For example, Christians have frequently abstained from red meat, with monks classically avoiding it altogether and laypeople being required not to eat it on particular days. As a result, Christians have promoted the eating of fish as an alternative (Grumett, 2011b). In the United States meat has sometimes been avoided in Christian communities, especially among millenarian groups such as the Shakers (Puskar-Pasewicz, 2006). Discourses linking bodily health with redemption, or at least with preparedness for redemption, can be traced back to Methodist founder John Wesley and have persisted in evangelical dietary discourse (Griffith, 1999). Moreover, in mid-nineteenth-century Britain, Christians were instrumental in the birth of modern secular vegetarianism (Calvert, 2007), which spread rapidly from Britain to the United States. More recently, Seventh-Day Adventists (Shurtleff and Aoyagi, 1992) and other Christians have played key roles in promoting dietary reform in the United States, particularly via the marketing of healthy breakfast products such as cereals (Sack, 2001; Carson, 1959).

Studies such as these suggest that Christianity possesses a distinctive dietary tradition and explanations for that tradition. Important points of divergence from secular dietary traditions may be identified. The widespread secular understanding of vegetarianism as entailing abstention from all animal, avian, and aquatic flesh, and even as tending towards veganism, is problematic for a Christian tradition that has tended to view quadrupeds (four-footed mammals) as the primary contested food category on the grounds that their life force is, like that of humans, red blood, and because they inhabit the land in close proximity to humans (Grumett and Muers, 2010: 74–76). Christian abstention is, moreover, frequently periodic rather than permanent, and as such is situated within a very different theological cosmology (Khalil, 1990). By rediscovering and rearticulating their distinctive dietary traditions, theologians may therefore bring distinctive critical resources to bear on current debates about food.

Theological engagements with ritual and liturgical studies

Food is a central part of the ritual of many religions. This is most obviously the case with meat. The teachings of both Judaism and Islam require that animals that are to be slaughtered for consumption as meat be killed humanely and suffer as little pain as possible. The animal's blood, recognized as the life force given to it by God, must be drained and not consumed. Rabbinic tradition imposes three specific requirements for Jewish slaughter (*shechitah*): a qualified slaughterer (*shochet*), the correct instrument (*halaf*), and the right procedure (Cohn-Sherbok, 2006). Islamic teaching requires a defined method of slaughter (*dhabh*), the cleansing of the carcass (*tadhkiyah*), and invocation of the name of God (*tasmiyah* and *takbīr*) (Masri, 2007).

In Judaism, fasting has been linked with the liturgical cycle following both the destruction of the first Temple and especially the leveling of the second Temple (Diamond, 2004). In Islam, the rules surrounding fasting may also be considered as ritual. With likely origins in the strict Lenten fasting of Syriac Christians, the observance of Ramadan is mandated by the Qu'ran (Wagtendonk, 1968). Fasting can be seen as a collective "pathway to Paradise" by which Muslims are cleansed from their sins and gain merit in the eyes of Allah (Buitelaar, 1993). Moreover, dining could even be viewed as itself governed by ritual, in so far as mindful practice and hospitality codes are central to it (Al-Ghazālī, 2000).

In the Christian eucharist a basic foodstuff, bread, is given a central representative function. But it would be wrong to infer from this that no other foods possess ritual or liturgical significance. In the early church, eucharists were celebrated with other foods including fish, cheese, vegetables, and fruits (McGowan, 1999). This suggests that the boundaries of the "liturgical" were not so clearly demarcated as in the present day, and that everyday food items acquired theological significance liturgically. Furthermore, contrary to common assumption, rituals and liturgies of animal sacrifice have persisted in several Oriental and Eastern Orthodox Churches (Grumett and Muers, 2010: 107–27), enacting the belief that an animal to be slaughtered is a gift of God to the whole human community. The best-known of these liturgies is the *madagh* of the Armenian Orthodox Church (Findikyan, 1992). There is evidence of less codified Christian sacrificial rituals continuing in Greece (Georgoudi, 1989).

Avenues for future research

Because Christianity has been the world religion most deeply implicated in the rise of modernity, the mechanization of production and consumption processes, and the erosion of traditions of localized and embodied living, the effort of retrieval required of Christian theologians is greater than the effort required by theologians of other confessions. Several stages of future work may be identified.

First, present-day theologians must *critically reappraise the theological tradition* in order to understand how and why food has come to be marginalized from their discipline. For instance, Augustine of Hippo was uneasy with dietary rules within Christianity because of his earlier membership of the Manichean religion, which had strict food rules founded on the belief that its elect members, by eating vegetal matter, were able to liberate light particles imprisoned within it. This led Augustine to employ eating imagery metaphorically in order to communicate supposedly more fundamental theological truths than those about real, everyday food items (Ferrari, 1979, 1978). His contention that dietary issues are *adiaphora* permeated much of the subsequent Christian tradition, preparing the way for the later devaluation of dietary discipline in Western monasteries, in which abstention from red meat by healthy adults was anciently accepted without question. But theologians also need to reappraise figures who are sometimes assumed to endorse modern vegetarianism uncritically, above all Francis of Assisi, who contrary to common supposition was not vegetarian. In fact, Francis embraced a dietary flexibility in order both to give and receive hospitality and to avoid being labelled a heretic (Grumett, 2007).

In parallel with the critique and re-evaluation of their own tradition, theologians need to *engage current non-theological interest in food*, both in other intellectual disciplines and in secular society. Theologians need to learn from discourses and communities in which food is taken seriously. There is already a growing body of literature that seeks to find spiritual inspiration for vegetarianism and other forms of mindful eating across a range of religious traditions (Sapontzis, 2004; Altman, 1999; Berry, 1998). These studies show that new forms of engagement are both possible and fruitful, not least in bringing theology to a wider audience than would normally engage it.

Having begun to reappraise their theological inheritance and engage secular interest in food, theologians will be able to begin to *shape ecclesial practice and witness*. This part of their task has implications for mission. Current interest in many churches in Fairtrade reveals a desire to examine food purchasing and consumption as spiritually significant facets of human life. Nevertheless, Fairtrade discourse is based on a far too uncritical acceptance of ecologically unsustainable patterns of consumption, production, and transportation. Churches need theological help in order to relate their own authentic food practices to those of the wider world in a process of mutual reflection and discovery (Grumett, 2011a). Part of this process is likely to involve the contextual reading of scripture (Grumett, 2011c; Barclay, 2010). This will enable, in turn, an invigorated theological critique of culture that employs doctrine to unmask its dietary pathologies (Grumett, Bretherton, and Holmes, 2011).

By combining critique of their own tradition with societal and ecclesial engagement, theologians will equip themselves to *establish a new practice-focused theology*. Foundations for this project may be found in the work of David Brown (esp. 2007: 120–84). Moreover, in philosophical theology there is the work of Philip Lyndon Reynolds on how views of soul and body in later medieval theology may be seen through the lens of beliefs about how food was assimilated, or not assimilated, into the physical human body (1999). In systematic theology Norman Wirzba has authored an excellent study (2011) that addresses key topics such as sin, grace, communion, and sacrifice through the lens of food, as well as considering food's ultimate ontological status by reflecting on its place in heaven. Wirzba also reflects on pressing contemporary issues such as justice and ecology. Notwithstanding the feminist critiques discussed earlier in this chapter, theology also offers resources to people on weight-loss programs (Soza, 2009). Furthermore, Angel F. Méndez Montoya has produced a study (2009) in which eucharistic motifs are central. This draws heavily on critical theory but does not offer many concrete proposals for everyday food choices.

In attempting to develop systematic accounts such as these, theologians might well need to rethink doctrinal suppositions that have gained acceptance in more fragmentary approaches. For instance, the popular idea that abstention from animal flesh might intimate a return to a paradisiacal condition in which humans and animals live in harmony rests on contestable assumptions about human origins. Abstention might find a firmer grounding in an eschatological account of what the world will, in Christ, in due time become (Southgate, 2008).

If scholars are to make their full intellectual contribution to addressing pressing issues in current human life, new disciplinary engagements will be urgently needed. As such engagements develop, however, it will be necessary for theologians to undertake ongoing self-reflection of a kind that enables them to understand not only the traditional disciplinary approaches from which they have emerged, but equally how they might return to those core disciplines with new sources, methodologies, and narratives to offer back to them.

What prospects might study and research into food and theology bring to the *renewal of theology*? They are likely to draw on a range of subdisciplines that normally interact infrequently. As seen in this chapter, systematic theology, biblical studies, Patristics, church history, ritual studies, liturgical studies, and feminist theological hermeneutics all provide tools and insights needed to understand the complex reality of food. In theology such intersubdisciplinary engagement needs to be promoted, with the rigorous enquiries of scholars with diverse expertise combined to make far greater advances in understanding than would be possible were the methods of just one subdiscipline employed. Theologians could fruitfully apply this intersubdisciplinary model of enquiry to other complex topics in material human life.

Moreover, when studying food and theology it becomes clear that sources and topics that Christian theologians sometimes regard as unimportant, such as church history and the Mosaic law, in fact contain material of central relevance to the questions being addressed. When studying food, theologians should be encouraged to continue to make direct reference to unfamiliar sources such as these, allowing their selection of sources to be guided by the evidence and imperatives of the research being undertaken.

Finally, the study of food and theology should cause theologians, as well as scholars in religious studies, to rethink the unfortunate divide that has opened between their respective disciplines. In reality, theologians can no more avoid the anthropological, cultural, and ritual dimensions of human life than religious studies scholars can rest content with neutral, ahistorical, unsystematic description. There is a need for closer working between scholars in these disciplines and for mutual acknowledgement of need and debt.

Practical considerations for getting started

A large volume of literature on food and spirituality exists aimed at the general reader. Although this might provide useful orientation, it is essential that anyone wishing to pursue the academic study of food and theology seek out serious scholarly sources, such as those cited in this chapter. An excellent entry-level survey is Stephen H. Webb's *Good Eating* (2001). This examines biblical and subsequent Christian teaching on food and considers why modern Christianity has failed to take food seriously. Webb challenges his readers to integrate food into their worldview, as well as providing the means for Christians who take diet seriously to develop their personal reflection on it.

The topic of food and theology is insufficiently evolved to have dedicated postgraduate programs. Students interested in working in the field should identify a potential advisor who is sympathetic to it and who has published relevant or related theological research, and approach them directly. Faculty working in biblical studies, Patristics, and church history often have theological interests and such people might also be approached.

As in some other areas of food studies, the placing of articles in discipline-specific journals can be difficult. Not all editors of theology journals yet regard food and theology as a topic worthy of attention. Journals that have published articles on food include *The Expository Times* and the *Evangelical Quarterly*. Another possible destination is the interdisciplinary *Journal for the Study of Religion, Nature, and Culture*. Food studies journals also accept articles on food and theology. Nevertheless, it is vital that the field comes to be recognized as part of mainstream theology, and if this is to happen theologians working on food will need to rise to the challenge of publishing in theological journals. Food and theology nonetheless has considerable potential as a research field because it is innovative and addresses issues of pressing public concern. This is likely to make it attractive to potential publishers and funders.

Key reading

Grumett, David and Rachel Muers (2010) *Theology on the Menu: Asceticism, Meat and Christian Diet.* London: Routledge.
Soza, Joel R. (2009) *Food and God: A Theological Approach to Eating, Diet, and Weight Control.* Eugene, OR: Wipf & Stock.

Webb, Stephen H. (2001) *Good Eating*. Grand Rapids, MI: Brazos.
Wirzba, Norman (2011) *Food and Faith: A Theology of Eating*. New York: Cambridge University Press.

Bibliography

Al-Ghazālī (2000) *On the Manners Relating to Eating*. Cambridge: Islamic Texts Society.
Altman, Donald (1999) *Art of the Inner Meal: Eating as a Spiritual Path*. New York: Harper.
Barclay, John M. G. (2010) "Food, Christian Identity and Global Warming: A Pauline Call for a Christian Food Taboo." *The Expository Times* 121(12): 585–93.
Bazell, Dianne M. (1997) "Strife among the Table-Fellows: Conflicting Attitudes of Early and Medieval Christians toward the Eating of Meat." *Journal of the American Academy of Religion* 65(1): 73–99.
Bell, Rudolph M. (1985) *Holy Anorexia*. Chicago, IL: University of Chicago Press.
Berry, Ryan (1998) *Food for the Gods: Vegetarianism and the World's Religions*. New York: Pythagorean.
Brown, David (2007) *God of Grace and Body: Sacrament in Ordinary*. Oxford University Press.
Buitelaar, Marjo (1993) *Fasting and Feasting in Morocco: Women's Participation in Ramadan*. Oxford: Berg.
Calvert, Samantha (2007) "A Taste of Eden: Modern Christianity and Vegetarianism." *Journal of Ecclesiastical History* 58(3): 461–81.
Carson, Gerald (1959) *Cornflake Crusade*. London: Gollancz.
Cohn-Sherbok, Dan (2006) "Hope for the animal kingdom: a Jewish vision." In *A Communion of Subjects: Animals in Religion, Science, and Ethics*, Paul Waldau and Kimberley Patton, eds., pp. 81–90 New York: Columbia University Press.
De Vogüé, Adalbert (1989) *To Love Fasting: The Monastic Experience*. Petersham, MA: Saint Bede's.
Diamond, Eliezer (2004) *Holy Men and Hunger Artists: Fasting and Asceticism in Rabbinic Culture*. Oxford: Oxford University Press.
Douglas, Mary (1999) *Leviticus as Literature*. Oxford: Oxford University Press.
——1966; revised edition 2002. *Purity and Danger: An Analysis of Concepts of Pollution and Taboo*. London: Routledge.
Fabre-Vassas, Claudine (1999) *The Singular Beast: Jews, Christians, and the Pig*. New York: Columbia University Press.
Feeley-Harnik, Gillian (1981) *The Lord's Table: Eucharist and Passover in Early Passover*. Philadelphia: University of Pennsylvania Press.
Ferrari, Leo (1979) "The Gustatory Augustine." *Augustiniana* 29: 304–15.
——1978) "The 'Food of Truth' in Augustine's Confessions." *Augustinian Studies* 9: 1–14.
Findikyan, Michael (1992) "A Sacrifice of Praise: Blessing of the Madagh." *Window Quarterly* 2, 4.
Georgoudi, Stella (1989) "Sanctified slaughter in modern Greece: the 'kourbánia' of the saints." In *The Cuisine of Sacrifice among the Greeks*, Marcel Detienne and Jean-Pierre Vernant, eds. Chicago, IL: University of Chicago Press, 183–203.
Gregory, James R.T.E. (2008) "'A Lutheranism of the Table': religion and the Victorian vegetarians." In *Theology on the Menu: Asceticism, Meat and Christian Diet*, David Muers and Rachel Grumett, eds., pp. 135–51 London: Routledge.
Griffith, R. Marie (1999) "Fasting, dieting and the body in American Christianity." In *Perspectives on American Religion and Culture*, Peter W. Williams, ed., pp. 216–27 Oxford: Blackwell.
Grimm, Veronika (1996) *From Feasting to Fasting, the Evolution of a Sin: Attitudes to Food in Late Antiquity*. London: Routledge.
Grumett, David (2011a) "Digesting the Word: A Triptych and Proposal on Dietary Choice." *The Other Journal* 19, at www.theotherjournal.com (accessed on March 29, 2012).
——(2011b) "Dining in the kingdom: fish eating and Christian geography." In *Emerging Geographies of Belief*, Catherine Leyshon *et al.*, eds., pp. 255–71 Newcastle: Cambridge Scholars.
——(2011c) "Eat Less Meat: A New Ecological Imperative for Christian Ethics?" *The Expository Times* 123(1): 54–62.
——(2008) "Mosaic food rules in Celtic spirituality in Ireland." In *Theology on the Menu: Asceticism, Meat and Christian Diet*, David Muers and Rachel Grumett, eds., pp. 31–43 London: Routledge.
——(2007) "Vegetarian or Franciscan? Flexible Dietary Choices Past and Present." *Journal for the Study of Religion, Nature and Culture* 1(4): 450–67.
Grumett, David and Rachel, Muers (2010) *Theology on the Menu: Asceticism, Meat and Christian Diet*. London: Routledge.

Grumett, David, Luke Bretherton, and Stephen R. Holmes. (2011) "Fast Food: A Critical Theological Perspective." *Food, Culture & Society* 14(3): 375–92.

Harvey, Barbara F. (1993) "Diet." In *Living and Dying in England, 1100–1540: The Monastic Experience*. Oxford: Clarendon, 34–71.

Henisch, Bridget Ann (1976) *Fast and Feast: Food in Medieval Society*. University Park: Pennsylvania State University Press.

Horrell, David G. (2005) *Solidarity and Difference: A Contemporary Reading of Paul's Ethics*. London: T&T Clark.

Houston, Walter (1993) *Purity and Monotheism: Clean and Unclean Animals in Biblical Law*. Sheffield: JSOT Press.

Kelhoffer, James A. (2005) *The Diet of John the Baptist: "Locusts and Wild Honey" in Synoptic and Patristic Interpretation*. Tübingen: Mohr Siebeck.

Khalil, Issa J. (1990) "The Orthodox Fast and the Philosophy of Vegetarianism." *Greek Orthodox Theological Review* 35(3): 237–59.

Kunin, Seth D. (2004) *We Think what we Eat: Neo-Structuralist Analysis of Israelite Food Rules and other Cultural and Textual Practices*. London: T&T Clark.

Leyerle, Blake (2004) "Monastic formation and Christian practice: food in the desert." In *Educating People of Faith: Exploring the History of Jewish and Christian Communities*, John Van Engen, ed., pp. 85–112 Grand Rapids, MI: Eerdmans.

MacDonald, Nathan (2008a) *Not Bread Alone: The Uses of Food in the Old Testament*. Oxford: Oxford University Press.

——(2008b) *What Did the Ancient Israelites Eat? Diet in Biblical Times*. Grand Rapids, MI: Eerdmans.

Masri, Al-Hafiz Basheer Ahmad (2007) *Animal Welfare in Islam*. Markfield: The Islamic Foundation.

McGowan, Andrew (1999) *Ascetic Eucharists: Food and Drink in Early Christian Ritual Meals*. Oxford: Clarendon.

Miller, William Ian (1997) "Gluttony." *Representations* 60: 92–112.

Montoya, Angel F. Méndez (2009) *The Theology of Food: Eating and the Eucharist*. Malden, MA: Blackwell.

Muers, Rachel and David Grumett (2008) *Eating and Believing: Interdisciplinary Perspectives on Vegetarianism and Theology*. London: T&T Clark.

Puskar-Pasewicz, Margaret (2006) "Kitchen sisters and disagreeable boys: debates over meatless diets in nineteenth-century Shaker communities." In *Eating in Eden: Food and American Utopias*, Etta M. Madden and Martha L. Finch, eds., pp. 109–24 Lincoln: University of Nebraska Press.

Reynolds, Philip Lyndon (1999) *Food and the Body: Some Peculiar Questions in High Medieval Theology*. Leiden: Brill.

Rousselle, Aline (1998) *Porneia: On Desire and the Body in Antiquity*. Oxford: Blackwell.

Sack, Daniel (2001) *Whitebread Protestants: Food and Religion in American Culture*. Basingstoke: Palgrave.

Sapontzis, Steve ed. (2004) *Food for Thought: The Debate over Eating Meat*. Amherst, MA: Prometheus.

Sharon, Diane M. (2002) *Patterns of Destiny: Narrative Structures of Foundation and Doom in the Hebrew Bible*. Winona Lake, IN: Eisenbrauns.

Shaw, Teresa M. (1998) *The Burden of the Flesh: Fasting and Sexuality in Early Christianity*. Minneapolis, MN: Fortress.

Shurtleff, William and Akiko Aoyagi (1992) *Bibliography and Sourcebook on Seventh-Day Adventists' Work with Soyfoods, Vegetarianism, and Wheat Gluten, 1866–1992*. Lafayette, CA: Soyfoods Centre.

Simoons, Frederick J. (1998) *Plants of Life, Plants of Death*. Madison: University of Wisconsin Press.

——(1961) 2nd edition 1994. *Eat Not this Flesh: Food Avoidances from Prehistory to the Present*. Madison: University of Wisconsin Press.

Soler, Jean (1979) "The semiotics of food in the Bible." In *Food and Drink in History*, Robert Forster and Orest Ranum, eds., pp. 126–38. Baltimore, MD: Johns Hopkins University Press. Reprinted 1997 in *Food and Culture: A Reader*, Carole Counihan and Penny Van Esterick, eds., pp. 55–66. New York: Routledge.

Southgate, Christopher (2008) "Protological and eschatological vegetarianism." In *Theology on the Menu: Asceticism, Meat and Christian Diet*, David Muers and Rachel Grumett, eds., pp. 247–65. London: Routledge.

Soza, Joel R. (2009) *Food and God: A Theological Approach to Eating, Diet, and Weight Control*. Eugene, OR: Wipf and Stock.

Twigg, Julia (1983) "Vegetarianism and the meanings of meat." In *The Sociology of Food and Eating: Essays on the Sociological Significance of Food*, ed., pp. 18–30 Anne Murcott. Aldershot: Gower.

——(1981) "The Vegetarian Movement in England, 1847–1981: With Particular Reference to its Ideology." University of London PhD thesis, at www.ivu.org/history/thesis/index.html (accessed July 11, 2011).

——(1979) "Food for Thought: Purity and Vegetarianism." *Religion* 9: 13–35.

Vandereycken, Walter and Ron Van Deth (1994) *From Fasting Saints to Anorexic Girls: The History of Self-Starvation*. New York: New York University Press.

Wagtendonk, Kees (1968) *Fasting in the Koran*. Leiden: Brill.

Walker Bynum, Caroline (1987) *Holy Feast and Holy Fast: The Religious Significance of Food to Medieval Women*. Berkeley: University of California Press.

Webb, Stephen H. (2001) *Good Eating*. Grand Rapids, MI: Brazos.

Wirzba, Norman (2011) *Food and Faith: A Theology of Eating*. New York: Cambridge University Press.

15

Food and art

Travis Nygard

This chapter discusses food within the discipline of art history. Methodologies of close looking are covered. Theories of iconography, symbolism, and design are discussed in relation to food. Art is considered as a data set useful in the interrogation of food-related social history. The question of whether the display of and debates about images of food can be a factor that causes social change is presented. Practical suggestions are included for undertaking image-related research, finding secondary literature, and securing funding. Ultimately, the chapter presents strategies for treating food and art symbiotically, rather than as two separate bodies of knowledge.

Introduction

Scholarship about the intersection of food and art can be undertaken by art historians, who see their mission as qualitatively interpreting and historicizing visual material. Indeed, scholars in this discipline sometimes study images of food, tools for preparing and serving food, and food products themselves. The discipline of art history took its modern form during the nineteenth century, when scholars began to classify the paintings and sculptures produced in Western Europe in rigorous ways, focusing on variables such as style, media, subject matter, and craftsmanship. The discipline celebrated "masterpieces"—the most skilfully produced art of each era. Although art-historical scholarship during the early twenty-first century embraces non-Western art, as well as some vernacular creativity, the discipline remains driven by the so-called "major" arts of painting, sculpture, and architecture produced in Europe and the Americas. Indeed, art historians most frequently scrutinize skilfully made objects that are visually complex, produced to bolster the agendas of powerful people and institutions or as items of luxury for elite members of society. Folk art, commercial art, and non-art imagery can also be interrogated by art historians, but scholarship in these areas rarely draws widespread attention within the discipline.

The discipline of art history has long embraced insights from other academic disciplines when interpreting imagery, and incorporating insights from food studies in no way undermines standard modes of inquiry about art. That said, art historians almost always forefront a specific work of art, the oeuvre of an artist, the art patronage of a specific person, or the history of an art movement in their scholarship rather than forefronting a type of food, food preparation technique, or idea about cuisine. A scholar interested in thinking art-historically about food would thus be well advised to begin with a well-known work of art or artist, and then contextualize it with ideas from across the field of food studies. During the course of analysis, insights from philosophers, psychologists, historians, critics, and theorists can also be brought into play. Like scholars from across the humanities, art historians often contextualize cultural phenomena by engaging with bodies of theoretical inquiry that expose power relationships. Some of these include Marxism, feminism, post-colonialism, queer theory, eco-criticism, theories of nationhood, theories of ability, and critical race theory.

Historical background of food scholarship in art history and major theoretical approaches in use

Food itself has traditionally fallen outside the realm of scrutiny by art professionals, but images of food are often analyzed carefully. That said, the best treatments of food by art historians working today start with the premise that the stories of art and food can be intertwined. Such scholarship shows that there was sometimes a symbiotic relationship between art and food making, and that considering the history of food concurrent with the history of art produces insights that would be impossible in treatments that studied art or food alone.

One of the most sustained and rigorous treatments of art and food together is the book by the art historian John Varriano, titled *Tastes and Temptations*. His work is an analytical and scholarly treatment of Renaissance Italy, in which he makes professional parallels between artists and cooks. He discusses ways to analyze images of food, from the symbolic to the sacred to the sensual. He considers ties between food making and art making on a literal level, including why eggs, butter, lard, and oils are used in both endeavors. He considers how people used both art and food to help them think, and he even considers art made from food products, such as sugar sculpture. The art historian Jocelyn Hackforth-Jones's book *Dining with the Impressionists* presents a similarly intriguing intertwined story of food and art history. Although her book lacks a full scholarly apparatus of footnotes, she presents a fascinating argument. She notes that the rise of impressionism was concurrent with the rise of modern cooking techniques in France, as bolstered by the revolutionary chef and writer Auguste Escoffier, and that impressionism can be understood as an obsessive celebration of new and modern foods. Within modernity, Cecilia Novera's book *Antidiets of the Avant-Garde* focuses on twentieth-century artists who radically questioned the roles of food in our lives. Although it is common for art historians to mention an anecdote about an artist's relationship to food in passing, it is rare for the subject to be given a full-blown analytical treatment. Alexandra Leaf and Fred Leeman's book *Van Gogh's Table at the Auberge Ravoux* is a rare example of scholarship on an artist that places more emphasis on how food fit into a painter's life rather than how art fit into it.

A theoretical approach that many art historians use when looking at food-related imagery is iconography. In the strictest sense of the word, iconography refers to the relationship of imagery ("icono") to written texts ("graphy"). An iconographic analysis of a biblical painting that shows people eating might compare the types of food and people in the image to scriptural accounts of the Last Supper, the Feast in the House of Levi, and the Wedding at Cana. A scholar would argue that the image fits one of these narratives better than others by articulating parallels between the image and text. The best iconographic analyses press the analysis further, into the realm of "iconology"—arguing that a more complete understanding of the image can be achieved by analyzing the norms and values of the era in which the painting was created. The most profound iconographic scholarship starts from the assumption that art is not simply an *illustration* of written sources, nor does it provide an objective window onto the past. Art, rather, presents ideas that may not be apparent by looking at the original textual story. To undertake an iconological analysis with an emphasis on food, a scholar might discuss how an artist has made strategic choices about which foods are depicted, how they are being served, if they are shown partially eaten, and whether they have symbolic meanings. In the case of Leonardo da Vinci's celebrated *Last Supper* from 1495–98 CE, for example, a scholar might note that it is well known that the mural was created for a refectory (dining hall) in a monastery, and it is commonly assumed that the monks were meant to empathize with the disciples as they consumed their meals. A food-related iconological analysis might strive to understand whether it is important that the rolls of bread on the table are shown uneaten, that empty plates and bowls are shown carefully placed in front of disciples, that wine glasses are all shown half full, that some fruits and vegetables are shown scattered on the tablecloth, and that two platters appear to contain the main course. The scholar would ultimately argue that the artist used the biblical text as a starting point, but that the painting also represents a new understanding of food geared toward the patron and viewer.

Perhaps the most directly food-related scholarship on art focuses on sculpture, painting, and mosaics that uses food as a medium. Using food to make art has been common, both in recent history and in the deep past. That said, because of the ephemerality of art that is often created to be consumed, it becomes increasingly more challenging to scrutinize this type of art farther back in time. Textual sources and prints, nonetheless, confirm that artists as far back as the Middle Ages in Europe made high quality sculptures from foodstuff. Indeed, the anthropologist Sidney Mintz explained in his groundbreaking book *Sweetness and Power* that sculptures, and sometimes even architecture, could be created from a marzipan-like paste of sugar mixed with ground nuts. Molds that were used to make visually spectacular desserts seem to have been strikingly similar to those used to make bronze sculpture, and the history of food presentation during pre- and early-modern history can thus be linked together. Analyses of food as a creative media are not linked to desserts either. Decorative molds for casting butter were common during the nineteenth century, and at its height this craft merged with the fine-art establishment. As the art historian Pamela Simpson has explained in her book *Corn Palaces and Butter Queens*, artists carved, cast, and exhibited sculptures made from butter across America, as well as made mosaics from grain and other grasses. Although art made from food may seem unusual, when the focus of the imagery was also food related it was in fact a form of experimental *design*.

Another theoretical approach common in art history is to scrutinize the relationship of *form* to *function* in food-related decorative arts, such as dishware and cutlery. Such an approach is usually described as the analysis of artistic *design*. Good design is when form is merged with function in a simple but thoughtful way. Form includes the actual shapes of objects, as well as decorations on them. Ancient Greek wine cups are often good examples of design, as they commonly contain painted scenes of drunken revelry or the god Dionysus. Extending the analysis to the actual shape of the cups, François Lissarrague demonstrated in his excellent book *The Aesthetics of the Greek Banquet* that ancient artists manipulated the shape of cups and serving vessels to control temperature, to prevent accidental sloshing, and to appear to hold less than they did in reality.

Research methodologies

Art historians are storytellers, who present research in analytical and narrative form, situating imagery in the context of a specific moment or era of a specific place. Original research consists of presenting previously unknown information about works of art, or interpreting well-known work in a new way. Art historians most frequently write about the intents and social perspectives of artists, but can also write from the perspectives of critics, other art historians, collectors, institutions, politicians, the general public, or anyone else who has been interested in art at a specific time and place.

The core data used by scholars of art are visual, and the basic methodology employed by all art historians is careful visual scrutiny of art objects. When this methodology is applied to a single work of art in a sustained way it is called "close looking," and the goal is usually to understand how an artist used the formal properties of art—such as color, line, composition, light, and texture—to make a visual statement. In the case of a still life painting showing fruit, we might start by asking whether the food is shown in saturated or muted colors, whether literal or implied lines direct our attention to some fruits more than others, if the foods are juxtaposed with each other in a thoughtful way, if some pieces of fruit are better illuminated than others, and if the food is rendered with clarity or with loose brushwork. Combined with a discussion of the subject matter, such as what types of fruit are present and whether they appear ripe, we would come to a conclusion about the meaning of this specific work of art, and how it speaks for itself. In the case of still lifes depicting luscious fruit such meaning is commonly assumed to be a celebration of exotics or a metaphor for sexual pleasure. Extending this methodology of close looking across many works of art, while seeking out visual patterns, is a strategy used to identify motifs and themes, which can together compose "visual cultures." Such an approach is often useful for embedding art into social history.

Pinpointing specific examples of art that changed how people understood their food, cooking, and eating is the type of questioning that is at the core of rhetorical and social art history. This is in contrast to scholarship that assumes art played a passive role in social history—reflecting societal norms and values but not steering them in new directions. Scholars pursuing this approach seek out images that were publicly debated, contributing to shifts in food-related policies, practices, and traditions. For example, a scholar could seek out evidence of whether the widespread cultural awareness during the twentieth century of Vincent van Gogh's *The Potato Eaters* from 1885—a painting that shows a peasant family so impoverished that they eat nothing but tubers in the winter—inspired conversations that ultimately resulted in the enactment of social welfare programs. Similarly, seeking out artistic representations of foods that were used as surrogates for actual food—due to specific items being out of season or otherwise unavailable— could be a step toward framing art as a central component of the rituals of eating. If foods depicted in paintings, sculptures, prints, or books were commonly used as the inspiration for the creation of real dishes, then an argument could be made that the imagery is just as important as the ingredients. Lastly, if it can be demonstrated that eaters sometimes evaluated the quality or significance of their food, not by contextualizing it amidst actual foodstuffs, but by comparisons to artistic representations of food, photographs of food in advertising, fake foods in store windows, and other visual representations of edible goods, then art could be framed as at the core of decisions that people make about their eating.

Analyses of art often also include discussion of food-related signs and symbols. This approach can be particularly useful when looking at emblems, portraits, and other highly contrived images that were meant to serve rhetorical purposes. Examining how foods create meanings in art, due to their symbolic nature, in ways that would not otherwise be apparent, is at the core of this approach. While some scholarship takes a piecemeal approach to symbols in imagery, proceeding from motif to motif, the best scholarship synthesizes meanings into a coherent whole, exploring how the art uses specific symbols to convey a total message.

Although most art historians do not work with living human subjects, scholars who study contemporary art often gather their data directly from artists, visiting their studios, corresponding with them, and conducting interviews. Some of the most compelling food-related art made in recent years is by artists who engage with foodstuff on a conceptual level and as a media. Rolando Briseño has drawn on the visual traditions of indigenous Mexico by making a sculpture from chocolate of a human heart and sculptures of Aztec deities from corn and wheat. Other well-known examples of contemporary art made from food include assemblages by Joseph Beuys created from margarine, fantastic foodscapes by Carl Warner, and a bust made from chocolate by Janine Anconi. Modern and contemporary artists have also critically engaged with eating utensils and packaging. Meret Oppenheim's fur-covered tea cup, Andy Warhol's Coke bottles and soup cans, and Judy Chicago's *Dinner Party* installation are some of the better-known examples.

Avenues for future research

As of 2011, all periods of art history remain understudied using food as a critical framework. Art historians typically define their fields of expertise by culture and time period. One might specialize, for example, in modern American or medieval Spanish art. Successful careers could be formed in any such field of art history by using food as an anchor, modeling inquiry on some of the trailblazing studies discussed above.

Because profound innovation can occur when disparate bodies of knowledge are put into conversation, increased collaboration between art historians and food professionals could be exciting. Some precedents in this spirit already exist. Art curator Yoshio Tsuchiya wrote *A Feast for the Eyes*, which explores the aesthetic norms of food presentation in Japan. Along with the food arranger Masaru Yamamoto, he interrogated seasonality, normality, functionality, aesthetics, and utensils. The fact that cooking is often viewed as women's work is a theme that was explored in an exhibition produced by the advocacy organization Girls Incorporated titled *Women of Taste*. The project paired chefs with textile artists, and the result was a series of innovative fine-art quilts that used food as their subject matter. People have sometimes recreated food that appears in art, or used art as inspiration for developing modern recipes. Claire Clifton, for example, wrote a book titled *The Art of Food*, which juxtaposes works of art with snippets of culinary history and newly developed recipes. *Eat Art*—a project sponsored by the National Gallery of Australia—featured the work of 31 chefs who were inspired by paintings in the collection. *Foodculture*, edited by Barbara Fischer, is also noteworthy as a collection of essays that attempts to bring the study of food and art together in innovative ways. An analysis of buying, preparing, and eating food in art, as well as food symbolism, is in the book by the art historian Kenneth Bendiner titled *Food in Painting*.

Large-scale and systematic projects geared toward identifying and cataloging works of art that focus on food, and subsequently solidifying a canon of great works of food-related art, is a task that remains to be undertaken. Certainly there have been attempts to gather food-related images together, and these resources are valuable. However, when compared to some of the large-scale, long-term, and in-depth thematic projects that have been undertaken in art history, it is clear that our cataloging of food in art has been modest in scope. As a contrast, note that The Image of the Black in Western Art, for example, is a project housed at the W. E. B. Du Bois Institute for African and African American Research at Harvard University, and it has been systematically collecting, cataloging, analyzing, and publishing images of black people since the 1960s (www.imageoftheblack.com, accessed on March 29, 2012). Similarly, the Index of Christian Art—an initiative that began at Princeton University in 1917—has amassed and published an immense amount of information about art produced by Christians of the Middle Ages (ica.princeton.edu, accessed on March 29, 2012). A parallel food-related project could potentially be undertaken by a research institute or university.

Using theoretical frameworks that are common in food studies, either in a literal or metaphorical way, has the potential to push art historical scholarship forward. Major concepts from across the field of food studies, such as food systems, could by applied to imagery. For example, the celebrated Warka Vase, carved in about 3000 BCE, seems to depict an ancient food system in Mesopotamia—from field to consumer. On the bottom of the vase beasts of burden are shown above a grain field; in the middle register baskets of foodstuff are being brought to a central location; and on the top register food is being redistributed with the oversight of temple officials. We might ask if the questions that scholars have posed about modern food systems can inform a reinterpretation of such historical imagery. Many other concepts from food studies have the potential to enrich the art-historical discourse. Scholars might ask, for example, if art making is similar to or different from following a recipe, whether artistic traditions are comparable to cuisines, and whether the highly developed taste of art and food connoisseurs are comparable.

Scrutinizing food itself as visual art, in a tight way, using art-historical theories and methodologies, is another area for further research. Since the mid-twentieth century art historians have increasingly broadened our definition of art, in light of the realization that art-historical questions, methods, and theories can be applied to many forms of creative expression besides masterpieces of painting and sculpture. Today it is common, indeed, to see art historians publish studies of "visual cultures" that include photography, diagrams, illustrations, cinema, and advertisements. It is also common for art historians to scrutinize the visual properties of "material cultures," such as everyday furniture, dishes, and other functional objects. Using these studies of visual and material culture as models, art historians could undertake studies of how food's visual properties can be aesthetically pleasing or revolting, rhetorically meaningful or vacuous, and stylistically traditional or innovative.

Practical considerations for getting started

Art historians undertake archival research to locate the primary source material needed for our historically grounded analyses. This can be a daunting task if it is begun without strategic prioritizing. When researching art masterpieces commissioned by wealthy patrons that are now in major museum collections, the task of working in archives tends to be easier than researching lesser-known works of art or artists. The types of archival material available vary widely from project to project, but scholars commonly look at letters, diaries, and legal records. One type of archival resource that could be fruitful for a scholar of food and art is the household inventory. These have often been located for well-known artists and patrons, and they are usually part of legal inheritance records. Such inventories are usually consulted by art historians because they itemize the art in a household, but they can also be useful for food historians when the contents of kitchens are inventoried. Revisiting household inventories in conjunction with information from scholarly biographies of well-known artists could reveal what an artist usually ate, and this could be used as a critical framework. It would be germane, for example, when the art of someone like Leonardo da Vinci is scrutinized—who we know followed a near-vegetarian diet and owned a cookbook—to use this information as part of the analytical framework when interpreting his images of eating. When researching a specific work of art in a museum collection, institutional archives can also be used by art historians. Objects in the permanent collections of museums often have corresponding files, which can be accessed by appointment.

There are four major bibliographic databases in the discipline of art history. Two of them, the Bibliography of the History of Art (BHA) and the Répertoire de la litterature de l'art (RILA), index scholarship published from 1975–2007. Free public access to BHA and RILA is provided by the Getty Research Institute on its website (www.getty.edu, accessed on March 29, 2012). Another database is the International Bibliography of Art, which covers scholarship published since 2008. ARTbibliographies Modern covers scholarship published since

1974 on art made since the nineteenth century. Both of the latter databases are accessible only at institutions whose libraries pay to license them.

Unfortunately, finding images of specific foods, or food-related activities, can be frustrating when using image databases. This is because imagery is notoriously difficult to catalog by theme. Nonetheless, numerous institutions have developed image databases to facilitate research. A leading database, which is available by license, is ARTstor. It contains over a million photographs of art and artifacts. Many art museums have also digitized their collections, and they usually make them available on their websites for free. Institutions that are particularly friendly toward scholars include the Metropolitan Museum of Art, the Brooklyn Museum, the British Museum, the Victoria and Albert Museum, and the Prints and Photographs Division of the Library of Congress. Each of them has a high-quality online catalog, and their positions toward scholarly non-profit publishing of art in their collections are less restrictive than average.

Because of the limitations of image databases for thematic research, most scholars continue to browse printed books and periodicals to find compelling imagery. Books that systematically document food as a subject matter for painting, sculpture, and photography are therefore valuable references. For scholars interested in Western imagery from ancient times through the eighteenth century, the book *Food in the Louvre* by chefs Paul Bocuse and Yves Pinard is notable. Scholars seeking examples of visual ephemera from the nineteenth and twentieth centuries, including popular prints and advertisements, should refer to *Food Mania* by Nigel Garwood and Rainer Voigt. In photography a book by Sarah Tanguy is notable, *Taken for Looks*. James Yood wrote a book about paintings in the collection of the Art Institute of Chicago, titled *Feasting*. Gillian Riley's *A Feast for the Eyes* similarly catalogs the works in the National Gallery of London. Silvia Malaguzzi's *Food and Feasting in Art* is a superb reference book on Western painting. It addresses common iconography, allegories, settings, dishware, and cutlery. A catalog created by Linda Weintraub titled *Art What Thou Eat* contains a substantial number of American paintings that focus on food.

Individuals considering advanced study and research in art history should refer to resources published by the College Art Association (CAA), which is the leading academic organization for art professionals. Of particular note are the CAA directories of graduate programs in art history and related fields, such as visual studies, museum and curatorial studies, and art education. They include detailed information on curricula, admissions requirements, and opportunities for funding. Scholarships, fellowships, internships, grants, and awards programs are prevalent in the visual arts, and the CAA also publishes information about such opportunities on its website (www.collegeart.org, accessed on March 29, 2012).

Key reading

Barnes, Donna (2002) *Matters of Taste: Food and Drink in Seventeenth-Century Dutch Art and Life*. Syracuse, NY: Exhibition catalog from the Albany Institute of History and Art published by Syracuse University Press.

Bendiner, Kenneth (2004) *Food in Painting: From the Renaissance to the Present*. London: Reaktion Books.

Bocuse, Paul and Yves Pinard (2009) *Food in the Louvre* (Paris: Musée du Louvre Éditions in association with Flammarion.

Cantú, Norma E., ed., (2010) *Moctezuma's Table: Rolando Briseño's Mexican and Chicano Tablescapes*. College Station: Texas A&M University Press.

Clifton, Claire (1988) *The Art of Food: Culinary Inspirations from the Paintings of the Great Masters*. Secaucus, NJ: The Wellfleet Press.

Fischer, Barbara (1999) *Foodculture: Tasting Identities and Geographies in Art*. Toronto: YYZ Books.

Garwood, Nigel and Rainer Voigt, (2001) *Food Mania*. London: Thames and Hudson.

Girls Incorporated (1999) *Women of Taste: A Collaboration Celebrating Quilt Artists and Chefs*, Jen Bilik, ed. Lafayette, CA: Exhibition catalog from the Smithsonian Institution Travelling Exhibition Service released by C&T Publishing.

Hackforth-Jones, Jocelyn (1991) *Dining with the Impressionists*. New York: Konechy and Konechy.

Leaf, Alexandra and Fred Leeman (2001) *Van Gogh's Table at the Auberge Ravoux*. New York: Artisan.

Lissarrague, François (1990) *The Aesthetics of the Greek Banquet: Images of Wine and Ritual*, Princeton, NJ: Princeton University Press.

Malaguzzi, Silvia (2006) *Food and Feasting in Art*, translated by Brian Phillips. Los Angeles, CA: J. Paul Getty Museum.

Mintz, Sidney (1985) *Sweetness and Power: The Place of Sugar in Modern History*. New York: Viking.

National Gallery of Australia (2004) *Eat Art*. Canberra: The Gallery.

Novera, Cecilia (2010) *Antidiets of the Avant-Garde: From Futurist Cooking to Eat Art*. Minneapolis: University of Minnesota Press.

Riley, Gillian (1997) *A Feast for the Eyes*. London: National Gallery Publications distributed by Yale University Press.

Simpson, Pamela (forthcoming 2012) *Corn Palaces and Butter Queens: A History of Crop Art and Diary Sculpture*. Minneapolis: University of Minnesota Press.

Tanguy, Sarah (2006) *Taken for Looks: Imaging Food in Contemporary Photography*. Exhibition catalog from the Southeast Museum of Photography at Daytona Beach Community College.

Tsuchiya, Yoshio (1985) *A Feast for the Eyes: The Japanese Art of Food Arrangement*, food arranger Masaru Yamamoto, translated by Juliet Winters Carpenter. Tokyo: Kodansha International.

Varriano, John (2009) *Tastes and Temptations: Food and Art in Renaissance Italy*. Berkeley: University of California Press.

Weintraub, Linda, ed. (1991) *Art What Thou Eat: Images of Food in American Art*. New York: Exhibition catalog from the Edith C. Blum Art Institute at Bard College published by Moyer Bell Limited.

Yood, James (1992) *Feasting: A Celebration of Food in Art*. New York: Universe in association with the Art Institute of Chicago.

16

Food in film

Anne Bower and Thomas Piontek

This article introduces theories and methods for exploring the representation of food in films; provides examples of existing scholarship (in print and online journals); and emphasizes the interdisciplinarity necessary for discussions of food in film. The authors suggest that interdisciplinary academic training is advantageous, since no universities offer graduate degrees (or funding) in food in film. Yet there's plenty of potential in this field. Beyond further analyses of feature films, scholars can investigate the evolving food film genre, food-focused documentaries, animated films, and online/computer games and videos, along with cooking shows.

Historical background and major theoretical approaches

Throughout cinematic history, food has played a part in all kinds of films, frequently revealing aspects of characters' emotions, identities, cultural backgrounds, fears, and aspirations. In fact, one of the very first short films ever made by the Lumière Brothers, *Repas de bébé* (*Baby's Dinner* or *Feeding Baby*) consists of one single shot of Auguste Lumière, his wife, and their baby daughter having dinner in a rural setting. Although the film is only 17 meters long and runs for less than a minute, it is of considerable historical significance, for it was part of the original Lumière brothers film program shown on December 28, 1895 in a room at the Grand Café in Paris and thus marks the official beginning of cinema as a theater-going experience. And while the short in itself may be completely banal, it derives power from the fact that it shows us living people, in motion, and in a real setting. Not only was this quite a novelty more than 110 years ago, it is also noteworthy for the way in which it interjects a new technology into people's lives while balancing the newness of that technology with the reassuring familiarity of what it depicted: the domestic scene, a baby being fed.

Since that first groundbreaking introduction of food *and* film, food has been put to many cinematic services. To start with, food can indicate setting—frequently revealing the national, regional, urban, rural, and class aspects of a film's location. Simultaneously, food may propel a film's plot and reveal a great deal about characters, as viewers perceive who cooks, who serves the food, who pays, who eats, who doesn't, who gags on food or hoards it. Food's elemental nature allows film makers to use it in myriad other ways. Gaye Poole points out that "it is possible to 'say' things with food—resentment, love, compensation, anger, rebellion, withdrawal. This makes it a perfect conveyor of subtext; messages which are often implicit rather than explicit, but surprisingly varied, strong, and sometimes violent or subversive" (Poole, 1999: 3).

As James R. Keller argues, whether food plays a major or a minor role in a particular film, "the culinary is highly suggestive of abstract cultural processes, such as class, race, gender, ethnicity, history, politics, geography, aesthetics, spirituality, and nationality, as well as more subjective conditions, such as obsession, indifference, depression, elation, rage, meditation, neurosis, psychosis, mental illness, mystical ecstasy, carnal desire, and love" (Keller, 2006: 1). Likewise, in any kind of movie, food imagery heightens sensory involvement, provoking taste and smell powerfully, and sometimes taking on (or contributing to) sexual messages. Then too, as has been remarked by a number of writers, when chefs and cooks are at the center of a film, they can be stand-ins for the movie director, just as the on-screen eaters of that food can be compared to those of us in the audience—gobbling up the movie. Sometimes the way the food is cooked can even relate to the artistry of how the director puts the film together.

As a discipline film studies preceded food studies by several decades, yet the two disciplines have much in common. Currently 155 colleges offer a major program in film studies (www. collegeboard.com/csearch/majors_careers/profiles/majors/50.0601.html, accessed on March 29, 2012), and that number continues to grow every year. In spite of this trend, the vast majority of classes dedicated to the analysis of film in the American academy today are being offered by departments that do not make film their primary subject—English, communications, history, foreign languages, to name a few.

Scholars in these disparate fields draw on their disciplines not only to develop their understanding of the films they analyze but also to show how the analysis of films contributes to their respective fields, expanding and revitalizing the study of history and English, for instance. In a recent critical essay Justin Philpot refers to this phenomenon as "studies with films," which he distinguishes from *film studies*, without however privileging one over the other (Philpot, 2010).

Being practiced in myriad academic departments, studies with film have necessitated and promoted an interdisciplinary approach to film analysis. In light of this development Philpot, among others, has advocated a comprehensive film studies methodology that "demands textual, historical and cultural analysis." Such an approach, he argues, could "lead to adoption and adaptation across a number of different fields and disciplines within the academy, forcing scholars to make new personal, theoretical and political connections in an attempt to better understand and order the world around them."

Along similar lines it could be argued that to date "studies with food" as practiced in various academic fields still vastly outnumber "food studies," even though a handful of colleges and universities in the US currently offer food studies degrees. However, at the present time, there is no degree program devoted to food in film (or food and film). So, of necessity, scholars working in this area bring the theories, vocabularies, and perspectives of their home disciplines to discussions of food in film—their literary, historical, cinematic, media studies, anthropological, gender studies, cultural studies, sociological, agricultural, economic, political, religious, and culinary backgrounds.

A literature professor, for instance, might explore a movie like George Tillman's *Soul Food* (1997) in terms of African-American literary history, looking at race, class, the legacy of slavery, and the nineteenth-century migration of Blacks from south to north. A scholar in gender studies could use theoretical approaches from that discipline, focusing on the traditional and nontraditional roles of the women in the film and the assumptions both the director and the male characters seem to bring to their relations with those women, all playing out around who prepares what food, how it is served and eaten, and whether or not the food scenes depict any changes in these male and female roles. A nutritionist might take an entirely different approach, applying the science of nutrition, public health principles, and knowledge of African-American foodways to his or her analysis. However, all these scholars would probably find themselves sliding in and out of their "home" disciplines to incorporate insights that come from other areas.

For a representative example of the way an interdisciplinary approach is basically *required* for anyone discussing food in film, one can look at Michael Nottingham's "Downing the Folk-Festive: Menacing Meals in the Films of Jan Svankmajer." In his discussion of the Czech surrealist filmmaker's work, Nottingham uses Michael Bakhtin's theory of the carnivalesque but combines that with his considerable knowledge of surrealism, folklore, and communism (Nottingam, 2004). Perhaps it is this necessary interdisciplinarity that makes food in film scholarship so fascinating. What follows is a brief and partial discussion of some of the commonly used theoretical approaches.

Structuralism and semiotics

Structuralism and semiotics frequently provide basic, underlying theoretical approaches to the study of food in film. Cinema functions, as Teresa de Lauretis first argued in her 1984 seminar study as "a signifying practice, a work of semiosis; a work that produces effects of meaning and perception, self-images and subject positions for all those involved, makers and viewers" (p. 38). A good example of a mainly semiotic approach to the study of food in film is Jane Ferry's analysis of the eight dinner scenes in Martin Scorsese's film adaption of Edith Wharton's *The Age of Innocence* (Ferry, 2003: 11–27). It is important to note, however, that Ferry also interweaves considerable historical research about nineteenth-century New York City (social customs, consumer patterns, fashions in dinnerware, typical upper-class menus, etiquette rules, and more) into her semiotic analysis.

For other examples of how semiotic theoretical underpinnings can be used in different productive ways, consider the combination of semiotics, gastronomic knowledge, and food history in Michael Ashkenazi's "Food, Play, Business, and the Image of Japan in Itami Juzo's *Tampopo*" (in Bower, 2004: 27–40), or the combination of semiotics and gender studies in Keller's "Four Little Caligulas: *La Grande Bouffe*, Consumption and Male Masochism" (in Keller, 2006: 49–59).

Cultural studies

As cultural studies gained credibility in the 1970s, film scholars began to incorporate cultural theory into their work while scholars in other fields began to study film. Philip Rosen describes this as "the emergence of a generation of thinkers about film who [had] in common a basic core bibliography regarding theories of culture and criticism" (Rosen, 1986: vii). A cultural studies perspective informs much of the current work on food in film, but is highly variable. Often this form of analysis focuses on genre, but can equally well delve into ethnicity, "high" culture vs. popular and mass culture, nation building, migration, changing economic and social patterns, pluralistic societies, and even spiritual values. And as film scholar E. Ann Kaplan points out, cultural studies scholars "have precisely appreciated popular culture's ability to bring forth what is repressed and what cannot be said," that is, the released voices of "certain ideological, minority, and female voices/positions/subjectivities" (Kaplan, 1991: 20).

While not explicitly stating that part of her approach to food in films is based on cultural studies, Parley Ann Boswell's critical concerns certainly derive from this approach, for her exploration of popular Hollywood films touches on issues of class, ethnicity, moral standing, repression of women, racial conflict, and more, as she looks at eating scenes in such movies as *Saturday Night Fever, Driving Miss Daisy, The War of the Roses,* and many more (Boswell, 1993: 7–23).

Gender studies

Broadly speaking, gender studies is concerned with the social and cultural construction of masculinities and femininities; it challenges the idea that there is any necessary connection between the biological states of being male or female on the one hand and the social constructs of gender, gender identity, and gender roles on the other. When applied to discussions of food in film, gender studies focus primarily on the role that food plays in the construction of different kinds of femininity (and, more rarely, alternative types of masculinity).

A fine example of gender studies propelling a food-in-film essay is Ellen J. Fried's "Food, Sex, and Power at the Dining Room Table in Zhang Yimou's *Raise the Red Lantern*" (in Bower, 2004: 129–46). Fried, like most scholars discussing food and film, intertwines information from other fields, in this case, primarily a most useful exploration of Chinese foodways. However, she remains focused on how these foodways and customs relate to the oppression of women in the culture depicted in the film.

For a different use of gender theory, one might consider Steve Zimmerman's chapter, "Someone's in the Kitchen" (in Zimmerman, 2010: 151–81.) Sweeping through a huge variety of films, and using his extensive knowledge of Hollywood movies, Zimmerman combines an interest in gender formation/representation with social history and popular culture analysis. In this sense, his chapter slides somewhat into the next category—historical criticism.

Historical criticism

Food in film scholarship frequently positions itself at the intersections of social history, film history, and different aspects of food history, often yielding insights we might never have otherwise gleaned. "Chickens, Cakes, and Kitchens: Food and Modernity in Malay Films of the 1950s and 1960s" (in Bower, 2004: 75–85), written by Timothy P. Barnard (a history professor at the National University of Singapore), highlights aspects of Malay cultural identity and nation building, culinary history, and the history of Malay film. In fact, Barnard concludes that Malay film is a "source for the cultural history of postwar Malay" (p. 83).

Another and very different example of such interdisciplinary yet history-focused work can be found in French scholar Anne Lair's essay "*Ratatouille*: An Historical Approach toward Gastronomy," which places the animated film *Ratatouille* (2007) in a broad historical context. Here is how Lair summarizes her approach:

> This paper will first examine how Paris has been favored as the center of France, the capital of gastronomy, and the city of pleasures. It will then examine gastronomic literature, which can be divided into several categories: cookbooks, etiquette literature, and restaurant guidebooks. We will also focus on 20th century gastronomy [which] due to changes in society, evolved towards lighter preparations while still maintaining excellent quality and standards. As we shall see, the movie *Ratatouille* illustrates the essence of French culinary art.
>
> *(Lair, 2009: 121)*

Research methodologies

Single film analysis

While food has always been an essential element in both life and film, it is perhaps food's very ordinariness that accounts for the fact that until recently food's role in movies has been given so little attention. But food's powerful representational, metaphoric, and even narrative power eventually became recognized by scholars who noticed food's central importance to both films that are not predominantly *about* food and films in which food takes center place. Examples of the analysis of food's significance in a particular film include Jane Ferry's previously cited analysis of the eight dinner scenes in Martin Scorsese's film adaption of Edith Wharton's *The Age of Innocence* (in Ferry, 2003: 11–27) and Michael Ashkenazi's "Food, Play, Business, and the Image of Japan in Itami Juzo's *Tampopo*" (also cited earlier). Dealing in depth with just one movie is often a comfortable way to begin one's exploration of food in film

Multiple film comparisons/discussions

When more than one movie is discussed within an article or essay, it becomes necessary to clearly state one's reasons for the specific selection of the films being discussed and to highlight the focal themes their comparison produces. Zimmerman is masterful at covering a wide selection of films while emphasizing a particular idea, as chapter headings in *Food in the Movies* suggest: "Romantic and Unromantic Meals," "Belly Laughs," and "Killer Meals."

Three movies are under discussion in Jane Ferry's chapter, "Boundaries of Purity and Pollution: The Dining Space" (in Ferry, 2003: 59–75), for what interests Ferry is how "the powers of communal bonding and psychological nurturance now come from eating in fast food establishments, and, by extension, restaurants" (p. 60). She discusses *Mystic Pizza*, *Better Off Dead*, and *Ordinary People*, in a sandwich-like format, with discussion of all three films and their themes, methods, etc. beginning and ending the essay, and a center portion devoting space to a separate exploration of each film.

Film adaptation

While comic books, television series, theatrical productions, non-fiction books, and even video games are now commonly adapted for the big screen, short stories and novels have served as the basis for screenplays from the earliest days of cinema. As early as the mid-1910s, stories derived from celebrated literature were seen as one way to lend prestige to a new medium struggling to gain both respectability and market share.

Nowadays most film scholars regard adaptations as *interpretations*. Arguing that change in adaptation is essential and practically unavoidable, they attempt to avoid the at-times absurd question of "accuracy" in a given adaptation and arguments as to a film's fidelity to its literary source. This more open way of looking at film adaptations allows us to appreciate that at times the shift from a literary to a visual medium can add a dimension to the adaptation that was missing from the source material. In terms of food studies perhaps the best example of such enhancement is Tony Richardson's 1963 adaption of Fielding's classic novel *Tom Jones*, which arguably contains the sexiest food scene in all movies. It is the visual medium that quite literally lets a piece of (chicken) meat appear so luscious that we immediately recognize food as an obvious and delicious stand-in for sex.

Auteurism

Auteur theory, first developed in France in the 1950s and imported to the US in the early 1960s, holds that the director is the primary creative force behind a film and can thus be considered its author or *auteur*. Since then auteurism has been subjected to considerable criticism. Critics and scholars alike have argued that, as a collaborative art, film is often simply too complex to be

Anne Bower and Thomas Piontek

attributed to one single person. Thus auteur theory was charged with elevating the position of a film's director at the expense of its studio, writer, producer, or more recently, its special effects supervisor. While some have subsequently rejected auteurism altogether others have argued for its limited usefulness in the study of a select few directors. Thus Bernard F. Dick maintains: "Just as a literary scholar can discuss *Hamlet* within the broader context of Shakespeare's plays, we can approach *Psycho* within the context of Hitchcock's work instead of viewing it merely as a horror film or as the prototype of the modern slasher film" (Dick, 2005: 328). A film director's repetition of certain themes, compositions, framings, or types of shots may comprise his unique style or "signature," which will reveal itself only by comparing a particular film to other films by the same author.

Of course, not every director can be considered an author in the sense of possessing a distinctive, recognizable style; yet most critics would agree that Alfred Hitchcock clearly fulfills the criteria of the auteur. In some food in film discussions, the auteurist approach makes great sense. A perfect example is David Greven's "Engorged with Desire: The Films of Alfred Hitchcock and the Gendered Politics of Eating" (in Bower, 2004: 297–310), which focuses on the primacy and prevalence of eating in Hitchcock's American films, analyzing the competing cinematic tensions that inform the depiction of food in Hitchcock and give his films "their distinctive aftertaste" (298).

For additional examples of auteurist food in film criticism see Michael Nottingham's analysis of the significance of meals in the work of surrealist filmmaker Jan Svankmajer cited above, and Eric L. Reinholtz's "Supper, Slapstick, and Social Class: Dinner as Machine in the Silent Films of Buster Keaton" (in Bower, 2004: 267–80). Borrowing the title of Walter Benjamin's famous essay, Reinholtz argues that the way food is used in Keaton's films forces audiences to confront the truth of the modern condition: "Keaton's representation of foodways promises to fulfill our appetite for comedy while its problematic consumption obliges us to rethink our assumptions about film, food, and society in 'the age of mechanical reproduction'" (p. 279).

Genre studies

What makes a group of films a genre is the sense, shared by filmmakers, critics, and audiences, that these films resemble each other in significant ways. This resemblance can be defined in terms of the films' topic or theme, setting, manner of presentation, plot pattern, distinctive emotional appeal, or to a lesser extent, their target audience. What then are the shared conventions that define the emerging "food film" genre?

To begin with, food has to play a star role no matter whether the film's protagonists are cooks (professional or domestic) or not. The central significance of food in film may be marked by any or all of the following: The camera will focus on food preparation and presentation, so that in close-ups and panning shots food fills the screen; a restaurant, dining room, kitchen, or a shop where food is made and/or sold will be the primary setting; and the film's narrative will depict characters negotiating questions of identity, power, culture, spirituality, or relationship through food. Films that quite obviously fit this definition include *La Grande Bouffe* (Ferreri, 1973), *Babette's Feast* (Gabriel Axel, 1987), *Chocolat* (Claire Dennis, 1988), *Like Water for Chocolate* (Alfonso Arau, 1992), *Eat Drink Man Woman* (Ang Lee, 1994), *Big Night* (Campbell Scott and Stanley Tucci, 1996), *Soul Food* (George Tillman Jr., 1997), and *Tortilla Soup* (Maria Rípoll, 2001).

Other films in which food plays a significant role, however, are not as easily categorized. Take, for instance, Marc Caro and Jean-Pierre Jeunet's *Delicatessen* (1991). Can this film, in which cannibalism is such a central issue, be considered a "food film"? In *Food, Film and Culture*, the only book-length genre study to date, James R. Keller seems to have no qualms about placing another cannabalistic film within the food film genre, opening his book with a chapter on Peter Greenaway's *The Cook, The Thief, His Wife, and Her Lover* (1989). As worldwide cinema continues to evolve, so too may our definition of the food film undergo change.

Avenues for future research

Rich opportunities lie ahead in working with the ever-increasing number of food documentaries. Such work will appeal to scholars with interests in how the food industry operates (growers, processors, distributors); organic foods; farmers' markets; and the localvore movement—all of which can have economic, political, social, and environmental implications. A useful website for those interested in food documentaries is Serious Eats: A Food Blog and Community (www. seriouseats.com), where one can find, among many other useful things, the article "Serious Green: Movies That Go Beyond Food Inc.," which features a list of recent and not-so-recent food documentaries.

In a very different vein, the animated film *Ratatouille* may inspire scholars to look back over decades of animated films to see what cultural, gender, nationalist, and other ideologies those films have promulgated through their use of food or how the characters are depicted through their relationship to food, or how the use of food tells us something about the film directors, studios, and other components. Many animated movies are directed at children, which raises the question of how the use of film relates to a society's vision of child health, child sexuality, child agency, family relations, and community relations.

James R. Keller defines the food film genre quite straightforwardly as a collection of films in which "food production, preparation, service, and or consumption play an operative and memorable role in the development of character, structure, or theme" (Keller, 2006: 1). However, future research may want to complicate this definition. For instance, the fact that food may play an "operative and memorable role" in any number of film genres raises the question of whether the food film itself can be classified as a genre. Perhaps it could be understood more productively as a collection of generic elements that operates trans-generically, something along the lines of what Chris Straayer first referred to as a "generic system" or "generic discourse" in her study of the temporary transvestite film.

Film scholars interested in the representation of food in film are unavoidably implicated in the continuing conflict between general film criticism and film theory. As we have seen, it is the scholar, dedicated to in-depth analysis, who can best bring a variety of theoretical and disciplinary approaches to elaborate what part food plays in a particular film. At the same time, "foodies" the world over have created blogs listing their favorite food movies or favorite food scenes, and some of these blogs offer useful insights. Movie reviewers get in the act too. It behooves scholars to take their work into consideration, for both bloggers and reviewers have valuable information and insights to offer.

A newer area that may yield interesting fodder for food in film scholars concerns the prodigious number of online, DSL, and other types of computerized games; online blogs, which include videos (home movies, if you will); and if one considers television and movie advertisements as films, there is plenty of room to discuss how these commercials (whether for food or for kitchens or for restaurants, hardware, or cars, etc.) shape and encode our consumerist desires and our culture.

How to get started

A few universities offer graduate degrees in food studies, wherein a student might be able to incorporate his or her interest in film. As of this writing, for example, New York University's

Steinhardt School of Culture, Education and Human Development offers an MA in Food Studies, which permits a focus on cultural aspects. At Chatham University, in Pittsburgh, PA, the MA in Food Studies includes one concentration (consisting of four courses) in communication and writing that includes film. Boston University has a Master of Liberal Arts in Gastronomy, with a History and Culture concentration, and the University of Indiana–Bloomington's unique PhD program in Anthropology of Food might allow for explorations of food in film as part of the overall program. New Mexico State University has a graduate minor in food studies, and the New School (New York City) has a Food Studies Continuing Education Program. At Dillard University in New Orleans, a new Institute for the Study of Culinary Cultures, focusing on foodways of the African diaspora, may offer opportunities for students and scholars at many levels. It is likely that the growing interest in food in film in particular and food studies in general will result in the creation of new graduate programs in the future.

While opportunities for graduate work in food studies, and more specifically in food and film, are extremely limited, it is quite possible to work within other graduate disciplines and develop a specialty focus concerning food in film. Whether film studies, media studies, literature, foreign languages, women's studies, history, or some other field, the scholar with critical interest in food in film can find a path to develop his or her critical abilities and achieve recognition. After all, this has been the path of most scholars who have written (and taught) about food and film, and it continues to work well.

Regardless of one's home discipline, one way to try out one's food-in-film abilities is to present papers at suitable conferences and symposia. The Annual Student Food Symposium held at UNC-Chapel Hill includes a section on the depictions of food in popular culture, the Association for the Study of Food in Society has been holding an annual conference since 1987, and both the American Culture Society and Popular Culture Society are open to food/film topics. Many other societies and scholarly associations have accepted papers relating to food and film. The annual Oxford Symposium on Food and Cookery changes its overall theme each year; depending on that theme a food in film topic might be appropriate. A newer group, The International Conference on Food Studies, may also provide opportunities for food-in-film academics. As we write this article, the group's website for the 2012 conference is food-studies. com/conference-2012 (accessed on April 3, 2012). The annual meetings of the Modern Language Association, American Comparative Literature Association, the joint meeting of the Popular Culture and American Associations, and similar professional conferences frequently include individual papers or entire sessions on the representation of food, including food in film.

Publishing in journals (print and online)

The Association for the Study of Food and Society (ASFS) website (www.food-culture.org, accessed on April 3, 2012) lists journals publishing food studies of various kinds. More specifically, one can find articles about food in film in such journals as the *Massachusetts Review*, *Food and Foodways*, and *Gastronomica*. Other publications to try are the *Journal of Popular Film and Television*, *Food, Culture, and Society*, *Film Quarterly*, *The Journal of Popular Culture*, and *The Journal of American Culture*. When approaching a journal that has not previously (or recently) published articles on food in film, it may be necessary to form a strong critical argument as to why an article being submitted is appropriate for that particular publication.

For certain kinds of articles or essays, online journals and blogs may be suitable, as with Critical Studies in Food and Culture (foodandculture.blogspot.com, accessed on April 3, 2012), a blog that posts information of interest to researchers investigating food and cultural studies, and has occasional calls for papers on set topics. Although internet sites come and go, when consistently available they can be a great boon, whether for publication or research. Most are devoted to discussion, to listing resources, or to republishing print (and online) articles. One site containing useful theoretical materials, lists, and articles is www.londonfoodfilmfiesta.co.uk/FILMMA~1/Rotana_Issue%2024_Food%20&%20Film%20Feature.pdf (accessed on April 3, 2012).

Another website, containing a very fine bibliography, along with an extensive list of films with notations about their content, is www.lib.berkeley.edu/MRC/foodmovies.html (accessed on April 3, 2012).

Key reading

Major work on food in film, like food studies itself, is of fairly recent vintage. The following books provide excellent background for food in film scholars, with many examples of film criticism.

Boswell, P. (1993) in "Hungry in the Land of Plenty: Food in Hollywood Films," *Beyond the Stars III,* Paul Loukies and Linda K. Fuller, eds., pp. 7–23. Bowling Green, OH: Bowling Green State University Popular Press.

Bower, Anne, ed. (2004) *Reel Food: Essays on Food and Film.* New York and London: Routledge.

Contains overview introduction plus 21 essays divided into three categories: "Cooking Up Cultural Values"; "Focus on Gender—the Body, the Spirit"; "Making Movies, Making Meals." Wide variety of theoretical approaches and writing styles.

de Lauretis, Teresa (1984) *Alice Doesn't: Feminism, Semiotics, Cinema.* Bloomington: Indiana University Press.

Dick, Bernard F. (2005) in *Anatomy of Film.* 5th edn, Boston, MA: Bedford/St. Martins.

Ferry, Jane (2003) *Food in Film: A Culinary Performance of Communication.* New York: Routledge.

Explores the representation of food and eating in selected films to demonstrate food's role in constructing meaning; argues that, within the narrative framework of films, food scenes reveal "powerful, coded cultural meanings" that structure complex social relation.

Kalpan, (1991) "Popular Culture, Politics, and the Canon: Cultural Literacy in the Postmodern Age," in *Cultural Power/Cultural Literacy: Selected Papers from the Fourteenth Annual Florida State University Conference on Literature and Film,* Bonnie Braendlin, ed., p. 20. Tallahassee: Florida State University Press.

Keller, James R. (2006) *Food, Film and Culture: A Genre Study.* Jefferson, NC and London: McFarland & Company.

Defines the food film genre and analyzes the relationship between the cinematic representation of food and a number of cultural constructs, including identity, race, ethnicity, family, gender, and nationality.

Lair, Anne (2009) "*Ratatouille*: An Historical Approach Toward Castronomy." In *Diverse By Design*: Carolyn Gascoigne and Melaine Bloom, eds. 2009 Report of the Central States Conference on the Teaching of Foreign Languages. Richard, VA: Robert Terry. www.csctfl.org/documents/CSCTFL_Report_2009.pdf#page=136, (accessed on April 3, 2012).

Loukides, Paul and Linda K. Fuller, eds. (1993) *Beyond the Stars: The Material World in American Popular Film,* Vol. III. Bowling Green, OH: Bowling Green State University Popular Press.

The first section of this volume is devoted to "Food and Other Consumables," and contains four interesting articles, three dedicated to food, one to the portrayal of marijuana in films. The book's introduction gives some useful thoughts on the "conventions" of presenting the material world in popular movies.

Nottingham, Michael (2004) "Downing the Folk-Festive: Menacing Meals in the Films of Jan Svankmajer." *Enter Text: An Interactive Interdisciplinary E-Journal for Cultural and Historical Studies and Creative Work,* 4, 1: 126–50, Winter, http://arts.brunel.ac.uk/gate/entertext/4_1/nottingham.pdf, (accessed on August 22, 2011).

Philpot, Justin (2010) "The Intent of Methodology: Cultural Studies, Film Studies and Challenging the Corporate Demands of the Academy," *The Projector* 10, 1, Spring: 46–54. www.bgsu.edu/departments/theatrefilm/projector/page81338.html (accessed on April 3, 2012).

Poole, Gaye (1999) *Reel Meals, Set Meals: Food in Film and Theatre.* Sydney: Currency Press.

Poole investigates how food in theatrical performances and in films carries social and symbolic meaning. Her range is extensive, from early theatre through the contemporary stage; from very early films to such food-in-film favorites as *Babette's Feast* and *Tampopo*.

Rosen (1986) *Narrative, Apparatus, Ideology: A Film Theory Reader,* New York: Columbia University Press, p. vii.
Zimmerman, Steve (2010) *Food in the Movies,* 2nd edition, Jefferson, NC: McFarland.

Contains scores of brief film summaries arranged in chapters that elaborate central notions, encapsulated in the chapter titles, such as "Missing Meals and Missing Appetites" and "Belly Laughs." In the chapter, "Food for Thought" Zimmerman deals thoughtfully with the food film genre. The book's voluminous coverage of films serves to introduce any number of possibilities for those interested in exploring movies for their deployment of food imagery and themes.

17

Food and television

Sarah Murray

This chapter on food and television defines an area of study found primarily within the humanities, which focuses on the social, cultural, and political implications of food's presence within the medium of television. A literature review offers an introduction to the theory and method of scholarship on food television, dividing the work among historiographic approaches, industry studies, and critiques of gender and class, noting the predominance of ideological analyses. The chapter encourages future research in all areas of this young subfield, especially those focused on race as well as food television audiences. The chapter ends with resources for graduate programs, funding, and archival research.

The history of food on television is as old as the history of television itself. Descending from the cookery broadcasts of the radio era, food's enduring presence on television has been iterative yet varied, ranging from segmented on-air cooking demos and educational "how-to" programs to celebrity-infused food competitions and narrowcasted lifestyle television for the foodie niche. Building from this rich history of programming is a meteoric rise in contemporary food television. The US cable channel Food Network launched in 1993. Its purchase by E. W. Scripps Company in 1997 and subsequent rise in popularity is generally agreed upon as one catalyst – along with heightened social and political interest in food – for a renewed and concentrated investment in food programming. Although initially scattered across niche cable and broadcasting markets in the mid-to-late 1990s, an increased focus on food has been televisually pervasive in the first decade of the twenty-first century.

Despite this longevity and recent proliferation of food programming, there remains a sparse body of academic research on food and television, and on food and media more broadly. Although limited in depth, the scope of research on food and television has significant breadth, housed within a vast array of disciplines, including sociology, women's and gender studies, American studies, cultural studies, policy and urban planning, and the broad rubric of media and communications (media studies, communication studies, visual and moving image arts, and rhetoric). Studies of food and television are also occasionally present in the fields of nutrition, environmental studies, agriculture, anthropology, history, and English. This chapter summarizes the burgeoning area of food and television, assessing theoretical and methodological approaches and bridging disciplines with the thematic consistencies of a humanities-focused body of literature.

Work on food and television coalesces around a primary objective to clarify the broad social, cultural, and political implications of food's presence within the medium of television. Research is motivated to determine how and why food is deployed discursively and formally in televisual spaces, and more specifically, how food programming is raced, classed, and gendered. Scholarship on food and television also interrogates the long-held binary of public–professional–masculine and private–domestic–feminine, as well as the ever-present culinary dichotomies of good/bad, healthy/junky, epicure/novice. Further, since television and food are both consumed, merging these consumptive practices highlights the process of what Warren Belasco and Philip Scranton call "culinary differentiation," or, the connection between food, consumption, and identity (2002: 2). Identity and consumption are subsequently linked to class-based notions of taste hierarchies, cultural distinction, and good consumer citizenship through lifestyle-based food television.

"Food and television" necessitates some clarification at the onset of this chapter. First, this is an overview of research stemming primarily from the perspective of media studies and its place within the larger humanities tradition. Research on food and television in the social scientific fields – much of which considers the effects of food programming on children or other vulnerable populations or the implications of food-related television advertisements – falls beyond the scope of this chapter. There also exists a significant history of research on food and communication within the field of anthropology; because the vast majority of this work does not attend to *media*, it is also not considered here. Moreover, this overview specifically aggregates the research on food and television, although other media (i.e., radio, film, internet, and new media technologies) are alluded to throughout. Although there is nascent work on other media not included here due to the focus on television, this chapter can be read as indicative of the state of a more broadly encompassing focus on food and media. Finally, the phrase *food television* is used interchangeably with the more common *cooking show* or *cooking program*. *Food television* intends to include all programming that directly incorporates food preparation, food information, or food-related entertainment as its main focus.

Historical background of food and television scholarship and major theoretical approaches in use

Scholarship addressing food and television is at once relatively consistent and vastly interdisciplinary. Although this work spans many disciplines, as discussed above, the literature is driven by a cluster of themes informed by broad theories of gender and class. More narrowly, the theoretical backdrop includes sociological gender theory, feminist television theory, Bourdieuian theories of distinction, theories on consumer citizenship and neoliberalism, ideological debates on the meaning of binaries such as public/private and masculine/feminine, and theories considering the formal and aesthetic properties of television. The extant body of research can be loosely organized into four interconnected areas: historiography; industry, formal, and aesthetic studies; ideological–textual analyses of gender; and ideological–textual analyses of class, taste, and cultural distinction.

A few truncated histories serve as suitable introductions to the literature. These surveys are not analytically driven; however, their broad overviews map the course of food and television and provide informal content analyses (Kackman, 2004; Lurie, 1999). Several scholars offer more in-depth chronologies of food programming on US television, whether via a peripheral focus of a more narrow thesis (Polan, 2011), as a portion of a more diverse collection (Ashley *et al.*, 2004), or as the primary objective of the research (Collins, 2009). This historical work – and most research on food and television to date – has focused nearly exclusively on the traditional domestic instructional format of the stand-and-stir televised cooking show. The *when* and *where* of cooking shows (i.e., as educational programming on Public Broadcasting Service versus commercial broadcasting on network television), as well as the *who* (e.g., hosts like Julia Child and James Beard) dominate the food and television landscape.

A limited few delve into discussions of the television and media industries as they pertain to food programming. Literature in this area is diffuse and explores a variety of theses, including: How early food television was produced and the broadcast networks that participated (Collins, 2009; Williams, 1999); the practice of time slotting in the construction of programming schedules (primarily in Britain) (Brunsdon, 2003; Brunsdon *et al.*, 2001); the formal and aesthetic properties of food as televised entertainment, education, or eroticization (Bell, 2010; Ray, 2007; Ketchum, 2005; Chan, 2003; Miller, 2002; De Solier, 2000; Finkelstein, 1999); the consideration of food television and the genres of "how-to," hobbyist, and lifestyle (Brunsdon, 2003; Ketchum, 2007, 2005); and the industrial and ideological problematics of repackaging non-Western food television for US audiences (Gallagher, 2004). Notably, most of this work focuses on US or British food television.

A significant portion of the scholarship on food and television is concerned with gender. Like the cookery radio broadcasts made famous by on-air personalities like Betty Crocker, television often perpetuates the relationship among women, domestic expertise, and food while reifying men's professional alignment with food in public spaces. However, contemporary scholarship convincingly argues that television complicates these gendered binaries by blurring public and private spaces and shifting men's and women's associations with food (Sanders, 2009; Hollows, 2007, 2003a, 2003b; Andrews, 2003). This research most often focuses on the television *chef* or *host*, as they are the on-screen focal point of food programming; thus, their presence as anchors of food television mediates and is mediated by the gendered spaces of televisual kitchens.

Although men and women have long shared the duty of hosting, there are studies that highlight the invisibility of women's roles as hosts and producers of popular food television shows (Marks, 2007; Bullaro, 2006; Chao, 1998). Most scholarship in this area, however, is more interested in critiquing food television's dependence on normative notions of domestic femininity and debating its subversive potential for women. These studies often consider the relationship between women hosts and their audiences (Shapiro, 2005), women hosts who hate to cook or have little experience in the kitchen (Williams, 1999), or women who operate outside the conventions of feminine performativity (Williams, 1999; Polan, 2011; Hollows, 2007).

One of the more well-developed strands of research on food television critiques cooking programs that feature women as overtly sensual, eroticized, and/or hyper feminine hosts. This, for some scholars, occurs through women's prominent relationship with food – the exhibition of "carnivalesque feasting" – as well as through "sexual double entendre in the titles, a sensual visual style, and sexual verbal references" (Andrews, 2003: 189–95; Chan, 2003). Other scholarship is more explicitly concerned with the place of feminism in female-hosted food programming. Some writers exercise caution, concerned that popular discursive definitions of *postfeminism* – the notion that we have progressed beyond "a particular moment of feminist activity and a particular set of feminist concerns" – are reductively linked to women's presence on food television (Gill, 2007: 251). For these writers, the eroticized host is a dangerously postfeminist performance of contemporary female consumption and consequently becomes the "single trope through which feminism is most often invoked in popular culture" (Brunsdon, 2005: 113; Gill, 2007).

Conversely, other scholars find positive feminist potential in women's televisual appearances in the kitchen. This literature asserts that women's use of irony, humor, and sensuality on cooking shows reshapes the relationship to the domestic and consciously utilizes the "ambivalence inherent in ironic discourse" to highlight both the pleasures and containments of the kitchen space (Sanders, 2009: 152). This approach also suggests that some food television is able to bring together the feminist and the cook in a way that treats food preparation as pleasure, not domestic work (Hollows, 2003a).

A subset of food and television scholarship on gender focuses on men. Much of this work is concerned with how men negotiate the televisual domestic kitchen (Hollows, 2003b; Attwood, 2005; Julier and Lindenfeld, 2005). This research suggests that men distance themselves from the traditionally feminized labor of the home kitchen via modern masculinities that associate food preparation with individualized and aesthetically driven lifestyles (Hollows, 2003b; Attwood, 2005). Along similar lines, food television hosted by men is often argued to be anchored by the energized, personality-driven "charismatic male" figure (Ketchum, 2004: 225). Other scholarship considers how Japanese masculinities are conveyed on television in Japan, a country where competitive food programming is pervasive (Holden, 2005).

Discussion of men as hosts of food television leads directly to a broad literature on class, taste, and processes of cultural distinction. A handful of scholars, for example, present intersectional research on working-class masculinities in the televisual kitchen, through considerations of the "regular guy" image (Ray, 2007: 55; Adema, 2000; Miller, 2002) or performances of regional masculinities (Smith and Wilson, 2004). Notably, this research recognizes the vital exchange that occurs when women's domestic food knowledge is transferred to men on cooking programs. Men's places in the domestic televisual kitchen has also been discussed within the context of how industry decisions to air food programming in certain time slots disseminates meaning about class and gender (Brunsdon *et al.*, 2001). Other scholarship argues that male hosts are freer to move about class-based genres of food television – travel, leisure, professionalization, and competition – while women are much more anchored to televised food preparation as "domestic work for family and friends" (Swenson, 2007: 9–10; Strange, 1998).

Much of the work that can be placed under the broad umbrella of class, taste, and distinction takes contemporary lifestyle television as its frame. Here, British, Australian, and US programming are again lumped together in a Westernized notion of lifestyle television as reflecting:

> changes in [a] national imaginary, whereby lifestyle "projects", such as home improvement and personal styling, are becoming increasingly important markers of self-identification, with these programmes providing key information regarding lifestyle consumption.
>
> *(Gorman-Murray, 2006: 229)*

Scholars theorizing within the context of lifestyle television recognize food programming as a raced, classed, and gendered blueprint not only for broad class-based taste hierarchies, but also for highly individualized cultural distinction. This research elucidates the process by which televised culinary education – how to purchase, cook, and consume as a foodie – offers directives for customized style and identity that sustains important class signifiers (De Solier, 2008, 2000; Gorman-Murray, 2006; Palmer, 2004; Strange, 1998). As many scholars point out elsewhere, this process of communicating cultural distinction through food is certainly not limited to television (Johnston and Baumann, 2010).

Further complicating this notion of distinction is scholarship that envelopes food television into the larger body of work on citizenship, gender, class, and consumption. Drawing again from the lifestyle television frame, this research conceptualizes food television as part and parcel of "trends in the way we understand ourselves as citizen and consumer" (Ouellette and Hay, 2008: 14). Food television is often implicated as neoliberalistically charged; that is, it ostensibly encourages less dependence on the governing state and more on the makeover – the personal, individual change that keeps you in good standing as a consumer citizen in a capitalistic economy and becomes "the key to social mobility, stability, and civic empowerment" (McCarthy, 2010: 17; De Solier, 2000, 2008). For many scholars, this translates to the discourses through which food television encourages particular eating habits, body sizes (as controlled through food), recipes, restaurants, and general food-related lifestyle choices. Taking a slightly different perspective, other work has considered how competitive food television (e.g., *Iron Chef America*) is constructed upon and further reifies the rituals and ideals of contemporary US citizenship (Bell, 2010).

What follows from the convergence of lifestyle television, consumer citizenship, and neoliberalistic individualism is niche television – television branded for highly targeted demographics; in this case, the niche would take shape around those with a vested interest in food. Although existing literature often makes an indirect connection between niche television and food (Ray, 2007; Ketchum, 2005; Brundson, 2003; De Solier, 2000), no studies explicitly consider niche food television via cultural or ideological analyses. Niche television is considered, however, in scholarship that assesses the political economy of the US cable channel Food Network (Ketchum, 2007, 2005; Banet-Weiser *et al.*, 2007). Food Network's launch created the first cable mainstay for television chefs and cooking shows and a concentrated site for "24/7" food television; consequently, the structure, content, and style of the channel has been of interest to scholars looking at niche media production, audiences, and branding.

Food is frequently peripheral to the primary objectives of research in media studies and within the humanities at large. It is not uncommon for scholarship on television to reveal key insights about its relationship to food. Thus, food and television scholars would be remiss to ignore research simply because food is not the focal point. Studies on 1950s and Cold War television (Boddy, 1993; Spigel, 1992), 1990s television (Becker, 2006), post-network television and cable narrowcasting (Lotz, 2009; Banet-Weiser *et al.*, 2007; Mullen, 2003), educational broadcasting (Ouellette, 2002), and reality television (Ouellette and Hay, 2008) are valuable resources. Similarly, bypassing work that is not readily about television or media is arguably even more prohibitive, as contemporary food studies – especially anthologies on food and culture – speak volumes about the relationship between food and television (Counihan and Van Esterik, 2008; Ashley *et al.*, 2004; Belasco and Scranton, 2002).

Research methodologies

Contemporary media studies research in the humanities tradition attends most readily to the triad of text, audience, and industry. Understanding these as the focus of this area facilitates a number of starting points for research on food and television that align with the field. As is evidenced by the literature review above, the vast majority of work on food and television takes the text – the actual food-related program – as its object of study. Thus, research methodologies in this area most frequently fall under the umbrella of *textual analysis*, a common method for humanities scholars. Textual analysis can initially be divided into two areas, *content analysis* and *interpretive textual analysis*, the latter further cascading into a number of submethodologies.

Content analysis is often descriptive in nature and thus rarely utilized as a singular method; instead, it is more frequently used as a supplement to more in-depth, analytical methods of textual analysis. For food and television scholars, content analysis is helpful for assessing the history of food programming on television (Collins, 2009; Kackman, 2004). Content analysis can also provide a quantitative assessment of representation; for example, scholars interested in determining the visibility of women as cooking show hosts or the number of shows that feature elimination-style competitions would benefit from this method.

191

Interpretive textual analysis remains the method of choice for food and television researchers. Within this frame, much of the literature can accurately be considered an amalgamation of semiotics, psychoanalytic analysis, rhetorical and discursive analysis, and, most prominently, ideological analysis. Most scholars are motivated to explicate the processes through which meaning making occurs and is disseminated via food's presence on television. Put another way, this research attempts to clarify our understanding of the ideologies of food as presented on television. Books and articles on food television assess the cultural norms of specific historical eras (Polan, 2011; Collins, 2009; Attwood, 2005; Brunsdon, 2003; Miller, 2002; Williams, 1999), the potency of political discourses like feminism (Gillis and Hollows, 2009; Hollows, 2007, 2003a; Brunsdon, 2005), and the meaning of food in relation to the sociocultural moment of contemporary television (De Solier, 2008; Ouellette and Hay, 2008; Ketchum, 2005; Palmer, 2004; Adema, 2000).

Ideological analysis is also an instrumental method for the large portion of research tackling issues of subject position and identity on food television. Gender analyses unpack connotative meaning in hosts' subversive on-screen performances (Sanders, 2009; Smith and Wilson, 2004), in their relationships to the binaries of public/private, domestic/professional (Hollows, 2003b), or in their suggestive dialogue and eroticized interactions with food (Andrews, 2003; Chan, 2003). This method is also the foundation for many class-based analyses that consider, for example, the discourses of culinary education (De Solier, 2000; Strange, 1998) or how food is integrated into the "lifestyle" of lifestyle television (De Solier, 2008; Ketchum, 2005; Palmer, 2004).

Industry and audience-based methodologies, while common in television and media research, are less prevalent within the subfield of food and television. Industry studies assess the economics of television production, the players involved (i.e., producers, actors, writers, advertisers, and media executives) as well as the construction, branding, marketing, and distribution of television and media products. Industry studies that attend to food television often consider the political economy of single television channels like Food Network (Ketchum, 2007), food programming's role in industrial shifts like cable narrowcasting and niche media (also Ketchum, 2007 and Banet-Weiser et al., 2007; Mullen, 2003), or how food television changes as it is repackaged for broader distribution (Gallagher, 2004). Audience studies – methods that consider viewer response to television via popular discourse, surveys, focus groups, or interviews – are effectively non-existent in the area of food and television, and are a suggested avenue for further research below.

Avenues for future research

Food studies and media studies share the distinction of being young fields informed by interdisciplinary underpinnings. Consequently, there is abundant opportunity to build from existing literature and fill sizable research gaps. First, the above survey of established research indicates a conflation of British, US, and Australian scholars and their researched texts. British scholars have historically led the charge in the area of food and television; consequently, a significant portion of the television studied is produced in the United Kingdom. While this scholarship has been foundational to the advancement of research in the US and elsewhere, there are cultural and industrial variables that are too often glossed over. Future research should consider the value of comparative analyses of regional, national, and global approaches to food and television. Closely related to this gap is the tendency to repeatedly focus on popular contemporary food television, such as widely distributed programs (e.g., *Iron Chef*) or celebrity chef hosts (e.g., Jamie Oliver, Nigella Lawson, Emeril Lagasse). These shows and figures provide scholars with accessible and plentiful material; however, given today's abundance of food programming there are innumerable texts in need of academic attention.

Food and television research similarly suffers from a dangerously narrow focus on *cooking shows*. Although the term *cooking show* is used interchangeably with *food television* throughout this chapter, little research has pushed beyond analysis of the traditional instructional stand-and-stir format, despite the proliferation of food-inflected game, travel, talk and trivia shows as well as elimination-based and documentary-style reality television. There is an imperative to produce work that differentiates among food television's varying formats, modes, and genres. The consequences of the current umbrella approach are generic categories that are hastily constructed and far from streamlined. Directly related to format and style is a lack of research on food television production and the mechanics of the television industries that operate behind these texts. There is a need for historical and contemporary discussions that consider *what* food television looks like and *how* it is created, branded, and distributed.

Moving to the front of the television set, virtually no one has undertaken research with the sole purpose of studying the food television audience. Questions of reception – the when, where, why, how, and with whom of people watching food television – are wide open and ripe for interrogation. Further, there are plenty of avenues for practical application, such as elucidating how viewers obtain, interpret, and utilize information from television about food, food industries, and food policies. Whether in the audience, behind the camera, or on-screen, the dearth of literature on race and food television is distressing, as is the lack of research on gender liminality, queer representation and queer aesthetics in food programming. Scholars entering the food and television field will find these two areas of representation and identity severely underdeveloped. Finally, although it may appear trivial, few scholars actually study the *food* of food television. While food programming and television chefs are frequently considered, the food itself – what is prepared, sold, and consumed and how it is framed visually and discursively on television – is mostly ignored.

Media studies has witnessed a growth in integrated approaches to the study of television through recent research that works to more holistically incorporate the text, industry, and audience into every project. This is a challenging and respected approach to media research and not without its limitations, as any project that takes a comprehensive aim runs the risk of diluting the expertise that comes with specificity. However, given food's established interdisciplinarity, future research may certainly benefit from this emerging methodology.

Practical considerations for getting started

Students interested in the study of food and television enter the field at a promising moment. While no graduate programs currently exist with a singular focus on food and media, many established departments welcome this research. Food has a rich history in many disciplines and with its contemporary social and political salience, there are plenty of well-funded and supportive programs from which to choose. Graduate programs in media studies, communications, cultural studies, American studies, and sociology are often productive homes for food and television scholars, while those interested in the practical application of this research might consider public policy, nutrition, urban studies/planning, environmental studies and even agriculture. As is the case with any narrowly focused or understudied topic, it is often more helpful to connect to leading scholars with recognized contributions in the area rather than specific programs or departments.

For established scholars and graduate students building on the extant food and television scholarship, there is impressive research support and sufficient – albeit sporadic – funding available. A number of archives in the US hold food and/or television materials. Any well-known media archive may contain at least some food-related programming, including: the UCLA Film and Television Archive, the University of Wisconsin Center for Film and Theater Research, the Museum of Broadcast Communications, the Library of American Broadcasting at the University of Maryland, the Paley Center for Media, the Walter J. Brown Media Archives and Peabody Awards Collection, the University of Wyoming American Heritage Center, the online Media History Digital Library, and even the Motion Picture, Broadcasting and Recorded Sound Division of the Library of Congress.

Although culinary archives rarely house digital or recorded collections, their print collections are certainly worth an initial inquiry for television scripts and the private papers of actors, producers, and advertisers. A short list includes: the Janice Bluestein Longone Culinary Archive at the University of Michigan, the Culinary Collection at Harvard University's Schlesinger Library, the Culinary Arts Museum at Johnson and Wales University, the National Archives, and the James Beard Foundation. Funding for research and education in the area of food and television is variable, although the contemporary cultural interest in food yields impressive intermittent opportunities. For example, one of the Andrew W. Mellon Postdoctoral Fellowships – a renowned fellowship in the humanities – took food as its theme in 2012–13. Like the majority of academic research in search of financial support, work on food and television can be funded if one is diligent, flexible, and attentive to a diverse array of opportunities.

As many food studies scholars will attest, food often becomes an object of study after the fact – an indirect path that begins with "what food can tell us about something else" and ends with the realization that "food issues matter in themselves" (Belasco, 2007: x). This is occasionally true of work on food and television, as scholars pursue other aspects of television and media as their principal focus and subsequently take up an interest in food. In these instances – as is the case with anyone delving into work on food and television – professional academic organizations offer a host of unparalleled resources. Organizations like the National Communications Association, the Society for Cinema and Media Studies, the International Communication Association, and the Association for the Study of Food and Society host annual conferences, publish academic journals, offer inclusion in email LISTSERVs and online forums, and provide invaluable social networks for researchers. Finally, as food remains a key touchstone for the contemporary cultural and political moment of the early twenty-first century, scholars are indebted to the internet and social networking sites, where timely and accurate information on television (e.g., ratings, audience response, programming schedules, media mergers) is available for the next research project on food television.

Key reading

Adema, Pauline (2000) "Vicarious Consumption: Food, Television, and the Ambiguity of Modernity." *Journal of American and Comparative Cultures* 23(3): 113–24.

Brunsdon, Charlotte (2005) "Feminism, Postfeminism, Martha, Martha, and Nigella." In *Cinema Journal*. 44(2): 110–16.

Collins, Kathleen (2009) *Watching What We Eat*. New York: Continuum.

Cramer, Janet M., Greene, Carlnita P. and Lynn M. Walters eds. (2011) *Food as Communication/Communication as Food*. New York: Peter Lang Publishing.

De Solier, Isabelle (2000) "TV Dinners: Culinary Television, Education and Distinction." In *Continuum*. 19(4): 465–81.

De Solier, Isabelle (2008) "Foodie Makeovers: Public Service Television and Lifestyle Guidance." In *Exposing Lifestyle Television: The Big Reveal*, edited by Gareth Palmer, 65–82. Hampshire: Ashgate.

Finkelstein, Joanne (1999) "Foodatainment." In *On Cooking*, special issue of *Performance Research*. 4(1): 130–36.

Gillis, Stacy and Joanne Hollows, eds. (2009) *Feminism, Domesticity and Popular Culture*. New York: Routledge.

Ketchum, Cheri (2007) "Tunnel Vision and Food: A Political Economic Analysis of *Food Network*." In *Cable Visions: Television Beyond Broadcasting*, edited by Sarah Banet Weiser, Cynthia Chris, and Anthony Freitas, 158–76. New York: New York University Press.

Holden, T. J. M. (2005) "The Overcooked and Underdone: Masculinities in Japanese Food Programming." In *Food and Foodways*. 13(1): 39–65.

Hollows, Joanne (2003a) "Feeling Like a Domestic Goddess: Postfeminism and Cooking." In *European Journal of Cultural Studies*. 6(2): 179–202.

Miller, Toby (2002) "From Brahmin Julia to Working-Class Emeril: The Evolution of Television Cooking." In *High-Pop: Making Culture into Popular Entertainment*, edited by Jim Collins, 75–89. Oxford: Blackwell.

Polan, Dana (2011) *Julia Child's The French Chef*. Durham, NC: Duke University Press.

Ray, Krishnendu (2007) "Domesticating Cuisine: Food and Aesthetics on American Television." In *Gastronomica*. 7(1): 50–63.

Smith, Greg M. and Pamela Wilson (2004) "Country Cookin' and Cross-Dressin': Television, Southern White Masculinities, and Hierarchies of Cultural Taste." In *Television & New Media*. 5(3): 175–95.

Strange, Niki (1998) "Perform, Educate, Entertain: Ingredients of the Cookery Programme Genre." In *The Television Studies Book*, edited by Christine Geraghty and David Lusted, 301–12. London: Arnold.

Williams, Mark (1999) "Considering Monty Margett's *Cook's Corner*: Oral History and Television History." In *Television, History, and American Culture: Feminist Critical Essays*, edited by Mary Beth Haralovich and Lauren Rabinovitz, 36–55. Durham, NC: Duke University Press.

Bibliography

Adema, Pauline (2000) "Vicarious Consumption: Food, Television, and the Ambiguity of Modernity." *Journal of American and Comparative Cultures* 23(3): 113–24.

Andrews, Maggie (2003) "Nigella Bites *The Naked Chef*: The Sexual and the Sensual in Television Cookery Programmes." In *The Recipe Reader: Narratives, Contexts, Traditions*. Janet Floyd and Laurel Forster, eds. Burlington, VT: Ashgate, 187–204.

Ashley, Bob, Joanne Hollows, Steve Jones, and Ben Taylor, eds. (2004) *Food and Cultural Studies*. London: Routledge.

Attwood, Feona (2005) "Inside Out: Men on the 'Home Front'." *Journal of Consumer Culture* 5(1): 87–107.

Banet-Weiser, Sarah, Cynthia Curtis, and Anthony Freitas, eds. (2007) *Cable Visions: Television Beyond Broadcasting*. New York: New York University Press.

Becker, Ron (2006) *Gay TV and Straight America*. New Brunswick, NJ: Rutgers University Press.

Belasco, Warren J. (2007) *Appetite for Change: How the Counterculture Took on the Food Industry*. 2nd updated ed. Ithaca, NY: Cornell University Press, Cornell Paperbacks.

Belasco, Warren and Philip Scranton, eds. (2002) *Food Nations: Selling Taste in Consumer Societies*. London: Routledge.

Bell, Christopher (2010) "Tonight's Secret Ingredient Is … *Iron Chef America* as Media Ritual." In *Journal of Media and Communication* 2(1): 20–32.

Boddy, William (1993) *Fifties Television: The Industry and its Critics*. Urbana: University of Illinois Press.

Brunsdon, Charlotte (2005) "Feminism, Postfeminism, Martha, Martha, and Nigella." In *Cinema Journal* 44(2): 110–16.

——(2003) "Lifestyling Britain: The 8–9 Slot on British Television." In *International Journal of Cultural Studies* 6(5): 5–23.

Brunsdon, Charlotte, Catherine Johnson, Rachel Moseley, and Helen Wheatley (2001) "Factual Entertainment on British Television: The Midlands TV Research Group's '8–9 Project'." In *European Journal of Cultural Studies* 4(1): 29–62.

Bullaro, Grace Russo (2006) "Beer, Sweat and 'Cojones': The Masculinization of Cooking and the Food TV Network." In *Columbia Journal of American Studies* 7(1): 1–19.

Chan, Andrew (2003) "*La Grande Bouffe*: Cooking Shows as Pornography." In *Gastronomica* 3(4): 46–53.

Chao, Phebe Shih (1998) "TV Cook Shows: Gendered Cooking." In *Jump Cut* 42: 19–27.

Collins, Kathleen (2009) *Watching What We Eat*. New York: Continuum.

Counihan, Carole and Penny Van Esterik, eds. (2008) *Food and Culture*. 2nd ed. New York: Routledge.

De Solier, Isabelle (2008) "Foodie Makeovers: Public Service Television and Lifestyle Guidance." In *Exposing Lifestyle Television: The Big Reveal*, edited by Gareth Palmer, pp. 65–82. Hampshire: Ashgate.

——(2000) "TV Dinners: Culinary Television, Education and Distinction." In *Continuum* 19(4): 465–81.

Finkelstein, Joanne (1999) "Foodatainment." In *On Cooking*, special issue of *Performance Research* 4(1): 130–36.

Gallagher, Mark (2004) "What's So Funny About Iron Chef?" In *Journal of Popular Film and Television* 31 (4): 177–84.

Gill, Rosalind Clair (2007) *Gender and the Media*. Cambridge: Polity Press.

Gillis, Stacy and Joanne Hollows, eds. (2009) *Feminism, Domesticity and Popular Culture*. New York: Routledge.

Gorman-Murray, Andrew (2006) "Queering Home or Domesticating Deviance?: Interrogating Gay Domesticity Through Lifestyle Television." In *International Journal of Cultural Studies* 9(2): 227–47.

Holden, T. J. M. (2005) "The Overcooked and Underdone: Masculinities in Japanese Food Programming." In *Food and Foodways* 13(1): 39–65.

Hollows, Joanne (2003a) "Feeling Like a Domestic Goddess: Postfeminism and Cooking." In *European Journal of Cultural Studies* 6(2): 179–202.

——(2003b) "Oliver's Twist: Leisure, Labour, and Domestic Masculinity in *The Naked Chef*." *International Journal of Cultural Studies* 6(2): 229–48.

——(2007) "The Feminist and the Cook: Julia Child, Betty Freidan and Domestic Femininity." In *Gender and Consumption: Domestic Cultures and the Commercialisation of Everyday Life*, edited by Emma Casey and Lydia Martens, 33–48. Hampshire: Ashgate.

Johnston, Josée and Shyon Baumann (2010) *Foodies: Democracy and Distinction in the Gourmet Foodscape*. New York: Routledge.

Julier, Alice and Laura Lindenfeld (2005) "Mapping Men onto the Menu: Masculinities and Food." *Food and Foodways* 13(1–2): 1–16.

Kackman, Michael (2004) "Cooking Shows." In *Encyclopedia of Television*, edited by Horace Newcomb, 584–85. 2nd ed. Chicago: Fitzroy Dearborn.

Ketchum, Cheri (2007) "Tunnel Vision and Food: A Political Economic Analysis of *Food Network*." In *Cable Visions: Television Beyond Broadcasting*, edited by Sarah Banet Weiser, Cynthia Chris, and Anthony Freitas, 158–76. New York: New York University Press.

——(2005) "The Essence of Cooking Shows: How the Food Network Constructs Consumer Fantasies." In *Journal of Communication Inquiry* 29(3): 217–34.

——(2004) "Gender, Charisma and the Food Network." In paper presented at International Communication Association Annual Meeting. New Orleans, LA.

Lotz, Amanda D., ed. (2009) *Beyond Prime Time: Television Programming in the Post-Network Era*. New York: Routledge.

Lurie, Karen (1999) *TV Chefs: The Dish on the Stars of Your Favorite Cooking Shows*. Riverside: Renaissance Books.

Marks, Susan (2007) *Finding Betty Crocker: The Secret Life of America's First Lady of Food*. Minneapolis: University of Minnesota Press.

McCarthy, Anna (2010) *The Citizen Machine: Governing by Television in 1950s America*. New York: The New Press.

Miller, Toby (2002) "From Brahmin Julia to Working-Class Emeril: The Evolution of Television Cooking." In *High-Pop: Making Culture into Popular Entertainment*, edited by Jim Collins, 75–89. Oxford: Blackwell.

Mullen, Megan Gwynne (2003) *The Rise of Cable Programming in the United States: Revolution or Evolution?* Austin: University of Texas Press.

Ouellette, Laurie (2002) *Viewers Like You? How Public TV Failed the People*. New York: Columbia University Press.

Ouellette, Laurie and James Hay (2008) *Better Living Through Reality TV: Television and Post-Welfare Citizenship*. Oxford: Blackwell.

Palmer, Gareth (2004) "The New You: Class and Transformation in Lifestyle Television." In *Understanding Reality Television*, edited by Su Holmes and Deborah Jermyn, 173–90. London: Routledge.

Polan, Dana (2011) *Julia Child's The French Chef*. Durham, NC: Duke University Press.

Ray, Krishnendu (2007) "Domesticating Cuisine: Food and Aesthetics on American Television." In *Gastronomica* 7(1): 50–63.

Sanders, Lise Shapiro (2009) "Consuming Nigella." In *Feminism, Domesticity and Popular Culture*, edited by Stacy Gillis and Joanne Hollows, 151–63. New York: Routledge.

Shapiro, Laura (2005) "'I Guarantee': Betty Crocker and the Woman in the Kitchen." In *From Betty Crocker to Feminist Food Studies*, edited by Arlene Voski Avakian and Barbara Haber, 29–40. Amherst: University of Massachusetts Press.

Smith, Greg M. and Pamela Wilson (2004) "Country Cookin' and Cross-Dressin': Television, Southern White Masculinities, and Hierarchies of Cultural Taste." In *Television & New Media* 5(3): 175–95.

Spigel, Lynn (1992) *Make Room for TV: Television and the Family Ideal in Postwar America*. Chicago: University of Chicago Press.

Strange, Niki (1998) "Perform, Educate, Entertain: Ingredients of the Cookery Programme Genre." In *The Television Studies Book*, edited by Christine Geraghty and David Lusted, 301–12. London: Arnold.

Swenson, Rebecca (2007) "Kitchen Convergence: Televised Translations of Masculinity, Femininity and Food." In paper presented at *NCA 93rd Annual Convention*, Chicago, IL.

Williams, Mark (1999) "Considering Monty Margett's *Cook's Corner*: Oral History and Television History." In *Television, History, and American Culture: Feminist Critical Essays*, edited by Mary Beth Haralovich and Lauren Rabinovitz, 36–55. Durham, NC: Duke University Press.

Interdisciplinary food studies

18

Food studies programs

Rachel Black

This section will look at the development of food studies as an academic discipline. A brief history of this developing field is followed by a survey of the existing food studies programs. Food studies methods are extremely diverse but this chapter attempts to outline some of the current trends such as a systems approach and an emphasis on experiential learning. Potential directions for the future, such as applied research and a policy focus, are also discussed.

Historical background of food scholarship in food studies and major theoretical approaches in use

Food as an academic area of study has been around for quite some time. Ancient Greek philosophers such as Plato and Epicurus gave food a great deal of attention. They were particularly interested in diet and well-being. However, it took some time before scholars began to study food holistically from the field to the midden. Food and eating have not always been central to academic concerns; often devalued as a carnal pleasure, food fell to a lower priority as a biological necessity that was not particularly worthy of intellectual attention as a subject in its own right.

It was not until the late eighteenth century and early nineteenth century that a Frenchman decided to consider food beyond diet and medicine. A lawyer originally from Belley, Ain, Jean Anthelme Brillat-Savarin (1755–1826) devoted his spare time to not only the table, but to writing one of the first works on food and eating that moved beyond a focus on production, the body or the kitchen alone. Clearly a labor of love, Brillat-Savarin's treatise, *La Physiologie du gout* (*The Physiology of Taste*), was not published until 1825, a year before the author's death. This late publication was in part due to Brillat-Savarin's fear that his interest in food would undermine his professional reputation. However, this work was largely responsible for elevating culinary discourse and the role of food in society. Brillat-Savarin's ode to the pleasures of the table and the centrality of food in social life has not been out of print since its first publication and *The Physiology of Taste* is one of the quintessential works that has helped shape modern food studies.

Gastronomy or the gastronomic sciences, as Brillat-Savarin proposed, are the first areas of academic focus that focused on a truly holistic approach to studying food. Food studies is born out of this same tradition that brings an interdisciplinary approach to studying where food comes from, how it is prepared, consumed, and disposed of. It is this holistic approach that sets food studies apart from other academic pursuits that focus on food such as nutrition, food policy and agricultural studies. These topics are often included in the food studies curriculum, but they are seen as pieces of a larger mosaic that needs to be considered from a variety of perspectives.

Largely a North American development, food studies comes out of the same area studies tradition as gender studies and American studies. These studies programs paved the way for interdisciplinary academic units that gather together academics with diverse backgrounds, tools, and training. Studies programs have produced graduates with doctorates in American and gender studies but food studies is still in its infancy as far as professional training is concerned, and there is some resistance to training PhDs in such a specialized academic area. Some scholars feel that it is negligent to produce PhDs who will have difficulties finding an academic home. Others argue that doctoral training is critical for producing a new generation of thinkers who will go out and apply their knowledge, understanding, and critical thinking skills to changing the world's food systems.

The first challenge for anyone with a degree in food studies is to communicate their degree and qualifications. The term food studies is still being defined. Recent waves of degree holders from undergraduate and graduate programs are blazing the trail. This tech-savvy group is certainly well positioned to define their qualifications; food blogs are just one way in which the field of food studies is being defined and communicated. Brillat-Savarin's concern for being taken seriously about food is still part of the discourse surrounding food studies. Although we have made immense strides towards achieving academic recognition, the field is still in the phase where we, as food studies scholars, have something to prove. On one hand, the proliferation of popular literature surrounding food, from the biographies of well-known restaurant critics to the advice of scholars on what we should eat to better our health, has been beneficial in bringing attention to the field of food studies. On the other hand, the general population does not differentiate between works that are sometimes anecdotal and the rigorous research and review process behind academic food studies books and articles that are being published. The academic food studies world still has a ways to go in order to claim academic legitimacy in this immensely popular topic that is very much part of popular culture in North America. The proliferation of academic food studies programs in the past five years is a good sign that we are on our way.

A number of scholars have blazed the trail by defining food studies scholarship through their innovative research methods and approaches to writing about food. Anthropologist Sidney Mintz's *Sweetness and Power* (1985) was one of the first examples of the ways in which food studies scholarship crosses disciplinary boundaries and uses food as a way to look at larger issues of economics, taste, and power. Many consider historian and American Studies scholar Warren Belasco as the grandfather of food studies. Belasco's *Appetite for Change: How the Counter Culture Took on the Food Industry* (1990) and *Meals to Come: A History of the Future of Food* (2006) are also excellent examples of the interdisciplinary approach that has come to define food studies. Belasco served as the editor of the journal *Food, Culture and Society*, one of the first food studies journals that helped shape the field. Belasco has served as a tireless mentor to many young academics. Anthropologist Carole Counihan has also been a key figure in the development of food studies. Counihan's anthropological work focuses on food and mainly uses ethnographic methods, but she also delves deeply into gender studies. *Around the Tuscan Table: Food, Family and Gender in Twentieth-Century Florence* (2004) develops Counihan's concept of food voices, which is used to explore concepts of gender, the body, and social change in contemporary Italian society. Counihan also serves as the editor for *Food and Foodways*, another early interdisciplinary journal that has been critical in developing food studies as an academic field. There are many other pioneering scholars who have contributed to the development of food studies, but this chapter is too brief to be able to cite them all.

Scholarly journals have played an important part in the development of food studies. As mentioned above, *Food, Culture and Society* and *Food and Foodways* were some of the first interdisciplinary journals to support and bring together new approaches for the study of food. These peer-reviewed journals have provided a forum for the lively discussion of new scholarship and methods. *Gastronomica* is another food studies journal that straddles the world of academia and the popular press. Darra Goldstein, the journal's editor, has done a great deal to ensure the quality of the scholarship of this journal, while setting a tone that is engaging and accessible to a popular audience. In addition to academic journals, more and more academic publishers have taken an interest in bringing to press food studies scholarship. Some of the main publishers that have well-developed food studies lists include Routledge, Berg, and the University of California Press.

Another important forum for the development of food studies is the Association for the Study of Food and Society (ASFS). Their journal *Food, Culture and Society* is only one element of this flourishing association. Each year, the ASFS holds a joint meeting with the Agriculture, Food and Human Values Society (AFHVS). These conferences have been quintessential for the creation of an academic food studies community; they provide a forum for the exchange of academic ideas and debate. There are often roundtable discussions at ASFS conferences that discuss the current state and future of food studies scholarship, graduate education, and publishing. The ASFS has a largely American membership but it has become the leading food studies association with a growing international presence as well. There is also a Canadian Association for Food Studies (CAFS) that brings together Canadian scholars studying food.

There is some debate surrounding who had the first food studies program. Boston University claims to have one of the longest running programs with their Masters of Liberal Arts in Gastronomy. Started in 1993 by Julia Child and Jacques Pépin, this program was born out of a "Culture and Cuisine of France" course, proposed by Pépin. This was a class that was very heavy on food and cooking, drawing on the strengths of the existing Culinary Arts program at Boston University. Julia Child was a strong believer that there needed to be a place for the serious academic study of food if Americans were to change the way they thought about everyday cooking and eating. Both Child and Pépin felt that food studies should be centered on experiential learning; in this case, the kitchen became an extension of the library and the classroom. Influenced by his culinary training in France, for Pépin apprenticeship and hands-on learning remain one of the most import keys to understanding food.

The Boston University Gastronomy Program offers Liberal Arts training focused on tackling complex food issues that require creativity and critical thinking. In 2008, Warren Belasco was brought in to further develop the academic scope of the Gastronomy Program. Belasco recommended creating area concentrations that would help train graduates for specific job markets and academic pursuits. There are currently four tracks in the Boston University program: food policy; communications; business and entrepreneurship; history and culture. Most graduates find work in food-related industries or they have started their own food businesses. A number have also gone on to study in PhD programs in history, anthropology, and American studies.

New York University's Steinhart School is home to the other original food studies program. Started in 1996, this interdisciplinary program focuses on food culture and food systems. It first grew out of a nutrition curriculum but it has morphed into a very dynamic interdisciplinary program with an emphasis on scholarship and research. Unlike many other programs, New York University offers graduate and undergraduate degrees in food studies. At the undergraduate level, there is a Bachelor of Science with a concentration in food studies and a minor in food studies. At the graduate level, the Steinhart School offers both an MA and PhD in food studies. The MA is divided into two streams: food culture or food systems. New York University is one of the only universities in the United States with a doctoral program in this field.

This program's strengths are its focus on urban food systems and food policy. Marion Nestle's research and popular publications have also set a tone for the curriculum. The New York University program is home to some of the leading food studies scholars whose research has been playing a major role in defining this new field. With the presence of a PhD program, New York University has raised the academic bar and is now producing scholars who will populate the new food studies programs that are emerging now.

The only other PhD program in food studies is at Indiana University Bloomington. In 2007, the university announced the creation of a PhD in the Anthropology of Food that is grounded in a food studies approach. Studies of food and culture meet nutritional sciences to create a well-rounded program. Richard Wilk, the director of this program, has published cutting-edge research on post-colonial foodways in Belize, the political economy of food, and questions of identity and food. Wilk has been a key figure in shaping the anthropology of food as well as the field of food studies.

As interest in food grows and as food studies gains recognition as an academic area of study, new food studies programs are developing in universities in North America and abroad. One of the first major international efforts to develop food studies was the opening of the University of Gastronomic Sciences (UNISG) in Italy in 2004. Carlo Petrini, the founder of the Slow Food movement, felt that it was time to create an institution devoted to preparing a new generation of thinkers trained in the arts, humanities, and sciences with a focus on food. This is one of the few programs where agroecology and biochemistry as well as history and anthropology are part of the core curriculum. Field trips, called *stages,* are an important part of the curriculum. The *stages* are trips where students go to various parts of Italy and sometimes to other countries to meet farmers and engage in hands-on food production activities and tastings. UNISG currently offers a *laurea* (three-year bachelor's degree) and *specialistica* (additional two years after the *laurea*) in gastronomic sciences. These programs are offered in Italian and are recognized as degrees in the *Facoltà di Agraria* (Faculty of Agricultural Sciences) in the European university system. In addition to these undergraduate degrees, UNISG also offers three Masters in Food Culture and Communications: in human ecology and sustainability; food, place, and identity; and media, representations, and high-quality food. These courses are taught in English and are populated mainly by American and other foreign students. This university has become an important center for the study of food in Europe.

In 2009, the Open University of Catalonia (UOC), based in Barcelona, Spain, started a Food Systems, Culture and Society Masters degree. UOC offers a number of specializations within this degree, ranging from food security and policy to food, culture, and territory. All of the UOC degrees are offered online in English and some are now available in Spanish, Catalan, and French. The UOC also has a partnership with the Food and Agriculture Organization (FAO) and offers a certificate in food security.

A number of other European institutions have programs that approach food studies from the lens of a specific discipline. These have likely been discussed at length elsewhere in this volume. Briefly, a few of the more prominent programs include the School of Oriental and African Studies Masters in the Anthropology of Food in London, England; the Université François-Rabelais de Tours's Institut Éuropéen d'Histoire et des Cultures Alimentation; and the City University London's Center for Food Policy.

In Australasia, the University of Adelaide has a Masters in Food Studies. Students can pursue this program at the campus in Australia or online. Started by Barbara Santich, this program ran for a number of years before a brief hiatus and it is now back in full force.

Existing and new food studies programs continue to grow at an impressive rate. Chatham University started a food studies program in 2010. Headed up by sociologist Alice Julier, the Chatham program focuses on sustainable food production. Students have the opportunity to get their hands dirty and gain a better understanding of how food is produced at the 388-acre Eden Hall campus near Pittsburg. Chatham offers a Master of Arts in Food Studies with four possible concentrations: food politics; food markets and marketing; communication and writing; and sustainable agriculture. Core courses focus on teaching students about food systems, access, and culture. The systems approach and focus on sustainable agriculture are some of the main draws of this program.

It is becoming increasingly common to find food studies courses in a variety of disciplines but a number of undergraduate programs have also begun to pop up throughout the United States. In 2010, the New School in New York started an undergraduate program in food studies. Fabio Parasecoli is the coordinator of this program that offers undergraduates courses that can be taken as part of the bachelor's program in liberal arts. The University of Vermont has created a food studies research cluster and is now offering an undergraduate minor in food systems. In 2012, UVM plans to start offering a Master of Science in Food Systems.

As this book goes to press, there are numerous programs being founded throughout North America. Marylhurst University near Portland, Oregon is starting a Masters in Food Studies. Syracuse University is developing a food studies program as part of their Department of Public Health, Food Studies and Nutrition, and the University of Michigan is creating a food systems cluster. Oregon State University is also starting to develop a food studies curriculum headed up by anthropologists and other social scientists. Students at the University of Texas, Austin are calling for the development of a food studies program at their institution. The future of food studies looks bright as the field continues to grow and evolve.

Part of this evolution is the development of theoretical and didactic trends in existing and new programs. These include an emphasis on experiential learning. Boston University, the University of Gastronomic Sciences, and Chatham University all include hands-on elements in their curriculum. At Boston University, this can mean a full culinary arts course or lab experiments that are an integral part of core courses like "Experiencing Food through the Senses." At the University of Gastronomic Sciences, this might take the form of a cheese-making class or participation in the biodynamic teaching garden. At Chatham, students are encouraged to take classes in agriculture that include a hands-on element.

Another major trend in the food studies curriculum is a systems approach. Studying food requires the understanding of complex systems of production, distribution, and waste management. Borrowing from ecology, food studies attempts to show the interconnections between all areas of food production and consumption. It also focuses in on systemic issues such as disparities in food access and the environmental impact of agricultural production. By looking at food systems, food studies is moving beyond the often-limiting focus of specific disciplines.

Research methodologies

It is difficult to individuate specific research methodologies that characterize food studies due to the interdisciplinary nature of the field. What is particularly interesting is the variety of the food studies methodology toolbox. As food studies programs grow and draw in scholars from a number of disciplines, the methodologies being used are expanding. Due to the complex nature of food systems, this is particularly relevant. It is necessary to have a variety of tools to deal with food issues that can vary from the environmental impact of gastronomic tourism to the economic viability of specific food businesses. Food studies students need the tools to be able to evaluate environmental impact and to write the business plan in this situation. This is just one example of what a food studies graduate might encounter.

One of the challenges that food studies educators face is how to give students practical skills in such a broad area of study. For this reason, many programs focus on critical thinking and a systems approach because these are skills that are useful in all situations. At the same time, some programs are developing concentration areas that help students develop a specific skill set that will prepare them for careers in an area such as food policy. Students focusing on food policy need a good understanding of food systems as well as practical skills such as grant writing.

Food studies methods are not unified and this leads to a great deal of innovation and creative thinking. Both qualitative and quantitative methods are important in food studies scholarship. It is not uncommon to see ethnographic research accompanied by critical analyses of census data. Julie Guthman's recent *Weighing In: Obesity, Food Justice and the Limits of Capitalism* (2011) is a good example of this interdisciplinarity that brings new perspectives to current obesity issues by drawing on scientific findings, statistical data, and a critical food systems approach that moves beyond consumption to refocus the debate on production. Janet Poppendieck's *Free for All: Fixing School Food in America* (2010) is another monograph that combines anthropological methods and sociological approaches to address the systemic issues that plague many school food programs in the United States. Food studies demands the cross of disciplinary boundaries: nutrition, history, biochemistry, and anthropology can meet food science, sociology, and psychology in some works. Scholars adapt, adopt, and create methodologies that help them deal with the complex issues surrounding food. It is perhaps this creative *briocolage* that most characterizes food studies. Studying food requires this kind of creative thinking in order to solve complex problems and generate new understandings of food systems.

Avenues for future research

Apparent from the survey of food studies programs above, food policy and food systems are two areas of particular concern for food studies scholars. In North America, these focal points have really come into the light because of the growing public discourse surrounding the dysfunctional nature of the American food system. From government subsidies to unchecked neoliberal approaches to food as a business, the United States faces serious issues of food access and the nutritional implications of a popular diet that is based on processed foods. What is clear is that food-related problems in the United States are systemic issues—fixing one piece will not make the entire puzzle fall into place. A food systems approach and critical analysis of national and local food policy are helping scholars and government agencies better understand the shortcomings of food systems. However, there is still a great deal of work to be done in this area.

Related to food systems and policy, the sustainable production of food is another area that can benefit from a food studies and gastronomic sciences approach. It is not enough to understand the principles of organic agriculture, permaculture, and climate change; there is a need to disseminate this information so that people can understand what the larger systemic implications are of our current food systems. In addition, governments and citizens need to be able to imagine alternate systems and possibilities for feeding the nation and the world's populations. Many food studies students come into academic programs wanting to solve the world's food problems. Most of them leave these programs with a better understanding how they can contribute directly to changing their own food system and that of those around them. Whether the scope is big or small, food studies programs are changing the way people think about food and the political, economic, and personal choices that they make about food each day.

The applied aspects of food studies certainly have great practical appeal and the food industry is one of the few sectors of the North American economy that is still growing. However, there is also need for historical, cultural, and social research to better understand some of the base issues surrounding larger problems. For example, what are the cultural implications of the loss of biodiversity that we are seeing in almost all cultures? What does the deskilling of cooking and agriculture mean for social relations? What can the spatial relations created by foodways tell us about the social lives of migrants? Food is not just the focal point in food studies, it is also the lens through which we can see the world. It offers us an intimate view onto people's inner and outer worlds: family life; the way people think about their bodies; and it can be an expression of alternative political views.

Practical considerations for getting started

Students looking to pursue a degree in food studies should have a look at all of the available programs before applying and making a decision about which program to attend. At the undergraduate level, there are very few programs that are entirely dedicated to food studies. However, the New School, New York University, the University of New Hampshire, and a growing number of institutions in the United States offer undergraduate degrees and minors in food studies. At the graduate level, there are a number of distinct Masters programs. Students should consider their learning objectives and try to understand which program is the best fit. If you are considering becoming a food writer, the New York University or Boston University programs might be best. If you want to be a market manager or manage an organic farm, the Chatham University program has a lot to offer. If you are looking for a unique experience abroad, the University of Gastronomic Sciences will be of interest to you. Once you have your sights set on a few programs, you should visit if you can. Try to talk to students in the programs, meet with instructors and sit in on a class.

There are not many scholarships for terminal Masters degrees (a Masters degree that does not lead to a PhD) so prospective graduate students need to be resourceful. Some universities offer general school scholarships and the Casten family even set up a Fulbright Scholarship for the University of Gastronomic Sciences. Hopefully, there will be an increase in funding for food studies programs and scholarships for students in the future as programs grow.

If your university would like to start a food studies program, the first step is gathering interested parties from the various schools and departments at your institution. It is likely that there is a closet food studies person in almost every department. Many academics do work focused on food but do not necessarily associate it with the field of food studies. Many programs have grown out of nutrition, food science, and agriculture departments and schools. However, there is a new breed of program that straddles disciplines and brings together the arts, social sciences, and hard sciences. This may be the way of the future given the trend towards a systems approach. For this reason, building a broad network of supporters and resources at your institution is critical. With the interest in food-related issues, food studies is an academic field that is drawing great interest from the public, students, and university administrators.

When considering starting a food studies program, it is important to look at the resources you have available at your institution as well as in your community. Are there appropriate labs, gardens, greenhouses, or kitchen facilities? Are there local businesses, industries, or research centers that would support such a program? Can your program speak to local issues and engage in giving back to community? In addition to a strong academic program, food studies programs can differentiate and find an important applied scope if they engage in local agriculture and food access issues.

With the growing number of programs opening each year, differentiation is key. Thus far most of the food studies programs in the United States have managed to choose different focal points – from sustainable agriculture to a focus on food and communications. These programs are complementary rather than competing against each other. There are so many food issues that need to be addressed through academic research that there is plenty of room for new programs and new areas of specialization.

Internet resources

Association for the Study of Food and Society
food–culture.org
Boston University, Gastronomy Program
www.bu.edu/met/programs/graduate/gastronomy/
Canadian Association for Food Studies
www.foodstudies.ca/
Chatham University, Food Studies
www.chatham.edu/mafs
Food, Culture and Society
www.bergpublishers.com/BergJournals/FoodCultureandSociety/tabid/521/Default.aspx
Food and Foodways
www.tandf.co.uk/journals/titles/07409710.html
Fulbright, Casten Family Foundation Award at the University of Gastronomic Sciences
us.fulbrightonline.org/program_country.html?id=54#casten
Gastronomica
gastronomica.org/
New School, General Studies, Food Studies Program
www.newschool.edu/generalstudies/foodstudies.aspx
New York University, Steinhardt School, Department of Nutrition, Food Studies and Public Health
steinhardt.nyu.edu/e/h/nutrition/index.php
University of Gastronomic Sciences
www.unisg.it
Universitat Oberta de Catalunya, Food Systems, Culture and Society
www.uoc.edu/masters/eng/master/web/food_systems_culture_society/food_systems_culture_-society/

Key reading

Belasco, Warren (2008) *Food: The Key Concepts.* Oxford: Berg.
Counihan, Carole and Penny Van Esterik (2007) *Food and Culture: A Reader*, 2nd edition. New York: Routledge.
Miller, Jeffery and Jonathan Deutsch (2010) *Food Studies: An Introduction to Research Methods.* Oxford: Berg.
Mintz, Sidney (1985) *Sweetness and Power: The Place of Sugar in Modern History.* New York: Viking.
Wilk, Richard (2006) *Fast Food/Slow Food: The Cultural Economy of the Global Food System.* Walnut Creek, CA: Altamira Press.

19

Food and American studies

Margot Finn

This entry outlines three ways of thinking about the field of American studies and the implications of each one for studying food. As an area study of the US, American studies often takes the form of case studies that use multiple approaches to examine a particular event, object, place, or group of people. As an interdisciplinary cultural studies method, American studies promotes the analysis of ideology, hegemony, social hierarchies and forms of oppression and resistance. As a confederation of (inter)disciplines, American studies invites connections between disparate approaches and attention to the experiences of marginalized populations and subjects.

Historical background of food scholarship in American studies and major theoretical approaches in use

Most histories of American studies locate the origins of the field in the early twentieth century, when scholars like Frederic Jackson Turner and Vernon Parrington began to describe American thought and culture as distinct from English and European culture. The first institutional forms of American studies, including departments and degree-granting programs, professional academic organizations (most notably the American Studies Association or ASA), and scholarly journals like *American Quarterly* were founded in the 1940s. Most of the first generation of Americanists were trained as literary critics and historians, and many of the courses that made up new American studies curricula were located in English and history departments. Scholarship in the field initially focused largely on the creation and study of an American literary canon and the history of influential white men. However, some Americanists also called attention to the importance of social history, folkways, and the lives of everyday Americans. Even in the first few generations of American studies scholarship, the field was influenced by left-leaning political movements, the populist mobilizations of the 1930s, and New Deal cultural projects. The experiences of marginalized racial and ethnic groups in the US became increasingly central to the field after the social movements of the 1960s and "anthropological turn" in the 1970s (a move away from traditional canons and "high culture" and embrace of a wider range of texts and behaviors as legitimate objects of scholarship across the humanities and social sciences).

Despite the prevalence of critical accounts and popular culture in American studies, there was little scholarship or teaching on food in the field until the late 1980s. The growing interest in food in the last two decades was marked in 2008 by a brief mention in the presidential address at the annual meeting of the ASA. Phil Deloria listed food studies among the "emergent interdisciplines" that sometimes find an institutional home in American studies, along with sports studies, performance studies, disability studies, and queer studies. However, like all of those fields, only a subset of scholarship within the field of food studies can shelter under the "big tent" vision of American studies.

The limitations are both topical and methodological. American studies has expanded its purview considerably in the last few decades to encompass transnational or global understandings of the US and its influence. Nonetheless, the *Americanness* of American studies functionally excludes work on food histories and cultures that are not interested in the US at all. Thus, whereas the collection of essays *McDonald's in East Asia* edited by James Watson would fit easily into American studies conversations about the US in the world and the "glocalization" of US cultural products, Richard Wilk's work on food traditions in Belize might be more of a stretch. Methodologically, although American studies might theoretically embrace scholarship from any discipline as long as it tilts in the direction of the US, in practice it continues to be dominated by literary criticism, historiography, and other humanistic methods. Survey, experimental, and applied research are rarely represented on the program at ASA and very few scientists are part of American studies departments. Even scholars trained in the "soft" social sciences are rarer than humanists. Most research in the fields of nutrition, agriculture, food science, public health, and ecology would be out of place in the pages of *American Quarterly*. Despite these limitations, scholars interested in the history, culture, and politics of food have found American studies to be somewhat more welcoming than some of the traditional disciplines and other interdisciplinary fields like women's studies.

The growing relationship between food studies and American studies reflects changes in both fields. In food studies, the proliferation of humanistic and cultural studies approaches and increasing attention to US foodways (related in part to the grassroots social movement for safer, more "natural," or more ethical food) has made recent scholarship on food more legible to Americanists. In American studies, the increasing acceptance of food as a legitimate object of scholarly concern reflects the extent to which the field has always been influenced by social movements, interested in debased or mundane topics that the traditional disciplines may exclude, and attracted to topics that demand an interdisciplinary approach.

Research methodologies

As there is no one agreed-upon definition of American studies or how to do it, I explore three possible conceptualizations of the field and the implications of each for doing research on food: (1) the idea of American studies as an area studies of the US; (2) the idea of American studies as a methodology; and (3) the idea of American studies as an arena for interdisciplinary encounter and anti-disciplinary innovation.

American studies as US area studies

Like most area studies fields, American studies took institutional shape in the immediate aftermath of the Second World War. Many of the same foundations and corporations that poured funds into research on foreign regions where the US had political and economic interests also supported the scholarship aimed at defining what made America unique. The American Civilization Program at the University of Pennsylvania was established with the help of several large grants from the Rockefeller Foundation, the American Sociological Association and American studies at the

University of Minnesota were supported by funds from the Carnegie Corporation, and American studies at Yale received a large endowment from the railroad and insurance executive William Robertson Coe. Many early American studies scholars like John William Ward and Alan Trachtenberg received funding from newly constituted bodies like the American Council of Learned Societies. Both American studies and area studies fields have been critiqued for the work they did during this corporate-funded "Golden Age," which may have produced ideological justifications and strategic knowledge in support of imperialist projects abroad and racist, sexist, heteronormative, xenophobic policies at home. However, Cold War Americanists and area studiers also significantly broadened the scope of scholarship, especially in the humanities, which had until then focused primarily on European and English history and letters.

American studies departments are also similar to other area studies departments in that they are often composed primarily of scholars trained in the traditional disciplines and the graduate students they train often end up employed in the traditional disciplines. Thus, although the departments themselves might be interdisciplinary, sometimes the scholarship they produce might be better described as *multi*-disciplinary. American studies is slightly different than other area studies in that it skews more towards the humanities than social sciences. This may also be a legacy of their Cold War origins: the project of defining "us" against a Communist "them" (or the many other Others against whom scholars defined American exceptionalism) is more of an interpretive and narrative project than the international area studies' attempt to understand the political and economic development of foreign countries and regions. Thus, where area studies departments often include political scientists, economists, and anthropologists, American studies is still dominated by literary critics and historians and over half of American studies PhDs who get academic jobs are placed in English or history departments.

However, both area studies and American studies see themselves as interdisciplinary and promote the use of multiple approaches to understand particular times, places, populations, and cultural forms. Both emphasize detail, specificity, context, and thick description in contrast to empirical and applied methods that look to make generalizations and abstractions. The method that emerges from these priorities sometimes takes the shape of interdisciplinary case studies: close examinations of particular events, social or cultural movements, populations, trends, or institutions from many different angles using a broad assemblage of texts. The cases are not always limited to the political borders of the US. For example, Warren Belasco's *Meals to Come: A History of the Future of Food* can be seen as a case study of representations of the future of food with an emphasis on American writers and thinkers, but the book also includes many British writers who influenced or were in conversation with the Americans. Language, rather than geography, defines the limits of the texts included. The book is also an exemplar of interdisciplinarity. Belasco analyzes a stunning array of sources, including government and think tank papers, science-fiction novels, artifacts from world's fairs, movies, advertisements, and Disney's EPCOT Center. A growing number of interdisciplinary studies on particular foodstuffs are also emblematic of the case study approach, like Cynthia Ott's dissertation, *Squashed Myths: The Cultural History of the Pumpkin in North America*.

American studies as a methodology

The conceptualization of the field that Deloria favors is a set of "practices developed over time, that are truly interdisciplinary, that are expansive, open, and welcoming to an infinite number of idiosyncratic adaptations from all directions, and that have oppositional content and political power" (Deloria, 2009: 15). He lays out a program for American studies as essentially a variant of cultural studies that happens to focus on the US (and its transnational influences and global resonances), but has no necessary relationship to the geographical, political borders of the US or even the idea of "America."

The methodology he describes has four registers: Textual interpretation, archive building, institutional contextualization, and social theory. In interpreting texts, American studies uses the tools of literary critics, art historians, and ethnographers: close reading, semiotics, thick description. In contextualizing them, they work like historians, assembling a broad range of sources and documents to capture the nuances of genres and periods and considering the political economy of institutions that govern how texts are produced, distributed, and consumed and the circuits they move through. At the level of theory, they put their case studies in conversation with others, consider the broader structures of power, lines of oppression, and forms of resistance represented by their particular case that might be portable and illuminate broader truths. *Meals to Come* also exemplifies this approach. Belasco uses the techniques of close reading and thick description to analyze his texts, places them in historical context using a broad assemblage of archival documents, and constructs a coherent narrative based largely on theoretical abstractions—the distinctions between classical, modernist, or recombinant visions of the future, each of which has a "heyday" but all of which are present in some form throughout the 200 years he surveys.

As Deloria notes, this method is expansive and flexible. It aims for a balance between specificity (close attention to texts and objects) and generality (theory and the analysis of power). It may be particularly useful for the analysis of food because, as Warren Belasco argues elsewhere, food "require[s] that we think about matters political, historical, economic, sociocultural, and scientific *all at once*" (Belasco, 2008: 7). Indeed, the necessity of understanding at least some of the science involved in agriculture, nutrition, medicine, public health, and food chemistry in order to account for phenomena like the organic revolution in farming, the rise of fast food, the transformation of home cooking, and the "obesity epidemic" may push the method to include quantitative social science and natural science too, which American studies has not traditionally done. For example, Carolyn de la Peña's *Empty Pleasures: Artificial Sweeteners from Saccharin to Splenda* draws on the science of sweetness, the business of chemistry, the history of dieting and nutrition, and the evidence (or lack thereof) for claims about the dangers of artificial sweeteners in order to account for the cultural history of sugar substitutes.

Deloria is not the first to propose that American studies be defined less by its institutional forms or geographical area of study than by a method. Michael Denning (2004) argues in "'The Special American Conditions': Marxism and American Studies" that American studies developed as sort of US analog to British cultural studies, but without the Marxism. In both its chauvinist, nationalist form and the critical form described as "anti-American studies" by Hemingway biographer Kenneth Lynn, American studies provided alternative explanations for the rise of capitalism and the American way, serving first as antidote and then as substitute for the Marxist tradition of radical cultural critique. Denning argues that American studies should take up Marxism more directly, especially the concepts of commodity/reification, ideology, class/hegemony, and cultural materialism, because they provide an international vocabulary, thus avoiding American parochialisms like "Emersonianism," and offer a coherent but interdisciplinary method. This method is slightly different than Deloria's, consisting of four moves: (1) illuminating the social life of material objects and texts, especially commodity fetishism and reification; (2) analyzing the nature and function of ideology; (3) specifying the relations between class and culture, relying primarily on Gramsci's theoretical framework of hegemony, historical blocs, and the construction of common sense; and (4) focusing on the material production and consumption of culture, including the institutions, formations, conventions, and means of production and the relationships between Raymond Williams's categories of dominant, residual, oppositional, and emergent cultures.

There are many examples of work on food in American studies that fit the above description. One example is Psyche A. Williams-Forson's *Building Houses Out of Chicken Legs: Black Women, Food, and Power*. Williams-Forson (2006) examines the complexity of black women's relationship to chicken in the US from slavery to the present. From cookbooks to advertisements to personal interviews, she analyzes how chicken is fetishized and deployed in racist and sexist stereotypes—as in Chris Rock's HBO special *Bigger and Blacker*, when he talks about Daddy wanting "the big piece of chicken" and Mama being occasionally unwilling to give it to him. She shows how black women used chickens as a source of income and empowerment, but how their domestic labor and cultural work was often appropriated by others. For example, white women "borrowed" black women's recipes without crediting them and the food industry deployed racist representations to sell fried chicken. Throughout, she exposes the fraught relationships between the material realities of food production and labor, ideologies about race and gender, and competing forms of agency and oppression.

American studies as an arena of (inter)disciplinary encounter

Lastly, American studies is sometimes defined not by its institutional forms or patterns in the scholarly practices of people affiliated with those institutions, but instead by the field's openness to topical and methodological innovation. Another way to put this might be that American studies is defined less by *what* American studies scholars study or *how* they study it than by the approaches and topics they are willing to embrace or unwilling to exclude. For example, in an 1974 essay in *American Quarterly* on social science in American studies, Stanley Bailis writes: "[American studies] has thus emerged not as a discipline, but as an arena for disciplinary encounter and staging ground for fresh topical pursuits. It embraces America in a Whitmanish hug, excluding nothing and always beginning" (a quote that also serves as one of three epigraphs in Gene Wise's (1979) seminal history of the field, "'Paradigm Dramas' in American Studies"). Similarly, in his overview of the field in the recently published *Encyclopedia of American Studies*, Michael Cowan characterizes the field as a "collection of movements" aimed at "enlarging the content of the field" and "diversifying the theories and methods brought to bear on that content."

In practice, the embrace has not always been as expansive as the above quotes might suggest. The relationship between American studies and ethnic studies has been especially tense. Scholars who identify more with the latter have complained that their work has been co-opted for a less radical intellectual or political agenda, and scholars in both fields have resented being forced to share limited pools of funding and institutional resources. Nonetheless, American studies has become a field where inquiries about culture, power, and inequality, attempt to account for transnational cultural flows, and an engagement with the complexities of borderlands and marginalized perspectives are not only welcome but practically *mandatory*.

Especially compared to the traditional disciplines, American studies has been relatively open to issues of race, gender, and class diversity, which came to dominate the field in the 1980s and 1990s. More recently, it has also been open to the kinds of questions raised by disability studies, queer studies, environmental studies, and food studies. In *American Studies in a Moment of Danger*, George Lipsitz chronicles how social movements have repeatedly pushed American studies to expand its purview. The labor movements of the 1930s; the 1960s civil rights, anti-war, feminist, gay rights, Asian American, Chicano/a, and American Indian movements; the "culture wars" of the 1980s; and the anti-globalization (or anti-neoliberal) movement represented by the protests at the 1999 World Trade Organization (WTO) meeting in Seattle were each echoed by changes in the scope and composition of American studies. This receptiveness to grassroots social movements may also be why the field has been somewhat more sensitive or receptive to the study of topics like food, which have historically been excluded from the humanities as too mundane to merit serious scholarly attention.

In practical terms, this aspect of American studies means that its work on food is especially likely to be concerned with intersecting oppressions based on gender, race, ethnicity, sexuality, class, religion, immigration status, ability, and age. American food studies may define America broadly, implicitly or explicitly rejecting political borders or seeking to interrogate the category of Americanness. Additionally, it is likely to be critical of dominant power structures and prevailing modes of economic production, and may seek to imagine alternate futures and forms of resistance for historically marginalized and oppressed populations. One example of these tendencies is Vicki L. Ruiz's 2007 ASA presidential address, titled "Citizen Restaurant: American Imaginaries, American Communities." Ruiz examines "racial/ethnic foodscapes as markers of belonging and difference within a larger frame of US inequality," and seeks to "explore the ways in which race infuses ordinary acts of reaction, resistance, appropriation, and ambivalence as they have played out in relation to food, labor, and immigration."

The openness of American studies to "emergent interdisciplines" offers both possibilities and potential limitations for food studies. On the one hand, American studies might serve as a meeting place where food scholars can explore the links between food studies, ethnic studies, environmental studies, women's studies, disability studies, sports studies, material culture studies, children's studies, etc. In the past five years, there have been multiple sessions on food at the ASA annual meeting, often held on the same day and in the same room, which therefore becomes a sort of gathering place for scholars from many different backgrounds. On the other hand, using American studies as a primary institutional home might push more food scholars towards the study of US topics to the exclusion of other national, regional, or global imaginaries. Trying to fit within the scope of American studies might limit how scholars frame projects or cause them to emphasize privileged categories of difference, like race and ethnicity, to the exclusion of categories like class, religious affiliation, and age.

Avenues for future research

Recent dissertations and books in American studies on food point to the potential of projects that center on particular *food items* (like corn and squash), *particular racial and ethnic groups* (like Mexican Americans), *comparisons between multiple groups* (like African Americans, Italians, and Swedes in Chicago), *regions* (like Northwest Ohio or the American South), *genres of cultural production* (advertising, film, reality television, cookbooks, etc.), *industries* (restaurants, supermarkets, advertising, food chemistry, etc.), and *social movements and discourses* (like organic farming or the "obesity epidemic"). There is rich and nuanced work being done on the history and culture of urban gardening, home cooking, farming, eating, and starving in America; however, the human acts of growing, preparing, and sharing food are almost unimaginably complex and far-reaching. It is hard to imagine running out of topics anytime soon.

Even subjects that have already been addressed can be updated, framed in new ways, or approached using new archives and methods. For example, the most comprehensive cultural history of dieting in the US is probably Hillel Schwartz's *Never Satisfied: A Cultural History of Diets, Fantasies, and Fat*. Although it is still a useful resource and widely considered to be one of the foundational texts in fat studies, it was published nearly three decades ago. Updated cultural histories of dieting might reread the history in light of diet fads and discourses that have emerged since the 1980s, the global spread of US diet culture, resistance to diet practices in ethnic and racial minority populations, the growing size acceptance movement, mass-media weight-loss narratives like "The Biggest Loser" and "Celebrity Fit Club," online weight-loss communities, or theories about the body emerging from fat studies, queer theory, and disability studies. Three general areas that seem especially rich for future study on food in American studies: (1) global flows of foods, tastes, practices, people, products, and ideas into and out of the US; (2) the role of food practices and ideologies in the creation and reproduction of intersecting social hierarchies; and (3) how contemporary food trends and reform efforts are situated in broader historical, cultural, and political contexts.

Practical considerations for getting started – funding, programs, archival sources, tools, data sets, internet resources, scholarships and awards, etc. (where and how?)

The American Studies Association website lists 61 graduate programs in American Studies, 28 of which offer a PhD. Several of them have food concentrations or are involved in cross-departmental food studies initiatives, including the Critical Studies in Food and Culture research cluster at the University of California, Davis and the Food Cultures cluster at the University of North Carolina. The Multi-campus Research Group on Studies of Food and the Body, which includes University of California, Davis, Santa Cruz, Berkeley, Santa Barbara, and Los Angeles is proposing a Designated Emphasis in Studies of Food, Systems, and Culture to be established in 2012 at the Davis and Santa Cruz campuses. There are also at least 18 centers and programs for American studies outside of the US, including the Clinton Institute for American Studies at University College Dublin in Ireland, undergraduate and graduate programs in American studies at the University of Sussex and University of Nottingham in England, the Institute for US and Canadian Studies at the Russian Academy of Sciences in Moscow, the American Studies Center at the University of Bahrain in Sakhir, and the American Studies Leipzig program, which publishes the graduate journal *Aspeers* whose forthcoming fifth issue will focus on American food cultures.

Funding for graduate study in American studies in the US is the same as in most humanities disciplines. Upon acceptance to a PhD program, students are usually offered a funding package with guaranteed support in the form of tuition waivers and stipends for a limited number of semesters. Some programs offer fellowship support for the first year of course work and a year of dissertation writing. Others may require students to teach every term. Teaching usually involves leading discussion sections and grading exams and papers for large lecture courses, but in many programs, students also have the opportunity to design and teach their own courses. Additional opportunities to work as a grader, teaching assistant, research assistant, or instructional support staff may be available. Some terminal MA programs also offer teaching support. Competitive grants and fellowships are also available to support graduate student research, travel, writing, and language study. Johns Hopkins University maintains a searchable funding database at jhuresearch.jhu.edu/funding.htm (accessed on April 3, 2012), and the *Chronicle of Higher Education* lists grants and fellowships in the last few pages of each issue.

The MA (in American studies or a related field) is not a prerequisite for entering most PhD programs, although some programs are beginning to favor students with a Masters in an effort to reduce average time to degree. Terminal MA programs are typically designed to be completed in two to three years and usually require the completion of a thesis, consisting of original scholarly research ranging from 30–100 pages. PhD programs may be completed in as little as five years, but average time to degree is significantly longer. No data are available for American studies programs exclusively; for all humanities disciplines, the average time to degree in 2003 was nine years as a registered student and 11.3 years total (Hoffer and Welch, 2006: 2–3, in Menand, 2010).

There are a growing number of culinary archives with materials of interest to American studies scholars. The Schlesinger Library at Harvard's Radcliffe Institute for Advanced Study has 15,000 titles related to food and cooking, including complete runs of many culinary and gastronomic titles and the papers of many notable individuals in the culinary field, including Julia Child, M. F. K. Fisher, Alice Bradley, the Corner Book Shop/Eleanor Lowenstein, and Elizabeth David. The Janice Bluestein Longone archive at the University of Michigan's Clements Library has an extensive collection of cookbooks, etiquette manuals, gastronomy, advertising, maps, catalogs, magazines, and ephemera from the sixteenth to the twentieth centuries with particular strengths in the late eighteenth, nineteenth, and early twentieth centuries. The Peacock-Harper Culinary Collection at Virginia Tech includes photographs, cookbooks, nutrition literature, and social commentary about food with a particular strength in children's cookbook and nutritional literature. The Buttolph Collection in the New York Public Library's Rare Book Division includes one of the world's largest collections of historical menus. The Szathmary Culinary Arts Collection at the University of Iowa includes more than 4,000 promotional recipe pamphlets produced by food and appliance manufacturers from the late nineteenth century to the present and the papers of Hungarian-born Chicago restauranteur and food writer Louis Szathmary. The Culinary Arts Museum at Johnson and Wales University in Providence, Rhode Island contains over 250,000 items including over 60,000 cookbooks and extensive restaurant ephemera and museums and the reference library of the Retail Bakers of America.

A growing number of digital archives are also becoming available. The *Oxford Encyclopedia of Food and Drink in America*, edited by Andrew F. Smith, includes 770 articles on particular foods ("Coca-Cola," "Po'boy Sandwich"), events ("Clambake"), trends ("Community Supported Agriculture"), ethnic and religious groups ("Native American Foods"), biographies ("Beard, James," "Lagasse, Emeril"), and political and social movements ("Temperance," "Food and Drug Act"). A searchable online version is available to library subscribers. Food blogs, message boards, recipe websites, restaurant review sites, and online communities also constitute rich sources of data.

Key reading

Selected books and articles on food by scholars with an American studies affiliation

Belasco, Warren (2008) *Food: The Key Concepts*. Oxford: Berg.
——(2007) *Appetite for Change: How the Counterculture Took on the Food Industry*, 2nd edn. Ithaca, NY: Cornell University Press.
——(2006) *Meals to Come: The History of the Future of Food*. Berkeley: University of California Press.
Bentley, Amy (1998) *Eating for Victory: Food Rationing and the Politics of Domesticity*. Urbana: University of Illinois Press.
Biltekoff, Charlotte (2007) "The Terror Within: Obesity in Post 9/11 U.S. Life." *American Studies* 48:3 (Fall): 29–48.
de la Peña, Carolyn (2010) *Empty Pleasures: The Story of Artificial Sweeteners from Saccharin to Splenda*. Durham: University of North Carolina Press.
Kasson, John F. (1987) "Rituals of Dining: Table Manners in Victorian America," in *Dining in America, 1850–1900*, ed. Kathryn Grover. Amherst and Rochester: The Margaret Woodbury Strong Museum.
Pleck, Elizabeth, (1999) "The Making of the Domestic Occasion: The History of Thanksgiving in the United States." *Journal of Social History* 32: 773–89.
Poe, Tracy N. "Origins of Soul Food in Black Urban Identity: Chicago, 1915–47." *American Studies International* 37:1 (February 1999): 4–34.
Ruiz, Vicki L. "Citizen Restaurant: American Imaginaries, American Communities." *American Quarterly* 60:1 (March 2008): 1–21.
Smith, Andrew F. ed. (2004) *The Oxford Encyclopedia of Food and Drinks in America*. New York: Oxford University Press.

Williams-Forson, Psyche A. (2006) *Building Houses Out of Chicken Legs: Black Women, Food, and Power*. Chapel Hill: University of North Carolina Press.

Recent dissertations on food in American studies

Adema, Pauline (2006) *Festive Foodscapes: Iconizing Food and the Shaping of Identity and Place*. Austin: University of Texas.

Crook, Nathan (2009) *Foods That Matter: Constructing Place and Community at Food Festivals in Northwest Ohio*. Bowling Green: Ohio State University.

Dolan, Kathryn Cornell (2010) *Fruits of Expansion: Empires of Consumption in U.S. Literature, 1840–1910*. Santa Barbara: University of California.

Finn, S. Margot (2011) *Aspirational Eating: Class Anxiety and the Rise of Food in Popular Culture*. Ann Arbor: University of Michigan.

Liggett, Lori S. (2006) *Mothers, Militants, Martyrs, & "M'm! M'm! Good" Taming the New Woman: Campbell Soup Advertising in Good Housekeeping, 1905–1920*. Bowling Green: Ohio State University.

Lindenfeld, Laura Ann (2003) *Feasting Our Eyes: Food Films, Gender, and United States American Identity*. Davis: University of California.

Ott, Cynthia (2002) *Squashed Myths: The Cultural History of the Pumpkin in North America*. Philadelphia: University of Pennsylvania.

Poe, Tracey N. (1999) *Food, Culture, and Entrepreneurship Among African Americans, Italians, and Swedes in Chicago*. Harvard, MA: Harvard University.

Russek, Audrey (2010) *Culinary Citizenship in American Restaurants*. Austin: University of Texas.

Sisson-Lessens, Kelly (2011) *Master of Millions: King Corn in American Culture, 1861–1936*. Ann Arbor: University of Michigan.

Thompson-Hajdik, Anna (2011) *Constructing and Consuming Rural Life in Modern America*. Austin: University of Texas.

Selected anthologies, books, and articles about food in the US

Abarca, Meredith E. (2006) *Voices in the Kitchen: Views of Food and the World from Working-Class Mexican and Mexican American Women*. College Station: Texas A&M University Press.

Avakian, Arlene V. (1997) *Through the Kitchen Window: Women Explore the Intimate Meanings of Food and Cooking*. Boston, MA: The University of Massachusetts Press.

Avakian, Arlene V. and Haber, Barbara, eds. (2005) *From Betty Crocker to Feminist Food Studies: Critical Perspectives on Women and Food*. Amherst, MA: University of Massachusetts Press.

Bower, Anne, ed. (1997) *Recipes for Reading: Community Cookbooks, Stories, Histories*. Boston, MA: The University of Massachusetts Press.

Brumberg, Joan Jacobs (1997) *The Body Project: An Intimate History of American Girls*. New York: Random House.

——(2000) *Fasting Girls: The History of Anorexia Nervosa*. New York: Vintage Books.

Campos, Paul (2004) *The Obesity Myth: Why America's Obsession With Weight is Hazardous to Your Health*. New York: Gotham Books.

Carney, Judith (2002) *Black Rice: The African Origins of Rice Cultivation in the Americas*. Cambridge, MA: Harvard University Press.

Counihan, Carole M. (1999) "Food Rules in the United States: Individualism, Control, and Hierarchy." In *The Anthropology of Food and Body: Gender, Meaning, and Power*, Carole Counihan ed. New York: Routledge.

——ed. (2002) *Food in the USA: A Reader*. New York: Routledge.

Deutsch, Tracy. "Making Change at the Grocery Store: Government, Grocers, and the Creation of Chicago's Supermarkets, 1920–50." *Enterprise and Society* 5(4) (December 2004): 607–16.

DeVault, Marjorie L. (1991) *Feeding the Family: The Social Organization of Caring*. Chicago, IL: The University of Chicago Press.

Diner, Hasia R. (2003) *Hungering for America: Italian, Irish, and Jewish Foodways in the Age of Migration*. Cambridge, MA: Harvard University Press.

DuPuis, Melanie (2002) *Nature's Perfect Food: How Milk Became America's Drink*. New York: New York University Press.

DuPuis, Melanie and Julie Guthman. "Embodying Neoliberalism: Economy, Culture and the Politics of Fat.," *Environment and Planning D: Society and Space* 24(3) (n.d.): 427–48.

Edge, John T. (2007) *Southern Belly*. Chapel Hill, NC: Algonquin Books.

Elias, Megan J. (2009) *Food in the United States, 1890–1945*. Santa Barbara, CA: Greenwood Press.

Fine, Gary Alan (1996) *Kitchens: The Culture of Restaurant Work*. Berkeley: University of California Press.

Friedberg, Susanne (2009) *Fresh: A Perishable History*. Cambridge, MA: Harvard University Press.

Fromartz, Samuel (2006) *Organic, Inc.: Natural Foods and How They Grew*. Orlando, FL: Harcourt Books.

Gabbacia, Donna R. (2000) *We Are What We Eat: Ethnic Food an the Making of Americans*. Cambridge, MA: Harvard University Press.

Glassner, Barry (2007) *The Gospel of Food: Everything You Think You Know About Food Is Wrong*. New York: Harper Collins.

Goodwin, Lorine Swainston (1999) *The Pure Food, Drink, and Drug Crusaders, 1879–1914*. Jefferson, NC: McFarland & Co., Inc.

Guthman, Julie (2004) *Agrarian Dreams: The Paradox of Organic Farming in California*. Berkeley: University of California Press.

Haley, Andrew P. (2011) *Turning the Tables: Restaurants and the Rise of the American Middle Class, 1880–1920*. Chapel Hill, NC: University of North Carolina Press.

Hoganson, Kristin (2007) *Consumers' Imperium: The Global Production of American Domesticity*. Chapel Hill: University of North Carolina Press.

Inness, Sherrie, ed. (2000) *Pilaf, Pozole, and Pad Thai: American Women and Ethnic Food*. Amherst: University of Massachusetts Press, pp. 175–98.

Kamp, David (2006) *The United States of Arugula: How We Became a Gourmet Nation*. New York: Random House.

Korsmeyer, Carolyn (1999) *Making Sense of Taste: Taste, Food, and Philosophy*. Ithaca, NY: Cornell University Press.

Kurlansky, Mark, ed. (2009) *The Food of a Younger Land*. New York: Riverhead Books.

Laudan, Rachel (1996) *The Food of Paradise: Exploring Hawaii's Culinary Heritage*. Honolulu, HI: University of Hawaii Press.

LeBesco, Kathleen and Peter Naccarato, eds. (2008) *Edible Ideologies: Representing Food and Meaning*. Albany: State University of New York Press.

Levenstein, Harvey (1993) *Paradox of Plenty: A Social History of Eating in Modern America*. Berkeley: University of California Press.

——(1988) *Revolution at the Table: The Transformation of the American Diet*. New York: Oxford University Press.

Long, Lucy M., ed. (2004) *Culinary Tourism: Explorations in Eating and Otherness*. Lexington: University of Kentucky Press.

Miller, Daniel (1998) "Coca-Cola: A Black Sweet Drink From Trinidad." In *Material Cultures: Why Some Things Matter*, ed. Daniel Miller. Chicago, IL: University of Chicago Press.

Nestle, Marion (2002) *Food Politics: How the Food Industry Influences Nutrition and Health*. Berkeley: University of California Press.

Neuhaus, Jessamyn (2003) *Manly Meals and Mom's Home Cooking: Cookbooks and Gender in Modern America*. Baltimore, MD: Johns Hopkins University Press.

Oliver, J. Eric (2006) *Fat Politics: The Real Story Behind America's Obesity Epidemic*. New York: Oxford University Press.

Parkin, Katherine J. (2006) *Food is Love: Advertising and Gender Roles in Modern America*. Philadelphia: University of Pennsylvania Press.

Petrick, Gabriella M. (forthcoming) *Industrializing Taste: Food Processing and the Transformation of the American Diet, 1900–1965*. Baltimore, MD: Johns Hopkins Press.

Pinney, Thomas (2005) *A History of Wine in America: From Prohibition to the Present*. Berkeley: University of California Press.

Pollan, Michael (2006) *The Omnivore's Dilemma: A Natural History of Four Meals*. New York: Penguin.

Poppendick, Janet (2010) *Free for All: Fixing School Food in America*. Berkeley: University of California Press.

——(1999) *Sweet Charity? Emergency Food and the End of Entitlement*. New York: Penguin.

Probyn, Elspeth (2000) *Carnal Appetites: FoodSexIdentities*. London: Routledge.

Ray, Krishnendu (2004) *The Migrant's Table: Meals and Memory in Bengali-American Households*. Philadelphia, PA: Temple University Press.

Root, Waverly and Richard de Rochemont (1976) *Eating in America: A History*. New York: William Morrow and Company.

Rothblum, Esther, Sondra Solovay, and Marilyn Wann, eds. (2009) *The Fat Studies Reader*. New York: New York University Press.

Schlosser, Eric (2001) *Fast Food Nation: The Dark Side of the American Meal*. New York: Houghton Mifflin.

Schwartz, Hillel (1986) *Never Satisfied: A Cultural History of Diets, Fantasies, and Fat*. London: The Free Press.

Shapiro, Laura (1986) *Perfection Salad: Women and Cooking at the Turn of the Century*. New York: Random House.

——(2004) *Something From the Oven: Reinventing Dinner in 1950s America*. New York: Viking.

Strauss, David (2011) *Setting the Table for Julia Child: Gourmet Dining in America, 1934–1961*. Baltimore, MD: Johns Hopkins University Press.

Theophano, Janet (2002) *Eat My Words: Reading Women's Lives Through the Cookbooks They Wrote*. New York: Palgrave McMillan.

Veit, Helen (forthcoming) *Victory Over Ourselves: American Food in the Era of the Great War*. Chapel Hill, NC: University of North Carolina Press.

Watson, James L., ed. (1997) *Golden Arches East: McDonald's in East Asia*. Stanford, CA: Stanford University Press.

Watson, James L. and Melissa L. Caldwell (2005) *The Cultural Politics of Food and Eating*. Malden, MA: Blackwell.

Witt, Doris. (1999) *Black Hunger: Food and the Politics of U.S. Identity*. New York: Oxford University Press,.

Zafar, Rafia. "The Signifying Dish: Autobiography and History in Two Black Women's Cookbooks." *Feminist Studies* 25(2) (Summer 1999): 449–69.

Selected anthologies, books, and articles about American studies

Brantlinger, Patrick (1990) *Crusoe's Footprints: Cultural Studies in Britain and America*. New York: Routledge.

Davis, Allen F. "The Politics of American Studies," *American Quarterly* 41 (September 1989): 353–74.

Deloria, Phil. "Broadway and Main: Crossroads, Ghost Roads, and Paths to an American Studies Future." *American Quarterly* 61(1) (March 2009): 1–25.

Denning, Michael (2004) "The Special American Conditions: Marxism and American Studies." In *Culture in the Age of Three Worlds*. New York: Verso.

Hoffer, Thomas B. and Vincent Welch, Jr. (2010) "Time to Degree of U.S. Research Doctorate Recipients," *InfoBrief; Science Resources Statistics*. National Science Foundation, March 2006: pp. 2–3, quoted in Louis Menand, *The Marketplace of Ideas: Reform and Resistance in the American University*. New York: Norton.

Kaplan, Amy and Donald Pease, eds. (1993) *Cultures of United States Imperialism*. Durham, NC: Duke University Press.

Kerber, Linda. "Diversity and the Transformation of American Studies." *American Quarterly* 41 (September 1989): 415–31.

Lipsitz, George (2001) *American Studies in a Moment of Danger*. Minneapolis, MN: University of Minnesota Press.

Lucid, Robert E., ed. "Programs in American Studies." *American Quarterly* 22 (Summer 1970): 430–605.

Maddox, Lucy, ed. (1999) *Locating American Studies: The Evolution of a Discipline*. Baltimore, MD: Johns Hopkins University Press.

Menard, Louis (2010) *The Marketplace of Ideas: Reform and Resistance in the American University*. New York: Norton.

Orvell, Miles, ed. (2009) *Encyclopedia of American Studies*. Baltimore, MD: Johns Hopkins University Press.

Pease, Donald E. and Robyn Wiegman, eds. (2002) *The Futures of American Studies*. Durham, NC: Duke University Press.

Radway, Janice. "'What's in a Name?' Presidential Address to the American Studies Association." *American Quarterly* 51 (March 1999): 1–32.

Walker, Robert H., ed. (1975) *American Studies Abroad*. Westport, CT: Greenwood Press.

Wise, Gene (1979) "'Paradigm Dramas' in American Studies: A Cultural and Institutional History of the Movement." *American Quarterly* 31(3): 293–337.

20

Folklore

Lucy M. Long

Folklore (folkloristics, folklife studies) has existed as a discipline since the early 1800s. It has expanded immensely from its initial emphasis on documenting and preserving European orally transmitted narrative traditions to exploring the meanings and functions of expressive performances of any group that gives that group a sense of connectedness. Food and foodways (the system of activities and conceptualization surrounding eating) have always been included within its scope, and the discipline has contributed numerous ethnographies of foodways traditions as well as theoretical frameworks for understanding food's connection to ethnic and regional identity, the maintenance of group boundaries, the politics of identity, food as an aesthetic domain, and culinary tourism.

Introduction

Folklore, also known as folkloristics, folklife studies, and folklore studies, is a highly inter-disciplinary field with its own core of theory and methodology. It is related most directly to anthropology and literature, but has strong ties with most arts and humanities disciplines, par-ticularly religious and ritual studies, history, American studies, ethnomusicology, theater, cultural studies, and performance studies. It also has a strong applied component, usually referred to as public folklore. This branch deals with public policy, arts administration, community development, social justice, cultural interpretation, and education.

Folklore has existed as an academic discipline since the early 1800s, rooted in European Romantic nationalism. Its focus originally was on lore, tales existing in oral tradition and usually told among peasantry. It later included "popular antiquities," the leftover "relics" of past cus-toms, ways of living, artistic expressions, and beliefs. The definition of the field and of its subject matter have expanded since then to be the study of unofficial culture, "artistic communication in small groups" (Ben-Amos, 1971), traditional practices and expressions, vernacular forms, and skills, knowledge, and beliefs transmitted through informal oral and imitative (internet included!) media. Food is firmly included within its scope.

Folklore offers perspectives on food that approach it as a powerful site for meaning making, an arena in which individuals and communities express their identities and beliefs as well as construct relationships and boundaries. It explores the potential food has for connecting us to our pasts, place, and other people while also allowing for aesthetic engagement and creative innovation. As such, a folkloristic perspective enables us to examine how food traditions tie us both inwardly to our own experiences and interpretations and outwardly to the larger world of political, environmental, economic, and social concerns.

History of food scholarship in folklore

Scholars date the study of folklore to 1812 when the Grimm brothers published German "household tales" collected primarily from peasant women who worked as nursemaids. This set the stage for other European scholars who researched the oral narratives of their own cultures. Two questions were asked of these tales: (1) where did the tale itself or motifs within the tale originate; and (2) what commonalities amongst cultures did these tales display? These questions represented the growing interest in understanding the nature of culture and the reasons for diversity within humanity as well as political events shaping the concept of nation. Central to this last concern was the identification of unique characteristics of specific cultures. Food and eating were noted as characteristics and motifs.

The Romantic nationalism movement encouraged further collecting of traditional lore. The romantic dimension posited that peasantry had close spiritual ties to the land, so that their ways of living and expressive forms represented the "soul" of that land. Their dances, narratives, and art were thought to be spontaneous expressions uninformed by educated intellectualism or modernization, and their religious and health belief systems were based on superstition. Documenting peasant cultures, therefore, uncovered the unique essence of that land. Traditional forms could then be used to construct a national identity. The concept of nation emerged in Europe in the late 1700s and 1800s as a political entity based on commonalities such as language and culture. Nations were similar to extended families in that citizens shared a heritage, values, and ways of living. The lore of the folk, since it was unique to that place, could be used to construct new customs and arts that would help to define the nation. Food had a role in defining nation, and the French concept of *terroir* may have roots in this movement.

Romantic nationalism took a different slant in England since the English dominated global commerce and boasted numerous colonies. "Popular antiquities" referred to the quaint and colorful customs from the past that could still be seen among the rural, uneducated "folk." In 1846, W. J. Thoms coined the term "folk-lore." Although the emphasis was on lore—oral narratives—it included "ways" of the folk, such as superstitions, beliefs, customs, and practices surrounding aspects of everyday life, including food production, preparation, and consumption.

Folklore research was also popular in the US, but with a significant difference: there were no peasants. Scholars then looked for other groups of people who displayed strong connections to the land or who lived outside the mainstream culture. This included ethnic groups (non-English-speaking ones), Native Americans, religious sects (such as the Amish), and people tied to the land through their occupations (fishermen, lumberjacks). Work by Robert Redfield in Mexico in the 1940s encouraged scholars to see these "little traditions" as part of the larger culture, rather than isolated pockets of culture immune to modernity and outside influence.

Scholars studying folklore in the nineteenth century developed systematic ways of collecting and cataloguing it, attempting to establish it as a science. Scholarly organizations developed throughout Europe, and universities offered courses and degrees in the subject, encouraging further documentation and the development of archives and museums. In the US, the American Folklore Society was established in 1888, with the purpose of recording the "fast-vanishing relics" of those groups untouched by industrialization. Closely aligned with anthropology and literary studies, it did not become its own university program until the 1950s when departments of folklore were established at the University of Pennsylvania, Indiana University, and the University of California at Los Angeles. All three contributed significantly to the study of food.

Today there are numerous departments of folklore throughout the world, and courses in folklore are oftentimes found within other disciplines. Food and foodways are commonly included in those courses.

The earliest folklore scholarship on food emphasized it as an aspect of peasant life, and in Europe it was an integral part of folklife ethnology. In the US the emphasis was on foods that were endangered by modern, industrial foods. John G. Bourke's article in the 1895 *Journal of American Folklore*, "Folk-Foods of the Rio Grande Valley and of Northern Mexico," is typical of the descriptive ethnographic approach most of these studies took.

In the 1960s and 1970s, a paradigm shift in folkloristics changed the way food was studied. The paradigm moved the focus of study from the text or product itself to the context and processes surrounding the performance of that text. The theories of functionalism and structuralism within anthropology had impacted folklore studies, so that the questions being asked now included the role, purpose, and meaning of traditions. Interpretation of folklore data was emphasized, and folklorists drew heavily from sociolinguistics in developing performance theory, an approach that sees meaning as dependent upon context and personal resources for participation. For example, an individual eating turkey on Thanksgiving could mean a wide variety of things—patriotism, pride in New England heritage, celebration of abundance, hunger, curiosity, family togetherness, etc. To understand the meanings it has for that individual, and the motivations behind that eating, we need to understand what choices that individual has as well as his or her personal background and the contexts in which he is eating. Food traditions, then, are shaped by historical and political forces, but also represent personal and aesthetic experiences and social relationships. The everyday or mundane is as significant as the public, iconic, and elite, and communities and the food traditions representing them are dynamic in that individuals are constantly constructing them anew. These understandings of food were then used in the emergence of other strands within folklore to explore ethnicity, feminist theory, region and place, cultural politics, identity construction, and critical theory.

A significant catalyst in this shift was Dr Don Yoder at the University of Pennsylvania who, although not writing about theory per se, established folklife, which included food, as a part of folklore studies. His article "Folk Cookery" in Richard Dorson's 1972 anthology, *Folklore and Folklife: An Introduction*, was seminal in introducing into folklore studies the term foodways, which he defined as the totality of practices and beliefs surrounding eating and food. He also inspired a generation of students, including Jay Anderson (1971), Janet Theophano (1984), Charles Camp (1989), Amy Shuman (1983), Angus Gillespie (1984, 1999), Leslie Prosterman (1995), Mario Montano (1997), Kathy Neustadt (1992), and Lucy Long (1998, 2004) who went on to develop foodway theory. Also in the early 1970s, Michael Owen Jones at the University of California, Los Angeles, Alan Dundes at the University of California, Berkeley, and the folklore programs at Indiana University and the University of Texas, Austin established food as part of its subject matter. Much of this work interpreted food as an expression of identity, as well as a means by which communities both construct their own identities and maintain group boundaries. Publications by Yvonne Lockwood, Susan Kalcik, and others represent these schools.

The late 1970s saw a surge in the folkloristic study of food with the establishment of a journal, *Digest: An Interdisciplinary Review of Food and Foodways*.[1] A number of anthologies followed that are seminal to food studies, as well as to furthering folklore theory: *Foodways and Eating Habits: Directions for Research* (Jones et al., 1983), *Ethnic and Regional Foodways in the United States* (Brown and Mussel, 1984), and "*We Gather Together:" Food and Festival in American Life* (Humphrey and Humphrey 1988). These works established a body of scholarship firmly grounded in ethnographic research that both celebrated the creativity of individual tradition bearers and their communities.

Later scholarship continued to explore the role of folklore in identity construction and cultural production, recognizing that tradition ties us to larger issues of colonialism, commodification of culture, and globalization: the 1998 special issue of *Southern Folklore* on culinary tourism and *Rooted in America: Foodlore of Popular Fruits and Vegetables* (Wilson and Gillespie, 1999). The former introduced the term, defining it as "eating out of curiosity." It was expanded and republished as *Culinary Tourism: Eating and Otherness* (Long, 2004), which emphasized that the meanings of eating and of tourism shift according to the individuals involved. It also expanded on the concept of foodways, an idea further developed by Long (2004) as a theoretical and methodological framework approaching food as product, processes, and performances. Foodways, in this sense, demonstrates the connectedness of all activities surrounding eating and identifies the ways in which it acquires meaningfulness for an individual. An "ethnography of eating" model developed by Long offers a similar approach. In 2009, a special issue of the *Journal of American Folklore* examined food and identity in the Americas, emphasizing the role cultural, economic, social, and political power play in the meanings we attach to foodways traditions.

Meanwhile, folklorists in the 1970s also began developing an applied branch, now referred to as public folklore, that focuses on folklore methods and theories being used in museums, arts agencies, festivals, and educational settings. Food was oftentimes used in such settings as a way of teaching about a specific culture or as a means of creating a sense of community around an activity. The Smithsonian Institution's Folklife Festival featured food traditions along with other expressive forms of cultural groups, and folklorists there developed foodways as a working theory and interpretive framework (Rahn, 2006). This work overlapped with using foodways concepts in folklore and education, emphasizing that eating is a universal and everyday activity so that it provides a commonality we all share. Exploring the wide variety of forms it takes is a way to exploring difference and conflicts arising from that difference. It also suggests that foodways can be fruitfully used for teaching a wide variety of skills and concepts. The Smithsonian Institution also sponsored a traveling exhibit on American food, called Key Ingredients and curated by folklorist Charles Camp, that was shown throughout the country and inspired numerous local foodways documentation projects and programs (Smithsonian Institution Traveling Exhibition Service 2003).

The study of food within folklore studies now ranges from recognition of its aesthetic nature and the ritualistic role it takes in our lives to using it to explore critical issues in health, sustainability, and social justice. Rather than romanticizing food traditions, folklore sees foodways as central to how individuals find and create meaningful lives.

Research methods

As a humanities discipline, folklore uses primarily qualitative and ethnographic research. It draws from anthropological and literary methods, but also has a distinctive approach in its attention to the individual and aesthetic experiences in specific contexts. It focuses on questions of what traditions are practiced within a group, what those practices and forms mean to the individuals participating in them, how artistic creativity is displayed, and how that participation is shaped by historical forces, cultural contexts, current circumstances, and personal choices. Such questions are best answered through ethnographic fieldwork – by observing people and then discussing with them their own motivations, intentions, values, and emotions. Those individuals are then understood within their larger cultural and social contexts. Archival or library research is usually necessary for comparison with other traditions or contexts.

Such research is qualitative in that it produces interpretive and experiential data. It is highly rigorous, though, in the required attention to details, personalities of individuals interviewed, and sensitivity to the nuances of social interactions between the researcher and the subjects. It also requires a full understanding of the contexts within which individuals are participating in their cultural forms. This translates into gaining familiarity with the scholarship on that culture as well as on the specific forms being emphasized. For example, research on Chinese-American restaurants would be grounded in studies of Chinese immigration history, Asian–American ethnicity, the development of restaurants in the US, Chinese as well as American culinary history, and theories shedding light on ethnicity, commercialization of food, food and identity, public vs. private spaces, and so on.

There are two primary approaches used in undertaking folklore ethnography. The first examines a group of people who seem to share a sense of community. The folklorist identifies the commonalities drawing the individual members together, then examines the expressive traditions growing out of those commonalities, assessing how those traditions give a cohesiveness to the group. Since folklorists emphasize the unofficial, informal culture, they oftentimes find groups within larger groups. For example, a town may have numerous restaurant owners who all belong to the chamber of commerce. They could be seen as constituting an official group; however, they probably do not feel a sense of commonality and camaraderie unless they meet informally and develop social relationships and traditions. These in turn enable them to come up with their own ways of dealing with competition for customers and the normal stresses of running restaurants.

Once the group is selected, an overview ethnography is done identifying the oral, material, and customary forms being practiced. Food and food habits would be one aspect of the culture as a whole. This enables the researcher to pinpoint those practices that either emotionally connect the members of the group or are being used intentionally to express identity and interests. It is frequently the informal and unofficial practices of the group that are the most meaningful to its members by allowing them to feel that they have a personal role in that practice and have traditionalized it for their own circumstances. This means that the researcher should not assume which traditions will be the most significant expressions of that community prior to research but should follow the lead of the community itself. For example, in an ethnography of a small Midwestern town, I found that while traditional home cooking was considered important, it was pizza and the rituals surrounding it that many of the residents felt were the most meaningful expression of their community.

Another important aspect of ethnography is selecting individuals to be interviewed. It should be a mixture of people representing the diversity as well as any divisions within the group. Also, a variety of skill and experience levels should be represented. Oftentimes, non-participants can shed insights on the value and functions of a tradition that "experts" in the group might miss because they assume that value. Similarly, groups oftentimes have an unofficial representative (someone who has been involved for a long time or has a special role of authority) as well as an officially designated leader. Scholars should make sure that they talk to both in order to get the public statement on the group as well as the more informal expressions of identity. In this way, the researcher gains a holistic perspective on the group as a dynamic unit shaped by external forces as well as by the vagaries of personalities and social interactions. A restaurant chef, for example, should be placed within several contexts in order to understand the meanings of cooking in a commercial, public space: the cultural attitudes towards food and cooking; the role of commerce in the valuing of activities; the family background and ethnicity, class, and gender of the chef as well as his or her own personal experiences and motivations.

A second approach in folklore ethnography is to focus on a specific genre, traditional form, or practice. Food is easily accessible for research since it is found in public contexts as well as private, and is an integral part of everyday lives of everyone in the community (whether they realize that or not). The ethnography should then be both "deep" and "wide." Deep refers to close attention to the details of the product or text. This involves description and cataloguing of its components and comparison with components of similar products in other contexts, enabling identification of what is unique to that product, what variations are possible, and what those variations might represent. Anthropologist Clifford Geertz termed this concept as "thick description," but it is integral to folklore methodology. It is particularly useful in exploring the creative and personal variations that occur with every "enactment" of a genre, demonstrating the ways in which tradition is a dynamic, "lived" experience. It also helps in identifying recurring motifs or themes that can then characterize that food tradition.

"Wide" in ethnography refers to an overview of the community surrounding the product. It not only describes the broader contexts shaping it, but it explores the processes behind its production. This enables the researcher to see how external forces (economics, politics, class, etc.) are shaping these processes. It also identifies the choices available in each specific performance of the product. A useful framework for an ethnographic overview of food in a specific group would be that of identifying oral, material, and customary forms related to food. The concept of foodways also provides a methodological framework: Product (recipes, ingredients, deals, meals), processes (procurement, preservation, preparation, presentation, consumption, disposal), and performance (conceptualizations, symbolic performances, contexts). This framework can be applied on a variety of levels from an ingredient to a dish to a meal to an individual's food habits to an entire culture.

An important aspect of fieldwork is the development of a mutually respectful relationship of trust between the folklorist and community. The researcher should be clear about their intentions and interests and ask permission before documenting by recording, photographing, or videotaping. Since folklore focuses on understanding the group's perspective and placing that perspective in context in order to understand its logic, this type of research is usually welcomed by a community once it is understood. Some folklorists, similar to anthropologists, speak of "giving voice" to people who otherwise would not be heard or understood. The ethics of ethnography are therefore fundamental to folklore methodology, not only in the way in which fieldwork is conducted, but also in the presentation of findings and the preservation of documentation.

Not all folklore research is ethnographic, however. Primary documents such as diaries, journals, and letters are a specific type of "voice" giving an individual's perception of their life. Cookbooks are read as cultural and communal expressions, not so much of what people actually eat as what they think they should eat and how they can cook their way into certain strata of society. Literature, films, music, and art frequently use food or eating as motifs. These forms are part of the larger cultural context, but they can also be the focus of the study, shed light on resources and concerns. For example, many traditional songs from the southern Appalachian Mountains tell of eating beans, cornbread, and fatback, drinking corn liquor, and hunting groundhogs, rabbits, and squirrels—all significant components of the traditional food culture. Similarly, the current popularity of vampire and zombie movies show varieties of cannibalism, possibly reflecting contemporary fears of losing our humanity and "civilization" in the face of frightening political and ecological times.

Avenues for furthur research

There are endless possibilities for future research on food in folklore studies. The focus on the individual's experience of tradition has relevance to understanding how personal food choices are tied to larger issues, particularly those relating to sustainability.

Understanding the meaningfulness of traditions and how they connect us through food helps in identifying changes that can be made that will be more compatible with sustainability. Individuals can better see how those traditions give them a sense of connection and therefore better select components to change or dismiss.

Similarly, the folklore emphasis on aesthetic experience can be useful in understanding current concerns simplifying our lives, living with "mindfulness," and downsizing our lifestyles. In this way, folklore is compatible with movements such as Slow Food, which emphasize the quality of the eating experience, but it also emphasizes the validity of everyday foodways. This moves society away from the emphasis on high-priced gourmet foods and also makes us aware of all the processes involved in eating a meal.

Folklorists also frequently work in the public sector, shaping public policy concerning the arts and humanities. A heightened awareness of the potential for food's power to evoke memories and emotions and to connect us with larger political issues could be very useful in those areas. Also, deeper understandings of food in museums and educational settings can be used to explore other topics, such as a regional culture, histories, political conflict, and so on. Intellectual property rights, intangible heritage, and cultural sustainability are difficult issues being addressed in the face of globalization. Food can be used to better understand them. Similarly, folklore perspectives on food can be used in community building and economic development, particularly at the local level.

Folklorists tend to be excellent documentaries of all aspects of a food culture and its contexts. Fieldwork collections contain numerous interviews, photographs, artifacts, and ephemera that are relevant to food studies. Some of these can be found in archives and libraries, particularly those that focus on traditional cultures of specific regions. The Library of Congress' Archive of Folk Culture is one such resource with many state and university archives also containing relevant materials. While these collections rarely specify foodways, they frequently include food as one aspect of traditional culture or as an aside in discussions of everyday and celebratory life. Cataloguing of these collections would provide a rich source for further research.

Practical considerations for getting started

Most academic folklore programs include food as an area of study, and students can focus on the subject if they wish to. See the American Folklore Society website for listings of programs. The website also lists public folklore organizations, museums, archives, libraries, and arts and culture centers that are amenable to student internships around food. The non-profit Center for Food and Culture, established in 2010, approaches food from a folkloristic perspective and offers a website (www.foodandculture.org, accessed on April 4, 2012) that serves as a networking clearinghouse for projects concerning food.

The Smithsonian Institution's annual Folklife Festival includes foodways in some form and offers internships and temporary positions. This festival, and others based on it around the country, is an excellent way to get a taste of how folklorists document food traditions and then present them to the public.

The Foodways Section of the American Folklore Society is another resource. Members are involved in a variety of aspects of food study. The Section also offers awards for student papers, sponsors panels and forums at the meetings, and publishes the *Digest*, a publication featuring ethnographic projects on foodways.

Note

1 Several studies in folklore address structural inequalities and imbalances and disjunctures in power structures with regard to food. See among them, Psyche Williams-Forson (2010) "Other Women Cooked for My Husband: Negotiating Gender, Food, and Identities in an African American/Ghanaian Household." *Feminist Studies* 36.2 (Summer): 435–61; and, Williams-Forson (2006) *Building Houses Out*

of *Chicken Legs: Black Women, Food, and Power*. Chapel Hill: UNC Press; LuAnn Roth (2006) "Beyond Communitas: Cinematic Food Events and the Negotiation of Power, Belonging, and Exclusion," *Western Folklore* 64. 3-4: 163–87; Amy Bentley (2002) "Islands of Serenity: Gender, Race, and Ordered Meals During World War II." In *Food in the USA: A Reader*, Carole M. Counihan, ed. New York: Routledge, pp. 171–92; Sidney Mintz (1985) *Sweetness and Power: The Place of Sugar in Modern History*. New York: Penguin Books.

Key reading

Brown, Linda Keller and Kay Mussel, eds. (1984) *Ethnic and Regional Foodways in the United States: The Performance of Group Identity*. Knoxville: The University of Tennessee Press.

Camp, Charles (1989) *American Foodways: What, When, Why and How We Eat in America*. Little Rock, AR: August House.

Georges, Robert A. (1984) "You Often Eat What Others Think You Are: Food as an Index of Others' Conceptions of Who One Is." *Journal of Folklore Research* 43: 249–56.

Gutierrez, C. Paige (1992) *Cajun Foodways*. Jackson: University Press of Mississippi.

Humphrey, Theodore C. and Lin T. Humphrey, eds. (1988) *"We Gather Together": Food and Festival in American Life*. Ann Arbor: University of Michigan Press.

Jones, Michael Owen, Bruce Giuliano, and Roberta Krell, eds. (1983) *Foodways and Eating Habits: Direction for Research*. Los Angeles: California Folklore Society.

Lockwood, Yvonne R. and William G. Lockwood (1991) "Pasties in Michigan's Upper Peninsula: Foodways, Interethnic Relations, and Regionalism." In *Creative Ethnicity: Symbols and Strategies of Contemporary Ethnic Life*, Stephen Stern and John Allan Cicala, eds. Logan: Utah State University Press. pp. 3–20.

Long, Lucy (2009) *Regional American Food Culture*. Nestfield, CT: Greenwood Press.

——(2007) "Greenbean Casserole and Midwestern Identity: A Regional Foodways Aesthetic and Ethos." *Midwestern Folklore* 33(1): 29–44.

——ed. (2004) *Culinary Tourism*. Lexington: University of Kentucky Press.

Montano, Mario (1997) "Appropriation and Counterhegemony in South Texas: Food Slurs, Offal Meats, and Blood." In *Usable Pasts: Traditions and Group Expressions in North America*, ed. Tad Tuleja, pp. 50–67. Logan: Utah State University Press.

Neustadt, Kathy (1992) *Clambake: A History and Celebration of an American Tradition*. Boston: University of Massachusetts Press.

Shuman, Amy (1981) "The Rhetoric of Portions," *Western Folklore* 40: 72–80.

Theophano, Janet (2002) *Eat My Words: Reading Women's Lives through the Cookbooks They Wrote*. New York: Palgrave.

Tye, Diane (2010) *Baking as Biography: A Life Story in Recipes*. Montreal: McGill-Queen's University Press.

Wilson, David S. and Angus K. Gillespie, eds. (1999) *Rooted in America: Foodlore of Popular Fruits and Vegetables*. Knoxville: University of Tennessee Press.

Yoder, Don (1972) Folk Cookery. In *Folklore and Folklife: An Introduction*, ed. Richard M. Dorson, pp. 325–50. Chicago, IL: The University of Chicago Press.

References

Anderson, Jay Allan (1971) "The Study of Contemporary Foodways in American Folklife Research." *Keystone Folklore Quarterly* 16: 155–63.

Camp, Charles (1989) *American Foodways: What, When, Why and How We Eat in America*. Little Rock, AR: August House.

Gillespie, Angus K. (1984) "A Wilderness in the Megalopolis: Foodways in the Pine Barrens of New Jersey." In *Ethnic and Regional Foodways in the United States: The Performance of Group Identity*, Linda Keller Brown and Kay Mussell, eds., pp. 145–68. Knoxville: University of Tennessee Press.

Goode, Judith, Janet Theophoano, and Janet Curtis (1984) "A Framework for the Analysis of Contiuity and Change in Shared Sociocultural Rules for Food Use: The Italian–American Pattern." In *Ethnic and Regional Foodways in the United States: The Performance of Group Identity*, Linda Keller Brown and Kay Mussel, eds., pp. 66–88. Knoxville: University of Tennessee Press.

Long, Lucy (1998) "Culinary Tourism: A Folkloristic Perspective on Eating and Otherness." *Southern Folklore* 55(3): 181–204.

——ed. (2004) *Culinary Tourism*. Lexington: University of Kentucky Press.

Montano, Mario (1997) "Appropriation and Counterhegemony in South Texas: Food Slurs, Offal Meats, and Blood." In *Usable Pasts: Traditions and Group Expressions in North America*, ed. Tad Tuleja, pp. 50–67. Logan: Utah State University Press.

Neustadt, Kathy (1992) *Clambake: A History and Celebration of an American Tradition*. Boston: University of Massachusetts Press.

Prosterman, Leslie (1995) *Ordinary Life, Festival Days: Aesthetics in the Midwestern County Fair*. Washington, DC: Smithsonian Institution Press.

——(1981) "Food and Alliance at the County Fair." *Western Folklore* 10: 81–90.

Shuman, Amy (1981) "The Rhetoric of Portions." *Western Folklore* 40: 72–80.

Wilson, David S. and Angus K. Gillespie, eds. (1999) *Rooted in America: Foodlore of Popular Fruits and Vegetables*. Knoxville: University of Tennessee Press.

Bibliography

Bendix, Regina (1997) *In Search of Authenticity: The Formation of Folklore Studies*. Madison: The University of Wisconsin Press.

Brunvand, Jan Harold (1998) *The Study of American Folklore*. 4. New York: W.W. Norton & Company, Inc.

Georges, Robert A. and Michael Owen Jones (1995) *Folkloristics: An Introduction*. Bloomington and Indianapolis: Indiana University Press.

Hollis, Susan Tower, Linda Pershing and M. Jane Young, (1993) *Feminist Theory and the Study of Folklore*. Urbana and Chicago: University of Illinois Press.

Jackson, Bruce (1987) *Fieldwork*. Urbana and Chicago: University of Illinois Press.

Jordan, Rosan A. and Susan J. Kalcik (1985) *Women's Folklore, Women's Culture*. Vol. 8. Philadelphia: University of Pennsylvania Press.

Oring, Elliott, ed. (1989) *Folk Groups and Folklore Generes*. Logan: Utah State University Press.

——ed. (1986) *Folk Groups and Folklore Generes An Introduction*. Logan: Utah State University Press.

Paredes, Americo and Richard Bauman (2000) *Toward New Perspectives in Folklore*. Bloomington, IN: Trickster Press.

Radner, Joan Newlon, ed. (1993) *Feminist Messages: Coding in Women's Folk Culture*. Urbana and Chicago: University of Illinois Press.

Sims, Martha C. and Martines Stephens (2005) *Living Folklore: an Introduction to the Study of People and Their Traditions*. Logan: Utah State University Press.

Tuleja, Tad, ed. (1997) *Usable Pasts: Traditions and Group Expressions in North America*. Logan: Utah State University Press.

Wilson, William A. (2006) *The Marrow of Human Experience: Essays on Folklore*. Jill Terry Rudy and Diane Call, eds. Logan: Utah State University Press.

21

Food museums

Elizabeth Williams

Until very recently museums did not seem to acknowledge that food was eaten in the historic period. Although natural history museums spend much energy and exhibit space exploring the food of the people of prehistoric times, they tend to concentrate their energies and material culture collection on art, government, war, and religion in the time where a written record is available. The food museum, whether completely standalone, or partially incorporated into other museums, is a fairly modern attempt to remember and explore the fact that people continue to eat. This essay explores the importance of and reasons for the existence of food museums today.

Historical background of food museums and how they have developed

Some people imagine that a food museum will contain faux food on a plate, like assorted dishes of possible selections in the storefronts of restaurants. Others expect to see wax or plastic effigies of asparagus and cauliflower or the like, and perhaps real vegetables and fruit in refrigerated cases. The more nostalgic people anticipate old signs, old jars and cans, and vintage tools on display. Perhaps they imagine photographs of older agricultural methods or postcards of uncanny tomatoes. A food museum might contain all of those things. But it is not a warehouse or a kitschy collection of cute paraphernalia. Given the broadest interpretation, food museums can be found in many forms and food has its place in many types of museums.

Before there was a specialized museum of food and drink, there was the natural history museum. The exhibits in these museums reflected the way that archeologists studied and researched prehistoric animals and peoples. A primary way to conduct this research was through food, since so much of the lives of early people was spent finding food, eating food, and preserving food. Thus, the natural history museum would contain exhibits that explored the food eaten by animals and people; the tools used to hunt, gather, fish, and store food; and the trash these activities left behind. Implements, vessels and their decoration and special ways that food was eaten and preserved all were studied by archeologists based on the evidence unearthed. Thus, vessels were studied and exhibited in these museums along with baskets and fish hooks.

Some of this organic material blends unidentifiably back into the environment. Sometimes this blending has meant that the more biodegradeable materials were lost, unable to be exhibited or unable to yield clues to prehistoric foodways. Hardier implements of earthenware, stone, and bone or even of leather, reed, or cloth yielded the most clues and made for the best display.

Vessels, baskets, and netting have changed so little since prehistoric times that they form a palpable link between the modern day and the past. Being able to see the artifacts – one of the contributions of museums – makes that link more real than merely making the statement does.

With more modern scientific technology, we find additional clues today in archeological sites. Evidence of bones in middens, vessels full of vegetable matter, can be analyzed bio-chemically, and even residue of seeds and early fermentation can be DNA tested, thus adding additional clues to the general body of knowledge. A natural history museum explaining the interplay between humans and other animals relates to the museum visitor how the geography and other environmental elements such as climate, available fauna and flora, size of population, technology, religion, social structure, and culture affect food and foodways.

The study of foodways shines a light on the development of agriculture and trade. Unlike the study of mining or other industry, food and eating are a universal constant in all climates and geographies. Starting from that given, the pattern of life in a particular location can be studied. Differences in climate, availability of certain types of flora and fauna, and geographic conditions might change the telling of the story, but the underlying story – the need to find and eat food – remains a constant. Natural history museums also usually strip away the present and explain the material available at different periods, making the layering of different foods and their devel-opment more evident, and creating a visual chronological record. The Agropolis Museum in Montpelier, France, is a modern day museum that uses the methods of the natural history museum to explain food and agriculture in a world context.

But when natural history museums begin to present the shift to agriculture paving the way to the growth of complex societies and a growth in population, they mirror the archeologists' shift in their studies to the larger body of cultural indicators, such as art, religion, and the social structure of governance. Food is no longer the center of their study. The culture of agricultural practices, its social hierarchy and governance, the serving of food, the preparation of food, and the meaning of food in an agricultural economy becomes secondary to the study of wars, governors, economy, and art. Thus food loses its central place in museums. Only when food is tangentially involved in economic or historical study – as in the explanation of a potlatch – does food re-enter the discussion or the exhibit. This loss of realization of how food continues to drive human culture is unfortunate. It means that the thread of continuity from past food-based explorations to the present is lost. In *Hungry City*, Carolyn Steel explains the development of the city of London through the need to feed the city. Natural history museums could have done the same thing: Presenting the visual imagery that could make the story come alive.

Another type of museum that focuses on food, the agricultural museum, takes a look at the crops of a region, the many aspects of the rural ways of life, agricultural techniques, and foodways. Often using tools and techniques of the past, the agricultural museum makes agriculture come alive through a combination of living exhibits – such as actual heirloom crops, real harvesting, and processing of foods – and more inanimate exhibits of implements, cookware, and explanatory materials.

Agricultural museums so often are not complete in that they deal with the land. They pointedly do not include fishing and hunting and gathering. So the agricultural museum's embrace of food is not complete. And of course, agriculture encompasses things beyond food, such as cotton or corn for ethanol, so agricultural museums include food, but are not exclusively about food. As the developed world has become more disconnected from food and its preparation with the continued growth of cities, the growth of commercial agriculture, and the use of manufactured foods, there has been a rise in agricultural museums. The Association for Living History, Farm and Agricultural Museums was founded in 1970. The need for an association to support these museums in 1970 indicates the maturity of the agricultural museum movement by that time.

Museums that focus on local histories, which might include fishing, aquaculture, or other food-producing techniques, and also food processing, like canning or freezing, and wine making, may be found around the world. They often showcase the local food-related industry for its economic value. But they are nonetheless instructive as indicators of food culture, as well as the economic importance of food in those particular communities.

Historic house museums have traditionally emphasized architecture and decoration in their explication of the historic structure. In early renovations, kitchens were often sacrificed and turned into storage space or offices, as the kitchen was not considered important to the story. Instead of talking about life in the house, docents would explain about the design of the house, the types of furniture, the artists whose works appeared on the walls, the genealogy of the primary owners of the house. Occasionally dining room tables were set with china and silver, but often this was to illustrate the beauty of the china and silver, as well as the wealth of the family, rather than the culture of eating.

The hearth, the servants, and the general operations of a house were considered uninteresting. Only recently have kitchens and the people who staffed them been connected to the beautiful table settings displayed in the dining room. The trend today allows the daily life that took place in the historic homes to be seen through the rhythm of the kitchen. Some homes have gone so far as to perform archeological digs to explore bones and other household waste in order to speculate more accurately about the life in the house.

Through expanded cultural interpretations there are programs both demonstrating or allowing participation in open hearth cooking or other techniques performed in these houses. In larger houses with separate pastry kitchens, the work of providing elaborate meals can be demonstrated by the equipment and the spaces where the work took place.

Kitchen buildings, the outdoor work spaces, wells, storage cellars, smoke houses, and even ice houses all contribute to an understanding of daily life in historic homes as well as to the layout of the entire sites. And the aesthetic beauty of silver and china can be augmented by an understanding of its use.

The opening of the kitchen as an area of interpretation in historic homes also expanded the appeal of the historic home to people beyond those with an interest in architecture. While appealing to a wider embrace of interests the house itself can expose the visitors to the cultural context of the house and its architecture, expanding the understanding of its aesthetics and also its place in time and culture. And since we all eat, this connection to food and the life and culture of the historic house is made open to the classes of people who may have served, worked in or supported the house. Laura Plantation in Vacherie, Louisiana, an early sugar plantation, emphasizes the crop grown at the historic site as well as the daily lives of all the inhabitants at all social levels.

In France, where the restaurant was invented, and iconic chefs are credited with the artistry equivalent to the other traditional fine arts – music, visual arts, theatre, literature, etc. – the homes of chefs were turned into shrines honoring them – a twist on the idea of a house museum. The childhood home of August Escoffier in Villeneuve, for example, displays the place that influenced him as well as notes, recipes, and menus that he developed. Europe has included cultural aspects of food production, including the kitchen, in history museums where there are important foods manufactured in the region. Sometimes these are exhibits, if not museums, devoted to a single food, like a particular cheese, or mustard, in those towns where these foods play an important role.

Today there has been a re-emergence of interest in food and foodways. In spite of the abundance of food in the Western world or because of it, there have developed philosophical debates about good food, sustainable food and other questions. With that popularity has developed an interest in the artifacts and art of food in museums that are not directly involved with food. For example, modern design and art museums have exhibited design for the kitchen and table, exploring the intersection of culture, design, and function. Art museums, which have historically viewed ethnic objects – which often are food related – as objects of art and decoration, are beginning to expand the idea of esthetics to embrace other practical items. Thus baskets, vessels, and other common objects can be seen and displayed as both art and utilitarian items simultaneously. When its purpose is known, a decorated pottery vessel can be described as a cooking pot or an olive oil storing jar and not just a generic vessel. Today, acknowledging its usefulness does not denigrate its artistic value.

Determining mission and scope of the museum

A food museum, like any museum, is not only defined by space. It can exist within a corporate building, telling the story of the company and its products. It can exist only virtually, and sometimes it may have programs and exhibits in a temporary space. It can exist as a gallery within another museum. Or a food museum can be a traditional museum that is a nonprofit or governmental organization with collections, archives, and libraries. A food museum can exist by appointment in a room in someone's home or garage, showcasing a collection of whatever has struck the fancy of the collector.

Fascination with objects and ephemera associated with certain iconic foods is a phenomenon that has been exploited by marketers who have created museums and collections. Corporate museums, which have superior access to documents and artifacts about themselves are, of course, excellent marketing tools. But beyond that these museums tell a story about a product that is both historical and preservative. These museums are designed to be instruments of promotion and to maintain and nurture the corporate or product mythology, but when well done, can also place the products and the company in historical perspective and tell a broad and interesting story.

There is enormous historical value to these museums, which – because of their unique access to material – create a historical bridge that illuminates the time and context of the company's foundation and spotlights what other products and environments contributed to the development of the product. Foodways using the product are also memorialized. And often monetary constraints that might limit other museums are not present at a corporate museum. Many are quite modern and use interactive techniques to engage the visitor in an entertaining way. For many it is the entertainment and samples that are the very reason to visit. The World of Coca-Cola, located in Atlanta, Georgia, tells the story of the development of Coca-Cola with the opportunity to see an early fountain and watch the brand populate the world. The Museum on Chocolate Avenue in Hershey, Pennsylvania, escorts the visitor through the vision of Milton Hershey and the founding of the company, the town and the vision, as well as telling the story of American chocolate.

Single food museums that are generic as opposed to corporate have also developed. These can be supported by government or by individuals. The local boosterism museum can be part of a promotion of a state or local product, thus having a marketing purpose similar to that of a corporate museum. An example of this type of food museum is the Idaho Potato Museum in Blackfoot, Idaho. This museum not only tells about the early potato and its New World origins, but explicates as well the history of the potato industry and its modern incarnation, including production and manufacturing.

Non-corporate or governmental museums, which are museums focused on a single food or product, may often have grown from personal collections stemming from personal interests and curiosity. These museums may be available only by appointment or have regular, but limited, hours of operation. They may be co-located with other businesses such as shops or a home. But they form an important function of preserving artifacts, educating the public and creating interest in the subject. The charming and informative Absinthe Museum in New Orleans, Louisiana, now closed, was located in two rooms of a shop that sold items imported from France. (The Absinthe Museum was reincarnated as La Galerie d'Absinthe inside of the Southern Food and Beverage Museum.) Some private collections are so extensive, the display so professional, and the associated ephemera so complete that the transition to museum is the only difference between private and public.

The Longone Culinary Archive at the University of Michigan at Ann Arbor is an example of a culinary theme that is woven through an existing archive, giving another aspect to the collection that had been hidden before. In addition to giving her collection of historic American cookbooks and ephemera to the university's archive, Janice Longone and a group of culinary historians have combed the archive noting culinary references on cartouches of maps, as well as in diaries and journals, and in general finding culinary materials and references in the non-culinary recesses of the archive, thus expanding the usefulness of and an exponential increase in the ease of searching the existing materials and creating a culinary museum within the larger context of the archive. This remarkable feat was accomplished without additional materials (except for the Longone collection).

Another interesting development is the web museum. These virtual museums take advantage of the limitless space that the web offers. They can be a combination of text and multimedia offerings. They are open 24 hours per day. The virtual museum allows the visitor to create a personal experience at the site without the limitations in space and reality. The depth of material can be greater than can be presented in an actual physical space. The drawback is that actual objects cannot be seen, only a photograph of an object. Interestingly the World Carrot Museum has designed a floor plan of the virtual museum with exhibits in the various galleries of the virtual building. The New York Food Museum supplements its online offerings with actual programming in the form of a pickle festival.

Our fascination with food and eating also has created a desire to learn how food is prepared, since this may no longer be learned at home. This fascination has led to the rise in television and web-based food programs and blogs. Food is lovingly documented by photo and in essays by people who care about the food that they eat, people who feel strongly that food is important. These people are not only documenting what they eat, exploring new foods like anthropologists, but are also collecting the accoutrements associated with the food. They have special tools, they have artfully designed eating implements, and they appreciate talent. These web tools and explorations go hand in hand with the virtual food museum.

All of this begs the question of how to define a museum that actually exists to document and exhibit food and foodways in all of its aspects. In an ideal state such a museum has exhibits that tell the story of food – its history, its processing, its way to the table, celebrations and other social components, and deal with the ephemeral nature of food through some means. These are places that may have different missions, but in some way mount exhibits. Their scope could be limited by geography or by type of food, but within that defined context, the museum can be as broad as the reach of the food itself. The museum at Johnson and Wales in Providence, Rhode Island, covers much of the world geographically through its displays of various places to eat from the classic diner to a historic room in an English pub. Its mission is to support the Culinary School at Johnson and Wales.

Only beautiful and curious objects were collected for cabinets of curiosities by travelers and by those who collected for geographical and anthropological societies. Thus an interesting and unusual basket or a beautiful pottery vessel might be rescued and displayed. A crude bone scraper might not be. Archeological digs that revealed cooking vessels and tools were important in preserving these artifacts, often when there were few other tangible objects left of the society. Today both the professional collector – the historian and archeologist – and the amateur understand the importance of the artifacts, both beautiful and merely utilitarian, in telling the complete story.

Agricultural museums; historic house museums with kitchens and dining rooms; libraries and archives with menu and cookbook collections; museums with special collections that are related to the table; open air museums like rural life campuses; single food museums; single collection museums; virtual museums; all reflect some aspect of the food museum. A place that collects artifacts and archival materials, in the broadest sense, about food and drink for preservation and displays this material in a way that interprets the story for the public is a food museum.

Practical considerations for getting started – funding, programs, archival sources, tools, artifacts, internet and technology resources

In order to create a food museum the most important factor is the evaluation of resources. This means resources of all kinds: funding, artifacts, and capable people. Whether the museum to be created is completely virtual or located within a wonderful facility, funding will be the first consideration. Funding will be necessary to support the person who is organizing the museum. Even when that initial person is a volunteer, there will still be expenses that must be covered. And once the planning process is implemented, the need for funding increases. Money is fundamental to support personnel, maintain artifacts, create exhibits, and to pay for space.

Sources of funding for a food museum include private donations of time and money. In the beginning these may be the only funding sources available. A great deal can be accomplished with a little money and many in-kind donations of services and goods. People will often be willing to get together to paint, build, or clean just on the basis of participating in a compelling idea. As the idea begins to materialize and the leap of imagination necessary to understand the concept becomes smaller, the easier it becomes to explain the idea and obtain small donations. It is also the case that donations of artifacts become more common when the public can see exhibits. The public becomes more trusting of the care that will be taken with the artifact when it sees the respect with which artifacts are treated in an exhibit. And the exhibits trigger memories of long-forgotten items in attics and garages that can find a new home at the museum.

Grant funding, start-up funding, and corporate sponsorship are other common sources of funding. Grants may be made by foundations or by a government entity. There are several aspects of food museums and start-ups that make grant funding problematic. One is that a museum must usually be two years old before grantors are willing to make grants to the institution. The second issue is that most mission statements of grantors cannot identify a way to classify a food museum. Is it more like a natural history museum, or does it qualify as one of the arts? Many agencies can interpret their rules and mission to allow a food museum to qualify as a folk art, but since food museums generally include aspects of the humanities and the arts, finding a neat solution to compartmentalization is often difficult.

Creating a museum with food at its core presents particular problems, because of the ephemeral nature of food and because food involves all of the senses. Creating exhibits that convey historical and mechanical information calls on the techniques that are generally applicable to history and natural history museums. But to explain in an experiential manner the way a flavor experience has influenced the development of food and foodways requires the serving of food and the demonstration of its preparation. Both of these events require the museum to set its priorities, but also to deal with the perishable and ephemeral nature of fresh food.

In order to have continuous demonstration a museum must deal with equipment and storage, as well as personnel. The practicalities of having a person demonstrate during all of the hours of operation are very expensive. Not only are there personnel costs, but also the cost of the food. Making the theme of the demonstration also reflect current exhibits creates the added issue of constantly changing the demonstration and retraining. The solution is often to limit the demonstrations to specified and advertised times, which may cause some visitors to miss the demonstrations, but it is a practical solution. But any regular demonstrations require a place to demonstrate and the appropriate equipment, a place to store food, and a place to clean up. If samples are provided, then the food must be prepared in the appropriate manner according to local health codes. It is not necessary that the samples be the same food that is demonstrated. A food museum must decide whether demonstrations and tastings are a regular part of the exhibitions of the museum or whether they constitute special programming. The choice will affect the cost of admission and the cost of running the museum.

Guest demonstrations by chefs, anthropologists, and home cooks as a part of special programming can also enhance the visitor's experience. The Southern Food and Beverage Museum in New Orleans has chosen to have regular weekly programming that includes demonstrations instead of daily demonstrations. This decision was based on cost factors and its early experience with the objections of casual museum goers to paying for the actual cost of daily demonstrations.

Food safety issues also affect the ability of visitors to handle food to learn about how it feels, smells, and looks. Food attracts insects and vermin that are not only a hazard in themselves, but which might also threaten other artifacts. If a technique requires the use of a tool, having the tool handled and available may threaten the safety of the visitor, if the tool is used incorrectly. The artifact – when used in a demonstration – itself might be threatened, if it is mishandled by the visitor, even if the mishandling is unintentional.

Another policy question that faces the food museum is the use of and the condition of its artifacts. Objects change with use, as do buildings. The questions that face those in historic preservation also face the restorer and the preserver. Does the museum only want "museum-quality" pieces that look unused, or does it want those pieces that obviously have been used and have a story to tell? Even if worn and broken artifacts do not have to function in the museum, should they be repaired and to what degree should repair be part of the story? Take a basket, for example. The top of the basket may be worn and frayed from use. If the basket is to be displayed in an exhibit, should it be repaired? Should the repairs be made obvious? Should it be displayed as is to indicate the typical wear that the basket would receive with use, perhaps beside a photo or drawing of a basket that is intact? Each of these options can be defended. Each affects the visitor's experience, thus knowing how the museum wishes to shape the visitor's experience is an important element of the philosophy and mission of the museum.

Besides the philosophical question raised by the issue of appropriate repairs and display, there is the more practical question to be decided. Can the artifact, especially one that is old, rare or fragile, be used as a part of a demonstration? Is it ever appropriate to use artifacts in demonstrations or must replica items be created for demonstration? Do questions of rarity, fragility or age affect the issue? Do we continue to use the artifact and let it further deteriorate and let its story change and evolve with use? The museum needs to create a policy to address this question. These are just some of the questions affecting food museums, but general questions that apply to any museum also apply to the food museum and must be addressed as well – for example, location and size of the museum.

What a museum provides for visitors and others and the future

As societies became more complex, the nature of what was being eaten was not recorded by the scribes of the day. Eating and food were relegated to the area of other personal needs such as sleeping and bathroom functions. It was ordinary and unremarkable, so there was no need to be so vulgar as to discuss it or record it. Although house accounts of the wealthy might be preserved and lend insight into the day-to-day life of a group, the day-to-day life of the poorest folk – who were probably illiterate – goes undocumented. Even in diaries where meals might be recorded, it is only the special meals that are remarked on. Because food was so ordinary and basic, the tools used to prepare it were not preserved, probably partly because they were worn and well used, but also because they were not deemed important enough to save. This lack of interest in the documentation of food and its preparation, especially the area of home cooking and eating, means that early tools and implements are often not available for current study. With the increased interest in food and eating that is seen today – in such things as the rise of the Food Network and the explosion of food blogs – the presentation of both the everyday and the special aspects of modern eating and their historical perspectives creates an opportunity for food museums to reach and teach its visitors.

Framing, in museum parlance, refers to the way a museum presents its material to the public. While it does refer to the traditional frame around a work of art, it also more generally refers to how something is introduced and laid out for the public. Immanuel Kant, in his explication of the beautiful, defines the role of the frame as the limits of the work within, but not part of the art, however decorative it may be. The frame is the subliminal indicator of the end of the art. Jacques Derrida considers it more than that. In his 1987 essay, "Parergon," Derrida defines *parerga* as a by-product of the underlying work that has its own tangential meaning.

Post-modern museums acknowledge that they are manipulating the viewer's perspective. No matter how straightforward a presentation may be, it still reflects a point of view. Adding sound evokes mood and is a framing device. The food museum also adds taste, smells, texture, and drink, including alcoholic drinks, to create a framing that evokes all of the senses. In determining size, the types of cabinetry in which to display and present, through the choice of artifacts, through wall text and through color, the museum is interpreting its story. It is creating myth and message. Even deciding what artifacts to leave exposed without benefit of glass or stanchions makes a statement. The statement may be, "This is accessible." But it might just as easily be, "This isn't important enough to protect."

Whether in the real or virtual world, the food museum preserves and interprets the material culture of all of the aspects of food and drink. Implements, vessels, and their decoration and special ways that food was eaten and preserved all were studied by archeologists based on the evidence unearthed. The museum takes those artifacts and interprets them for the public. But the food museum also collects and interprets more recent history, reminding older visitors of their own past experiences and introducing younger visitors to those experiences, thus forming a bridge to the future.

Material culture can be made up of large machinery and huge buildings or it can be made of the ephemera that are discarded every day. By deciding what to collect, how to interpret it, and how and when to present it, the food museum preserves and interprets the past. This preservation is of both the distant past and the emerging past. And the mythos and facts merge through the telling of the story and the decisions and the vageries of the collection.

Authenticity in food is very hotly debated currently. Determining what is authentic may not be possible. Authenticity in the museum is equally as unobtainable, but it is something that must be acknowledged. The exhibit cannot be authentic, because it is an exhibit and not the real thing. But even given those limitations, the interpretation of the authentic, the attempt to capture it, and the attempt to reproduce it will change the experience and the exhibit given even the most sincere, knowledgeable, and native curator. The museum cannot give up its attempt to at least reflect the authentic, but must also be aware that displaying instead of living the moment renders the moment inauthentic.

The future of the food museum is a mixture of technology that is developing in all museums that will allow the story to be told in a more interactive manner. This technology recognizes that the food museum is after all a museum. But equally important is that food and food culture is being recognized as important in all museums in a way that has not been recognized since the early exhibits in natural history museums. This phenomenon is making all museums potential sources of information for those in food studies.

As the examination of food and foodways grows there will also be more food museums in the future. And with the growth of new museums with new attitudes toward interpretation and different artifacts and points of view, the preservation and documentation of foodways will be ever greater, creating new avenues of study and more varied experiences for museum visitors.

Food is tangible and ephemeral at the same time. Objects in a museum are not ephemeral. It is the special role of the food museum to evoke the ephemeral nature of food, while remaining tangible. This means using the tangible artifact to evoke identity, meaning, history, and memory. It means using the tangible artifact to evoke all of the senses that form our taste sensation – touch, sight, smell, taste, and hearing. The future of the food museum will be to perform this evocation with increasing success and imagination.

Key reading

Diamond, Jared (2005) *Guns, Germs and Steel: The Fates of Human Societies*. New York: W.W. Norton and Company.

Derrida, Jacques (1987) "The Parergon" published in *The Truth in Painting*. Chicago: University of Chicago Press.

Dudley, Sandra (2009) *Museum Materialities: Objects, Engagements, Interpretations*. London: Routledge.

Genoways, Hugh and Andrei, Mary Anne (2008) *Museum Origins: Readings in Early Museum History and Philosophy*. Walnut Creek,CA: Left Coast Press.

Kant, Immanuel (1978) *The Critique of Judgement*, translated by James Creed Meredith. Oxford: Oxford University Press.

Kirshenblatt-Gimblett, Barbara (1998) *Destination Culture: Tourism, Museums, and Heritage*. Berkley: University of California Press.

Lavine, Steven D. (1991) *Exhibiting Cultures: The Poetics and Politics of Museum Display*. Washington, DC: Smithsonian Books.

Macdonald, Sharon (2002) *Behind the Scenes at the Science Museum*. Oxford: Berg Publishers.

Steel, Carolyn (2008) *Hungry City: How Food Shapes Our Lives*. New York: Chatto & Windus.

Online resources

www.museum.agropolis.fr
www.hersheystory.org
www.clements.umich.edu/longone-archive.php
www.foodmuseum.com
www.foodhistorynews.com/directory.html
www.nyfoodmuseum.org

22

Food and law

Baylen J. Linnekin and Emily Broad Leib

This chapter discusses the field of food law, including both describing existing areas of law pertinent to food law and identifying burgeoning subjects for research within the field. Topics include the history of food safety law in the United States; the regulation of food conducted by the Food and Drug Administration, United States Department of Agriculture, and other federal agencies; increasing food regulation at the state and local level; food and the environment; old and new conceptions of public health, including the growing focus on obesity and diet-related disease; food access, food insecurity and food deserts; and alternative food systems such as local, organic, and sustainable foods.

Introduction

The impact of law on the broad range of food we grow, raise, buy, sell, cook, and eat is an increasingly important and prevalent academic topic. Legal scholars who focus on food seek to define and clarify the rules that apply—or that should apply—to society's increasingly complex relationship with food. Scholarly debates over legal responses to pressing issues like obesity, food safety, genetically modified organisms (GMOs), local foods, food vendors, and access to food are both vibrant and vital to deciding future outcomes in these areas.

While these debates are ongoing, laws governing food have existed at least since the dawn of recorded history. Jewish, Christian, and Muslim traditions each dictate certain rules that apply to food. The Bible claims that shortly after God created Adam and Eve, the first humans, he forbade them from eating the apple. The sacred texts of Muslims and Jews forbid adherents from consuming pork, among other foods. Hence, ancient biblical and religious scholars are likely also some of the earliest scholars of the various laws that apply to food.

Laws pertaining to food have existed in what is now the United States since colonial times. British mercantilist laws impacted colonial trade in a wealth of food and drink, including molasses and its derivative, rum. The colonies themselves regulated trade in food between one another, most often in the form of inspections (Hutt 1984). The colonies also had in place various laws regulating the sale of food and (especially) drink in taverns.

In spite of a history stretching back thousands of years—hundreds in this country—the development of a scholarly approach dedicated specifically to food and law ("food law") is a relatively new phenomenon. The field of food law owes its birth to an American food system and regulatory structure that have become increasingly interstate and modernized over the last 100 years.

Early food law scholarship focused on nationwide problems like the need to limit the presence of pathogens and filth in the areas of food processing and production, and the challenge of ensuring honesty in food labeling (Litman and Litman, 1981). Recent food law scholarship at the national level has also dealt with an enormous array of issues, including obesity (Gostin *et al.*, 2009), the environmental impact of agricultural production (Ruhl, 2000), and conservation of fisheries (Carr and Scheiber, 2002). While these national (and even international) issues are still lively sources of scholarship, a significant portion of recent academic food law research focuses on more local food issues, including debates over the right to raise one's own livestock in an urban environment (Wood *et al.*, 2010) or the scope and impact of state and local regulations pertaining to farmers' markets (Coit, 2008).

Historical background of food justice scholarship and major theoretical approaches in use

Food law scholarship traces its roots to a variety of legal traditions. These include food and drug law, agricultural law, administrative law, constitutional law, environmental law, animal law, and health law. The study of food-related policies—the principles that undergird laws—also plays a key role in food law scholarship. Academic food law research represents a growing body of work that both informs and responds to developments in the laws and regulations that apply to food.

Prior to the turn of the twentieth century, the study of food and law was disjointed and was focused largely on the study of patchwork state and local regulations and on the absence of a system of federal oversight (Pratt, 1880). The field of food law did not yet exist. While courts heard and decided legal disputes in which food was a central issue (The Samuel, 1816), little evidence suggests discussion of these cases made its way to the classroom in the form of food law courses, or into academic food law journals dedicated to their discussion. While food law scholars and others today may, with the value of hindsight, look back at the nation's early history as an important period in the development of food law scholarship—whether in viewing the American Revolution as a rebellion spurred in large part by increasingly onerous British food laws, or by exploring particular case law and other legal history as presenting rich examples worthy of debate from a food law perspective—food law as we know it is in fact a modern conception.

Food and drug law

The field of food and drug law traces its roots to the Pure Food and Drugs Act of 1906 and its successor, the Federal Food, Drug, and Cosmetic Act of 1938 (FDCA), which respectively led to the establishment and strengthening of the federal government's Food and Drug Administration (FDA). Harvey W. Wiley, a chemist and former academic who had advocated since the 1880s in favor of stronger food regulations, spearheaded passage of the 1906 Act (FDA Consumer, 2006). The purpose of the act "was to prevent injury to the public health by the sale and transportation in interstate commerce of misbranded and adulterated foods" (United States v. Lexington Mill & Elevator Co., 1914). It put into place a system of federal inspection and oversight in the overlapping areas of food safety, public health, and the prevention of fraud vis-à-vis food.

After passage of the 1906 Act, a body of scholarship—often grounded in case law—arose in these areas (McDermott v. Wisconsin, 1913). Some early food and drug law scholars were strong critics of what they saw as the act's shortcomings—including ironically, Wiley, the so-called "Father of the Pure Food and Drugs Act" (Wiley, 1929). Some of the chief areas of concern included expansion of the FDA's mission beyond that originally intended (Wiley, 1929), the lack of FDA inspectors available to enforce the existing law (Herring, 1934–35), and unsafe food additives (Schlink, 1935). Together, this criticism helped spur passage of the FDCA.

An overwhelming amount of food and drug law scholarship since passage of the act has analyzed existing FDCA provisions and resultant FDA regulations or suggested improvements to the FDCA or to FDA regulations. For example, beginning in the 1950s, postwar food law scholarship began to embrace what some consider to be a more scientific regulatory approach (Hutt, 1985). This fact, along with rising concerns about increased rates of cancer (Fortin, 2009), helped usher in the so-called Delaney Clause, an amendment to the FDCA, in 1958. The Clause, one of several important changes to the FDCA that year, banished from the food supply substances shown to cause cancer in laboratory animals or humans (Fortin, 2009). By the following year, though, commentators were already sharpening their knives on the Delaney Clause (Oser, 1959).

Agricultural law

Another major approach to the study of food law is agricultural law, which examines the system of laws and policies that apply to farms and farming. The field of agricultural law rose in scope and significance alongside food and drug law as the result of passage of the Meat Inspection Act of 1906, which solidified the role of the US Department of Agriculture (USDA) in monitoring the nation's agricultural production, processing, and sales. The act, signed into law the same day as the Pure Food and Drugs Act, was largely the result of public pressure arising from the publication of *The Jungle* (Sinclair, 1906), a novel that depicted horrific food-safety conditions in and around the Chicago stockyards and slaughterhouses—the gateway through which the majority of the nation's animals were slaughtered and packed for food.

The field of agricultural law broadly includes everything from the contents of the federal "Farm Bill," a quinquennial law that supports and subsidizes a variety of agricultural activities, to regulations concerning USDA grading of meat, poultry, pork, dairy, eggs, and produce. Recent examples of agricultural law scholarship demonstrate the breadth of the field, including journal articles on factory farming and food safety (Follmer and Termini, 2009), farm subsidies and the Farm Bill (Windham, 2007–8), USDA organic certification (Traher, 2010), the negative impact of the USDA's commodity crop system on the nation's school lunch program (Dillard, 2008), and crafting policies that encourage sustainable agriculture (Schneider, 2009).

Administrative law

Administrative law, the body of law that governs the activities of executive agencies like the FDA and USDA, plays an important role in food law scholarship. Numerous federal agencies aside from the FDA and USDA regulate the food system, including the Environmental Protection Agency (EPA) and Federal Trade Commission (FTC). These agencies, like the FDA and USDA, are subject to the Administrative Procedure Act (APA), which catalogs the manner in which agencies may make, carry out, and enforce regulations. Administrative law scholars analyze the rulemaking process (the manner in which an agency crafts regulations), the interpretation and implementation of rules, the process of adjudication (in cases where an agency or a party regulated by the agency is alleged to have violated a particular regulation), and other facets of the administrative law. Scholars have analyzed agency authority to regulate the food system in areas as disparate as FTC regulation of food marketing to children (Pomeranz, 2010; Redish, 2011), EPA regulation of non-point source water pollution (Adler, 1999), and disputes between administrative agencies over beer-labeling jurisdiction (Cooper, 1979).

Constitutional law

Constitutional law governs the distribution and exercise of federal, state, and local government power and the protection of individual rights. Constitutional law plays a key role in the area of food law because it provides, for example, a context through which scholars may analyze whether food laws promulgated by the federal government are authorized by one of the enumerated powers of the federal government (Epstein, 1987). Laws passed by Congress and regulations implemented by federal agencies generally rely on the Commerce Clause, which authorizes the federal government "to regulate Commerce with foreign Nations, and among the several States" (US Constitution, Art. 1, Sec. 8). The Supremacy Clause, meanwhile, bars states from acting in areas expressly reserved to or occupied by the federal government. Taken together, the Commerce Clause and the Supremacy Clause (US Constitution, Art. 6) imply a "Dormant Commerce Cause," which courts have held prohibits states from passing regulations that either discriminate against or place an "undue burden" on out-of-state businesses (Tribe, 2000). This has led some scholars to question the legality of state laws that favor in-state or local food products (Denning *et al.*, 2010; Harrington, 2007).

Many other constitutional law principles impact food law. Debate over the scope of the First Amendment's protection of "freedom of speech" often arises in the context of commercial food marketing and labeling (Kamp *et al.*, 1999; Shaffer *et al.*, 2006; McNamara, 1982; Pomeranz, 2010). For example, the Supreme Court has held that beer manufacturers have the right to display truthful alcohol content on bottles and cans (Rubin v. Coors Brewing Co., 1995). The First Amendment's Free Exercise Clause has also been raised in the context of the food to be provided to prisoners with religious dietary constraints (Nelson, 2009). The right to hunt plays a key role in the ongoing discussion over the Second Amendment (Halbrook, 2010–11). The Twenty-First Amendment, which repealed alcohol prohibition in 1933, is also a frequent subject of scholarship (Woodard, 2004–5; Stanzione, 2011; Perkins, 2010).

Environmental law

Environmental law analyzes laws that protect the environment and natural resources. Environmental laws have traditionally contained many loopholes for agricultural activities (Ruhl, 2000), which some scholars believe have thwarted environmental law policy goals. Scholars have identified special protections for agricultural activities within environmental law and several other areas of law as a form of "agricultural exceptionalism" stemming from the original vision of the United States as an agrarian society (Schneider, 2010). Some recent environmental law scholarship focuses on renewed efforts to bring agricultural activities under existing or new environmental regulations (Minan and Frech, 2010).

Animal law

Animal law, which is linked to environmental law but is viewed as a separate field, analyzes the rights and welfare of companion animals, wildlife, animals raised for food, and animals used for research (Sunstein, 2000, 2003). In recent years, animal law scholars have assessed a host of topics, including the legality and morality of raising and slaughtering livestock in today's industrial agricultural system (Schlosser, 2002; Welty, 2007).

Health law

Health law scholars study laws impacting human health and the provision of healthcare services. They increasingly focus their research on the repercussions of high rates of obesity and diet-related disease on human health, and on the propriety and efficacy of legal mechanisms to address these problems (McMenamin and Tiglio, 2006; Gostin *et al.*, 2009; Monroe *et al.*, 2009; Fleischhaker *et al.*, 2009; Must *et al.*, 2009).

Other areas

Numerous other areas of law help shape the debate and laws that impact food. Labor law scholarship is a rich area of research impacting food law, as many scholars have analyzed the treatment and condition of farm laborers in the US and abroad (Luna, 1998). Intellectual property law has also emerged as a key area of food law in recent years, as patenting of seeds and use of GMOs have been considered by various scholars and courts (J. E. M. Ag Supply v. Pioneer Hi-bred International, 2001; Monsanto Co. v. Geertson Seed Farms, 2010). Recent antitrust law scholarship has focused on whether and how to reduce market consolidation in the food system (Shively and Roberts, 2010). Scholars conduct research in food law in dozens of other legal fields, notably land use law, property law, natural resources law, human rights law, and international trade law.

Research methodologies

Legal scholars have focused their research in the area of food law on a variety of longstanding and emerging issues. Owing to the contributions of scholars from food and drug law, constitutional law, agricultural law, and the other food law fields described earlier, food law research—like the field of food studies—is interdisciplinary, multidisciplinary, and transdisciplinary (Miller and Deutsch, 2010). Thus, the research methodologies applicable to food law span diverse fields within the study of law.

Food safety and public health have long been part of the food law literature (Wiley, 1929). Many food law advocates have argued that the nation's food safety and inspection system is broken (DeWaal, 2007a, 2007b; Durbin, 2004). They cite numerous incidences of dangerous pathogenic contamination of food—including E. coli and salmonella—transmission of those pathogens to humans, and resulting human illness. These food law scholars often suggest that additional funding and resources be allocated to the FDA and USDA.

Another longstanding area of interest to and debate among food law scholars is product labeling. Discussion of mandatory FDA ingredient labeling (Hauser, 1972), the FDA's Nutrition Facts panel (McCutcheon, 1994), USDA organic labeling (Friedland, 2005), and country-of-origin (COOL) labeling (Chang, 2009) are just some of the many product-labeling issues that food law scholars have debated over the years. Notably, the impact on the consumer of this information as it appears on food labels is also a rich topic (McCabe, 2008–9).

In recent years some food law scholars have begun to argue for a more aggressive style of public health advocacy: What some call a "new" public health (Epstein, 2002). Whereas traditional notions of public health—such as those that spurred passage of the Pure Food and Drugs Act of 1906 and the Meat Inspection Act of 1906—centered on preventing pathogens from appearing in food, food laws based on the "new" public health include "any matter of general public interest or concern" (Epstein, 2002). The banning of foods that may be subjectively unhealthy but are neither poisonous nor pathogenic—such as trans fats, Happy Meals, or caffeinated beer—are examples of laws justified by such a "new" public health approach. While some in the food law community support this approach, critics of this "new" public health are numerous (Thaler and Sunstein, 2008; Burnett, 2006–07; Linnekin, 2009–10; Whitman and Rizzo, 2006–7).

In recent years, a new branch of scholarship in food law has cemented its place in the literature. This new research strand is concerned with examining and proposing changes to legal structures at the federal, state, and local level to improve the outcomes of the food system in terms of a variety of goals, including everything from public health to social justice to the economy. Critics in this area have drawn attention to the legal and political mechanisms behind the food and agricultural system in this country, and detailed what they perceive as negative impacts on human and animal health, the environment, human rights, food safety, and other areas (Nestle, 2003; Pollan, 2006; Schlosser, 2002; McWilliams, 2009). Food law scholars have called increasingly on lawmakers, meanwhile, to craft laws that foster and encourage the production of healthy, sustainable foods (Schneider, 2010).

Avenues for future research

Food law is a field in flux. Regardless of a scholar's ideological bent, few are content with the current state of our food system. The future of food law scholarship therefore rests in the need to challenge existing statutes and regulations, either by tearing them down or by improving upon them.

The expanding field of food law offers many rich areas for scholarship, within both the existing legal fields and along new frontiers. Three broad and sometimes overlapping foci that will likely guide future food law scholarship are the public health impacts of the food system in the areas of food safety and obesity; the regulation and promotion of alternative food systems, including local foods; and food access and the prevalence of food insecurity.

Public health impacts of the food system in the areas of food safety and obesity

The Food Safety Modernization Act (FSMA), which granted a host of new powers to the FDA, is considered by many to be the most important food safety law passed in more than 70 years (Food Safety Modernization Act of 2010, Pub. L. No. 111–353). Food law research into the FSMA will focus on the expansion of FDA authority, the impacts of the law on overall food safety, increased costs to food producers, and consumer health and welfare.

The fastest growing area of food law concerns responses to the epidemics of obesity and diet-related disease that have arisen over the past 50 years. Recent studies put the combined rates of overweight and obesity in the United States at more than two-thirds of the population (Flegal et al., 2010). In response, recent laws at the federal, state, and local level have expanded nutrition labeling to include food served in certain restaurants (New York City Health Code, 2011; Patient Protection and Affordable Care Act of 2010). While early public health research into the efficacy of these laws has not shown promise (Hoefkens et al., 2011; Finkelstein et al., 2011), additional research from food law scholars is needed to determine both the legality and potential impacts of nutrition labeling for restaurant food.

Food marketing, especially as pertains to children, is another emerging issue. In response to studies suggesting an impact of food marketing on the food choices of children (Institute of Medicine, 2006), an Interagency Working Group on Food Marketed to Children, made up of representatives from the Centers for Disease Control (CDC), FTC, FDA, and USDA, recently issued preliminary guidance on marketing food to children. At the local level, some municipalities have banned restaurants from giving away an "incentive item," such as a toy with a Happy Meal, unless the meal meets certain nutritional guidelines (San Francisco Municipal Code, 2011).

Federal, state, and local governments have also banned or sought to attach excise taxes to certain foods and food ingredients, based on the contentious claim that certain foods—like sweetened beverages or foods containing trans fats—are so "obesogenic" (prone to causing obesity) that access to them should be denied or limited. Some local governments have also recently amended zoning codes to limit access to fast food restaurants. For example, Detroit prohibits fast food restaurants from opening within 500 feet of a school (Detroit Municipal Code, 2011), while Los Angeles has banned any new standalone fast food restaurant from opening within a mile of existing fast food restaurants in certain parts of the city (Los Angeles Council File, 2010). Additional research is needed into the legal mechanisms and outcomes of bans and taxes on unhealthy foods, as well as potential legal methods to incentivize the purchase of healthy foods.

Alternative food systems

A second emerging area of food law concerns the promotion and regulation of alternative food systems and methods of food production. Such alternatives include organic foods, which now have a separate set of regulations at the federal level; sustainable foods; and local foods. Popular books like *The Omnivore's Dilemma* (Pollan, 2006) and *Fast Food Nation* (Schlosser, 2002) and films like *Food, Inc.* (Kenner and Schlosser, 2009) have begun to spur a response from the food law community regarding the mainstream industrial agricultural food system. Research is also just beginning to suggest ways to regulate, promote, and improve alternative food systems.

A variety of legal and policy solutions have been proposed or piloted at the federal, state, and local level in hopes of reversing the trend on obesity, increasing access and affordability of healthy food products, and improving legal regimes for alternative food systems. For example, several states now require state agencies and officials to give preference to foods produced within their state, even when those food items are more expensive (Mass. Gen., 2011). A recent USDA rule clarifies that states can authorize or require schools to use a geographic preference mechanism in purchasing food products using federal school food dollars (7 CFR, 2011).

Some municipalities have used zoning codes in an effort to increase access to healthy foods and improve the capacity of alternative food systems. Cleveland amended its zoning code to clarify that agricultural activities are allowed in urban areas, to designate and protect spaces for urban gardens and community gardens, and to make clear that agriculture is permitted on vacant lots, even those zoned for residential areas (Cleveland, Ohio, Zoning Code, 2011). Many states, such as Ohio, have created so-called "cottage food" laws, which allow for the sale of certain non-potentially hazardous foods produced in a home kitchen (Ohio Rev. Code Ann., 2011). Other states, such as Vermont, have funded the purchase of mobile food processing and slaughter units (in this case for poultry) in order to assist local farmers and promote the local food system (Vermont Legislature, 2007). Additional research is needed to examine the impacts of these geographic preference laws, zoning amendments, and other mechanisms on the reduction of unhealthy food options, the increase of healthy food options, and the promotion of alternative food systems.

Food insecurity and food access

A distinct new area of food law research (though linked with obesity) concerns food insecurity, food access, and food deserts. Food insecurity is the metric used to determine hunger in the United States. The USDA defines food security as "access, at all times, to enough food for an active, healthy life for all household members" (USDA Economic Research Service, 2010). Food insecurity can result from either an inability to afford food or from a lack of access to food. Scholars and practitioners have identified a new metric used to describe a lack of food access: "Food deserts." According to the 2008 US Farm Bill, a food desert is an "area in the United

States with limited access to affordable and nutritious food, particularly such an area composed of predominantly lower income neighborhoods and communities" (Food, Conservation, and Energy Act of 2008). Those living in food deserts have limited access to fresh produce and often must pay a premium for such produce, as travel to a supermarket is limited due to distance or cost and groceries in smaller stores can cost 10 percent more than items in full supermarkets (US Department of Agriculture, 2009). Thus, individuals living in food deserts often subsist on fast food or unhealthy food purchased from convenience stores, which many studies have found correlates with high obesity rates within food deserts (USDA Report to Congress, 2009; Larson *et al.* 2009). A few recent studies have called into question this link between food deserts and obesity, evidencing this as an emerging and as-yet unsettled area of knowledge, though it is likely that law and policy approaches to increase access in food deserts will continue to play a role in the field (An and Sturm, 2012; Lee, 2012). One approach to increasing food access—healthy food financing initiatives—offers loans and grants to individuals seeking to provide healthy food in food deserts. Since Pennsylvania created its Fresh Food Financing fund in 2004, other states and the federal government have followed suit. Future research will likely continue the focus on legal mechanisms to increase access to healthy foods and eliminate food deserts in order to both alleviate hunger and malnutrition and reduce rates of overweight and obesity.

Practical considerations for getting started – funding, programs, archival sources, tools, data sets, internet resources, scholarships and awards, etc. (where and how?)

Persons interested in pursuing a career in food law will likely first pursue a Juris Doctor (JD) degree. While a student pursuing a JD does not typically have the opportunity to specialize in any one area, many law schools today offer a food and drug law course. The website of the nonprofit Food and Drug Law Institute (FDLI) (www.fdli.org) lists several dozen such schools around the country. Many schools also offer coursework in agricultural law, environmental law, animal law, and other fields that focus to varying degrees in the area of food law. Additionally, a small but growing number of law schools now offer transdisciplinary coursework outside of the traditional food and drug law framework (combining, for example, discussion of agricultural law and food and drug law).

Law students have the opportunity to serve as editors of law reviews and journals at their respective law schools. There is often strong competition to serve on these publications. Most law reviews focus on general legal topics, though articles selected for publication may include food law scholarship. Several journals, including the *Journal of Food Law & Policy* at the University of Arkansas School of Law, focus largely or exclusively on food law. In addition to serving as editors of scholarly work by accomplished outside writers (practicing lawyers, legislators, advocates, and others), students who serve on a law review or journal often have the opportunity to submit their own work for publication. In some cases, students who do not serve on a law review or journal may still have the opportunity to publish work. Another opportunity for publication is through the FDLI, which holds an annual writing contest in the area of food and drug law. Winners of the H. Thomas Austern Memorial Writing Competitions win both a cash prize and the opportunity to publish their work in the FDLI journal.

Current or prospective law students seeking information about the style, substance, and breadth of student writing in the area of food and drug law may wish to consult *Food and Drug Law: An Electronic Book of Student Papers* (www.law.harvard.edu/faculty/hutt/book_index.html, accessed on April 4, 2012), an online collection of student work from Harvard University Law School professor Peter Barton Hutt's food and drug law course, dating back to 1994.

Students who have earned a JD and who wish to pursue food law further have several options. Drake University Law School offers a Food and Agricultural Law Certificate, while the Institute for Food Laws and Regulations at Michigan State University offers an International Food Law Internet Certificate. For those wishing to pursue a higher-level academic degree in food law, the University of Arkansas School of Law offers a one-year Master of Laws (LLM) degree in agricultural and food law.

Key reading

Hutt, M. and L. Grossman (2007) "Food & Drug Law," 3rd. ed. Eagan, MN: Foundation Press.
Hutt, P. and P. Hutt (1984) II "A History of Government Regulation of Adulteration and Misbranding of Food." 39 *Food Drug Cosm. L.J.* 2.
Jackson, W. and W. Berry (2009) A 50-Year Farm Bill, *New York Times*, January 5, A21.
McWilliams, J. E. (2009) "Just Food," New York: Little, Brown and Company.
Nestle, M. (2003) "Food Politics: How the Food Industry Influences Nutrition and Health. Berkeley and Los Angeles: University of California Press.
Paarlberg, R. (2010) "Food Politics: What Everyone Needs to Know," Oxford: Oxford University Press.
Pollan, M. (2006) "The Omnivore's Dilemma: A Natural History of Four Meals," New York: Penguin Press.
Poppendieck, J. (2010) "Free for All: Fixing School Food in America," Berkeley: University of California Press.
Ruhl, J.B. (2000) "Farms, Their Environmental Harms, and Environmental Law," 27 *Ecology Law Quarterly* 263.
Salatin, J. (2007) "Everything I Want to Do Is Illegal: War Stories from the Local Food Front," Swoope, VA: Polyface.
Schlosser, E. (2002) "Fast Food Nation: The Dark Side of the All-American Meal," New York: Perennial.
Schneider, S. (2011) "Food, Farming, and Sustainability: Readings in Agricultural Law," Durham, NC: Carolina Academic Press.
Sinclair, U. (1906) "The Jungle," New York: Doubleday, Jabber, & Co.
Singer, P. (2001) "Animal Liberation," New York: Ecco Press.

Bibliography

7 C.F.R. (2011) § 210, 215, 220, 225, 226.
Adler, R. W. (1999) "Integrated Approaches to Water Pollution: Lessons from the Clean Air Act", 23 *Harv. Envtl. L. Rev.* 203.
An, R. and R. Sturm (2012) "School and Residential Neighborhood Food Environment and Diet Among California Youth," *American Journal of Preventive Medicine* 42, 2.
Burnett, D. (2006–07) "Fast-Food Lawsuits and the Cheeseburger Bill: Critiquing Congress's Response to the Obesity Epidemic," 14 *Va. J. Soc. Pol'y & L.* 357.
Carr, C. J. and H. N. Scheiber, (2002) "Dealing with a Reasource Crisis: Regulatory Regimes for Managing the World's Marine Fisheries", 21 *Stan. Envtl. L.J.* 45.
Chang, P. (2009) "Comment," "County of Origin Labeling: History and Public Choice Theory," 64 *Food & Drug L.J.* 693.
Cleveland, Ohio (2011) "Zoning Code" Ch. 336-37.
7 C.F.R. (2011) § 210, 215, 220, 225, 226.
Coit, M. (2008) "Jumping on the Next Bandwagon: An Overview of the Policy and Legal Aspects of the Local Food Movement," 4 *J. Food L. & Pol'y* 45.
Cooper, I. P. (1979) "The FDA, the BATF, and Liquor Labeling: A Case Study of Interagency Jurisdictional Conflict," 34 *Food Drug Cosm. L.J.* 370.
Denning, B., Graff, S., Wooten, H. (2010) "Laws to Require Purchase of Locally Grown Food and Constitutional Limits on State and Local Government: Suggestions for Policymakers and Advocates," 1 *J. of Agricultural and Community Dev't* 139.
de Schutter, O., "Countries Tackling Hunger with a Right to Food Approach," Briefing note by the Special Rapporteur on the right to food, May 2010.
Detroit, Mich., (2011) Mun. Code § 61-12-91.
DeWaal, C. S. (2007a) "Food Safety and Security: What Tragedy Teaches Us about Our 100-Year-Old Food Laws," 40 *Vand. J. Transnat'l L.* 921.
——(2007b) " Food Protection and Defense: Preparing for a Crisis," 8 *Minn. J.L. Sci. & Tech.* 187.

Dillard, J. A. (2008) "Sloppy Joe, Slop, Sloppy Joe: How USDA Commodities Dumping Ruined the National School Lunch Program," 87 *Or. L. Rev.* 221.

Durbin, R. J. (2004) "Food Safety Oversight for the 21st Century: The Creation of a Single, Independent Federal Food Safety Agency," 59 *Food & Drug L.J.* 383.

Epstein, R. (1987) "The Proper Scope of the Commerce Power," 73 *Va. L. Rev.* 1387.

Epstein, R. A., "In Defense of the "Old" Public Health: The Legal Framework for the Regulation of Public Health," John M. Olin L. and Econ. Working Paper No. 170 12 (2nd Series) (2002), ssrn.com/abstract_id=359281 (accessed on April 4, 2012).

FDA Consumer, "Harvey W. Wiley," January–February, 2006, www.fda.gov/AboutFDA/WhatWeDo/History/CentennialofFDA/HarveyW.Wiley/default.htm (accessed May 1, 2012).

Finkelstein, E. A., Strombotne, K. L., Chan, N. L., and Krieger, J. (2011) "Mandatory Menu Labeling in One Fast-Food Chain in King County, Washington," 40 *Am. J. Prevent. Med.* 2.

Finkelstein, E. A., Trogdon, J. G., Cohen, J. W., and Dietz, W. "Annual medical spending attributable to obesity: Payer- and service-specific estimates." 28 *Health Affairs* 5 (2009), content.healthaffairs.org/content/28/5/w822.short (accessed on April 4, 2012).

Flegal, K. M., Carroll, M. D., Ogden, C. L., and Curtin, L. R. "Prevalence and trends in obesity among US adults, 1999–2008." *Journal of the American Medical Association*, 303 (2010) 3, jama.ama-assn.org/content/303/3/235.full (accessed on April 4, 2012).

Fleischhacker, S., Ammerman, A., Purdue, W. C., and Miles, J. (2009) "Improving Legal Competences for Obesity Prevention and Control," 37 *J.L. Med. & Ethics* 76

Follmer, J. and Termini, R. B. (2009) "Whatever Happened to Old Mac Donald's Farm … Concentrated Animal Feeding Operation, Factory Farming and the Safety of the Nation's Food Supply," 5 *J. Food L. & Pol'y* 45.

Food, Conservation, and Energy Act of 2008, Pub. L. No. 110-246, §7527(a).

Food Safety "Modernization Act of 2010," Pub. L. No. 111–353.

Fortin, N. D. (2007) "Food Regulation: Law, Science, Policy, and Practice," Hoboken, NJ: Wiley.

Friedland, M. T. (2005) "You Call That Organic – The USDA's Misleading Food Regulations," 13 *N.Y.U. Envtl. L.J.* 379.

Gostin, L. O., Pomeranz, J. L., Jacobson, P. D., and Gottfried, R. N. (2009) "Assessing Laws and Legal Authorities for Obesity Prevention and Control," 37 *J.L. Med. & Ethics* 28.

Halbrook, S. P. (2010–11) "The Constitutional Right to Hunt: New Recognition of an Old Liberty in Virginia," 19 *Wm. & Mary Bill Rts. J.* 197.

Harrington, A. R. (2007) "Not all It's Quacked up to Be: Why State and Local Efforts to Ban Foie Gras Violate Constitutional Law," 12 *Drake J. Agric. L.* 303.

Hauser, J. N. (1972) "The Proposal to Require Label Listing of All Ingredients in Standardized Foods: A Critique," 21 *J. Pub. L.* 301.

Herring, E. P. (1934–35) "The Balance of Social Forces in the Administration of the Pure Food and Drug Act," 13 *Soc. F.* 358.

Hoefkens, C., Lachat, C., Kolsteren, P., Van Camp, J., and Verbeke, W. (2011) "Posting point-of-purchase nutrition information in university canteens does not influence meal choice and nutrient intake," 94 *Am J Clin. Nutr.* 2.

Hutt, P. B. (1985) "The Importance of Analytical Chemistry to Food and Drug Regulation," 68 *J. Ass'n Off. Analyt. Chem.* 147.

Hutt, P. B. and Hutt, P. B. II (1984) "A History of Government Regulation of Adulteration and Misbranding of Food," 39 *Food, Drug, and Cosmetic Law Journal* 2.

Institute of Medicine, "Food Marketing to Children and Youth – Threat or Opportunity," 2005. www.iom.edu/Reports/2005/Food-Marketing-to-Children-and-Youth-Threat-or-Opportunity.aspx (accessed on May 1, 2012).

J. E. M. Ag Supply, Inc. v. Pioneer Hi-bred International, Inc., (2001) 534 U.S. 124.

Kamp, J., Troy, D. E., and Alexander, E. (1999) "FDA Marketing v. First Amendment: Washington Legal Foundation Legal Challenges to Off-Label Policies May Force Unprecedented Changes at FDA," 54 *Food & Drug L.J.* 555.

Kenner, R. and Schlosser, E. (2009) "Food, Inc.," Magnolia Home Entertainment, November 3.

Larson, N. I., Story, M. T., and Nelson, M. C. (2009) "Neighborhood Environments: Disparities in Access to Healthy Foods in the U.S.," 36 *American Journal of Preventive Medicine* 1.

Lee, H. (2012) "The Role of Local Food Availability in Explaining Obesity Risk Among Young School-Aged Children," 74 *Social Science & Medicine* 8.

Linnekin, B. J. (2009–10) "California Effect and the Future of American Food: How California's Growing Crackdown on Food and Agriculture Harms the State and the Nation," 13 *Chap. L. Rev.* 357.

Litman, R. C. and Litman, D. S. (1981) "Protection of the American Consumer: The Muckrakers and the Enactment of the First Federal Food and Drug Law in the United States," 36 *Food Drug Cosm. L.J.* 647.

Los Angeles Council File No. 10–1843 (December 8, 2010). clkrep.lacity.org/onlinedocs/2010/10-1843_ca_12-08-10.pdf (accessed on May 1, 2012).

Luna, G.T. (1998) "An Infinite Distance? Agricultural Exceptionalism and Agricultural Labor," 1 "U. Pa. J. Lab. & Emp. L." 487, 489.

Mass. Gen. Laws ch. 7, § 23B (2011).

McCabe, M. S. (2008–09) "Loco Labels and Marketing Madness: Improving How Consumers Interpret Information in the American Food Economy," 17 *J.L. & Pol'y* 493.

McCutcheon, J. (1994) "Nutrition Labeling Initiative," 49 *Food & Drug L.J.* 409.

McDermott v. Wisconsin (1913) "228 U.S. 115."

McMenamin, J. P. and Tiglio, A. D. (2006)"Not the Next Tobacco: Defenses to Obesity Claims," 61 *Food & Drug L. J.* 445–518.

McNamara, S. H. (1982) "FDA Regulation of Labeling and the Developing Law of Commercial Free Speech," 37 *Food Drug Cosm. L.J.* 394.

McWilliams, J. E. (2009) "Just Food," New York: Little, Brown and Company.

Miller, J. and Deutsch, J. (2010) "Food Studies: An Introduction to Research Methods," London: Berg Publishers.

Minan, J. H. and Frech, T. M. (2010) "Pesticides as Pollutants under the Clean Water Act," 47 *San Diego L. Rev.* 109.

Monroe, J. A., Collins, J. L., Maier, P. S., and Merrill, T. (2009) "Legal Preparedness for Obesity Prevention and Control: A Framework for Action," 37 *J.L. Med. & Ethics* 15.

Monsanto Co. v. Geertson Seed Farms, (2010) 130 "S. Ct. 2743."

Must, A., Bennett, G., Economos, C., and Goodman, E. (2009) "Improving Coordination of Legal-Based Efforts across Jurisdictions and Sectors for Obesity Prevention and Control," 37 *J.L. Med. & Ethics* 90.

Nelson, J. D. (2009) "Incarceration, Accommodation, and Strict Scrutiny," 95 *Va. L. Rev.* 2053.

Nestle, M. (2003) "Food Politics: How the Food Industry Influences Nutrition and Health," Berkeley and Los Angeles: University of California Press.

New York City Health Code, "Title" 24, § 81.50, (2011).

Ohio Rev. Code Ann. §3715.025 (2011) (LexisNexis 2011).

Oser, B. L. "Current Problems Posed by the Food-Additives Amendment," 14 *Food Drug Cosm. L.J.* 574 (1959).

Patient Protection and Affordable Care Act of 2010, "Pub. L." No. 111–48, § 4205.

Perkins, R. M. (2010) "Wine Wars: How We Have Painted Ourselves into a Regulatory Corner," 12 *Vand. J. Ent. & Tech. L.* 397.

Pollan, M. (2006) "The Omnivore's Dilemma: A Natural History of Four Meals," New York: Penguin Press.

Pomeranz, J. L. (2010) "Television Food Marketing to Children Revisited: The Federal Trade Commission Has the Constitutional and Statutory Authority to Regulate," 38 *J.L. Med. & Ethics* 98.

Pratt, J.T. (1880) "Food Adulteration, or, What We Eat, and What We Should Eat" Chicago: P. W. Barclay & Co.

Redish, M. H. "Childhood Obesity, Advertising, and the First Amendment: A White Paper," 2011. www.gmaonline.org/file-manager/Health_Nutrition/childhood_advertising_firstamendment.pdf (accessed on May 1, 2012).

Rubin v. Coors Brewing Co., (1995) 514 U.S. 476.

Ruhl, J. B. (2000) "Farms, Their Environmental Harms, and Environmental Law," 27 *Ecology Law Quarterly* 263.

San Francisco Municipal Code (2011) 8–417.4.

Schlink, F. J. (1935) "Eat, Drink and be Wary" New York: Covici, Friede.

Schlosser, E. (2002) "Fast Food Nation: The Dark Side of the All-American Meal," New York: Perennial.

Schneider, S. A. (2010) "A Reconsideration of Agricultural Law: A Call for the Law of Food, Farming, and Sustainability," 34 *Wm. & Mary Envtl. L. & Pol'y Rev* 935.

——(2009) "Reconnecting Consumers and Producers: On the Path toward a Sustainable Food and Agriculture Policy," 14 "Drake J. Agric. L." 75.

Shaffer, A., Vallianatos, M., Azuma, A. M., and Gottlieb, R. (2006) "Changing the Food Environment: Community Engagement Strategies and Place-Based Policy Tools That Address the Influence of Marketing," 39 *Loy. L. A. L. Rev.* 647.

Shively, J. D. and Roberts, J. S. (2010) "Competition Under the Packers and Stockyards Act: What Now?," 15 *Drake J. Agric. L.* 419.

Sinclair, U. (1906) "The Jungle," New York: Doubleday, Jabber, & Co.

Stanzione, N.J. (2011) "Granholm v. Heald: Wine In, Wit Out," 17 "Widener L. Rev."" 95.

Sunstein, C. (2000) "Standing for Animals (With Notes on Animal Rights)," 47 *UCLA L. Rev.* 1333.

——"The Rights of Animals," 70 *U. Chi. L. Rev.* 387 (2003).

Thaler, R. H. and Sunstein, C. R. (2008) "Nudge" New Haven, CT: Yale University Press.

The Samuel (1816) 14 U.S. 1 Wheat. 9.

Traher, M. (2010) "USDA Organic Certification for the Innovative Farmer," 19 *J. Contemp. Legal Issues* 254.

Tribe, L. H. (2000) "American Constitutional Law," 3d ed., vol. 1, New York: Foundation Press.

Trust for America's Health (2010) "F as in fat: How obesity threatens America's future," healthyamericans.org/reports/obesity2010/Obesity2010Report.pdf (accessed on April 4, 2012).

United States v. Lexington Mill & Elevator Co., (1914) 232" *U.S. 399,"* 409.

USDA Economic Research Service, (2010) "Food security in the United States: Key statistics and graphics." Citing, Nord, M., Coleman-Jensen, A., Andrews, M., and Carlson, S., Household Food Security in the U.S., 2009. Economic Research Report No. (ERR-108), www.ers.usda.gov/Briefing/FoodSecurity/stats_graphs.htm (accessed on April 4, 2012).

USDA Report to Congress, (June 2009) "Access to Affordable and Nutritious Food: Measuring and Understanding Food Deserts and Their Consequences," www.ers.usda.gov/Publications/AP/AP036/AP036fm.pdf (accessed on April 4, 2012).

US Department of Agriculture, (2009) "Access to affordable and nutritious food: Measuring and understanding food deserts and their consequences."" Report to Congress. www.ers.usda.gov/publications/ap/ap036/ap036.pdf (accessed on April 4, 2012).

Vermont Legislature, "Budget Bill," Act 65 of 2007, Sec. 82(a).

Welty, J., (Winter 2007) "Humane Slaughter Laws," 70 *Law & Contemp. Probs.* 175.

Whitman, D.G., Rizzo, M. J. (2006–07) "Paternalist Slopes," 2 *N.Y.U. J.L. & Liberty* 411.

Wiley, H. W., "The History of a Crime Against the Food Law," New York: Arno Press (1929 [1976]), see esp. p. 354.

Windham, J. S., "Putting Your Money Where Your Mouth Is: Perverse Food Subsidies, Social Responsibility and America's 2007 Farm Bill," 31 "Environs: Envtl. L. & Pol'y J." 1 (2007–08).

Wood, M., Pyle, J., Rowden, N., and Irwin, K. (2010) "Promoting the Urban Homestead: Reform of Local Land Use Laws to Allow Microlivestock on Residential Lots," 37 *Ecology L. Currents* 68.

Woodard, L. P. (2004–05) "Comment, Shipping Directly to Consumers ... Wine Not," 32 *W. St. U. L. Rev.* 63.

23

The intersection of gender and food studies

Alice McLean

This article covers the history of feminist food studies as well as recent contributions to the study of gender and food by scholars of masculinity, LBGT studies, and queer theory. Key themes include: food as voice; eating problems; eating pleasures; women's empowerment through food; caregiving; feeding; cooking; essentialism; post-colonial foodways; gender performance; material bodies; culinary masculinity; culinary autoethnography; culinary auto-biography; recipes; community cookbooks; domestic cookbooks; culinary colonialism; non-heteronormativity; female appetite; private vs. public spheres; domesticity; lesbian appetite; women as gatekeepers; female identity; female self-expression; patriarchy; multiple masculinities; second-wave feminism; third-wave feminism; women's studies; ethnic heritage.

While feminist scholars have been examining women's relationship with food since women's studies first formed into a field of its own in the 1970s, feminist food studies has only begun to cohere into a self-referential field of study within the past 15 years. As it has done so, key sites of investigation have come firmly and repeatedly into relief. In keeping with women's studies at large, feminist food studies has locked onto the domestic sphere as a conflicted site, one that simultaneously reproduces patriarchal values and, hence, the physical, intellectual, and ideological subordination of women *and* that serves as a space where women enjoy an amount of power and control far surpassing that which they exert over the public and political realms. Feminist food studies likewise focuses intently on the female body and the myriad ways in which its appetites are nourished or suppressed by cultural forces. Beginning in the 1980s, feminists from a range of fields including anthropology, history, folklore, sociology, literature, and medieval studies began to conceptualize appetite and food choice (or food refusal) as "an important voice in the identity of a woman" and to explore cookery and recipe writing as crucial forms of self-expression (Brumberg, 1988: 168; Bynum, 1987; Kirshenblatt-Gimblett; Ireland, 1981; Leonardi, 1989; Michie, 1987; Schofield, 1989). Toward that end, scholars not only claimed domestic and community cookbooks as rich sources for academic investigation but also established women's culinary autobiography as essential to the study of contemporary women's literature.

In the 1990s the work of such scholars began to coalesce within and alongside the burgeoning field of food studies, ultimately emerging into a recognizable subfield of its own, an emergence marked by the publication of several anthologies that serve as foundational texts in feminist food studies—Anne Bower's *Recipes for Reading* (1997); Carole Counihan and Steven L.

Kaplan's *Food and Gender: Identity and Power* (1998); selected essays on gender and women's studies from Carole Counihan and Penny Van Esterick's *Food and Culture* (1997); Dean Curtin and Lisa Heldke's *Cooking, Eating, Thinking* (1992); Marjorie DeVault's *Feeding the Family* (1991); Mary Anne Schofield's *Cooking by the Book* (1989); and Arlene Voski Avakian's *Through the Kitchen Window* (1998).

Within the past decade scholars of masculinity studies, LBGT studies, and queer theory have made invaluable contributions to the study of gender and food, expanding and reconfiguring the bounds of feminist food studies to account for gender as "a dynamic and purposeful accomplishment: Something people produce in social interaction" (Carrington, 1999: 50). Toward that end, scholars have begun to theorize "eating and feeding" as acts that "enable modes of cultural analysis that are attentive to ... sex, ethnicity, wealth, poverty, geopolitical location, class and gender. Eating ... makes these categories matter again: it roots actual bodies within these relations" (Jarvis, 2000: 784; Probyn, 2000: 9; Ehrhardt, 2012). Post-colonial and poststructural scholars have likewise begun to dismantle "the ideological boundary between home and marketplace" in order to illuminate the ways in which women bridge "public (productive) and (private) reproductive spaces" (Julier, 2005: 169; Abarca, 2012: 109; Allen and Sachs; Barndt; Schroeder, 2002; Sharpless; Williams-Forson). Examining how women move between and interweave the public and private realms, feminist food studies strives to jettison the remnants of dualistic thinking in order to illuminate, challenge, and destabilize the classist, racist, sexist, and "heterosexist cultural mechanisms that discipline and gender the 'female' body" (Jarvis, 2000: 775).

Historical background of feminist food studies and major theoretical approaches in use

Eating problems, eating pleasures

Since the 1970s feminist scholars have focused intently on the ways in which patriarchal culture deforms women's relationships with food. Such work targets sexism by illuminating pervasive ideological constructs that align a woman's appetite for food, for public voice, and for economic, political, or social power with greed and moral corruption (Bruch, 1978; Brumberg, 1988; Chernin, 1981; Michie, 1987; Orbach, 1978). Such an alignment, scholars have argued, fuels an ideal of femininity that lauds subservient, demure, and domesticated behavior. Such ideals encourage women to stifle their physical and intellectual hungers, a repression that results in eating disorders ranging from bulimia and anorexia to obesity. Historically Western women have used food refusal, both unconsciously and consciously, as a means of expressing their protest against the patriarchal forces that subordinate them within the private realm and deny them agency within the public sphere. As anthropologist Carole Counihan explains: "Patriarchal Western society not only restricts women's economic and political opportunities but also defines their role within the family as nurturer and food provider, a role compatible with the use of food as voice" (1999: 107). As a result, feminist scholars study the ways in which women use food refusal to voice their protest against "the general rule governing the construction of femininity: that female hunger—for public power, for independence, for sexual gratification—be contained, and the public space that women be allowed to take up be circumscribed, limited" (Bordo, 1993: 171).

By the 1980s, post-colonial feminists had begun to critique the essentialism that characterized much early scholarship, an essentialism built on a notion of womanhood that often elided race, class, ethnicity, and sexuality from the equation. In an attempt to rectify such essentialism,

Becky Thompson expanded the scholarship on women's eating disorders beyond the white, middle-class, heterosexual woman to include "African-American women, Latinas, and lesbians." In her research, published in *A Hunger So Wide and So Deep* (1994), Thompson discovered that "the particular constellation of eating problems among the women did not vary with race, class, sexuality, or nationality." Across the spectrum, they arose "as sensible acts of self-preservation—in response to myriad injustices including racism, sexism, homophobia, classism, the stress of acculturation, and emotional, physical, and sexual abuse" (221). As Counihan explains: "[T]hat Western women strive for power and identity through closing off the body and denying their own physicality and penetrability is a clear statement that their bodies are source and symbol of their subordination," a fact clearly borne out by Thompson's study, which unearthed sexual abuse as the most pervasive cause of eating problems among the women she studied (1999: 62).

Whereas the eating problems women develop as a response to injustice both arise from and attest to their subordinate place within society, the history of British and American suffragists demonstrate food refusal as a means of political empowerment. When British and American suffragists were imprisoned for picketing, many of them chose to go on hunger strike. Officials responded with force-feeding. As scholars have shown, the figure of the force-fed hunger striker replicates the dynamics of patriarchal suppression, yet, at the same time, public outrage over her treatment helped earn women the vote. In such cases, women performed their culturally scripted role of self-denial, yet successfully transformed its significance from a gesture of deference to the needs of others into a powerful venue for political self-expression and cultural transgression. Because the force-fed suffragist simultaneously embodied woman's oppression, her self-empowerment, and her vociferous hunger for a public voice, she became the focus of much scholarly attention in the late 1980s and 1990s, a time when food studies scholars began to expand their focus beyond women's eating problems in order to construct a more nuanced conception of women's relationships with food (Betterton, 1996; Howlett, 1996; Schlossberg, 2003; Tickner, 1988).

Like scholars of the hunger-striking suffragist, medievalist Caroline Walker Bynum took on the self-starving figure. In researching the renunciation of food by medieval women for her book *Holy Feast and Holy Fast*, Bynum (1987) relied heavily on the written and spoken words of female mystics to uncover "women's use of food as symbol, putting it into a cultural context" (xiv). She found that the women themselves, as well as hagiographers, did not perceive of fasting as a renunciation of the flesh. "Rather they spoke of abstinence as preparatory to and simultaneous with true feeding by Christ. It was identification with Christ's suffering. It was affective, even erotic, union with Christ's adorable self" (120). Bynum's findings on the cultural meaning of medieval fasting as well as the self-perception of the fasters themselves provide a stunning contrast to contemporary food refusal. As Bynum reflects: "Medieval people saw food and body as sources of life, repositories of sensation ... In contrast, modern people see food and body as resources to be controlled. Thus food and body signify that which threatens human mastery" (300).

Bynum's work on medieval women would signal the beginning of a monumental shift in feminist scholarship on women and food. Whereas early scholars focused almost exclusively on women's eating problems as symptomatic of cultural constraints on female appetite and on the kitchen as a site of women's oppression, within the last 15 years feminist food studies has revalued women's considerable appetite—for food, for knowledge, for power, and for creative self-expression—reclaiming women's hunger as a source of empowerment. In so doing, scholars have begun to conceptualize food in women's lives as a "vehicle for artistic expression, a source of sensual pleasure, an opportunity for resistance" (Avakian, 1997: 6; Abarca, 2006; André, 2001;

Bower, 1997; Beoku-Betts, 2002; Black, 2010; DeSalvo and Giunta, 2002; Heller and Moran, 2003; McLean, 2012; Randall, 1997; Sceats, 2000; Schaffer, 2003; Scott, 1997; Theophano, 2002; Upton, 1989; Williams-Forson, 2006; Yaeger, 1988; Zafar, 2002).

Writing as late as 1997, however, Barbara Haber could still lament the fact that feminist scholars focused almost exclusively on "eating disorders and the victimization of females," reflecting that "[i]t will be a great relief to me when feminists ... can see food as a way in which women have historically sustained and celebrated life" (Avakian, 1997: 68, 73). Haber's commentary appears in Arlene Voski Avakian's pioneering anthology of women's writing *Through the Kitchen Window*, an anthology that would prove an invaluable step toward rectifying the imbalance noted by Haber. Including celebratory essays by such feminist icons as Dorothy Allison, Margaret Randall, and Gloria Wade-Gayles, *Through the Kitchen Window* took part in a change that would help cohere feminist food studies into a subfield of its own. "Provocative, questioning, and destabilizing of essentialist stereotypes," collections such as *Through the Kitchen Window*, *Cookin' With Honey: What Literary Lesbians Eat* (Scholder, 1996); and *Milk of Almonds: Italian American Women Writers on Food and Culture* (DeSalvo and Giunta, 2002) "have foregrounded the psychological, economic, social, and political implications of food-making and eating" in contemporary women's lives (DeSalvo and Giunta, 2002: 7).

Fifteen years after Haber lamented the relative lack of scholarship on women's empowerment through food, studies exploring the topic abound, including several essays that appear in the anthology that Haber coedited with Avakian in 2002, *From Betty Crocker to Feminist Food Studies: Critical Perspectives on Women and Food*. Other contributions include anthologies of literary criticism, which "explore how women write about food and oral pleasure, and, in so doing, negotiate their relation to the body as well as to language and culture" (Heller and Moran, 2003: 2; André, 2001; Floyd and Forster, 2003; Schofield, 1989), and projects that conceptualize women's cookery as a form of community building and self-expression and explore women's cookery instruction and recipe writing as a means of recording and preserving the values and traditions that characterize familial, social, ethnic, racial, and national foodways (Abarca, 2006; Avakian; Beoku-Betts, 2002; Blend, 2001; Bower, 1997; Counihan, 2009; DeSilva, 1996; Goldman, 1992; Inness, 2001; Leonardi, 1989; Pilcher; Sharpless; Theophano, 2002; Williams-Forson; Witt, 2004). Studies such as Meredith Abarca's "*Charlas Culinarias*" and Carole Counihan's "Mexicanas Taking Food Public" examine the interstices of the private and public realms to uncover how women bring their considerable cooking and community-building skills into the public realm in order to support themselves and their families, working to "rescue and revive many of the silenced voices omitted in the official discourse of history" (André, 2001: 18). Laura Shapiro's *Perfection Salad* traces the rise of the domestic science movement, which worked to transform food preparation and other household duties into a science. The movement's success led to the rise of home economics departments at the university level, bringing the realm of domestic management into the field of public education. In "Recipes for *Patria*," Jeffrey Pilcher explores how Mexican women helped to secure Indian foods as an integral part of their national cuisine, resisting the effort of Mexican leaders to adopt a decidedly Western European model of cookery.

Scholars likewise blend field research with activism in order to make visible and correct the injustices of the agri-food business, which institutionalize and perpetuate the subordination of women. Through the "Tomasita Project," which traces the journey of a corporate tomato from Mexico, through the United States and into Canada, Deborah Barndt "gathers the stories of the most marginalized women workers in the food chain" and, in so doing, implements the principles of popular education, integrating "research, learning, and organizing for social change" (1999: 79). Like "The Tomasita Project," Carole Counihan's *A Tortilla is Like Life* gives voice to Mexicanas "who have been previously excluded from the pages of history" and draws inspiration from and methodological grounding in ecofeminism. In keeping with "Chicano environmentalism," Counihan "seeks to promote just and sustainable communities and to document Mexicano food production and land and water use" (xiii).

Post-colonial scholars examine the role of food in the construction and maintenance of empire and the gendering of colonial bodies (Chaudhuri, 1992; Goldman, 1992; Roy, 2010; Zlotnick, 1996). In "Domesticating Imperialism: Curry and Cookbooks in Victorian England," Susan Zlotnick (1996) demonstrates how "British women helped incorporate Indian food into the national diet and India into the British Empire" (63). In "'I Yam What I Yam: Cooking, Culture, and Colonialism," Anne Goldman (1992) explores how writers of the culinary auto-ethnography are driven "to represent the relation between subjectivity and ethnicity as a conscious, practiced one … Without sacrificing an acknowledgement of the physical and emotional burdens imposed by imperialism, these writers recuperate a sense of agency for people who, in traditional political and literary theory, have often been subject in name only" (192).

Masculinity studies has joined the field, often exploring how men negotiate and perform masculinity when taking on (or refusing to take on) the culturally coded feminine task of cooking for others (Deutsch, 2005; Mechling, 2005; Parasecoli, 2008). Scholars have likewise begun to analyze dietary practices as a means of masculine performance—ranging from Ghandhi's hunger strikes in India to Progressive Era male fasting and the Atkins diet in the United States (Roy, 2010; Griffith, 2000; Bentley). In *Alimentary Tracts*, Parama Roy (2010) explores "carnality, including alimentation, [as] an important theater for the soul making of Indians as well as for the self-making of Anglo-Indian," finding that "[m]eat eating or a kind of culinary masculinity … would nourish, in the most literal sense, not just Indian resistance to British rule but an entry into modernity and a condition of postcoloniality" (80–81). In "The Other Atkins Revolution," Amy Bentley (2004) examines the "masculinization of dieting" brought about by the Atkins regimen, which enables men to ingest an abundance of foods— namely meat and fat—that are culturally coded masculine (35).

Within the past five years, LBGT studies has actively extended and reconfigured the investigative strategies that have preoccupied women's studies scholars since the 1980s. Expanding our understanding of the kitchen as a space where heterosexually gendered subjects are produced, LBGT scholars have begun to conceptualize the kitchen as a site where individuals can effectively queer—challenge, bring into question, destabilize—the very same heteronormative ideology upon which the traditional family structure and, in turn, patriarchal ideology, depends. As Anita Mannur reflects, scholars have begun to "highlight the powerfully affective potential of food, and its ability to engender anti-normative forms of desire that challenge the notion that the home, as microcosm of the nation, is a necessarily heterosexual formation designed to reproduce citizens that will uphold tradition and its concomitant values" (237). A foundational queer cookbook, *The Alice B. Toklas Cookbook*, for example, has garnered critical attention as a work that destabilizes and reconfigures the rigidly gendered boundaries of the domestic kitchen as well as the domestic cookbook (Toklas, 1954). By inserting recipes into a gastronomic travelogue, Toklas effectively "queers" the bounds of the domestic food writing tradition, creating a text that moves freely between the private and the public realms. Dorothy Allison's "Lesbian Appetite" has likewise inspired scholarship that explores the importance of eating and feeding to the construction of "sexual identities, personal histories and lesbian communities" (Lindenmeyer 19). In particular, Christina Jarvis (2000) demonstrates how Allison's story showcases the performance of a "variety of lesbian roles and identities through the very material realm of eating and sexual practices," thereby countering "the heterosexist fiction that sex, gender, and desire are coherent, interrelated, biologically determined elements" (775).

Cooking, caring, feeding

Masculinity and LBGT studies have done much of late to complicate the work of feminist food scholars, particularly in illuminating the rigidly gendered act of feeding or cooking for others.

As anthropologist Carole Counihan explains: "The predominant role of women in feeding is a cultural universal, a major component of female identity, and an important source of female connection to and influence over others" (1999: 46). Until the 1990s, woman's domestic role as food provider was understood to provide her with an amount of power; she acted as gatekeeper of the household's food provisions (Allen and Sachs: 25). Recent scholarship by sociologists Marjorie DeVault, Alex McIntosh, Mary Zey, and Jeffrey Sobal has significantly challenged this notion. In *Feeding the Family*, DeVault (1991) traces the modern conception of family to the Industrial Revolution and the rise of separate spheres, which designated men's work as wage earning outside the home and women's work as focused on "transforming wages into the goods and services needed to maintain the household" (15). Such a bifurcation constructed a notion of "family" patterned on "women's service for men." As DeVault argues, however, such "patterns are not 'natural'; they are produced by characteristic ways of understanding the family" (18). When Alex McIntosh and Mary Zey (1998) re-examined the notion of women as gatekeepers, they found that "although women have generally been held responsible for these roles, men, to varying degrees, control their enactment" (126). In turn, "family meals are masculine meals" in that "men's food preferences dominate family food choices" (Sobal, 2005: 142).

Since such dynamics produce and reinforce a patriarchal structure, scholars have begun to research the caring work within LBGT households in order to uncover the patterns that occur within same-sex families. In his study of gay and lesbian households, Carrington discovered that the traditional gendering of caring work greatly impacted the self-presentation of the couples whom he studied. Lesbian families worked to present both partners as caregivers and gay-male families worked to downplay the domestic work of the main caregiver. In other words, his findings uncover "an abiding concern about maintaining traditional gender categories, and particularly of avoiding the stigma that comes with either failing to engage in domestic work for lesbian families or through engaging in domestic work for gay-male families" (Carrington, 1999: 59). Among the participants in Carrington's study, those individuals earning the least money or with less prestigious careers were far more likely to act as the main caregivers, a finding that replicates the dynamic found in most heterosexual families.

Extending the scholarship on caring work, masculinity scholars have begun to explore the tensions that arise when heterosexual men take on domestic cookery. Findings show that men cooking for other men will "draw upon multiple versions of masculinity" and work to masculinize their actions through crude humor and gender play (Deutsch, 2005: 93). Men also underscore—consciously or unconsciously—cooking for others as a "noble gesture of affection and brotherhood" (Mechling, 2005: 86). As Jonathan Deutsch has demonstrated in his study of firehouse cookery, however, despite the fact that the firefighters perform the act of cooking for one another "in a decidedly self-conscious way, a proverbial winking over one's shoulder," the meals they cook are inspired by and materialize the concerns of the domestic, or female, cook—a concern with economy, health, pleasing the group, and cooking with efficiency.

Research methodologies

Largely structuralist in approach, early feminist scholarship focused on uncovering the ways in which patriarchal structures subordinate, silence, and devalue women physically, intellectually, and psychologically. Beginning in the 1980s, third-wave feminist scholars began to take much second-wave feminist scholarship to task for essentializing women's experiences, effectively articulating a feminist agenda that speaks from, of, and to a white, middle-class, heterosexual positionality. Taking part in the theoretical shift from structuralism to post-modern and post-colonial thought, third-wave feminism jettisoned the dualistic thinking that essentialized the female experience, an essentialism built on a unified notion of womanhood that often elided race, class, ethnicity, nationality, and sexuality from the equation. Scholars began to shift feminist thought from its monolithic conception of womanhood toward a more nuanced, dynamic, and, ultimately, complex understanding of women.

As scholarship interweaving food, gender, and women's studies has grown, so too have the number of methodologies in use, although the majority of methodologies remain qualitative in nature. Reflecting the trend in scholarship at large, early feminist food studies tends to utilize the methodological approach(es) specific to a given field—anthropology, sociology, folklore, literature, history. As interdisciplinary fields—including women's studies, American studies, cultural studies, African-American studies, and food studies—have flourished, so too has multi-disciplinarian scholarship. While much leading scholarship in feminist food studies will inevitably continue to reflect the single disciplinarity of its author, innovative multidisciplinarian contributions have multiplied exponentially of late. In their nimble, provocative, and inventive investigations of how gender, sexuality, race, ethnicity, and nation are constructed through food, the authors of such scholarship provide one model for future feminist food studies—one that, refusing to be bound by field or methodology, enjoys a deep familiarity with the inter-disciplinary fields of food, gender, and post-colonial studies as well as an expertise in the myriad ways they overlap. Meredith Abarca's *Voices in the Kitchen*; Fabio Parasecoli's *Bite Me*; Parama Roy's *Alimentary Tracts*; Doris Witt's *Black Hunger*; and Psyche Williams-Forson's *Building Houses Out of Chicken Legs* provide just such models. Yet another model can be found in the work of scholars such as Carole Counihan and Lisa Heldke, whose work fits within the disciplinary bounds of their particular fields, yet comfortably approaches academics from a range of disciplines, while simultaneously working to effect broader social change.

Avenues for future research

The self-destructive relationship between Western women, the body, and food is, I contend, significantly different from that of women in many non-Western cultures, for reasons that bear continuing investigation by both historians and anthropologists.

(Counihan, 1998)

The divide between the public and private sphere is no longer feasible or desirable for most men and women. Identifying individual and institutional-level solutions is in the best interest of both [parties], and to do this, it is necessary to continue examining the masculinities and femininities constructed around specific household tasks.

(Swenson, 2009)

We suggest that weaving the strands of feminist studies together with political economy and sociology can provide strong theoretical grounding for a feminist food studies that would illuminate causes, conditions, and possibilities for change in gender relations in the agri-food system.

We need to understand much more about gender relations in the food system. We need to know much more about who women food activists are, their motivations, and their visions for the food system. We have much to learn about the possibilities for changing gender relations and the emerging field of feminist food studies can lead the way through weaving together feminist studies of food and the body with feminist work in the sociology and political economy of agriculture.

(Allen and Sachs, 2012)

Race and gender are often deployed as labels that describe only the experiences of women or people of color, as if these were not reciprocal, structural, and relational terms that define life circumstances for dominant groups, too. What if we saw the construction of race and gender, of the "devalued Other" as a *defining feature* of both the production and consumption of food?

Most emphatically, it seems essential that studies of food and social life must explore how gender and race and class collide to create both the local and the global. Such research would focus on how specific food behaviors and roles regarding commensality are given gendered and racial meanings, how paid and unpaid food labor is divided to express gender and race differences symbolically, and how diverse social structures—not just families or ethnic groups—incorporate gender and racial values and convey advantages. These books would analyze the *construction* of such packages, simultaneously emphasizing the symbolic and the structural, the ideological and the material, the interactional and the institutional levels of analysis.

(Julier, 2005)

Within a context where desire for contact with those who are different or deemed Other is not considered bad, politically incorrect, or wrong minded, we can begin to conceptualize and identify ways that desire informs our political choices and affiliations. Acknowledging ways the desire for pleasure, and that includes erotic longings, informs our politics, our understanding of difference, we may know better how desire disrupts, subverts, and makes resistance possible.

(hooks, 1998)

Against arguments that see in eating a confirmation of a predetermined identity, the point is to focus on the different forms of alimentary assemblages. It is here that we see glimpses of the types of intermingling of bodies that suggest other ways of inhabiting the world.

(Probyn, 2000)

As the nascent field of food studies takes shape, insights from queer studies have the potential to enrich our understandings of the interrelationships among food, gender and sexuality by encouraging us to rethink and refine our conceptions of these connections.

(Ehrhardt, 2012)

Practical considerations for getting started

Choosing a graduate program

Given that the number of scholars working in the fields of food and gender studies has grown exponentially over the past 15 years, those wishing to pursue a graduate degree in women's and gender studies with a focus in food studies, a food studies degree with a woman's studies focus, or a degree in another field entirely with an emphasis in gender and food studies would do well to connect directly with those scholars with whom you might like to work. If they do not teach in universities or colleges offering the graduate degree you wish to attain, they can, at the least, offer concrete advice. For those interested in completing a Masters thesis or dissertation that explores the intersection of gender and food within a single discipline, then seeking a degree program in the field of your choice at an institution with one or more scholars with research interests in food studies would be advisable.

Choosing a thesis reader with expertise in food studies

If you are already enrolled in a graduate program, just discovering an interest in completing a thesis significantly invested in food studies, and cannot locate a scholar at your particular institution to act as reader for the food studies portion of your research, locate and ask someone from another institution to act as an outside reader.

Networking

Because networking is an essential component of success at the graduate and post-graduate level, graduate students, faculty, and independent researchers currently working on gender and food studies should attend the annual conference for the Association for the Study of Food and Society, as it is an especially collegiate gathering, supportive of students and established faculty alike.

Funds for gender studies scholars are available through the following organizations:

American Association of University Women
Chicana/Latina Foundation
The National Council for Black Studies
National Women's Studies Association
Transgender Scholarship and Education Legacy Fund (TSELF)
Woodrow Wilson Doctoral Dissertation Fellowship in Women's Studies

Key reading

Abarca, Meredith (2006) *Voices in the Kitchen: Views of Food and the World from Working-Class Mexican and Mexican American Women*. College Station: Texas A&M University Press.
——(2012) "*Charlas Culinarias:* Mexican Women Speak from Their Public Kitchens." In *Taking Food Public*. Carole Counihan and Psyche Williams-Forson, eds. New York: Routledge.
Adams, Carol J. (2010) *The Sexual Politics of Meat: A Feminst-Vegetarian Critical Theory*. New York: Continuum.
André, María Claudia (2001) *Chicanas and Latin American Women Writers Exploring the Realm of the Kitchen as a Self-Empowering Site*. Lewiston, NY: Edwin Mellen.
Appadurai, Arjun (1988) "How to Make a National Cuisine: Cookbooks in Contemporary India." *Contemporary Studies in Society and History* 30: 3–24.
Allen, Patricia and Carolyn Sachs (2012) "Women and Food Chains: The Gendered Politics of Food." *Taking Food Public*. Eds. Carole Counihan and Psyche Williams-Forson. New York: Routledge.
Avakian, Arlene Voski (1998) *Through the Kitchen Window: Women Writers Explore the Intimate Meanings of Food and Cooking*. Boston, MA: Beacon.
Avakian, Arlene Voski and Barbara Haber, ed. (2005) *From Betty Crocker to Feminist Food Studies: Critical Perspectives on Women and Food*. Amherst: University of Massachusetts Press.
Barndt, Deborah (2008) *Tangled Routes: Women, Work, and Globalization on the Tomato Trail*. Second Edition. Lanham, MD: Rowman and Littlefield.
——(1999) *Women Working the Nafta Food Chain: Women, Food & Globalization*. Toronto: Second Story Press.
Bentley, Amy (1998) *Eating for Victory: Food Rationing and the Politics of Domesticity*. Chicago: University of Illinois Press.

Beoku-Betts, Josephine (2002) "'We Got Our Way of Cooking Things': Women, Food, and Preservation of Cultural Identity among the Gullah." *Food in the U.S.A.* Ed. Carole Counihan. New York: Routledge.

Blend, Benay (2001) "I am an Act of Kneading": Food and the Making of Chicana Identity." *Cooking Lessons: The Politics of Gender and Food.* Ed. Sherrie Inness. Lanham, MD: Rowman & Littlefield.

Bordo, Susan (1993) *Unbearable Weight.* Berkeley: California University Press.

Bower, Anne L. (1997) *Recipes for Reading: Community Cookbooks, Stories, Histories.* Amherst: University of Massachusetts Press.

Bruch, Hilda (1978) *The Golden Cage: The Enigma of Anorexia Nervosa.* New York: Vintage.

Brumberg, Joan Jacobs (1997) "The Appetite as Voice." *Food and Culture: A Reader.* Eds. Carole Counihan and Penny Van Esterik. New York: Routledge.

——(1988) *Fasting Girls: The Emergence of Anorexia Nervosa as Modern Disease.* Cambridge, MA: Harvard University Press.

Bynum, Caroline Walker (1987) *Holy Feast and Holy Fast: The Religious Significance of Food to Medieval Women.* Berkeley: University of California Press.

Carrington, Christopher (1999) *No Place Like Home: Relationships and Family Life Among Lesbians and Gay Men.* Chicago, IL: University of Chicago.

Chaudhuri, Nupur (1992) "Shawls, Jewelry, Curry, and Rice in Victorian Britain." *Western Women and Imperialism: Complicity and Resistance.* Eds. Chaudhuri and Margaret Strobel. Bloomington: Indiana University Press.

Chernin, Kim (1981) *The Obsession: Reflections on the Tyranny of Slenderness.* New York: Harper and Row.

Counihan, Carole (1999) *The Anthropology of Food and Body: Gender, Meaning, and Power.* New York: Routledge.

——(2004) *Around the Tuscan Table: Food, Family, and Gender in Twentieth-Century Florence.* New York: Routledge.

——(2012) "Mexicanas Taking Food Public: The Power of the Kitchen in the San Luis Valley." *Taking Food Public.* Eds. Carole Counihan and Psyche Williams-Forson. New York: Routledge.

——(2009) *A Tortilla is Like Life.* Austin: University of Texas Press.

——(1998) "Western Women's Prodigious Fasting." *Food and Gender: Identity and Power.* Eds. Carole Counihan and Steven L. Kaplan. Newark, NJ: Gordon and Breach.

Counihan, Carole and Steven L. Kaplan (1998) *Food and Gender: Identity and Power.* Newark, NJ: Gordon and Breach.

Curtin, Deane W. and Lisa M. Heldke (1992) *Cooking, Eating, Thinking: Transformative Philosophies of Food.* Bloomington: Indiana University Press.

DeSalvo, Louise and Edvige Giunta (2002) *The Milk of Almonds: Italian American Women Writers on Food and Culture.* New York: The Feminist Press.

DeSilva, Cara (1996) *In Memory's Kitchen: A Legacy From the Women of Terezin.* Trans. Bianca Steiner Brown and David Stern. Northvale, NJ: Jason Aronson.

Deutsch, Jonathan (2005) "'Please Pass the Chicken Tits': Rethinking Men and Cooking at an Urban Firehouse." *Food and Foodways* 13, nos. 1–2: 91–114.

DeVault, Marjorie (1991) *Feeding the Family: The Social Organization of Caring and Gendered Work.* Chicago, IL: University of Chicago Press.

Ehrhardt, Julia C. (2012) "Toward Queering Food Studies: Foodways, Heteronormativity, and Hungry Women in Chicana Lesbian Writing." *Taking Food Public.* Eds. Carole Counihan and Psyche Williams-Forson. New York: Routledge.

Floyd, Janet and Laurel Foster (2003) *The Recipe Reader: Narratives—Contexts—Traditions.* Aldershot: Ashgate.

Gabaccia, Donna (1998) *We Are What We Eat: Ethnicity and the Making of Americans.* Cambridge, MA: Harvard University Press.

Gard, Michael and Jan Wright (2005) "Feminism and 'the obesity epidemic.'" *The Obesity Epidemic: Science, Morality, and Ideology.* New York: Routledge.

Goldman, Anne (1992) "'I Yam What I Yam': Cooking, Culture, and Colonialism." *Decolonizing the Subject: The Politics of Gender in Women's Autobiography.* Eds. Sidone Smith and Julia Watson. Minneapolis: University of Minnesota Press.

Heller, Tamar and Patricia Moran (2003) *Scenes of the Apple: Food and the Female Body in Nineteenth- and Twentieth-Century Women's Writing.* Albany: State University of New York Press.

hooks, bell (1998) "Eating the Other: Desire and Resistance." *Eating Culture.* Eds. Ron Scapp and Brian Seitz. Albany: State University of New York.

Hughes, Marvalene H. (1997) "Soul, Black Women, and Food." *Food and Culture: A Reader*. Eds. Carole Counihan and Penny Van Esterik. New York: Routledge.

Inness, Sherrie A. (2001) *Kitchen Culture in America: Popular Representations of Food, Gender, and Race*. Philadelphia: University of Pennsylvania.

——(2001) *Pilaf, Pozole, and Pad Thai: American Women and Ethnic Food*. Amherst: University of Massachusetts Press.

Jarvis, Christina (2000) "Gendered Appetites: Feminisms, Dorothy Allison, and the Body." *Women's Studies*. Vol. 29: 763–92.

Julier, Alice (2005) "Hiding Race and Gender in the Discourse of Commercial Food Consumption." *From Betty Crocker to Feminist Food Studies*. Eds. Arlene Voski Avakian and Barbara Haber. Amerst: University of Massachusetts Press.

Julier, Alice and Laura Lindenfeld (2005) "Mapping Men onto the Menu." *Food and Foodways*. Vol. 13: nos. 1–2, 1–16.

Kelly, Traci Marie (2001) "'If I Were a Voodoo Priestess': Women's Culinary Autobiographies." *Kitchen Culture*. Ed. Sherrie A. Inness. Philadelphia: University of Pennsylvania Press.

Kirshenblatt-Gimblett, Barbara (1987) "Recipes for Creating Community: The Jewish Charity Cookbook in America." *Jewish Folklore and Ethnology*. Vol. 9: 8–11.

Ireland, Lynne (1981) "The Compiled Cookbook as Foodways Autobiography." *Western Folklore*. Vol. 40: 108, 109.

Leonardi, Susan J. (1989) "Recipes for Reading: Summer Pasta, Lobster à la Riseholme, and Key Lime Pie." *PMLA*. Vol. 104: no. 3, 340–47.

Lupton, Deborah (1996) *Food, the Body, and the Self*. London: Sage.

Mannur, Anita (2012) "Feeding Desire: Food, Domesticity, and Challenges to Hetero-Patriarchy." *Taking Food Public*. Eds. Carole Counihan and Psyche Williams-Forson. New York: Routledge.

McFeely, Mary Drake (2000) *Can She Bake a Cherry Pie: American Women and the Kitchen*. Amherst: University of Massachusetts Press.

McIntosh, Alex and Mary Zey (1998) "Women as Gatekeepers." Eds. Carole Counihan and Steven L. Kaplan. *Food and Gender: Identity and Power*. Newark: Gordon and Breach.

McLean, Alice (2012) *Aesthetic Pleasure in Twentieth-Century Women's Food Writing: The Innovative Appetites of M. F. K. Fisher, Alice B. Toklas, and Elizabeth David*. New York: Routledge.

Mechling, Jay (2005) "Boy Scouts and the Manly Art of Cooking." *Food and Foodways* Vol. 13: nos. 1–2, 67–89.

Michie, Helena (1987) *The Flesh Made Word*. New York: Oxford University Press.

Neuhaus, Jessamyn (2003) *Manly Meals and Mom's Home Cooking: Cookbooks and Gender in Modern America*. Baltimore, MD: Johns Hopkins University Press.

Parasecoli, Fabio (2008) *Bite Me: Food in Popular Culture*. Oxford: Berg.

Parkin, Katherine J. (2006) *Food is Love: Advertising and Gender Roles in Modern America*. Philadelphia: University of Pennsylvania Press.

Pilcher, Jeffrey M. (1998) *Que Vivan los Tamales! Food and the Making of Mexican Identity*. Albuquerque: University of New Mexico Press.

Probyn, Elspeth (2000) *Carnal Appetites: FoodSexIdentities*. New York: Routledge.

Roy, Parama (2010) *Alimentary Tracts: Appetites, Aversions, and the Postcolonial*. Durham, NC: Duke University Press.

Sceats, Sarah (2000) *Food, Consumption and the Body in Contemporary Women's Fiction*. Cambridge: Cambridge University Press.

Schenone, Laura (2003) *A Thousand Years Over a Hot Stove: A History of American Women Told Through Food, Recipes and Remembrances*. New York: W. W. Norton & Company.

Schofield, Mary Anne (1989) *Cooking by the Book: Food in Literature and Culture*. Bowling Green, OH: Bowling Green University Press.

Shapiro, Laura (1995) *Perfection Salad: Women and Cooking at the Turn of the Century*. New York: North Point.

——(2004) *Something From the Oven: Reinventing Dinner in 1950s America*. New York: Viking.

Silver, Anna Krugovoy (2002) *Victorian Literature and the Anorexic Body*. Cambridge: Cambridge University Press.

Sobal, Jeffery (2005) "Men, Meat, and Marriage: Models of Masculinity." *Food and Foodways*. Vol. 13: nos. 1–2, 135–58.

Theophano, Janet (2002) *Eat My Words: Reading Women's Lives through the Cookbooks They Wrote*. New York: Palgrave.

Thompson, Becky W. (1994) *A Hunger So Wide and So Deep: A Multiracial View of Women's Eating Problems*. Minneapolis: University of Minnesota.

Van Esterik, Penny (1989) *Beyond the Breast-Bottle Controversy*. New Brunswick, NJ: Rutgers University Press.

——(2008) "The Politics of Breastfeeding: An Advocacy Update." *Food and Culture: A Reader*, Second Edition. New York: Routledge.

Williams-Forson, Psyche (2006) *Building Houses Out of Chicken Legs: Black Women, Food, & Power*. Chapel Hill: University of North Carolina Press.

Witt, Doris (2004) *Black Hunger: Soul Food and America*. Minneapolis: University of Minnesota Press.

Zafar, Rafia (2002) "The Signifying Dish: Autobiography and History in Two Black Women's Cookbooks." *Food in the USA: A Reader*. Ed. Carole M. Counihan. New York: Routledge.

Zlotnick, Susan (1996) "Domesticating Imperialism: Curry and Cookbooks in Victorian England." *Frontiers*. Vol. 16: nos. 2–3, 51–69.

Bibliography

Abarca, Meredith (2006) *Voices in the Kitchen: Views of Food and the World from Working-Class Mexican and Mexican American Women*. College Station: Texas A&M University Press.

——(2012) "*Charlas Culinarias:* Mexican Women Speak from Their Public Kitchens." *Taking Food Public*. Eds. Carole Counihan and Psyche Williams-Forson. New York: Routledge.

Acosta-Belén, Edna (2001) "Preface". In *Chicanas and Latin American Women Writers Exploring the Realm of the Kitchen as a Self-Empowering Site*. Lewiston, NY: Edwin Mellen.

André, María Claudia (2001) In *Chicanas and Latin American Women Writers Exploring the Realm of the Kitchen as a Self-Empowering Site*. Lewiston, NY: Edwin Mellen.

Appadurai, Arjun (1988) "How to Make a National Cuisine: Cookbooks in Contemporary India." *Contemporary Studies in Society and History*. Volume 30: 3–24.

Allen, Patricia and Carolyn Sachs (2012) "Women and Food Chains: The Gendered Politics of Food." *Taking Food Public*. Eds. Carole Counihan and Psyche Williams-Forson. New York: Routledge.

Avakian, Arlene Voski (2005) "Shish Kebab Armenians: Food and the Construction and Maintenance of Ethnic and Gender Identities among Armenian American Feminists." *From Betty Crocker to Feminist Food Studies: Critical Perspectives on Women and Food*. Arlene Avakian and Barbara Haber, eds. Amherst: University of Massachusetts Press.

——(1997) *Through the Kitchen Window: Women Writers Explore the Intimate Meanings of Food and Cooking*. Boston, MA: Beacon.

Avakian, Arlene Voski and Barbara Haber, ed. (2005) *From Betty Crocker to Feminist Food Studies: Critical Perspectives on Women and Food*. Amherst: University of Massachusetts Press.

——(2005) "Feminist Food Studies: A Brief History." *From Betty Crocker to Feminist Food Studies: Critical Perspectives on Women and Food*. Amherst: University of Massachusetts Press.

Barndt, Deborah (2008) *Tangled Routes: Women, Work, and Globalization on the Tomato Trail*. Second Edition. Lanham, MD: Rowman and Littlefield.

——(1999) *Women Working the Nafta Food Chain: Women, Food & Globalization*. Toronto: Second Story Press.

Bentley, Amy (1998) *Eating for Victory: Food Rationing and the Politics of Domesticity*. Chicago: University of Illinois Press.

——"The Other Atkins Revolution: Atkins and the Shifting Culture of Dieting." *Gastronomica* 4, 3 (August 2004): 34–45.

Beoku-Betts, Josephine (2002) "'We Got Out Way of Cooking Things': Women, Food, and Preservation of Cultural Identity among the Gullah." *Food in the U.S.A.* Carole Counihan, ed. New York: Routledge.

Betterton, Rosemary (1996) "'A Perfect Woman': The Political Body of Suffrage," *An Intimate Distance: Women, Artists and the Body*. London: Routledge, 56–78.

Black, Shameem (2010) "Recipes for Cosmopolitanism Cooking across Borders in the South Asian Diaspora." *Frontiers* 31, 1: 1–30.

Blend, Benay (2001) "I am an Act of Kneading": Food and the Making of Chicana Identity." *Cooking Lessons: The Politics of Gender and Food*. Sherrie Inness, ed. Lanham, MD: Rowman & Littlefield.

Bordo, Susan (1993) *Unbearable Weight*. Berkeley: California University Press.

Bower, Anne (1997) *Recipes for Reading: Community Cookbooks, Stories, Histories*. Amherst: Univerisity of Massachusetts Press.

Bruch, Hilda (1978) *The Golden Cage: The Enigma of Anorexia Nervosa.* New York: Vintage.

Brumberg, Joan Jacobs (1997) "The Appetite as Voice." *Food and Culture: A Reader.* Eds. Carole Counihan and Penny Van Esterik. New York: Routledge.

——(1988) *Fasting Girls: The Emergence of Anorexia Nervosa as Modern Disease.* Cambridge, MA: Harvard University Press.

Bynum, Caroline Walker (1987) *Holy Feast and Holy Fast: The Religious Significance of Food to Medieval Women.* Berkeley: University of California Press.

Carrington, Christopher (1999) *No Place Like Home: Relationships and Family Life Among Lesbians and Gay Men.* Chicago, IL: University of Chicago.

Chaudhuri, Nupur (1992) "Shawls, Jewelry, Curry, and Rice in Victorian Britain." *Western Women and Imperialism: Complicity and Resistance.* Chaudhuri and Margaret Strobel, eds., pp. 231–46. Bloomington: Indiana University Press.

Chernin, Kim (1981) *The Obsession: Reflections on the Tyranny of Slenderness.* New York: Harper and Row.

Counihan, Carole (1999) *The Anthropology of Food and Body: Gender, Meaning, and Power.* New York: Routledge.

——(2004) *Around the Tuscan Table: Food, Family, and Gender in Twentieth-Century Florence.* New York: Routledge.

——(2002) "Food as Women's Voice in the San Luis Valley of Colorado." *Food in the U.S.A.* Carole Counihan, ed. New York: Routledge.

——(2012) "Mexicanas Taking Food Public: The Power of the Kitchen in the San Luis Valley." *Taking Food Public.* Carole Counihan and Psyche Williams-Forson, eds. New York: Routledge.

——(2009) *A Tortilla is Like Life.* Austin: University of Texas Press.

Counihan, Carole and Steven L. Kaplan (1998) *Food and Gender: Identity and Power.* Newark: Gordon and Breach.

Counihan, Carole and Penny Van Esterick (1997) *Food and Culture: A Reader.* Oxford: Routledge.

Curtin, Deane W. and Lisa M. Heldke. (1992) *Cooking, Eating, Thinking: Transformative Philosophies of Food.* Bloomington: Indiana University Press.

DeSalvo, Louise and Edvige Giunta (2002) *The Milk of Almonds: Italian American Women Writers on Food and Culture.* New York: The Feminist Press.

DeSilva, Cara (1996) *In Memory's Kitchen: A Legacy From the Women of Terezin.* Trans. Bianca Steiner Brown and David Stern. Northvale, NJ: Jason Aronson.

Deutsch, Jonathan (2005) "'Please Pass the Chicken Tits': Rethinking Men and Cooking at an Urban Firehouse." *Food and Foodways* 13, nos. 1–2.

DeVault, Marjorie (1991) *Feeding the Family: The Social Organization of Caring and Gendered Work.* Chicago, IL: University of Chicago Press.

Ehrhardt, Julia C. (2012) "Toward Queering Food Studies: Foodways, Heteronormativity, and Hungry Women in Chicana Lesbian Writing." *Taking Food Public.* Carole Counihan and Psyche Williams-Forson, eds. New York: Routledge.

Ellmann, Maud (1993) *Hunger Artists: Starving, Writing, and Imprisonment.* Cambridge, MA: Harvard University Press.

Floyd, Janet and Laurel Foster (2003) *The Recipe Reader: Narratives—Contexts—Traditions.* Aldershot: Ashgate.

Forster, Laurel (2003) "Liberating the Recipe: A Study of the Relationship Between Food and Feminism in the early 1970s." *The Recipe Reader: Narratives—Contexts—Traditions.* Aldershot: Ashgate.

Furst, Lilian R. and Peter W. Graham (1992) *Disorderly Eaters: Texts in Self-Empowerment.* University Park: Pennsylvania State University Press.

Gabaccia, Donna (1998) *We Are What We Eat: Ethnicity and the Making of Americans.* Cambridge, MA: Harvard University Press.

Geis, Deborah R. (1998) "Feeding the Audience: Food, Feminism, and Performance Art." *Eating Culture.* Eds. Ron Scapp and Brian Seitz. Albany: State University of New York.

Goldman, Anne (1992) "'I Yam What I Yam': Cooking, Culture, and Colonialism." *Decolonizing the Subject: The Politics of Gender in Women's Autobiography.* Eds. Sidone Smith and Julia Watson. Minneapolis: University of Minnesota Press.

Goldstein, Darra (2005) "Women under Seige: Leningrad 1941–42." *From Betty Crocker to Feminist Food Studies: Critical Perspectives on Women and Food.* Arlene Avakian and Barbara Haber, eds. University of Massachusetts Press: Amherst.

Griffith, Marie (2000) "Apostles of Abstinence: Fasting and Masculinity During the Progressive Era." *American Quarterly* 4: 599–638.

Haber, Barbara (2005) "Cooking to Survive: The Careers of Alice Foote MacDougall and Cleora Butler." *From Betty Crocker to Feminist Food Studies: Critical Perspectives on Women and Food*. Arlene Voski Avakian and Barbara Haber, eds. Amherst: University of Massachusetts Press.

Hedlke, Lisa (2003) *Exotic Appetites: Ruminations of a Food Adventurer*. New York: Routledge.

Heller, Tamar and Patricia Moran (2003) *Scenes of the Apple: Food and the Female Body in Nineteenth- and Twentieth-Century Women's Writing*. Albany: State University of New York Press.

hooks, bell (1998) "Eating the Other: Desire and Resistance." *Eating Culture*. Ron Scapp and Brian Seitz, eds. Albany: State University of New York.

Howlett, Caroline J. "Writing on the Body? Representation and Resistance in British Suffragette Accounts of Force Feeding." *Genders* 23 (30 June 1996): 3–49.

Hughes, Marvalene H. (1997) "Soul, Black Women, and Food." *Food and Culture: A Reader*. Carole Counihan and Penny Van Esterik, eds. New York: Routledge.

Hyman, Gwen (2009) *Making a Man: Gentlemanly Appetites in the Nineteenth-Century British Novel*. Athens: Ohio University Press.

Inness, Sherrie A. (2001) *Kitchen Culture in America: Popular Representations of Food, Gender, and Race*. Philadelphia: University of Pennsylvania.

——(2001) *Pilaf, Pozole, and Pad Thai: American Women and Ethnic Food*. Amherst: University of Massachusetts Press.

Julier, Alice (2005) "Hiding Race and Gender in the Discourse of Commercial Food Consumption." *From Betty Crocker to Feminist Food Studies*. Arlene Voski Avakian and Barbara Haber, eds. Amherst: University of Massachusetts Press.

Julier, Alice and Laura Lindenfeld (2005) "Mapping Men onto the Menu." *Food and Foodways* 13, nos. 1–2: 1–16.

Kelly, Traci Marie (2001) "'If I Were a Voodoo Priestess': Women's Culinary Autobiographies." *Kitchen Culture*, Sherrie A. Inness, ed., pp. 228–51. Philadelphia: University of Pennsylvania Press.

Kirshenblatt-Gimblett, Barbara (1997) "The Moral Sublime: The Temple Emanuel Fair and its Cookbook, Denver, 1888." *Recipes for Reading: Community Cookbooks, Stories, Histories*. Anne Bower, ed. Amherst: University of Massachusetts Press.

——(1987) "Recipes for Creating Community: The Jewish Charity Cookbook in America." *Jewish Folklore and Ethnology* 9: 8–11.

Ireland, Lynne (1981) "The Compiled Cookbook as Foodways Autobiography." *Western Folklore* 40: 108, 109.

Leonardi, Susan J. (1989) "Recipes for Reading: Summer Pasta, Lobster à la Riseholme, and Key Lime Pie." *PMLA*. 104, no. 3: 340–47.

Linzie, Anna (2006) *The True Story of Alice B. Toklas: A Study of Three Autobiographies*. Iowa City: University of Iowa.

Lupton, Deborah (1996) *Food, the Body, and the Self*. London: Sage.

Mannur, Anita (2012) "Feeding Desire: Food, Domesticity, and Challenges to Hetero-Patriarchy." *Taking Food Public*. Eds. Carole Counihan and Psyche Williams-Forson. New York: Routledge.

McFeely, Mary Drake (2000) *Can She Bake a Cherry Pie: American Women and the Kitchen*. Amherst: University of Massachusetts Press.

McIntosh, Alex and Mary Zey (1998) "Women as Gatekeepers." Carole Counihan and Steven L. Kaplan, eds. *Food and Gender: Identity and Power*. Newark: Gordon and Breach.

McLean, Alice (2012) *Aesthetic Pleasure in Twentieth-Century Women's Food Writing: The Innovative Appetites of M. F. K. Fisher, Alice B. Toklas, and Elizabeth David*. New York: Routledge.

Mechling, Jay (2005) "Boy Scouts and the Manly Art of Cooking. *Food and Foodways* 13, 1–2: 67–89.

Michie, Helena (1987) *The Flesh Made Word*. New York: Oxford University Press.

Neuhaus, Jessamyn (2003) *Manly Meals and Mom's Home Cooking: Cookbooks and Gender in Modern America*. Baltimore, MD: Johns Hopkins University Press.

Orbach, Susie (1978) *Fat is a Feminist Issue: The Anti-Diet Guide to Permanent Weight Loss*. New York: Paddington.

Parasecoli, Fabio (2008) *Bite Me: Food in Popular Culture*. Oxford: Berg.

Pilcher, Jeffrey M. (1997) "Recipes for *Patria*: Cuisine, Gender, and Nation in Nineteenth-Century Mexico. *Recipes for Reading*. Ed. Anne Bower. Amherst: University of Massachusetts Press.

——(1998) *Que Vivan los Tamales! Food and the Making of Mexican Identity*. Albuquerque: University of New Mexico Press.

Probyn, Elspeth (2000) *Carnal Appetites: FoodSexIdentities*. New York: Routledge.

Randall, Margaret (1997) *Hunger's Table: Women, Food & Politics*. Watsonville, CA: Papier-Mache Press.

Roy, Parama (2010) *Alimentary Tracts: Appetites, Aversions, and the Postcolonial*. Durham: Duke University Press.

Sceats, Sarah (2000) *Food, Consumption and the Body in Contemporary Women's Fiction*. Cambridge: Cambridge University Press.

Schaffer, Talia (2003) "The Importance of Being Greedy: Connoisseurship and Domesticity in the Writings of Elizabeth Robins Pennell." *The Recipe Reader*, Janet Floyd and Laurel Forster, eds. Burlington: Ashgate.

Schenone, Laura (2003) *A Thousand Years Over a Hot Stove: A History of American Women Told Through Food, Recipes and Remembrances*. New York: W.W. Norton & Company.

Schlossberg, Linda (2003) "Consuming Images: Women, Hunger, and the Vote," *Scenes of the Apple: Food and the Female Body in Nineteenth- and Twentieth-Century Women's Writing*, Tamar Heller and Patricia Moran, eds. Albany: State University of New York.

Schofield, Mary Anne (1989) *Cooking by the Book: Food in Literature and Culture*. Bowling Green, OH: Bowling Green Universtiy Press.

Scholder, Amy (1996) *Cookin' With Honey: What Literary Lesbians Eat*. Ithaca, NY: Firebrand.

Schroeder, Kathleen (2012) "A Feminist Examination of Community Kitchens in Peru and Bolivia." *Taking Food Public*. Carole Counihan and Psyche Williams-Forson, eds. New York: Routledge.

Scott, Nina M. (1997) "Juana Manuela Gorriti's *Cocina eclectic*: Recipes as Feminine Discourse." *Recipes for Reading*. Anne L. Bower, ed. Amherst: University of Massachusetts Press.

Shapiro, Laura (1995) *Perfection Salad: Women and Cooking at the Turn of the Century*. New York: North Point.

Silver, Anna Krugovoy (2002) *Victorian Literature and the Anorexic Body*. Cambridge: Cambridge University Press.

Sobal, Jeffery (2005) "Men, Meat, and Marriage: Models of Masculinity." *Food and Foodways* 13, nos. 1–2: 135–58.

Swenson, Rebecca (2009) "*Domestic Divo*? Televised Treatments of Masculinity, Femininity and Food." *Critical Studies in Media Communication*. Vol. 26: No. 1: 36–53.

Theophano, Janet (2002) *Eat My Words: Reading Women's Lives through the Cookbooks They Wrote*. New York: Palgrave.

Thompson, Becky W. (1994) *A Hunger So Wide and So Deep: A Multiracial View of Women's Eating Problems*. Minneapolis: University of Minnesota.

Tickner, Lisa (1988) *The Spectacle of Women: Imagery of the Suffrage Campaign 1907–1914*. Chicago, IL: University of Chicago Press.

Toklas, Alice B. (1954) *Alice B. Toklas Cookbook*. New York: Harper and Brothers,

Upton, Lee (1989) "Eating Our Way Toward Wisdom: M. F. K. Fisher's Oysters." *Cooking by the Book: Food in Literature and Culture*. Ed. Mary Anne Schofield. Bowling Green, OH: Bowling Green University Press.

Williams-Forson, Psyche (2006) *Building Houses Out of Chicken Legs: Black Women, Food, & Power*. Chapel Hill: University of North Carolina Press.

——(2012) "Other Women Cooked for My Husband: Negotiating Gender, Food, and Identities in an African American/Ghanian Household." *Taking Food Public*. Carole Counihan and Psyche Williams-Forson, eds. New York: Routledge.

Witt, Doris (2004)*Black Hunger: Soul Food and America*. Minneapolis: University of Minnesota Press.

Yaeger, Patricia (1988) *Honey-Mad Women: Emancipatory Strategies in Women's Writing*. New York: Columbia University Press.

Zafar, Rafia (2002) "The Signifying Dish: Autobiography and History in Two Black Women's Cookbooks." *Food in the USA: A Reader*. Carole M. Counihan, ed. New York: Routledge.

Zlotnick, Susan (1996) "Domesticating Imperialism: Curry and Cookbooks in Victorian England." *Frontiers* 16.2–3: 51–69.

24

Culinary arts and foodservice management

Vivian Liberman and Jonathan Deutsch

It would seem obvious that opportunities exist for food studies scholars in the professional field of cooking and serving food, but these opportunities are relatively recent developments. This chapter considers three predominant career and practical opportunity areas for food studies scholars in culinary arts and foodservice management.

1. *Educating future cooks and chefs in cultural and social aspects of food, food systems and food policy. Most culinary schools now include coursework on gastronomy so that hands-on and management studies in cooking are contextualized in the history and culture of the profession.*
2. *Working with the foodservice industry to design and market products and services that will appeal to target markets. Food studies scholars can consider the cultural and social contexts of the markets and human behavior in relation to food. For example, foodservice operators on college campuses experience intense pressure to deliver sustainable food. Negotiating this commitment, communicating its advances and limitations to students, and being aware of consumer demands on the horizon is often assisted by a consultant food scholar.*
3. *Writing and communicating to industry. For example, the second author on this paper writes a weekly magazine advice column for restaurants[1] where industry research and best practices are summarized and made accessible to busy restaurant owners and chefs.*

Historical background and major theoretical approaches

For years, the foodservice and culinary industries merged art and craft, but it was not until recent times that academic studies began to align with the world of foodservice and culinary management. To be sure, nutrition departments had been studying foodservice for most of the twentieth century, as had its later spinoffs in hospitality management programs and hotel schools in the US (hotel schools were long established in Europe). But, to generalize, rarely was the lens reversed—cooks simply were not trained in the academic study of food; it was the rare tradesman who had access to higher education. Cooking was a trade whereas gastronomes and food scholars were not cooks by profession, though many no doubt knew their way around a kitchen. Even erudite "chefs' chefs" like Antonin Careme, Auguste Escoffier, and Fernand Point, leaders in the cooking trade, came up through apprenticeships rather than formal education in the study of food.

For a long time, people who entered the culinary industry, especially in the West, did so because it was a family tradition, because they (or their families) needed the financial security that an apprenticeship could offer, or because it was an industry that allowed for success with minimal formal education. The culinary industry was (and to a large extent remains) an environment filled with drugs, alcohol, and a schedule alternate to that of many formally educated workers. "My cooks, for one: every one of them came from the Fortune Society, guys who spent their off-hours in halfway houses, allowed out only to work." (Bourdain, 2000: 146). "If the restaurant industry was likened to a class hierarchy, we could think of the back of the house as the working, the front of the house as the middle, and the owners as upper strata" (Sen and Mamdouh, 2008: 122). Culinary skills, techniques, and knowledge were learned within the confines of the kitchen.

Many chefs learned their craft on the job, and not in a college. They worked with craftsmen (and they were mostly men) who took them under their wings and taught them what they knew. Once they had learned all there was to learn there, they would go to another place to learn more or to take over a kitchen. Thomas Keller, one of the best chefs in the United States, began his career in a restaurant managed by his mother and continued his education in Europe where he worked at numerous well-known restaurants (Thomas Keller Restaurant Group, 2007). Joe Bastianich, restauranteur, winemaker, and now celebrity, did the same, after leaving behind a formal education (Bastianich, 2011). Today, culinary and food education are more popular, and more academic institutions have begun to offer degrees within food preparation, food science, and more recently food studies.

The cooking trade stood in sharp contrast to academe, which focused more on nourishing the mind. When food was discussed it was often in the form of agriculture studies, nutrition or food science. The food studies field has managed to convene academics with culinarians and restaurateurs and join forces to allow academics to study food and chefs and restaurant managers to study food with academic lenses.

With the professionalization of the foodservice and culinary field, the ongoing formalizing of Western culinary education, and the media attention and celebrity status brought upon chefs over the last few decades, opportunities exist for food scholars to work with aspiring and established chefs and foodservice operations.

Teaching food studies in a culinary program

Formal culinary education (differentiating from schools of home economics and culinary apprenticeship programs) in the US began with the inception of the Culinary Institute of America, which opened in 1946 in New Haven, CT, poised to take advantage of returning Second World War veterans using their GI bill tuition. Two women, Frances Roth and Katharine Angell, decided that to make great cooks, a great training program was needed and the school was meant to graduate the best cooks. In the 1970s they moved to Hyde Park, NY, to build a better-suited school on the former campus of a Jesuit novitate (Culinary Institute of America, 2011). Meanwhile, the 1950s saw an emergence of interest in food technology in the United States. Colleges such as Rutgers (Rutgers, 2007), UC Davis (UC Davis, 2011) and many others were founded or expanded within this time, with research done on the chemistry of food. Food technology, culinary arts, and hospitality management became more standard offerings, closely aligned with the food industry. All of these related to the preparation, service, and processing of foods.

In the early 1990s, the emergence Food Network served to glamorize the foodservice and culinary industries. Emeril Lagasse, Giada de Laurentis, Rachael Ray and others made professional cooking look like a fun profession. As chefs and restaurateurs became more glamorized by TV, customers began to expect to see the chef at the restaurant, maybe even meet them. The customer expectations grew and food became more of a subject of interest through over 60 shows and many bestselling cookbooks that followed (Mitchell, 2010). This spotlight on the profession of the chef further demanded that chefs be well-versed not only in cooking skills but the general picture of food and the food system and be comfortable articulating an informed opinion. The study and practice of food became more acceptable, and cooking more approachable. Since its creation, the Food Network has continued to grow in viewership (there is now a separate cooking channel), as has the study of food and the number of culinary arts and food studies programs in the United States and around the world (Mitchell, 2010).

Education and food have merged in the practical sense with the opening of more culinary programs both in the public and the private sectors of education. Allculinaryschools.com lists close to 40 different private colleges (typically for-profit institutions) that offer culinary diplomas, certificates, associates and bachelors degrees. In addition, more community colleges such as Kingsborough Community College, Miami Dade College, Oakland Community College, and many more are in the limelight to offer affordable, high-quality education within the culinary, hospitality, and nutrition fields. According to the US Department of Education, there are 378 colleges offering culinary arts programs within the United States and Puerto Rico and 334 colleges offering hospitality programs, many of which include a cooking component, and of course prepare students for a career in foodservice (US Department of Education). These include private, public, and those offering all kinds of degrees and offering financial aid (US Department of Education). In addition to what are now known as traditional culinary degrees, offering culinary skills, cooking techniques, and all the necessary preparation required to enter a career as a line cook en route to become a chef, culinary and foodservice have merged with traditional science, journalism, writing, and other fields to focus on practical applications of the field, or use food to help study the field itself.

Science and food join forces to popularize molecular gastronomy. Hervé This, Ferran Adrià, and many more chefs and scientists have been studying the physical and chemical changes of food. With this understanding, they have been able to modify food and speed up the chemical processes. This has become such a central part of modern cuisine that many chefs are now more interested in the study of food, in order to help them achieve these techniques. On the other hand, scientists use food as a medium of study at Harvard University, where Chef Ferran Adrià has now become a guest faculty member at seminars in chemistry and physics, which have been a part of a series titled "Science and Cooking: A Dialogue" (Andrews, 2010).

Culinary and foodservice careers are no longer just about cooking and running hotels and restaurants. Moving up the ladder in a kitchen—and, increasingly, onto the television screen and newspaper pages—requires more than culinary technique. Due to the myriad opportunities a culinarian or hospitality professional can take, preparation beyond the technical became imperative to be able to compete within the field. The foodservice industry is shaped like a pyramid, where the people within higher positions are very few and the skilled workers at the bottom abound. To better prepare those chefs and entrepreneurs, the curriculum of these colleges is generally well rounded and will include courses in business, culinary arts, and gastronomy.

Culinary colleges include history and culture lessons within their cooking curriculum. The structure of the French-style professional kitchen, also known as the brigade system, is best understood through the culinary history that helped build the modern culinary world. In addition, the use and selection of ingredients and the ability to understand culinary cultures is impacted by the exchange of ingredients throughout history. Due to Department of Education requirements, accreditation requirements, as well as interest in providing a better-rounded education for the students, culinary colleges include general education courses within other liberal arts areas.

A food studies degree becomes valuable within culinary education because it becomes the link between the logical and the practical. Students within culinary colleges will need to be exposed to great chefs, who in turn will teach them how to successfully prepare dishes and hone their techniques. However, they will also need to learn the theoretical areas of the field. Teaching general education courses within culinary colleges is the perfect fit for candidates with a food studies degree, since it introduces the discipline through a food frame.

Colleges are in need of food studies experts, since when the programs are being developed, it is important to understand the practical needs of a graduate as well as the theoretical knowledge that will complement it. The curriculum should be developed in a manner that will incorporate both aspects: Practical and theoretical. Food studies has been a field that has elevated food education to an intellectual level, which allows for people with this background to have an education appropriate to consult for curriculum development in colleges, among other aspects.

Of special appeal are jobs in food studies for candidates who possess both a practical and theoretical understanding of food, to build credibility among students. This type of "scholar in whites" can model for students the value for cooks of having a well-rounded perspective. Relevant coursework common to culinary programs includes culinary math, food history, food and culture, international cuisine, cultural foods, food policy, and food product identification and selection.

Profile

Beth Forrest, a graduate of Boston University's history department, has dedicated her research to food. As a food historian, she has joined the ranks of food education, first at Boston University, where she taught a research methodologies course for the Food Studies Program. Understanding the impact of food history and gastronomy in the lives of culinarians, she has since begun teaching gastronomy at the renowned Culinary Institute of America. Her experience working in restaurants throughout her life allows her to demonstrate that combination of the practical and theoretical within the foodservice and food studies field.

Working with the foodservice industry

Large food companies rely on food scientists and engineers to create new products, but it is the marketing people who sell the product to the world of consumers. Gastronomy can include more than just a liberal arts perspective to food. Within the area of the business of food, as well as a sociological and anthropological approach of the study of people and their consumer behaviors, we are able to study trends and behavioral patterns.

Profile

Kara Nielsen, a graduate of the Boston University Gastronomy Program, has taken this direction and joined her degree in gastronomy with her prior culinary and management experience to the Center for Culinary Development, where she is a trendologist. The center develops products within the foodservice industry and relies on Nielsen's experience to discover the trends within the areas and study the community's consumer behaviors. What do people want to eat? What are they buying? What products are needed within the market to satisfy these needs? What will consumers want next? And years from now? These are some of the questions they seek to answer.

Most large food companies continue to innovate products to compete with other companies and maintain consumer loyalty. Food studies professionals who understand business, consumer behavior, and food, can be the perfect candidates for such a company. Understanding what people want to eat, and how to make a product with a competitive advantage over those already in the market that may be comparable, is important for the survival of a food company wanting to keep up in the highly competitive consumer packaged goods and foodservice markets.

Food corporations with research and development departments rely on people with research skills for market research, sensory and consumer analysis, and trend reports, to name a few. In addition, foodservice operations experience an ongoing struggle to stay in front of consumer needs—creating culturally relevant menus, communicating sustainability philosophies, introducing cultural foods to a new market, and projecting future trends and demands are all opportunities for the food scholar working with industry.

Improving upon a business sometimes is done best from the outside. Business consultants exist within every field, including foodservice. In order to consult for a business, a person must be equipped with practical and theoretical knowledge. Within foodservice, there are numerous areas of consulting: Restaurants, food companies, and universities are a few.

Consulting for restaurants can include creating a concept (menu, décor, service style, theme), writing a business plan, finding investors, and doing market research. All of these would require knowledge easily acquired within a food studies program. Food studies graduates who have taken a business approach or have industry experience can consult on the financial health of a company and how to improve it. This can be both a for-profit or non-profit food production or foodservice operation. Having a higher education and understanding social aspects of food make great grant writers, food journalists, and promoters.

Market research is one of the most important components of a business plan, financial success for a company, and its competitive advantage. Food companies compete with one another, oftentimes with the same type of product. Understanding what the competing companies are offering, about their products, and the demographic they promote to and target, will allow for new product development, better marketing, and sales.

Writing

Plenty of food magazines, television shows, blogs, and other media require people who have an understanding of food, research methodologies, and writing skills. Publications such as *America's Test Kitchen* and *Cook's Country* are research-driven from both the theoretical and practical perspectives. The test kitchen develops recipes through trial and error, while the editorial department thoroughly looks to find out the theoretical behind the practice, and explain it in layman's terms that will appeal to the regular home cook.

In addition, a number of trade magazines for the culinary and foodservice industry seek to make industry research accessible, inform readers of new trends and developments, showcase innovative practices, and provide advice. Food scholars, especially those with practical experience, often write for these publications. *Restaurant Business*, *Nation's Restaurant News*, and the American Culinary Federation's *The National Culinary Review* are just a few of the many publications within the trade.

The food sections in newspapers are a good entry into the world of food writing for students interested in food journalism. These serve as a platform to build a portfolio that can be expanded into feature writing within national magazines such as *Food and Wine* and *Saveur* and other consumer publications. Often these publications demand both the practical (recipe or instructional article) and the theoretical (history, culture, or folklore of the food), so work in this field is well suited to a food studies scholar with practical training.

Research methodologies

Research among food scholars in culinary arts and foodservice management is very much applied research, often serving industry or an organization. Examples of published research include program evaluations, studies of a practice used in the profession, or analysis of a program in culinary, foodservice, or hospitality education. Of course much of the research in culinary arts and foodservice is intended for market understanding and is not intended for publication. A wide range of qualitative and quantitative methodologies are drawn upon, with a prevailing guideline of using the methods that have the potential to best answer the research question.

An example of relevant research illustrating each of these areas follows:

Program evaluation: Raizman, Debra J.; Montgomery, Deanna H.; Osganian, Stavroula K.; Ebzery, Mary Kay; *et al.* "CATCH: Food service program process evaluation in a multicenter trial." *Health Education Quarterly* Vol. Suppl. 2, 1994, S51-S71.

> Excerpt from Abstract: "Describes the process evaluation system for Eat Smart, a component of the Child and Adolescent Trial in Cardiovascular Health (CATCH), which focuses on menu planning, food purchasing, food preparation, and program promotion within schools. Eat Smart aims to decrease total fat, saturated fatty acids, and sodium in school meals. The Eat Smart process evaluation assesses the intervention, contextual factors, and external and competing programs that may affect implementation and influence study outcomes."

A practice in the profession: Lisa Sheehan-Smith, "Key Facilitators and Best Practices of Hotel-Style Room Service in Hospitals." *Journal of the American Dietetic Association* Vol. 106, Issue 4, April 2006: 581–86.

> "This qualitative study sought to identify the features, advantages, and disadvantages of hotel-style room service; the barriers to, and facilitators for, implementing the process; and 'best practices.' The study took place in four heterogeneous hospitals. Participants included hospital administrators, managers, and room-service employees. Data-collection methods included semi-structured interviews, observations, and document analysis."

A program in hospitality education: Alison Morrison and G. Barry O'Mahony "The liberation of hospitality management education." *International Journal of Contemporary Hospitality Management*, Vol. 15 Iss.: 1 (2003): 38–44.

> "Hospitality management higher education's historic origins have resulted in a strong vocational ethos permeating the curriculum. Knowledge about hospitality has been drawn from the industry and the world of work rather than from the many disciplines or other fields of enquiry, which can help to explain it. By the late 1990s there was a strengthening international movement, driven by higher education hospitality academics towards the liberation of hospitality management higher education from its vocational base and to explore the inclusion in the curriculum of a broader and more reflective orientation. This paper investigates the historical evolution of hospitality management education, concepts associated with liberal education, and provides an illustrative case study that evaluates how a more liberal base was introduced into the curriculum at two universities located in Australia and Scotland respectively."

In all three of these "baskets" of research traditional research methods are enhanced by a researcher's understanding of the practical considerations of foodservice management and culinary arts or hospitality education and applied to practice, including for-profit, non-profit, and education. Venues for presenting and publishing work in this area include the meetings of the Association for the Study of Food and Society (ASFS) and Agriculture, Food and Human Values Society (AFHVS), the International Council of Hotel and Restaurant Industry Educators (ICHRIE), Foodservice Educators Learning Community (FELC), and the International Foodservice Executives Association (IFSEA). Relevant journals include the *Journal of Foodservice*; *Food, Culture and Society*; *Agriculture, Food and Human Values*; *Journal of Hospitality and Tourism Education*; *Ecology of Food and Nutrition*; and *Cornell Hotel Administration Quarterly*.

Avenues for future research

In addition to the types of research delineated above, the coming years will bring many more opportunities for food scholars in culinary arts and food management. Examples include:

- evaluations of sustainability programs in foodservice;
- policy research on ethical procurement;
- evaluation of cooks' role in improving public health;
- food processing methods, and ethical implications;
- using food as a teaching tool within other disciplines;
- food education and its impact on global health;
- consumer navigation/understanding of the food system;
- school foodservice as co-educator.

Practical considerations

A food scholar looking to have impact in the culinary and foodservice world is best served by having both practical and food studies education. Practical culinary training coupled with industry experience gives a candidate a strong footing to be a credible trusted source when working with industry. In addition, graduate study in any discipline with a focus on food or in an interdisciplinary food studies or gastronomy program can provide the research and writing skills and food studies and food systems knowledge needed for success in this field.

Both food studies and culinary programs often make available scholarships for study. These scholarships are often funded by individual hospitality or foodservice companies (such as Hilton or Aramark), or industry associations (such as the National Restaurant Association Education Foundation or Les Dames d'Escoffier). Often, universities will also offer assistantships for the students within these departments to work in their administrative offices or teach, in exchange for tuition reimbursement. Some departments offer limited funding for students and sponsor their graduate education as well.

Many trade associations host conferences where graduate students can compete by submitting their papers. Oftentimes these competitions will offer a cash prize to the students who place within the competition. Many departments will fund the student's registration fee and travel expenses to these conferences, offering scholarships for their advancement within the field. These conferences are also a great networking tool for students trying to integrate their practical background into the theoretical realm of food studies. Membership within an association such as the American Culinary Federation and participation in their events, competitions, and expositions, will allow for the honing of practical skills and the building up of a network of skilled workers. In addition, medaling at their competitions will usually include cash prizes and scholarship opportunities, depending on the type of membership held.

Trade associations are a great source of educational resources and networking opportunities. Some associations focus on the practical needs of the industry. The National Restaurant Association gathers information needed for restaurant business owners to run a successful operation. They publish educational resources that provide training materials for the most important certifications and applications of the foodservice industry.

The American Culinary Federation is divided in regional chapters where chefs, cooks, and culinary students can get to know each other and use each other as resources. They promote furthering education through their certification programs, which range from certified culinarians through Certified Master Chefs and Certified Master Pastry Chefs. Those certifications require practical examinations as well as theoretical courses and tests that will mark the levels of accomplishment of chefs moving up the ranks. In addition, they have the CCE (Certified Culinary Educator), which requires the educator to film a class in which they are performing specific culinary skills in front of a class of students. Based on the video coupled with a written evaluation, the chef will achieve that level of certification (American Culinary Federation).

The above mentioned are just two of the many associations within the culinary and foodservice field from a practical perspective. Others include the Bread Bakers Guild, the Hotel Lodging Association, Research Chefs of America, International Association of Culinary Professionals, among many more. All of these require membership.

Many academic disciplines also have their own trade associations. However, for more academic participation, some of the interdisciplinary organizations become a more obvious choice for foodservice professionals. Membership in associations such as the Association for the Study of Food and Society (ASFS) and the Association for the Study of Food and Human Values Society (AFHVS) allow practical and theoretical approaches to be intertwined. The members of these associations are widespread in their experience and expertise and their joint conference invites a wide variety of subjects and lenses of the study of food and agriculture.

Each of the before-mentioned associations have their unique publication that allows for readership and contribution from their members. The culinary associations generally have a less academic approach to their journals, with more of a newspaper/newsletter style to their publication. These publications are weekly or monthly, allowing for frequent updates on the happenings within the industry. The interdisciplinary and academic associations, however, publish quarterly journals, which are more academic in style. Portions of papers and reviews of academic books are featured within them, making the readership smaller than the ones previously mentioned.

Note

1 monkeydish.com/ideas/advice-guy (accessed on April 5, 2012).

Key reading

Belasco, W. (2008) *Food: The Key Concepts*. Oxford: Berg.

Brizek, M. G. and M. A. Khan (2002) "Ranking of U.S. Hospitality Undergraduate Hospitality Programs: 2000–2001." *Journal of Hospitality and Tourism Education* 14 (2): 4–8.

Deutsch, J. and A. Hauck-Lawson, eds. (2004) "Food Voice in the Classroom: A Collection of Teaching Tools." *Food, Culture and Society: An International Journal of Multidisciplinary Research* 1 (1): 108–133.

Deutsch, J. and J. Miller, (2010) *Food Studies*. Oxford: Berg.

Miller, J., J. Deutsch, and Y. Sealey-Ruiz (2005). "Food Studies as a Mechanism for Advancing Multicultural Education in Hospitality Programs." *Journal of Hospitality and Tourism Education* Winter.

Ruark, J. K. (1999). A Place at the Table. *Chronicle of Higher Education* 45 (44), A–7, chronicle.com/article/ More-Scholars-Focus-on/15471 (accessed on May 1, 2012).

Wolf, Marina (2001, May). "Food for Thought: Food-studies scholars pursue truth at the table." *MetroActive Dining* March 5, 2001, www.metroactive.com/papers/sonoma/.03.01/foodstudies-0118.html (accessed on October 13, 2003).

Bibliography

American Culinary Federation. www.acfchefs.org (accessed October 11, 2011).

Andrews, Colman (2010) "Gastronaut." *Bloomberg Business Week*, no. 4194: 62–67.

Association for the Study of Food and Society. www.food-culture.org (accessed October 11, 2011).

Bourdain, Anthony (1999) Don't Eat Before Reading This. *The New Yorker*, April 19.

——(2000) *Kitchen Confidential: Adventures in the Culinary Underbelly*. London: Bloomsbury.

Joseph Bastianich (2011) www.joebastianich.com (accessed October 11, 2011).

Mitchell, Christine M. (2010) "The Rhetoric of Celebrity Cookbooks." *Journal of Popular Culture*, 43 (3), 524–39.

National Restaurant Association. www.restaurant.org (accessed October 11, 2011).

Rutgers, the State University of New Jersey (2007) www.rutgers.edu (accessed September 20, 2011).

Sen, R., and F. Mamdouh (2008) *The accidental American Immigration and Citizenship in the Age of Globalization*. San Francisco, CA: Berrett-Koehler Publishers.

The Creative Kitchen. thecreativekitchen.com (accessed October 1, 2011).

The Culinary Institute of America (2011) www.ciachef.edu (accessed September 20, 2011).

Thomas Keller Restaurant Group (2007) www.tkrg.org (accessed September 20, 2011).

UC Davis (2011) www.ucdavis.edu (accessed September 20, 2011).

US Department of Education. ed.gov (accessed October 1, 2011).

25

Food, cultural studies, and popular culture

Fabio Parasecoli

Food studies shares with cultural studies its focus on the connections between lived bodies, imagined realities, and structures of power. Both disciplines acknowledge that not only material practices, but also desires, fantasies, fears, and dreams coagulating around food, its production, preparation, and consumption, deeply influence our development as individual subjects and as members of all kinds of social formations. Lived food experiences, including recipes, food-related traditions, cooking techniques, even daily shopping, should then be analyzed in their relations with power structures such as the food industry, marketing and advertising firms, political lobbies, academic institutions, and media.

Cultural studies, an academic field that developed from the late 1950s, aims to understand contemporary cultures by examining their internal dynamics, their everyday performances, and their media representations, including expressions of popular and mass culture. Grounded in Marxian and post-structuralist critical theory, cultural studies explores how meaning is generated, disseminated, reproduced, negotiated, and resisted through values, beliefs, symbols, practices, institutions, as well as economic, social, and political structures within a given culture. Acknowledging the fluidity and constant transformation of its object of study, especially under the acceleration imparted by technological innovations and globalization, cultural studies critiques any a priori hierarchies imposed on the various facets of a culture, based on aesthetic, moral, or historical values, which the discipline actually considers as part of what needs to be analyzed as expression of class and other social dynamics (Simon, 1999; Swirski, 2005).

Popular culture is sometimes referred to as mainstream culture, or that which is popular with the masses, and its study is at times considered as a subfield resulting from the combination of cultural studies and communication studies. However, for the purpose of this article, popular culture is defined as the totality of ideas, values, representations, material items, practices, social relations, organizations, institutions, and other phenomena that are conceived, produced, distributed, and consumed within a market- and consumption-influenced environment, with or without the specific economic goal of reaping a profit. This definition both includes the mainstream and all possible alternative or oppositional subcultures, as well as the dynamics through which the mainstream is established, opposed, and constantly evolving. For example, specific subgroups in a society may develop their own forms of expression, through which they may directly or indirectly criticize and oppose the mainstream. Yet, by so doing they inherently engage with it, often fueling the interest of the very cultural apparatuses that they initially aimed to undermine. As a consequence, aspects of their subculture may eventually be taken out of context, absorbed, and used in mainstream popular culture.

Cultural studies shares many common elements with food studies, which promotes and practices the analysis of cultural, social, and political issues concerning the production, distribution, representation, and consumption of food. However, they differ mainly in that while cultural studies has historically focused on specific communities and subcultures, exploring expressions and practices among which food might or might not be featured, food studies concentrates its attention on food in its material, representational, and symbolic aspects as they unfold across societies, communities, and subcultures.

The presence of food in everyday life is pervasive, permeating popular culture as a relevant marker of power, cultural capital, class, gender, ethnicity, and religion, which both cultural and food studies recognize as crucial. Consequently, both disciplines are well equipped to examine lived food experiences, including recipes, food-related traditions, cooking techniques, even daily shopping, in their relations with power structures such as the food industry, marketing and advertising firms, political lobbies, academic institutions, and media.

Food studies and cultural studies share a keen interest in the fraught and complex connections between lived bodies, imagined realities, and structures of power built around food. Both disciplines acknowledge that not only the material aspects of individual and communal practices, but also desires, fantasies, fears, and dreams coagulating around and in the body, deeply influence our development as individual subjects and as members of all kinds of social formations. However, the ubiquitous nature of the cultural elements relating to food makes their ideological and political relevance almost invisible, buried in the supposedly natural and self-evident fabric of everyday life. Meanwhile, our own flesh becomes fuel for all kinds of cultural battles among different visions of personhood, family, society, polity, and economics. Employing cultural studies' political sensibilities, its attention for lived experiences, and its critical approach towards cultural hierarchies, food studies can provide an accessible analytical framework to achieve a deeper comprehension of twenty-first-century globalized post-industrial societies.

Historical background of food scholarship in cultural studies and major theoretical approaches in use

Despite their similarity of approach and intellectual project, very little scholarship in food studies has explicitly acknowledged its debt to cultural studies in terms of attention to material culture and the way it is experienced by specific communities enmeshed in complex power structures. Probably due to the disciplinary provenance of its practitioners, most works in food studies locate themselves within more established traditions, especially history, geography, sociology, anthropology, American studies, and media analysis. As food studies grows in terms of popularity, academic respectability, as well as numbers of dedicated departments and students, it is likely that scholars will feel more comfortable in identifying themselves with the new field, and as a consequence will be more open to recognize food studies' debt to other multidisciplinary and relatively recent fields of research, including cultural studies. At the same time, cultural studies might more frequently include food among its topics of investigation, originating work that could fall under both disciplines. Due to the lack of research on food explicitly falling under cultural studies and presented by its practitioners as such, this section will first briefly introduce the origin of cultural studies, and then focus on food scholarship that presents common traits with cultural studies, despite its possible formal classification under other academic traditions.

The foundation of the theoretical approach that would be later defined as cultural studies is usually identified with Richard Hoggart's *The Uses of Literacy* (1957) and Raymond Williams's *Culture and Society* (1958) and *The Long Revolution* (1961), which in different ways point to the vitality and richness of contemporary "mass" culture and its expression through language, places of socialization and entertainment, new technologies, and popular media, among others. A living culture is not only made of its highest achievements and literary works, but also of all sorts of material artifacts, texts, representations, behaviors, attitudes, institutions, and places that constitute the framework of analysis of what Williams defined as "structures of feeling": the particular living result of all the elements in the general organization of a culture in a certain period (1961: 48). In 1964 the new discipline found a home in the newly launched Centre for Contemporary Cultural Studies at the University of Birmingham, directed by Hoggart and soon after by Stuart Hall. Drawing from critical theory, semiotics, and sociology, but also influenced by feminist theory, the Centre introduced the Gramscian concept of cultural hegemony, interpreted as the manipulation of the value system by the ruling class to establish its cultural dominance and to impose its world view as natural and beneficial to society as a whole, to understand the dynamics of power and dominance that shape popular culture. However, the Center tended to consider citizens not as defenseless dupes that accepted whatever was presented to them by the cultural industry, but rather as capable of producing their own interpretations and uses of any mass culture object. For example, in the essay "Encoding and Decoding in Television Discourse" (Hall, 1973) Stuart Hall argued that media producers often find their intended messages failing to get across to their audiences, who instead distort it or accept it quite selectively, depending on their cultural, social, and political environment and by doing so resist any attempt at dominating their worldview and sensibility.

Over time, researchers in cultural studies turned their attention to subcultures, delineated as social groups within a larger society that differentiated themselves through the adoption of specific behaviors, languages, dress codes, and modes of congregating. The discipline was also influenced by the work of the French theorist Michel Foucault, who focused on the analysis of discourse and the structures of power that at the same time it constitutes and expresses. Under the influence of French theory and upon its diffusion in the US and Australia, cultural studies lost some of its more political undertones and the concern about class that had characterized it in Birmingham, while shifting its focus on identity issues such as gender, sexuality, embodiment, ethnicity, race, nationality, status, and consumption, and maintaining a constant and productive interaction with similar developments in queer studies, performance studies, and media studies.

Food studies, as an interdisciplinary field that deals with a specific aspect of material culture, its representations, and its lived experiences, has often embraced subject matters, theoretical frameworks, research methodologies, and predilection for the qualitative that would also fall under the heading of cultural studies. Based on previous classificatory schemes elaborated in other disciplines by Goody (1982), Mennell, Murcott and Van Otterloo (1992) and Beardsworth and Keil (1997), in their volume on food and cultural studies – so far the only one explicitly dedicated to the relationship among the two disciplines – Bob Ashley (2004) and his colleagues at Nottingham Trent University identify three distinct approaches: Structuralist, Culturalist, and Gramscian.

The structuralist approach, inspired by the work of Claude Lévi-Strauss and Roland Barthes, analyzes food as a cultural system and as a code continuously producing signs that allow a specific community to engage in meaningful symbolic action. However, the meaning of food signs, generated by the differences between all the elements in the system as a whole rather than by pre-existing and defined signification, can never be fixed, revealing itself as variable, contested, and incomplete. Food does not have any intrinsic and natural meaning, if taken separately from the social and cultural habits that surround it, which at any rate are closely connected with it, to form a complex set of practices and representations. Examples of this approach would be Mary Douglas's "Deciphering a Meal" (1975), where the renowned anthropologist analyzes the structure of a meal in terms of acceptability and cultural communication, and Jean Soler's "The Semiotics of Food in The Bible" (1973), which interprets the dietary prescriptions of the Bible in terms of underlying cultural structures and the oppositions and differences that determine them. Structuralist frameworks have been often evaluated unenthusiastically because of their intrinsic difficulty in explaining change. Furthermore, they tend to highlight the preeminence of systems of meanings in which individuals are born into rather than the initiative and autonomy of individuals and communities.

Culturalist approaches, on the other hand, focus on the value of lived experiences of people and their agency, often underlining their resistance to power. Michel De Certeau's *The Practice of Everyday Life* (1984), for instance, theorizes that consumers' tactics are a form of struggle against the strategies put into place by economic and political powers. This kind of culturalism has been criticized for its tendency to essentialism and to romanticized representations of its subjects, the sensibility towards the transmission and the reproduction of culture. However, the emphasis on the creativity and autonomy of subcultures, including all kinds of marginal communities, and the participated description of their lives has generated excellent research not only on migrant communities, ethnic, and racial minorities, but also on the connection between memory and present-day customs (Adapon, 2008; Fine, 1996; Ray, 2004).

The necessity to take change into account has led to what Mennell (1996) and Beardsworth and Keil (1997) have defined as a developmental approach, corresponding to what Ashley *et al.* (2004) define as the Gramscian approach when its focus shifts to the constant negotiations between cultural groups and social classes, as well as to the hegemonic dynamics engendering ever-changing configurations of domination and subordination. While emphasizing the power of the leisure industries, media, government, advertisers, and politicians, this approach has also been influenced by cultural theory and post-structuralism, adopting the analysis of discourse, ideology, and frames, the theorization of contextual and multiple subjectivities in the absence of prevalent narratives, and the examination of consumption and lifestyles as identity markers, also as expressed in popular culture, media, and other kinds of performances (Belasco, 1989; Johnston and Bauman, 2010; Williams-Forson, 2006).

Research methodologies

Due to its inherent multidisciplinarity, food studies employs information, theoretical frameworks, and methodologies developed in academic traditions as diverse as social and political theory, political economy, nutrition, biology, agronomy, the culinary arts, history, philosophy, literary and art criticism, feminist and queer theory, performance studies, and media and communication studies. What can the research approaches developed so far in the exploration of food bring to cultural studies and its understanding of popular cultures and their connection with power structures? And what can cultural studies contribute to food studies in terms of methods?

Sharing with cultural studies its concern towards social differentiation, stratification, and inequality both in its synchronic and historical dimensions, food studies has often borrowed analytical tools and methods from sociology and history (Caldwell, 2004; Caldwell, Dunn and Nestle, 2009). At the same time, it underlines the importance of the lived aspects of these dynamics, which has led to the discipline's preference for qualitative research and its penchant for what Geertz (1973) called "thick description." Consequently, the food-related research that could also be considered under the cultural studies discipline has often had recourse to the anthropological method of ethnography, based on fieldwork and different forms of observation and participation, which are also integrated with an emphasis on the material and performative cultural forms that used to constitute the domain of research of folklorists (Adema, 2009; Bestor, 2004; Farquhar, 2002; Wenner, 2009).

At the same time, due to the globalized and instantly connected nature of contemporary pop culture, both in its mainstream and oppositional aspects, food studies and cultural studies have made frequent use of concepts and methods developed in post-colonial studies, global studies, ethnic studies, gender studies, semiotic, discourse analysis, media and communication studies. New conceptualizations of the connection among seemingly distant elements, influencing each other and surfacing in the most unexpected contexts, are being developed (Parasecoli, 2008). A given ingredient or food-related practice can be analyzed, embraced, or demonized by scientists and nutritionists, media gurus, politicians in search of visibility, and social activists in different parts of the world and different cultural and social contexts. Their diverse and often opposite conclusions may then be picked up in bits and pieces by newspapers, magazines, TV talk shows, and blogs, influencing consumers' expectations and behaviors, creating fads and fashions, generating new and always shifting practices and subcultures. At the same time these changes may influence the manufacture of novel products by the food industry, which translates into nutritional claims, advertising, marketing campaigns, and changes in distribution chains that in turn interact with consumers' perceptions and shopping habits, scientists' research, and myriad social and political agendas. Cultural studies, and the food-related research that gets its inspiration from it, are outlining methods to grapple with the connections, the mechanisms, and even the malfunctions in the extensive, intrusive, and all-encompassing web of meanings, practices, and values that constitute the contemporary food world. To respond to these stimulations, some authors have adopted the approach developed by Appadurai *et al.* in *The Social Life of Things* (1986). The essays in the collection suggest that, rather than focusing on specific communities and how they incorporate a variety of food in their lived experiences, it can be effective to look at how specific ingredients, dishes, and foods acquire different cultural, social, and political meanings depending on their context of consumption (Watson, 1997; Watson and Caldwell, 2005).

Avenues for future research

The food-related research in cultural studies has the potential to expand in many directions, applying scholarly analytical rigor and its emphasis on power and politics to phenomena in contemporary popular culture that so far have been the favorite domain of self-appointed cultural commentators, bloggers, and journalists.

Well-established subcultures sprouted around food issues, including foodies, vegetarians, vegans, locavores, dumpster divers, would deserve greater attention not only from the sociological and political points of view but also in terms of the lived experiences and the performances of newly built and shifting individual and collective identities. The same can be said of groups that embrace a diet as a permanent lifestyle out of religious or health motivations, or adopt a determined eating pattern to achieve specific physical goals, like athletes and body builders. While the symbolic, discursive, and psychological content of diets such as Weight Watchers and Atkins has been examined (Bentley, 2004; Hendley, 2003; Parasecoli, 2005a, 2005b; Stalker, 2009), the internal dynamics of the communities built around them have not been fully explored in terms of shared values, practices, and power relations.

Interesting subcultures also have grown around the symbolic and material negotiations around body images in their connection with food, in particular around fat. While foundational work in this direction has been produced in critical theory, gender studies, and media studies

(Bordo, 1993; Braziel and LeBesco, 2001; Rothblum, Solovay and Wann, 2009), cultural studies could give a unique contribution with its explicit analysis of how communities built around these issues create specific subcultures that may relate in diverse ways with the mainstream.

Both food studies and cultural studies could also find useful analytical tools to understand these aspects of food-related experiences in embodiment theory, which, starting from the 1980s, has underlined the interplay between brain, body, and world (Blackman, 2008). Building on Marcel Mauss's anthropological reflection the "techniques of the body" (1935) and Mikhail Bakhtin's work on Carnival and the grotesque in literary criticism (1965), this approach emphasizes how power and the principles it promotes are not always imposed on the subject from the outside, but are materialized through norms and regulations in the body itself. Although we perceive our body as natural – we are actually taught to categorize it as such – it would be naive to assume that these crucial elements of the embodied experience are irrelevant in terms of power relationship (as diffused as the power sources may be). We cannot exclude food and ingestion from hegemonic struggles. The way we categorize and experience our physical needs, the way we choose, store, prepare, cook, ingest, digest, and excrete food, are far from being neutral or innate.

Research has also highlighted the role of both sensory experiences and memory in the way individuals and communities experience and represent the consumption and distribution of food (Holtzman, 2006; Parasecoli, 2007; Sanchez Romera, 2007; Sutton, 2001, 2008). This approach disputes the understanding of bodies as pre-social, fixed, and static, but rather conceptualizes them as affective, permeable to the outside, always unfinished, and in process. They are not there just to be passively inscribed on by cultural and social norms, as malleable masses that cannot talk back. Through their connections with food, bodies show that nature and culture are deeply entangled, existing in complex relations that are contingent and mutable.

Practical considerations for getting started

Although the interest in food and food-related issues is growing rapidly, as the expansion of food studies as an academic field suggests, there are no cultural studies programs that focus specifically on food. However, since food studies is increasingly being recognized as a legitimate discipline and new departments are being established, students can apply to cultural studies programs in institutions where food studies is either present with its own department or practiced in other departments, and where students are allowed to focus on two areas of study rather than just one. However, since food studies is still a relatively recent field, especially when applying to a PhD program, students should make sure that there are advisors who share that particular interest.

Academic associations are important forums to network with other students and more established scholars, to explore possible directions of study, and to stay updated about recent research. The Association for the Study of Food and Society, the Association for Cultural Studies, the Cultural Studies Association (US), and the Popular Culture Association/American Studies Association organize yearly conferences and local meetings that accept graduate students' submissions for posters and panel presentations. They all have websites that provide helpful resources and links, and edit journals that can be useful for students' research and for the publication of their own work. Among the food studies journals that publish work that could fall under the heading of cultural studies we can mention *Food, Culture & Society*, *Food and Foodways*, and *Gastronomica*. Also journals focusing more specifically on cultural studies and popular culture accept food-related articles and essays, such as the digital journal *Lateral*, *Cultural Studies*, *The International Journal of Cultural Studies*, *Continuum* (with a specific interest also on media), the *Cultural Studies Review* (published in Australia), and *TOPIA: Canadian Journal of Cultural Studies*.

Fabio Parasecoli

Institutions that have cultural studies Masters and PhD programs offer frequent postdoctoral fellowships and scholarships. Announcement can be found on the websites and listservs of the above-mentioned associations, on university websites, and also on websites such as Humanities and Social Sciences Online (www.h-net.org), GoAbroad (scholarships.goabroad.com), and Free Scholarship Information (infoscholarship.net).

Key reading

Appadurai, Arjun (1986) *Social Life of Things: Commodities in Cultural Perspective*. Cambridge: Cambridge University Press.
Ashley Bob, Joanne Hollows, Steve Jones, and Ben Taylor (2004) *Food and Cultural Studies*. London and New York: Routledge.
Geertz, Clifford (1973) "Thick Description: Toward an Interpretive Theory of Culture". In *The Interpretation of Cultures: Selected Essays*. New York: Basic Books, pp. 3–30.
Swirski, Peter (2005) *From Lowbrow to Nobrow*. Montreal: McGill-Queen's University Press.

Bibliography

Adapon, Joy (2008) *Culinary Art and Anthropology*. Oxford: Berg.
Adema, Pauline (2009) *Garlic capital of the world: Gilroy, garlic, and the making of a festive foodscape*. Jackson: University Press of Mississippi.
Ashley Bob, Joanne Hollows, Steve Jones, and Ben Taylor (2004) *Food and Cultural Studies*. London and New York: Routledge.
Bakhtin, Mikhail (1984 [1965]) *Rabelais and his World*. Bloomington: Indiana University Press.
Beardsworth, Alan, and Teresa Keil (1997) *Sociology on the Menu*. London and New York: Routledge.
Belasco, Warren (2006 [1989]) *Appetite for Change: How the Counterculture Took on the Food Industry*. Ithaca, NY: Cornell University Press.
Bentley, Amy (2004) "The Other Atkins Revolution: Atkins and the Shifting Culture of Dieting." *Gastronomica* 4 (3): 34–45.
Bestor, Theodore C. (2004) *Tsukuji: The Fish Market at the Center of the World*. Berkeley and Los Angeles: University of California Press.
Blackman, Lisa (2008) *The Body*. Oxford: Berg.
Bordo, Susan (1993) *Feminism, Western Culture, and the Body*. Berkeley: University of California Press.
Braziel, Jana Evans and Kathleen Le Besco, eds. (2001) *Bodies out of bounds: fatness and transgression*. Berkeley: University of California Press.
Caldwell, Melissa L. (2004) *Not by Bread Alone: Social Support in the New Russia*. Berkeley and Los Angeles: University of California Press.
Caldwell, Melissa L., Elizabeth C. Dunn, Marion Nestle (2009) *Food and Everyday Life in the Postsocialist World*. Bloomington: Indiana University Press.
Crowley, Karlyn (2002) "Gender on a Plate: The Calibration of Identity in American Macrobiotics." *Gastronomica* 2 (3): 37–48.
De Certeau, Michel (1984) *The Practice of Everyday Life*. Berkeley and Los Angeles: University of California Press.
Douglas, Mary (1999 [1975]) "Deciphering a Meal." In Implicit Meanings: Selected Essays in Anthropology. London: Routledge, 231–51.
Farquhar, Judith (2002) *Appetites: Food and Sex in Post-socialist China*. Durham, NC and London: Duke University Press.
Fine, Gary Alan (1996) *Kitchens: The Culture of Restaurant Work*. Berkeley and Los Angeles: The University of California Press.
Goody, Jack (1982) *Cooking, Cuisine, and Class: A Study in Comparative Sociology*. Cambridge: Cambridge University Press.
Hall, Stuart (1980 [1973]) "Encoding/decoding." In Centre for Contemporary Cultural Studies (Ed.): *Culture, Media, Language: Working Papers in Cultural Studies*, 1972–79. London: Hutchinson, pp. 128–38.
Hendley, Joyce (2003) "Weight Watchers at Forty: A Celebration." *Gastronomica* 3(1): 16–21.
Hoggart, Richard (1957) *The Uses of Literacy: Aspects of Working Class Life*. London: Chatto and Windus.

280

Holtzman, Jon D. (2006) "Food and Memory." *Annual Revue of Anthropology* 35: 361–78.

Johnston, Josée and Shyon Bauman (2010) *Foodies: Democracy and Distinction in the Gourmet Foodscape*. New York: Routledge.

Mauss, Marcel (1973 [1935]) "Techniques of the Body." *Economy and Society* 2(1): 70–85.

Mennell, Stephen (1996) *All Manners of Food: Eating and Taste in England and France from the Middle Ages to the Present*. Urbana and Chicago: University of Illinois Press.

Mennell, Stephen, Anne Murcott, and Anneke H. Van Otterloo (1992) *The Sociology of Food: Eating, Diet, and Culture*. London: Sage.

Parasecoli, Fabio (2005a) "Feeding hard bodies: Food and nutrition in men's fitness magazines". *Food and Foodways* 13(1–2): 17–37.

——(2005b) "Low-carb Dieting and the Mirror: A Lacanian Analysis of the Atkins Diet." In *The Atkins Diet and Philosophy*. Lisa Heldke, Kerri Mommer, and Cynthia Pineo eds., pp. 196–212. Chicago, IL: Open Court.

——(2007) "Hungry Engrams: Food and Non-Representational Memory." In *Food and Philosophy*. Fritz Allhoff and Dave Monroe, eds., pp. 102–14. Malden, MA: Blackwell.

——(2008) *Bite Me: Food in Popular Culture*. Oxford: Berg.

Ray, Krishnendu (2004) *The Migrant's Table: Meals and Memories in Bengali-American Households*. Philadelphia: Temple University Press.

Rothblum Esther, Sondra Solovay, and Marilyn Wann, eds. (2009) *The Fat Studies Reader*. New York: New York University Press.

Sanchez Romera, Miguel (2007) *La neurogastronomia: la inteligencia emocional culinaria*. Madrid: Grupo Saned Ediciones-Verlag.

Simon, Richard Keller (1999) *Trash Culture: Popular Culture and the Great Tradition*. Berkeley: University of California Press.

Soler, Jean (1997 [1973]) "Semiotics of Food in the Bible." In *Food and Culture: A Reader*. Carole Counihan and Penny van Esterik, eds., pp. 55–66. London and New York: Routledge.

Stalker, Nancy (2009) "The Globalisation of Macrobiotics as Culinary Tourism and Culinary Nostalgia." *Asian Medicine* 5(1): 1–18.

Sutton, David (2001) *Remembrance of Repasts: An Anthropology of Food and Memory*. Oxford: Berg.

——(2008) "A Tale of Easter Ovens: Food and Collective Memory." *Social Research* 75(1): 157–80.

Swirski, Peter (2005) *From Lowbrow to Nobrow*. Montreal: McGill-Queen's University Press.

Watson, James L. (1997) *Golden Arches East: McDonald's in East Asia*. Stanford, CA: Stanford University Press.

Watson, James L. and Caldwell, Melissa L. (2005) *The Cultural Politics of Food and Eating*. Malden, MA: Blackwell.

Wenner, Lawrence (2009) *Sport, Beer, and Gender: Promotional Culture and Contemporary Social Life*. New York: Peter Lang.

Williams, Raymond (1958) *Culture and Society*. London: Chatto and Windus.

——(1961) *The Long Revolution*. London: Chatto and Windus.

Williams-Forson, Psyche (2006) *Building Houses out of Chicken Legs: Black Women, Food, and Power*. Chapel Hill: University of North Carolina Press.

26

Food and race

An overview

Psyche Williams-Forson and Jessica Walker

A rapidly evolving area of focus in food studies is the role of race and ethnicity. Using a number of methodological and theoretical approaches, this work holds race as central to examine such issues as the nature of race and ethnic relations in food systems and in food interactions; the ways in which race reveals inter-, intra-, and external group tensions in food relations; the structural processes that influence and contribute to the manifestation of racial and ethnic tensions; and the ways in which food can be a vehicle for identifying a community's responses to cultural and/or social maligning. This essay explores these tensions and considers also the ways that power dynamics are revealed in food and foodways when issues of race and ethnicity are held as central.

The last several years have witnessed efflorescence in the field of food studies with new work surfacing almost daily in every discipline and from every point of view. A rapidly evolving area of focus is the intersection of race and food. This work takes myriad approaches to placing race at the center of their analysis. These kinds of analyses include, for example, examining the nature of race and ethnic relations in food systems and in food interactions; ferreting out the ways in which race reveals inter-, intra-, and external group tensions in food relations; identifying the structural processes that influence and contribute to the manifestation of racial and ethnic tensions among communities; and studying how food can be a vehicle for identifying a community's responses to race and/or ethnic maligning. Additionally, food has been a lens for examining complex historical processes wherein power, race, class, and gender are central.

As an object, food offers us a way into cultural, political, economic, and techno-scientific history, and significant to these discussions, though often ignored or overlooked, is race, class, and gender. Food also offers a way to analyze race and gender relations from the standpoint of power because it is not limited to a single area of society but is implicit in the process of sharing cultural norms and values. Examining food from the standpoint of race reveals too how various groups exercise power in their everyday lives as well as the ways that influential institutions use food to monopolize power. Furthermore, we learn more how material and social relations are power-laden.[1]

In the main, what these arguments emphasize is that food is not value-free. Food, though it has plenty of nutritional relevance, is generally without any particular social value until it is placed in a certain political, economic, and cultural context. And when is food ever devoid of such contexts? It is in these instances that the meanings embedded in food are revealed to be much more than what meets the eye. Food then, is inextricably linked to the many variables of our identity—gender, class, ethnicity, region, able-bodiedness, and sexuality. Therefore, it stands to reason that food is also inseparably tied to race.

This discussion uses the framework of racial formation theory to define race as a socially constructed identity. From this point of view, in the United States, social, economic, and political forces rather than biology or physicality determine race.[2] Race, according to this definition, is also extremely fluid and changing, shaped by more than upbringing. How we view race and understand racial categories is influenced by where we see ourselves in the world and in relation to others. It is also influenced by the ways in which various ideologies operate in our lives and that of others.[3] From the ground to the table, this racial construct has always had an adverse affect on food producers, consumers, and workers manifesting in discriminatory practices, ideologies, stereotypes, and beliefs about people and their cultures.

In American society, race and ethnic relations refer to major race groups—white, black, Latina, and Asian. None of these blanket designations refer to the inherent differences between and among members of these groups. For example, "black" as a race includes a vast variety of ethnicities and peoples. Is the person from one of the many African countries or Caribbean nations? When we designate a person as "Asian" to whom are we referring—one who is Chinese, Taiwanese, Japanese, Korean, Filipino, Thai, Vietnamese, or Indonesian? Our tendency to reduce these very diverse ethnic differences to a mere racial designation has lent itself to very troubled pasts. Given this, a more diversified way of examining food can be exercised when not only race but also ethnicity is examined. Ethnicity relates to one's cultural attributes such as, but not limited to, nationality, culture, ancestry, language, customs, and beliefs.

The complexities and differences of foodways—or food practices—are better illuminated when these broader dimensions of our identity are considered. As it stands, we rely too often on biological perceptions of race to judge others in our society. Too often the biologically reduced variable of race and its consequent meanings of judgment are relied upon in US society. The implications of this for studying food and food practices are that the material lives of people can be divorced from the innumerable aspects of their identity; a misrepresentation that studies focusing on race have made clear.

Major theories and methods used to study food and race

Since most every study of food necessarily engages the study of race on some level, it can be said that a number of theoretical perspectives have been employed.[4] These include archeology, anthropology, history, literature, folklore, cultural studies, intersectionality, and critical race theory. What follows is a representative sample of some of the work in the field that has been undertaken using these methods.

Jeffrey Pilcher's body of research on Mexico and the Mexican identity has gone far to contribute not only to the food history of Latin America but also to a number of other areas of study including Mexican foodways generally and business history specifically.[5] Taking as its focus food and nationality—another aspect of race—as well as gender, class, and region, Pilcher's analysis is profound for the ways in which it teases out the evolution of Mexican identity formation through food. So insightful has been Pilcher's research and its resulting connections that the UN Educational, Scientific and Cultural Organization (UNESCO) recently conferred the status of Intangible Cultural Heritage on traditional Mexican cuisine.[6] Equally provocative is Pilcher's use not only of historical sources like archival research, but also cookbooks, fiction, and studies on consumer, and culinary history illustrating that a thorough study of food is best carried out using multidisciplinary methods. Frederick Douglass Opie's *Hog and Hominy* also makes use of historiography to explore identity, but from the perspective of African Americans and "soul food." Opie also uses archival research but also oral history, self-ethnography, and popular culture. Building off the work of culinary historians such as Karen Hess, Jessica Harris, Vertamae Smart Grosvenor, and Howard Paige, Opie illustrates the connections between African cultural elements and retentions and the evolutions of foods in African-American communities. Equally as important as the food history in Opie's analysis is the act of cooking. Important to Opie's thesis is a delineation of the resiliency of African Americans, as evident by their persistent food culture. In *Cooking in Other Women's Kitchens*, Rebecca Sharpless focuses on the tasks of cooking by also taking a narrative approach while using theories of history. What makes Sharpless's work distinctive from Pilcher and Opie is her primary concentration on gender as well as race. Theorizing from these perspectives, Sharpless provides a compelling composite of the lives of some of the African-American woman who worked as cooks. Giving voice to this often unnamed group of women, Sharpless reveals much about the unexplored personal lives of those who performed domestic work in the homes of others. For Sharpless, a focus on race reveals how it significantly shaped the labors of African-American women and cooking became a different form of domestic labor because of it.

Food has long been a part of literature, with food-related themes being common among all types of writing from narratives by and about women to children's literature, memoir, poetry, and critical analysis. While food is a major theme in literature generally, in the field of food studies race has been used as a lens to examine affinity, community, and belonging, illustrate resistance and affirmation, convey worldview, and reveal ritual and dining processes. For example, in *Eating Identities: Reading Food in Asian American Literature*, Wenying Xu makes central the ways that food is a signifier of identity serving "as a dominant site of economic, cultural, and political struggle."[7] Similar to other works of literary criticism, Xu draws on post-colonial theory, queer theory, psychoanalytical theory, and Marxist literary theory to provide a close reading of mostly Japanese and Japanese-Canadian, Chinese, and some Vietnamese texts. In all, Xu argues not only for the centrality of food in the everyday lives of Asian Americans, but also for the ways in which examining the centrality of food at particular social and historical junctures reveals psychic and emotional struggles of the self. Moving beyond gender and ethnicity to also consider race and sexuality, Wenying Xu expands the discourses with which to consider the geopolitical circumstances of Asian-American peoples.

Turning to another area of the Asian diaspora, Anita Mannur examines South Asian communities using theories from queer, feminist, and critical race studies. *Culinary Fictions: Food in South Asian Diasporic Culture* concerns itself with the cultural politics of consumption, production, difference, and citizenship. Taking an interdisciplinary approach to literature, popular culture, film, and other cultural products (i.e., cookbooks), Mannur explores the ways in which national identities are imagined and belonging is affirmed and resisted. Using race as a trope, Mannur explores the concept of immigrant nostalgia using a queer, non-heteronormative lens. In this, she reveals how immigrant cultural identities are negotiated and mediated by the complexities of not only diasporic but also sexual politics. For Mannur, food production offers potential routes to liberation from the constraints of heteronormativity.

Similarly exposing the limits of heterosexual gender ideologies using queer theories, Julia Ehrhardt explores food and race to think through the performance of identity in literature in her essays, "Towards Queering Food Studies: Foodways, Heteronormativity, and Hungry Women in Chicana Lesbian Literature," and "Meeting at a Barbecue: Dorothy Allison, Zora Neale Hurston, and Apocalyptic Literary Miscegenation." In "Towards Queering Food Studies," Ehrhardt reads the ways that food and foodways appear and are used in literature written by Chicana lesbians. In this analysis, foods often considered part of the "cornerstone of the

Chicano diet" like tortillas, biscochitos (Mexican anise-flavored cookies), chiles, and salsas are used symbolically and metaphorically to illustrate how Chicana women resist oppressive culinary cultures to exert self-definition and creative expression. Food is also used to demonstrate how their respective authors subvert "sacred" Chicano heterosexual rituals and the "constructions of the Chicana cook" to represent queer sexualities and lesbians as producers and consumers of good food.[8]

"Meeting at a Barbecue: Dorothy Allison, Zora Neale Hurston, and Apocalyptic Literary Miscegenation" considers one of the South's most enduring traditions—barbecuing. Yet, rather than conducting an analysis that lapses into revering this signature tradition, Ehrhardt argues for the ways in which barbecue functions as a literary trope to reinforce Southern race, gender, and class hierarchies. Further complicating the role of the pig in American culinary culture, but writing from the standpoints of anthropology, sociology, history, and literature, Andrew Warnes traces what he calls "this most American food" to illuminate how race, ethnicity, nationalism, and colonialism are imbricated in food. Beginning with the etymology of the term "barbacoa" to its evolution as "bbq," in *Savage Barbecue: Race, Culture, and the Invention of America's First Food*, Warnes richly details how the practice of roasting meat progressed from Native Americans and Indians of the Caribbeans during the era of Columbus to the present moment. Europeans, unfamiliar with the culinary practices of native peoples, decided this roasting was a form of cannibalism. As a result, barbacoa became synonymous with savagery. To expound upon his thesis of the ways in which imperialism and racism undergird the practice of barbecuing, Warnes interprets such literary texts as Ned Ward's "The Barbacue Feast," which was published in 1707. In his interpretation of the text, "the whipping of slaves goes hand in hand with the savage barbecuing of meat." As Warnes theorizes, "both belong to the production of a new imperial supremacy that can corrupt those it empowers." In all, what Warnes posits are the ways in which food is indelibly entangled in the economics of early world geopolitics and the Native inhabitants of the Americas.

A similar concern pervades Warnes' first book, *Hunger Overcome: Food and Resistance in Twentieth-Century African American Literature*, which argues for the ways in which Western cultures produce and normalize the idea of race. Similar to Ehrhardt, Warnes examines the literature of Zora Neale Hurston but also Richard Wright and Toni Morrison, along with popular fiction and film, Warnes argues that each author presents hunger not as a condition that could be avoided but rather as a weapon to extract and enforce docility and acquiescence from African-American people during enslavement and well beyond.

Writing from a multifocal perspective to link nativism, nationalism, and race privilege, Kyla Tompkins turns to the history of actually eating, rather than focusing on a specific food or foods, in *Racial Indigestion Eating Bodies in the 19th Century*.[9] Using a rare archive of children's literature, documents of architectural history, domestic manuals, dietetic tracts, novels, and advertising from the nineteenth-century United States Tompkins probes how eating was and is a political act—erotic yet violent—to reveal how eating produces political subjects by justifying the social discourses that create bodily meaning. With this claim, she moves forward our understanding of the deeply related connections between literature, gender, race, class, and food. Using close critical readings of classic literary works, Tompkins provides an interdisciplinary examination of the ways that the body politic informs the quotidian act of eating and more importantly the racial dynamics inherent therein. This work is particularly exciting in its explication of gendered and raced bodies as "things" of consumption in the historical imagination. More pointedly, Tompkins's work challenges the contemporary "foodie activist" to reexamine the "colonial, even imperialist, pathways" upon which food and food cultures rely.

Taking a different literary approach to centralize race as well as gender and class, Rafia Zafar in her seminal essay, "The Signifying Dish: Autobiography and History in Two Black Women's Cookbooks," explains how black women exhibited agency even as they worked to establish a sense of comfort both within their own homes and in their roles as domestic laborers to white employers. Furthermore, as she negotiates the intersections of memory, race, history, and food she pushes back against the pervasive image of African-American women as mammy and Aunt Jemima. Zafar questions whether when African-American women write recipes, they can, in the process, also *right* history? With this question, Zafar points to the ways in which groups like African Americans assume the process of redefining the foods that are a part of their culinary cultural experience.[10] Both Zafar and Doris Witt use soul food as a trope to conclude that a persistent set of ideologies link people, foods, and historical junctures. Because food is used to define boundaries—who is in-group and who is external to the group—racial groups contend with commercial and cultural representations of themselves by contesting and rejecting them while simultaneously laying claim to them.

In her study, *Black Hunger: Food and the Politics of U.S. Identity*, Doris Witt takes a cultural studies approach using psychoanalytic and literary theory, to engage in a similar task of deconstruction. Generally speaking, cultural studies combines a number of theories to understand the ways in which meaning is generated, disseminated, and produced through practices, beliefs, institutions, and political, economic, or social structures within a given culture. At its core *Black Hunger* argues for the importance of food in the development of personal, social, and national identity. Moving from Aunt Jemima to contemporary black women, Witt argues that food was a way of erasing black women and their labor even while Americans forged and developed a national identity.

Witt is one of many contributors to the collection of essays compiled by Ann Bower in *African American Foodways* wherein the food culture is explored from a multiplicity of perspectives. Stemming from the 1999 conference, "Grits, Greens and Everything in Between," the contributors to this volume apply varying approaches to the study of food and race, all of which are useful to future scholarly undertakings. Of particular note is Robert Hall's historical essay that focuses on the food crops like yam and other ingredients that were involved in the Columbian exchange, along with slaves, ideologies, and cultural practices. Like Doris Witt, who explores the concept of soul food in *Black Hunger*, William "Bill" Whit takes up the subject in this volume from a sociological perspective to argue that the production of the foods involved are "exemplary" of cultural performance. Anne Yentsch, one of the few archaeologists to focus on African women, uses faunal remains and excavations to discuss slave kitchens and other spaces where women worked. Like Zafar who is discussed above, Bower returns to her earlier work on cookbooks to focus specifically on the National Council of Negro Women, a middle-class organization of women who not only used their cookbook to celebrate cultural memory but also to participate in the project of racial uplift. Psyche Williams-Forson's essay conjoins and crosses disciplinary boundaries to argue for the importance of chicken as a pervasive cultural object in the everyday lives of African Americans.

Analysis of this argument is furthered by Williams-Forson in her book, *Building Houses out of Chicken Legs: Black Women, Food, and Power*, which takes a cultural studies approach incorporating black feminist theory, literature, popular and material culture along with personal interviews, folklore, and culinary history. Using a single-food analysis approach, Williams-Forson illustrates how power permeates objects and is used to exert psychological trauma and simultaneously functions as a tool of empowerment. The strength of the methodological and theoretical approach used is that it strives to understand what is experienced at the intersection of two or more axes of oppression at different historical moments and in different contexts.

As a social marker, food can be used to indicate cultural belonging and identity. Alternatively, it can be used to target a group for discrimination and prejudice. Stereotypes are often used to justify maligning a group or individuals. Stereotypes are widely accepted as fixed and oversimplified conceptions, images, or ideas. For example, Igor de Garine observed that even as late as the 1990s Italians were still known by the French as "macaroni eaters." Other groups have been similarly referenced in a derogatory manner with regard to food, perhaps most notably African Americans. As highlighted in *Building Houses out of Chicken Legs*, African Americans in the US have been negatively associated with eating fried chicken and watermelon. So pervasive is this stereotype that the forty-fourth president, Barack Obama, has not escaped association. Certain other foods, such as those consumed in the US South, have been referred to as "nigger foods." These include foods customarily also heralded by some as "soul food"—pork fat, chit'lins, greens, peas and beans, cornbread, and chicken parts.[11]

Advocating against such representations is one kind of food justice, even though the definition typically is used "to explore how racial and economic inequalities manifest in the production, distribution, and consumption of food, and the ways that communities and social movements shape and are shaped by these inequalities."[12] By employing a combination of cultural studies and intersectionality theories, Williams-Forson recognizes the multidimensional and relational nature of social locations, places and forces (economic, cultural, political), lived experiences, and overlapping systems of discrimination and subordination. Intersectional theories and approaches capture several levels of difference while simultaneously revealing how intersecting forms of oppression can be beneficial for those who identify as normative—(e.g. white, heterosexual, male, upper-class, Protestant).

Other scholars seeking to communicate a commitment to social justice by dismantling structures of power examining race in food studies have gravitated toward intersectional and critical race theories. An interdisciplinary and often grassroots movement, food justice advocates argue that the social construction of racial formations in the United States helps to organize material relations of capitalism leading to unequal access to various goods, including food.

Working within the realm of the sustainable agriculture movement, geographers, Julie Guthman, Rachel Slocum, and Aimee Harper, among others, argue that privileges borne from racial formations reproduce unequal relations of power that shape lives in indelible ways. Using a combination of ethnography, surveys, and focus groups these analyses argue that while race and issues of racism are persistent throughout the movement, it is often disregarded and overlooked. As a result of this ongoing marginalization and food insecurity, many of America's young, elderly, poor and low-income, as well as rural find themselves trapped in a cycle of health and environmental risks. A major culprit of which is the industrial food system. Unmasking the contradictions and restabilization of institutional racism is one of the aims in applying this body of theory to the study of food.[13]

Alison Alkon and Julian Agyeman have pushed these discussions further in their anthology *Cultivating Food Justice: Race, Class, and Sustainability*. Taking as its starting point the scrutiny of über-visible authors Michael Pollan, Barbara Kingsolver, and Eric Schlosser who urge us to consume foods primarily produced and distributed locally, thereby supporting the sustainable agriculture movement, this collection of essays explores "just alternatives" to exploitative food systems and the ways in which these alternatives are being explored by low-income communities. The studies offered in the book consider several important issues including, but not limited to, agricultural and land-use policies that systematically disadvantage Native-American, African-American, Latino/a, and Asian-American farmers and farm workers; food security and access in urban, suburban, and rural areas, and new directions of scholarship in this sub-field. The collection seeks to serve as a primer to ways of achieving a just and sustainable agriculture.[14]

New directions in race and food studies

Discussed up to this point has been, more or less, the work that has served to establish race as a viable area of focus in food studies. Using a multiplicity of theories and approaches new perspectives have entered the field of food studies. But it has been rightly noted in several contexts that food-related issues defy disciplinary assignment or boundaries. Thus, some of the best work has overlapped disciplines and sought out interdisciplinarity for its strengths and potentials in further advancing inquiries in food studies. Much has been done but more needs to be done.

Along these lines is the proliferation of scholarship focusing on the importance of foodways of ethnic communities in America. Started by the seminal anthology of Linder Keller Brown and Kay Mussell, *Regional and Ethnic Foodways: Performance of Group Identity* argues for a sustained analysis of symbolic group interaction. Taking a multidisciplinary approach to folklore and the ways in which culture operates in our everyday lives, Brown and Musell include essays from ethnic and regional groups ranging from Jewish communities to Tejano migrant communities to argue for the ways in which food acts as a system of communication identifying social group dynamics.

Not alone in this reach, there is also Donna Gabbacia's *We are What We Eat: Ethnic Food and the Making of Americans* and Hasia Diner's *Hungering for America: Italian, Irish, and Jewish Foodways in the Age of Migration*. Taking a historical approach, Gabbacia illustrates the ways in which ethnic culinary patterns have influenced and left their mark on American eating habits. Richly detailing the intermingling of recipes, foods, and spices, Diner looks at the ways in which ethnic entrepreneurship and connoisseurship have shaped our current consumption and taste. Diner, who also uses historical methods and approaches but also draws upon memoirs, cookbooks, newspaper accounts, surveys, films and studies of consumer culture, primarily teases out the ways that the culinary and cultural patterns of Italians, Irish, and Jewish immigrants were influenced by and influenced American culinary culture.

Other studies that have taken on ethnic food and foodways along with gender and identity include, among others, Sherrie Inness, *Pilaf, Pozole, and Pad Thai: American Women and Ethnic Food*, Meredith Abarca, *Voices in the Kitchen: Views of Food and the World from Working-Class Mexican and Mexican American Women*, Carole Counihan, *Around the Tuscan Table: Food, Family, and Gender*, and *A Tortilla is Like Life: Food and Culture in the San Luis Valley of Colorado*. Taken together, these studies expand our thinking on gender, resistance, agency and food in their respective ethnic communities. Perhaps more importantly they convey how food procurement, preparation, and consumption speaks to multi-generational cultural traditions and tastes and the ways in which these customs and beliefs have persisted and adapted despite appropriation and commodification by American commercial culture; in particular, restaurant culture.

The Migrant's Table: Meals and Memories in Bengali-American Households by Krishnendu Ray reminds us of the role of globalization and modernization in the life of the immigrant as they navigate the tumultuous waters to redefine notions of "home." Ray's study in particular points to the elisions that have occurred in studying other migrant groups—non-European and non-Latin American. More work, for example, needs to be done on Caribbean and African people around the diaspora, who have made America their home. The explosion of grocery stores in urban areas that cater to the Caribbean–West African–Latin American triad suggest that these foodstuffs are similarly shared and simultaneously differentiated. Understanding what and how these phenomena are experienced is critical to expanding the study of ethnic foodways in America.[15]

Analyses that examine the intersections of food and race usually, but not always, also examine power and privilege and are rooted in history. The roots of food insecurity for American indigenous nations, for example, are due in no small part to genocide and settler colonialism whereby their lands and many of their cultural practices were appropriated and/or decimated by migrants who executed sovereignty. These significant truths provide a necessary framework for understanding food insecurity among Native American communities, who, according to the US Department of Agriculture, have one of the highest incidents of hunger, lack access to basic and affordable foodstuffs, and consequently experience some of the most debilitating illnesses.[16] Further work on Native Americans along these lines would be a welcome addition to the field.

Deborah Gewertz and Frederick Errington have undertaken similar work in their anthropological study, *Cheap Meats: Flap Food Nations in the Pacific Highlands*. Flaps, or the cheap, fatty remainders of cut mutton and lamb, which are similar to fatback in American society, are said to represent the hazy post-colonial relations between those of the Pacific Islands—especially Papua New Guinea, Fiji, and Tonga—and Australian and New Zealand settlers. Nutritionally, flaps are viewed as the discarded foods of the wealthy. Flaps represent an interesting dilemma; on the one hand, they are a cheap source of food. On the other hand, the fattiness lends itself to unhealthy eating and thereby contributes to the diseases that accompany longstanding unhealthy diets—diabetes, high cholesterol, and high blood pressure. Either way, however, the food is illustrative of a particular kind of food insecurity.

A comparable kind of anthropological but also historical probing should ensue for African-American communities, which has its incidences of food insecurity rooted in the period of enslavement, Reconstruction, and the Jim Crow eras—each of which denied African Americans wholesale access to land. A 1999 case, *Pigford v. Glickman*, sought to redress some of this ill by bringing a class action lawsuit against the United States Department of Agriculture (USDA) alleging over a decade of racial discrimination in farm loans and assistance allocation. The lawsuit ended with a settlement on April 14, 1999. This case, and the reasoning behind it, is directly tied to the prevalence of food insecurity today for many African Americans. As Slocum nicely explains: "The history of slavery and the years of struggle that continue in the wake of slavery should be recognized as intimately tied to white privilege and to those communities of color that experience food insecurity, do not own land, are politically disenfranchised, and economically disadvantaged."[17] More work on African-American farmers historically and today would also go far toward advancing our understanding of community food insecurity.

There is still a great deal of work to be done around race, food, and technology. In her essay, "The History of Technology, the Resistance of Archives, and the Whiteness of Race," Carolyn de la Peña writes: "[M]uch scholarship [tends] to focus on big questions concerning the relationship between technology and cultural values or social change, rather than examining cultures and social relations embedded in the technologies themselves. Within this landscape there are few built-in mechanisms for producing scholarship that prioritizes race." Suggestions offered by de la Peña rightly include such new volumes as "Technology and the White-American Experience(s)" and "Technologies of Sameness." Added to this could be more work on spices, canning, kitchen culture, and dieting forms among other aspects of technology. Equally compelling are the ways that technology intersects with globalization and transnationalism, for instance through the intersection of new media, urban spaces, and gourmet food carts.

The field of disability studies is a venue ripe for discussions of food and race. In her essay, "Do the Hands that Feed Us Hold Us Back?" Denise Lance explores the challenges faced by those who need eating assistance and the ways they try to balance dependence, potential embarrassment, and intimacy of assisted eating. In what ways do meanings surrounding food assistance change when the recipient is living with disabilities? More importantly, in what ways can being assisted with food intake change or get highlighted when your race heightens the attention to your disability? These questions and many others like it can further enrich the field.

Research on the ways in which race is important to restaurant culture has received limited coverage in food studies. Beyond considering these establishments from the standpoint of atmosphere, ambience, and cuisine more research should be conducted on how this aspect of the food service sector is a culinary landscape of discrimination and disparity. Saru Jayaraman, co-founder of Restaurant Opportunities Center United, analyzes a pervasive scene in the restaurant industry: "[W]hite workers serving and bartending; workers of color clearing tables, preparing food, and washing dishes."[18] The restaurant sector is the second largest private-sector employer—retail being the first—but it is the largest part of the nation's food system employing the most workers. Yet, less than 0.01 percent of these workers are unionized meaning that the industry is able to offer mostly low- and poverty-wage jobs with little access to benefits. Even as most of our focus is on sustainability and food justice, it seems clear that broader definitions of sustainability need to be entertained in order to bring about changes in living wages and equal opportunities.

Practical considerations for getting started

As illustrated throughout this discussion, students interested in pursuing race in food studies have a number of theoretical approaches and methods from which to choose and with which to work. In looking at programs wherein you can undertake your research you should consider not only the strengths of the primary advisor with whom you will work but also the range of other scholars (academic and non-academic) with whom you can work.

It is important when planning to undertake interdisciplinary work that you have a plethora of sources and perspectives to use. Not only are you concerned for expertise but also access to libraries, archives, informants, media, and more. It is important, then, to consider situating yourself in a department that embraces interdisciplinarity. To this end, programs in cultural studies, food studies, women's and gender studies, and American studies are most likely the best fit. This does not, in any way, exclude the disciplines of literature, history, sociology, or anthropology. Rather, it simply pushes you to think broadly and beyond disciplinary boundaries and academic circles. Often, single disciplinary departments find it difficult or antithetical to embrace such a wide berth.

As with any program of study, it is most important that you find the department or program that will offer you the best fit.

Notes

1 Several studies in folklore address structural inequalities and imbalances and disjunctures in power structures with regard to food. See among them, Psyche Williams-Forson, "Other Women Cooked for My Husband: Negotiating Gender, Food, and Identities in an African American/Ghanaian Household." *Feminist Studies* 36.2 (Summer 2010): 435–61; and, Williams-Forson, *Building Houses Out of Chicken Legs: Black Women, Food, and Power.* Chapel Hill: UNC Press, 2006; LuAnn Roth, "Beyond Communitas: Cinematic Food Events and the Negotiation of Power, Belonging, and Exclusion." *Western Folklore* 64. 3-4 (2006): 163–87; Amy Bentley, "Islands of Serenity: Gender, Race, and Ordered Meals During World War II." In *Food in the USA: A Reader.* Carole M. Counihan, ed. New York: Routledge, 2002: 171–92; Sidney Mintz, *Sweetness and Power: The Place of Sugar in Modern History.* New York: Penguin Books, 1985.
2 Michael Omi and Howard Winant, *Racial Formation in the United States.* New York: Routledge & Kagan Paul, Inc, 1986: 61.
3 Omi and Winant, *Racial Formation*, p. 65-67.
4 Studies of white racial and ethnic groups have been primarily focused upon in food studies from almost every socioeconomic class. For this reason, this discussion is limited primarily to non-white groups, though race is all-encompassing. An excellent review of several topics pertaining to race and food studies from a different perspective is Doris Witt, "Global Feminisms and Food: A Review Essay." *Meridians* 1.2 (Spring 2001): 73–93.

5 This section begins with a disciplinary focus, but it should be noted that some of the most diverse studies on food and race in the communities of early American settlers, Native Americans, and African Americans originated in archeology.

6 Intangible cultural heritage is described as "oral traditions and expressions such as epics, tales, and stories, performing arts including music, song, dance, puppetry and theatre, social practices, rituals and festive events, knowledge and practices concerning nature and the universe—for example, folk medicine and folk astronomy, and traditional craftsmanship, as well as the sites and spaces in which culturally significant activities and events occur … It is the culture that people practice as part of their daily lives. It is beliefs and perspectives, ephemeral performances and events that are not tangible objects of culture like monuments, or paintings, books or artefacts." See also Richard Kurin, "Safeguarding Intangible Cultural Heritage in the 2003 UNESCO Convention: A Critical Appraisal." *Museum* 56, 1-2 (2004): 66–77.

7 Wenying Xu, *Eating Identities: Reading Food in Asian American Literature*. Honolulu: University of Hawai'i Press, 2007: 14.

8 Julia Ehrhardt, "Towards Queering Food Studies: Foodways, Heteronormativity, and Hungry Women in Chicana Lesbian Literature." *Food and Foodways* 14 (2006): 91–109. Barbecue has long been tied to race, gender, region, and class. It is not surprising then, that it is often the subject of scholarly work in literature and other disciplines. To this end, see also Ehrhardt's "Meeting at a Barbecue: Dorothy Allison, Zora Neale Hurston, and Apocalyptic Literary Miscegenation." *Critical Essays on the Works of American Author Dorothy Allison*. Christine Blouch and Laurie Vickroy ed. Lewiston, NY: Edwin Mellen Press, 2004: 71–90.

9 Kyla Tompkins, *Racial Indigestion Eating Bodies in the 19th Century*. New York: New York University Press, 2012.

10 The abundance of cookbooks that are available for consideration visually and anecdotally illustrate the ways in which people of all races, classes, and ethnicities produce food and practice food cultures. These cultural documents shed some light on how food factors into the process of identity formation. Not to be dismissed, some of these cookbooks place culinary habits within a political and social history context sharing the lived experiences and realities of those who have long since passed away. In some instances, these cookbooks are the last remaining cultural artifacts of their kind.

11 Igor de Garine, "Views about Food Prejudice and Stereotypes." *Anthropology of Food* 40, 3 (2001): 487–507. Williams-Forson, *Building Houses Out of Chicken Legs*. See also, among others, Jeff Weinstein, "'Obama Fingers'—Surprise, Food Has Race." *Arts Journal*, March 19, 2009. www.artsjournal.com/outthere/2009/03/obama_fingers_-_surprise_food.html (accessed on November 1, 2011); and Jesse Bering, "Culinary Racism: Trying to Explain the 'Obama Fried Chicken.' Incident and Others Like It." *Slate*, November 1, 2011. www.slate.com/articles/health_and_science/science/2011/11/obama_fried_chicken_incident_explaining_racist_food_stereotypes.html (accessed on November 28, 2011).

12 Alison Hope Alkon, "Food justice" (in this volume).

13 See Julie Guthman, *Agrarian Dreams: The Paradox of Organic Farming in California* and "If They Only Knew: Colorblindness and Universalism in Alternative Food Institutions." *The Professional Geographer* 60, 3 (2008): 387–97; Rachel Slocum, "Dismantling Racism in Community Food Work." www.foodsecurity.org/race/RacismFoodSystem.pdf (accessed on April 8, 2012), and "Anti-racist Practice and the Work of Community Food Organizations." *Antipode* 38, 2: 327–49; and Amie Breeze Harper, *Sistah Vegan: Food, Identity, Health, and Society: Black Female Vegans Speak*. New York: Lantern Books, 2010. For more on this body of work also see Alkon, "Food justice" (in this volume).

14 Alison Hope Alkon and Julian Agyeman, *Cultivating Food Justice, Race, Class, and Sustainability* Cambridge, MA: MIT Press, 2011.

15 See for example, Susan Kalcik, "Ethnic Foodways in America: Symbol and the Performance of Identity." In *Ethnic and Regional Foodways in the United States*. Linda Keller Brown and Kay Mussell, eds. Knoxville: University of Tennessee Press, 1984: 37–65; Williams-Forson, "Other Women Cooked for My Husband"; S. K. Lee, J. Sobal and E. A. Frongillo, Jr., "Acculturation, Food Consumption and Diet-related Factors among Korean Americans." *The Journal of Nutrition Education* 31, 6 (1999): 321–30.

16 See Lorenzo Veracini, *Setter Colonialism: A Theoretical Overview*. New York: Palgrave Macmillan, 2010.

17 Slocum, "Dismantling Racism in Community Food Work."

18 Saru Jayaraman, "Restaurants and Race: Discrimination and Disparity in the Food Service Sector." special issue, *Globalization Comes Home, Race, Poverty, Environment: A Journal for Social and Environmental Justice* 18, 1 (2011). urbanhabitat.org/18-1/jayaraman (accessed November 30, 2011).

Special topics in food studies

27

Food justice

An overview

Alison Hope Alkon

As popular attention to industrial agriculture's health and environmental risks rises, it becomes necessary to understand the ways that inequalities are embedded in food systems. Building on the fields of environmental justice, critical race theory, food studies, and sustainable agriculture, food justice research explores how racial and economic inequalities manifest in the production, distribution, and consumption of food, and the ways that communities and social movements shape and are shaped by these inequalities. As an emerging field, it has the potential to enrich both social theory and social change. This chapter provides an overview of food justice research, highlighting the connections and contributions it offers.

As popular media attention to the health and environmental risks embedded in the industrial agriculture system rises, it becomes increasingly important to understand the ways that inequalities are embedded in and reproduced by industrial food systems. Food justice research explores how racial and economic inequalities manifest in the production, distribution, and consumption of food, and the ways that communities and social movements shape and are shaped by these inequalities. This research program has been taken up by an interdisciplinary group of scholars including sociologists, cultural geographers, and anthropologists. It is also often conducted in coordination with activists, comprising what Michael Burawoy (2005) would call organic public sociology. Though it is a newly emerging field, it has the potential to bear fruit that can nourish both social theory and social change. This chapter provides an overview of the field of food justice research, highlighting connections and contributions offered by this nascent body of scholarship.

Food justice research responds to, builds upon, and at its best even helps to inspire a grass-roots movement for social change. Broadly, the movement consists of "communities exercising their right to grow, sell and eat food that is fresh, nutritious, affordable, culturally-appropriate and grown locally with care for the well-being of the land, workers and animals" (Just Food, 2010). Acknowledging that low-income people and people of color often lack access to healthy food, economic opportunities, and green space, the movement largely comprised a network of local projects creating local food systems and green jobs in, for, and with marginalized communities. Many food justice activists are particularly conscious of racial and economic inequalities. Detroit's African American D-Town Farmers, for example, argue that food justice necessitates that those who have been most marginalized by the agribusiness system need to "lead the movement to provide food for the members of their community" (White, 2010: 204).

The movement argues that the current, industrial agri-food system often prevents communities from producing and consuming food in an environmentally sustainable and socially just manner. In addition, food justice scholars and activists often argue that even progressive movements for food system reform do not engage with analyses of past and present inequalities, and that the benefits of these movements have accrued disproportionately to those who maintain race and class privilege. Food justice scholarship aims to understand how racial and economic inequalities shape and are shaped by the production, distribution, and consumption of food in the hopes of building a broader and more diverse movement to transforming the food system.

Historical background of food justice scholarship and major theoretical approaches in use

The field of food justice research can trace its roots to a variety of interdisciplinary traditions. These include environmental justice, critical race theory, sustainable agriculture, and food studies. Together, these literatures contribute to a growing field, which in turn offers insights into each of them.

The environmental justice literature has focused most clearly on the ways that low-income communities and communities of color have been disproportionately overexposed to the toxic consequences of environmental degradation, using statistical analyses to demonstrate associations between race, class, toxicity, and health outcomes (United Church of Christ, 1987; 2007; Pastor, Morella Frosch and Sadd, 2006; Mohai and Saha, 2003; Israel et al., 2005; Petersen et al., 2006). The academic literature has also followed communities as they have mobilized against incinerators (Cole and Foster, 2001), petrochemical facilities (Allen, 2003), and toxic waste (La Duke, 2004), and have organized transnationally against the export of hazardous waste to the global south (Pellow, 2007) and for a justice-based approach to global warming (Roberts, 2009). More recently, scholars have also begun to investigate lack of access among these same communities to environmental benefits. Several notable environmental justice scholars examine issues of food access from this perspective (Gottlieb and Joshi, 2010; Gottlieb and Fisher, 1996; Pinderhughes and Miner, 2002). Food, particularly fresh produce, can serve as an important subject through which to observe disparities in environmental privilege (Park and Pellow, 2011; Morland et al., 2002; Zenk et al., 2005). Moreover, activists have cited food justice projects' potential to create green jobs, which prominent environmental justice activists have highlighted as paramount to communities whose employment numbers have been decimated by the decline in domestic manufacturing jobs (Jones, 2008; Pinderhughes, 2006). Food justice projects can also provide access to healthy food, green space, and outdoor activities that are often missing from these neighborhoods (Kessel et al., 2009).

Arguing that an increasingly industrializing agriculture creates harmful conditions for food system workers, food consumers, and the natural environment, food justice activists work to create local, organic alternative mechanisms for the production, distribution and consumption of food. In seeking to understand these efforts, social scientists draw on the work of sociologists who take a political economy approach to industrial agriculture, highlighting its role in the creation of global economic inequality and the production of dependence on US food sources in formerly self-sufficient agricultural societies (Magdoff, Foster and Buttel, 2000; Buttel, Larson and Gillespie, 1990; Clapp and Fuchs, 2009; Friedman, 1982). Foster (1999) traces sociologists' interest in sustainable agriculture to Marx's concept of metabolic rift, which states that as capitalism creates conditions of material estrangement between humans and nature, it leads the former to unsustainable forms of resource extraction. British high farming, for example, had disastrous effects on soil fertility, necessitating the early import of Peruvian bird guano and synthetic fertilizer. The increased industrialization and consolidation of agricultural firms occurring since Marx's observations have held increasingly dire consequences for the soil and water on which food production depends (Buttel, Larson and Gillespie, 1990). Scholars have been particularly interested in the struggles of farm workers to better their situations through unionization (Ganz, 2000; Daniel, 1981). As will be covered in more detail below, coalitions between consumers and workers present an exciting future direction for food justice scholarship.

Like their counterparts in the sustainable agriculture movement, food justice activists seek to create what Lyson calls a civic agriculture, which links the agricultural and environmental to the "economic, social, cultural, and political dimensions of community life" and encourages community involvement in the creation of local food systems (Lyson, 2004: 28). Doing so certainly exemplifies and extends economic sociologists' claims that the market is embedded in social life (Granovetter, 1985). However, in choosing to create alternatives to industrial agriculture, rather than work to transform it, food justice activists ignore the warnings of more critical sociologists and fellow travelers. With regard to the sustainable agriculture movement, critics have argued that although its support is based largely on broad social values consistent with Dunlap and Catton's (1979) New Environmental Paradigm (Beus and Dunlap, 1990), the changes advocated by the movement come through specific techniques and practices that do not disrupt the agribusiness system (Buttel, 1997). These arguments are aligned with broader work critiquing consumption-based approaches to social change more generally (Szasz, 2007; Princen, Manites and Conca, 2002). Some food justice scholars offer related criticism targeted at efforts to increase the consumption of local and organic food (Guthman, 2008; Allen, 2004), while others focus on explaining how communities came to lack food access, or else emphasize non-market aspects of food justice activism, including the growing of food for an individual's consumption, the bartering of foods or the creation of links between food and individual and collective identity formation (Mares and Peña, 2010).

The food justice literature tends to draw on critical race scholarship to inform its analysis of unequal access to healthy food. Scholars examine the racialization of the food system from an institutional perspective, tracing the ways that racial and economic inequalities are built into the zoning ordinances, mortgage policies, and other institutions and policies that determine how industries, human communities, and goods and services come to exist in particular places, all of which affect question of food access (McClintock, 2011; Alkon and Norgaard, 2009; Massey and Denton, 1998; Lipsitz, 1998; Pellow, 2002). Food justice scholars also examine how various racial projects—political and economic undertakings through which racial hierarchies are established and racialized subjectivities are created—influence who gets to influence the food system, who has access to what kinds of food, and how communities decide which foods are appropriate for them (Omi and Winant, 1994). Federal immigration laws, for example, act as racial projects when they define who is a legitimate subject deserving of agricultural workplace protections, and who is regarded as an alien "other" (Brown and Getz, 2011). Similarly, city planning and mortgage lending policies become racial projects when they serve to shape built environments that lack access to basic amenities including grocery stores, and to restrict communities of color to those environments (McClintock, 2011). Additionally, the appropriation of Native American lands by white settlers and past- and present-day forced assimilation are examples of racial projects that have deprived some Native American tribes of both material wealth and cultural sovereignty, including access to traditional foods (Norgaard, 2011). While these communities' circumstances are widely divergent, racial projects such as these have led to widespread hunger and food insecurity. Food justice scholarship suggests that the food system itself can be seen as a racial project. The kinds of food and food system influence that a community has access to—certainly the result of political and economic structures—can be instrumental in shaping members' individual, cultural, and collective subjectivities.

Critical race theory also provides a basis for deconstructing the unexamined race and class privilege that pervade the sustainable agriculture movement. Scholarly critics of this movement argue that it serves to reproduce the abilities of whites and middle-class people to reap the economic and cultural benefits of their social location. Both ethnographic investigations (Slocum, 2006) and surveys (Guthman, 2006) have demonstrated that sustainable agriculture movement participants resist discussing issues of race, even though race certainly influences who is food insecure (Morland *et al.*, 2002), who can own farms (Gilbert, Sharp and Felin, 2002; Romm, 2001), and who becomes agricultural laborers (Legett, 2002). Indeed, by highlighting themes of community and self-sufficiency while ignoring the ways these ideals are mediated by race, sustainable agriculture practitioners further mask the impact of racial inequality on food systems (Slocum, 2006). Because this impact goes largely unrecognized, the above-described institutionalized racism of industrial agriculture can be reproduced, rather than contested, by alternative food systems. Making this reproduction visible is one of the key contributions of food justice scholarship.

Lastly, the field of food studies has devoted significant attention to the relationship between food, social structure, and culture. Classic food studies texts established the paramount role of the global food system in the development and perpetuation of global inequalities and the exploitation of laborers from and in the global South (Mintz, 1985). Food justice studies extend this analysis to material inequalities within the global North, examining the development of a community's foodways in the context of a racialized global food system. Moreover, food studies is concerned with how individuals participating in culturally defined proper ways of eating perform membership in particular groups while marking others as outsiders (Douglass, 1996; Witt, 1999). For example, Avakian (1997) noted that American-born descendents of Jewish and Chinese immigrants continue to cherish stigmatized foods such as matzoh or boiled chicken feet. In contrast, however, others have found that second-generation Jewish Americans in New York developed a love for Chinese food, much as the Chinese in Hong Kong embrace McDonald's, precisely because they see such foods as distinct from their cultural background (Tuchman and Levine, 1993; Watson, 1997). Food justice activists demand the right not only to adequate food, but to "culturally appropriate" food. How both communities and authorities construct notions of what food is appropriate for whom is a key question for food justice scholars. Similarly, food studies explores the processes through which individuals and communities construct notions of authenticity and exoticism, concepts that are particularly significant to the intersection of food and race and thus essential to understanding food justice (Johnston and Baumann, 2007; Heldke, 2003). Food studies offers us the insight that food and culture are deeply entwined, but that relationship is fluid and develops in accordance with particular cultural moments. Indeed, this body of work often traces the ways that particular foods come to be associated with particular groups, as well as the meanings groups derive from their food practices. Scholars have also examined the ways that food can reflect, reinforce, or even create social hierarchies, as foods come to be associated with members of various races, classes, and even genders (Goody, 1998; Albala, 2007).

The field of food studies has devoted significant attention to the relationship between food and cultural identity, but has not examined the ways that such a relationship is structured by institutionalized inequalities of material resources and decision-making power, which is a key strength of the environmental justice literature. Neither has this literature addressed the political economy of agriculture in the depth found in the sustainable agriculture literature, which is highly relevant to its analysis of local food traditions. On the other hand, the complexity and fine-grained analysis through which food studies understands the relationship between race, identity, culture, and hierarchy is precisely the reason that studies of food have so much to offer to the environmental justice literature, which has thus far rarely engaged with critical race theory's analysis of how race is not biologically determined, but learned, performed, and practiced through social interaction (cf Pulido, 1996, 2000; Park and Pellow, 2004; Sze, 2006). Put simply, *studies of food need justice and studies of justice need food*. It is only in this newly emergent body of work on food justice that the racialized political economy of food production and distribution meets the cultural politics of food consumption and its influence on individual and cultural identities.

Research methodologies

Researchers have approached food justice from a variety of directions. Perhaps the most foundational studies are quantitative and GIS-based work that documents disproportionate access to healthy food in communities of color and low income. Many studies have found that white and middle-class neighborhoods are more likely to contain supermarkets than working-class and African-American ones (Morland *et al.*, 2002; Beaulac *et al.*, 2009; Block and Kouba, 2005; Lee and Lim, 2009; Páez *et al.*, 2010), and that such supermarkets most often offer the highest quality and variety of fresh produce, whole grains, and other "healthy" foods. Conversely, Sloane (2004) found that inner-city supermarkets, when they can be found, have higher prices and smaller selections of "healthy" foods (produce, whole grains, etc). Raja *et al.* (2008), however, found extensive networks of small grocery stores in neighborhoods of color. Nearly every food justice organization has already conducted, or is interested in conducting, a food assessment of their local area, which can provide opportunities for graduate student training, particularly at the MA level. In addition, many of these studies deal with just one city or urban area. Opportunities also exist to "scale-up" these data, allowing for comparisons and searching for patterns.

A second set of food justice research are historical studies that investigate the political and economic circumstances that create this lack of access. Norgaard (2011), for example, offers a racialized environmental history of the Karuk Tribe, whose ancestral territory is on the California–Oregon border. Although they sustainably managed a complex ecosystem that provided ample salmon and other food sources prior to white settlement, the Karuk today experience some of the highest rates of diet-related diseases. Norgaard and her co-authors document how outright genocide, lack of recognition of land occupancy title and forced assimilation have resulted in both poor food access among the Karuk and severe environmental degradation of the region. Cultural geographers tend to undertake similar studies through the lens of political ecology. McClintock (2011), for example, takes on the question of how the Oakland flatlands, which are predominantly populated by low-income people and people of color, became a food desert. He locates his explanation in various processes through which capital unevenly shapes the built environment, including residential development, city planning, and racist mortgage lending. Similarly, Brown and Getz (2011) situate the striking rates of hunger faced by California farmworkers in the neoliberal domestic policies and international trade regimes that spur migration, depress farmworker wages, and exempt agricultural laborers from rights enjoyed by other workers.

In addition, researchers work closely with community-based food justice organizations to record their responses to the above circumstances. This results in a rich body of case studies seeking to understand the ecological, economic, and racial dimensions of food justice activism. At the Masters level, many of these studies are quite celebratory, documenting the various approaches taken by organizational leaders. Dissertation-level work tends to be more reflexive and critical, moving beyond questions of efficacy to examine the ways that inequalities are reproduced and contested. My own dissertation, for example, uses food justice to deconstruct neoliberal assumptions embedded in the idea of the green economy, specifically the notion that buying and selling local and organic food can create environmental protection and social justice (Alkon, 2008). In this way, food justice research, while sympathetic to the goals of the food justice movement, also pushes it to craft more structural and collective responses and to imagine possibilities for activism beyond the creation of alternative food systems. This kind of work requires ongoing and sustained relationships with activists and organizations, which can be difficult to negotiate but incredibly rewarding.

Avenues for future research

As a young field, there are many directions in which food justice scholarship might begin to move. First, food justice scholars can use their analyses to better deconstruct the relationships between race, class, and geography that inform food insecurity. Several historical studies offer finely grained analyses of the interplays between these factors (Brown and Getz, 2011; McClintock, 2011). However, the question remains as to how, in the present tense, to work from the nexus of multiple racial, spatial, and economic circumstances. I certainly do not mean to suggest that the food justice movement, or scholars associated with it, must partition out the various oppressions of race and class. To the contrary, all oppressions, but particularly those of race and class, are experienced and understood in tandem, and also that structural racism is a process through which racial exclusions create and reify economic inequalities. However, better attention to the dynamic interplays between race, class, and geography might better help us to tease out the various factors that can produce food insecurity, as well as the ways that our multiple social locations influence the various food environments we occupy.

Second, food justice scholarship can further explore the intersection of labor and the food system. Nationally, 75 percent of farmworkers are Mexican-born (Center for Social Inclusion, 2007) and in California, the nation's largest agricultural state, 97 percent are foreign-born (Philpott, 2008). On average, farmworkers garner half the wages paid to other manual labor occupations, experience high rates of work-related injuries and, ironically, are often food insecure (Center for Social Inclusion, 2007). Egregious cases of farmworker abuse can be seen in annual death rates of workers in California, as well as the enslavement of workers in Immokelee, Florida (Williams, 2008). In addition, food-processing plants in rural areas employ largely black or non-white immigrant labor, and their inflation-adjusted wages have fallen by half in the past 25 years (Philpott, 2008). The food movement tends to idealize family farms and unprocessed foods. For this reason, their writers and activists often serve to metaphorically erase the presence of these workers. Food justice scholarship would do well to examine the production of food insecurity among farm and food industry workers, as well as to think more deeply about the relationship between race, labor, and food.

In addition, there is a glaring gap in the literature on food justice and gender, as existing scholarship tends to follow activists' highlighting of race and class. Gender inequalities, however, intersect with the food system in a variety of ways ranging from the inclusion of women in farm ownership and management (Feldman and Welsh, 1995; Hall and Mogyorody, 2007; Meares, 1997; Trauger, 2004) to the ways that women's identities and economic opportunities are shaped and constrained by food provisioning strategies (Williams-Forson, 2006). A gendered food justice analysis could also help to illuminate sexual abuse and rape of women farmworkers (Morales Waugh, 2010), as well as investigate whether similar patterns occur in other sectors of the food system. Additionally, it is not uncommon for popular food writing to blame the feminist movement for decreases in home cooking and family meals (Pollan, 2010; Flammang, 2010), a subject that seems ripe for a food justice analysis. Food justice scholarship takes an intersectional approach to race and class, and integrating gender would help it to better capture the complexities of how inequality intersects with the food system.

Lastly, food justice scholars can compare the various strategies adopted by food justice activists in order not only to assess them, but to analyze what they tell us about the ways that people understand their power to create social change. Food justice activists overwhelmingly create local programs that develop food entrepreneurs, creating opportunities for low-income people of color to benefit from the growing interest in local food systems. Interestingly, most activism does not attempt to create limits on the exploitative power of industrial agriculture. Nor does it enlist state support, relying instead on some form of market response, or the non-market creation of goods. Scholars might begin to unpack the assumptions guiding activists to attempt to ameliorate the consequences of both state and market forces through the creation of local alternatives rather than by directly challenging the structural conditions they identify as barriers to a just and sustainable food system.

Practical considerations for getting started

There are no particular programs specializing on food justice per se, but students interested in the subject approach it from a wide variety of angles. Perhaps the most common are applied Masters programs in fields like community development or urban policy and planning. Colleagues in both fields report that many students are interested in food systems and food justice. As with any field, it is important to locate a potential advisor who is interested in the kind of work you want to do, and who may have ongoing connections to activists and organizations that you can work with.

Within the academy, the field of food studies is growing rapidly. Most students interested in pursuing PhDs in the field of food justice enter traditional PhD programs. Food justice scholarship seems to be most prominent in the field of cultural geography; literally hundreds of papers on the topic were presented at the 2011 annual meetings. There are also a growing number of anthropologists and sociologists interested in the topic, as well as those pursuing degrees in American, environmental, and urban studies. Because food justice is such a young field, not every PhD student works specifically with an advisor who shares that particular interest. Food justice is relevant to a variety of fields including urban and rural development, social movements, political economy/ecology, and environmental issues. It is possible to enter a program with a strong focus in one or more of these areas and to focus one's own work on food justice. One strength of this field is its interdisciplinarity, and scholars with a wide variety of tools have and will continue to make important contributions to it.

There are a number of scholarships and paid programming aimed at training food justice activists, particularly youth of color, to become movement leaders. There are no scholarships particularly aimed at food justice at the graduate level. However, students and scholars interested in this topic have benefited from a variety of funding sources including the National Science Foundation, the National Institute of Health, Departments of Public Health, and a wide variety of grants aimed at health, environmental, or racial inequalities. In addition, many smaller foundations seek to support partnerships between activists and researchers. Because of its public, engaged nature, food justice scholarship can often be supported in this way. Food justice is a topic of growing popular and academic interest, and students and scholars with competitive proposals have successfully obtained funding at a variety of levels.

Key reading

Slocum, Rachel (2006) "Anti-racist Practice and the Work of Community Food Organizations." *Antipode* 38(2): 327–49.

Alkon, Alison Hope and Julian Agyeman (2011) *Cultivating Food Justice: Race, Class and Sustainability.* Cambridge, MA: MIT Press.

Guthman, Julie (2008) "If They Only Knew: Colorblindness and Universalism in Alternative Food Institutions." *The Professional Geographer* 60(3): 387–97.

Gottlieb, Robert and Andrew Fisher (1996) "'First Feed the Face': Environmental Justice and Community Food Security." *Antipode* 28 (2): 193–203.

Gottlieb, Robert and Anupama Joshi (2010) *Food Justice.* Cambridge, MA: MIT Press.

Brown, Sandy and Christie Getz (2011) "Farmworker Food Insecurity and the Production of Hunger in California." In *Cultivating Food Justice: Race, Class and Sustainability*, Alison Hope Alkon and Julian Agyeman (eds). Cambridge, MA: MIT Press.

E. Melanie DuPuis and David Goodman "Should we go 'Home' to Eat? Toward a Reflexive Politics of Localism." http://dx.doi.org/10.1016/j.jrurstud.2005.05.011

White, Monica Marie (2010) "Shouldering Responsibility for the Delivery of Human Rights: A Case Study of the D-Town Farmers of Detroit." *Race/Ethnicity: Multidisciplinary Global Perspectives* 3(2): 189–211.

Allen, Patricia (2004) *Together at the Table: Sustainability and Sustenance in the American Agrifood System.* State College, PA: Pennsylvania State University Press.

Mares, Teresa and Devon G. Peña (2010) "Urban Agriculture in the Making of Insurgent Spaces in Los Angeles and Seattle." Jeffrey Hou (ed.) *Insurgent Public Space: Guerrilla Urbanism and the Remaking of Contemporary Cities.* New York: Routledge.

Bibliography

Albala, Ken (2007) *Beans: A History.* Oxford: Berg.

Alkon, Alison Hope (2008) *Black, White and Green: A Study of Farmers Markets.* PhD dissertation, Department of Sociology, University of California, Davis.

Alkon, Alison Hope and Julian Agyeman (2011) *Cultivating Food Justice: Race, Class and Sustainability.* Cambridge, MA: MIT Press.

Alkon, Alison Hope and Kari Marie Norgaard (2009) "Breaking the Food Chains: An Investigation of Food Justice Activism." *Sociological Inquiry* 79(3): 289–305.

Allen, Barbara L. (2003) *Uneasy Alchemy: Citizens and Experts in Louisiana's Chemical Corridor Disputes.* Cambridge, MA: MIT Press.

Allen, Patricia (2004) *Together at the Table: Sustainability and Sustenance in the American Agrifood System.* State College, PA: Pennsylvania State University Press.

Avakian, Arlene Voski, ed. (1997) *Through the Kitchen Window: Women Explore the Intimate Meanings of Food and Cooking*, Boston, MA: Beacon Press.

Beaulac, Julie, Elizabeth Kristjansson, and Steven Cummins (2009) "A Systematic Review of Food Deserts, 1966–2007." *Preventing Chronic Disease: Public Health Research, Practice, and Policy* 6 (3): 1–10.

Beus, Curtis E. and Riley E. Dunlap (1990) "Conventional Versus Alternative Agriculture: The Paradigmatic Roots of the Debate." *Rural Sociology* 55(4): 590–616.

Block, Daniel and Joanne Kouba (2005) "A Comparison of the Availability and Affordability of a Market Basket in two Communities in the Chicago Area." *Public Health Nutrition* (7): 837–45.

Brown, Sandy and Christie Getz (2011) "Farmworker Food Insecurity and the Production of Hunger in California." In *Cultivating Food Justice: Race, Class and Sustainability*, Alison Hope Alkon and Julian Agyeman, eds. Cambridge, MA: MIT Press.

Burawoy, Michael (2005) "204 American Sociological Association Presidential address: For public sociology." *British Journal of Sociology* 56(2): 259–94.

Buttel, Fredrick H. (1997) "Some Observations on Agro-Food Change and the Future of Agricultural Sustainability Movements." In *Globalizing Food: Agrarian Questions and Global Restructuring*, David David and Michael Watts, eds. New York: Routledge.

Buttel, Fredrick H., Olaf F. Larson, and Gilbert W. Gillespie, Jr. (1990) *The Sociology of Agriculture.* New York: Greenwood Press.

Center for Social Inclusion (2007) "Structural Racism and our Food." www.centerforsocialinclusion.org (accessed October 30, 2009).

Clapp, Jennifer and Doris Fuchs (2009) *Corporate Power in Global Agrifood Governance*. Cambridge, MA: MIT Press.

Cole, Luke and Sheila Foster (2001) *From the Ground Up: The Rise of the Environmental Justice Movement*. New York: New York University Press.

Daniel, Cletus E. (1981) *Bitter Harvest: A History of California Farmwokers*. Ithaca, NY: Cornell University Press.

Douglass, Mary (1996) *Purity and Danger: An Analysis of the Concepts of Purity and Taboo*. New York: Taylor.

Dunlap, Riley and William R. Catton (1979) "Environmental Sociology." *Annual Review of Sociology* 5: 243–73.

Feldman, Shelley and Rick Welsh (1995) "Feminist Knowledge Claims, Local Knowledge, and Gender Divisions of Agricultural Labor: Constructing a Successor Science." *Rural Sociology* 60: 23–43.

Flammang, Janet A. (2010) *The Taste for Civilization: Food, Politics, and Civil Society*. Bloomington, IL: University of Illinois Press.

Foster, John Bellamy (1999) "Marx's Theory of Metabolic Rift: Classical Foundations for Environmental Sociology." *American Journal of Sociology* 105(2): 366–405.

Friedman, Harriet (1982) "The Political Economy of Food: The Rise and Fall of the Postwar International Food Order." *American Journal of Sociology* 88: 248–86.

Ganz, Marshall (2000) "Resources and Resourcefulness: Strategic Capacity in the Unionization of California Farmworkers." *American Journal of Sociology* 105(4): 1003–62.

Gilbert, Jess, Gwen Sharp and Sindy Felin (2002) "The Loss and Persistence of Black-Owned Farms and Farmland: A Review of the Research Literature and its Implications." *Southern Rural Sociology* 18: 1–30.

Gottlieb, Robert and Anupama Joshi (2010) *Food Justice*. Cambridge, MA: MIT Press.

Gottlieb, Robert and Andrew Fisher (1996) "'First Feed the Face': Environmental Justice and Community Food Security." *Antipode* 28 (2): 193–203.

Goody, Jack (1998) *Food and Love: A Cultural History of East and West*. London: Verso.

Granovetter, Mark (1985) "Economic Action and Social Structure: The Problem of Embeddedness." *American Journal of Sociology* 91(3): 481–510.

Guthman, Julie (2008) "If They Only Knew: Colorblindness and Universalism in Alternative Food Institutions." *The Professional Geographer* 60(3): 387–97.

——(2006) "Neoliberalism and the making of food politics in California." *Geoforum* 39(3): 1171–83.

Hall, Alan and Veronika Mogyorody (2007) "Organic Farming, Gender and the Labor Process." *Rural Sociology* 72(2): 289–316.

Heldke, Lisa (2003) *Exotic Appetites: Ruminations of a Food Adventurer*. New York: Routledge.

Israel, B. A., E. A. Parker, Z. Rowe, A. Salvatore, M. Minkler, J. Lopez (2005) "Community-based Participatory Research: Lessons Learned from the Centers for Children's Environmental Health and Disease Prevention Research." *Environmental Health Perspectives* 113(10): 1463–71.

Johnston, Josée and Shyon Baumann (2007) "Democracy versus Distinction: A Study of Omnivorousness in Gourmet Food Writing." *The American Journal of Sociology* 113(1): 165–204.

Jones, Van (2008) *The Green Collar Economy: How One Solution can Fix our Two Biggest Problems*. New York: Harper One.

Just Food (2010) *Food Justice*. www.justfood.org/food-justice (accessed July 7, 2010).

Kessel, A., J. Green, R. Pinder, P. Wilkinson, C. Grundy, and K. Lachowycz (2009) "Multidisciplinary Research in Public Health: A Case Study of Research on Access to Green Space." *Public Health* 123(1): 32–38.

La Duke, Winona (2004) *Indigenous People, Power and Politics: A Renewable Future for the Seventh Generation*. Minneapolis, MN: Honor the Earth.

Lee, G. and H. Lim (2009) "A spatial statistical approach to identifying areas … foods in the City of Buffalo, New York." *Urban Studies* 46(7): 1299–315.

Legett, John C. (2002) "Race, Nationality, and the Division of Labor in U.S. Agriculture." *Labor and Capital in the Age of Globalization*, Berch Berberoglu, ed. New York: Rowman & Littlefield.

Lipsitz, George (1998) *The Possessive Investment in Whiteness*, Philadelphia, PA: Temple University Press.

Lyson, Thomas A. (2004) *Civic Agriculture: Reconnecting Farm, Food and Community*. Boston, MA: Tufts University Press.

Magdoff, Fred, John Bellamy Foster, and Frederick H. Buttel (2000) *Hungry for Profit: The Agribusiness Threat to Farmers, Food and the Environment*. New York: Monthly Review Press.

Mares, Teresa and Devon G. Peña (2010) "Urban Agriculture in the Making of Insurgent Spaces in Los Angeles and Seattle." Jeffrey Hou (ed.) *Insurgent Public Space: Guerrilla Urbanism and the Remaking of Contemporary Cities*. New York: Routledge.

Massey, Douglass and Nancy Denton (1998) *American Apartheid: Segregation and the Making of the Underclass*. Cambridge, MA: Harvard University Press.

McClintock, Nathan (2011) "From Industrial Garden to Food Desert: Demarcated Devaluation in the Flatlands of Oakland, California." Alison Hope Alkon and Julian Agyeman (eds). *Cultivating Food Justice: Race, Class and Sustainability*. Cambridge, MA: MIT Press.

Meares, A. (1997) "Making the Transition from Conventional to Sustainable Agriculture: Gender, Social Movement Participation, and Quality of Life on the Family Farm." *Rural Sociology* 62: 21–47.

Mintz, Sidney (1985) *Sweetness and Power: The Place of Sugar in Modern History*. New York: Penguin.

Mohai, Paul and Robin K. Saha (2003) "Reassessing Race and Class Disparities in Environmental Justice Research Using Distance-Based Methods." Paper presented at the annual meeting of the American Sociological Association, Atlanta Hilton Hotel, Atlanta, GA. www.allacademic.com/meta/p107607_index.html (accessed August 16, 2003).

Morales Waugh, Irma (2010) "Sexual Harassment Experiences of Mexican Immigrant Farmworking Women." *Violence Against Women* 16(3): 237–61.

Morland, Kimberly, Steve Wing, Ana Diez Roux, and Charles Poole (2002) "Neighborhood Characteristics Associated with the Location of Food Stores and Food Service Places." *American Journal of Preventive Medicine* 22: 23–29.

Norgaard, Kari (2011) "A Continuing Legacy: Institutional Racism, Hunger and Nutritional Justice on the Klamath." Alison Hope Alkon and Julian Agyeman, eds. *Cultivating Food Justice: Race, Class and Sustainability*. Cambridge, MA: MIT Press.

Omi, Michael and Howard Winant (1994) *Racial Formation in the United States: From the 1960s to the 1990s*. London: Routledge.

Páez, Antonio, Ruben Gertes Mercado, Steven Farber, Catherine Morency, and Matthew Roorda (2010) "Relative Accessibility Deprivation Indicators for Urban Settings: Definitions and Application to Food Deserts in Montreal." *Urban Studies* 47(7): 1415–38.

Park, Lisa Sun-Hee and David Pellow (2004) "Racial Formation, Environmental Racism, and the Emergence of Silicon Valley." *Ethnicities* 4(3): 403–24.

——(2011) *Slums of Aspen: Immigrant Labor, the Environment, and the Politics of Poverty*, New York: New York University Press.

Pastor, Manuel, Rachel Morello-Frosch, and James Sadd (2006) "Breathless: Air Quality, Schools, and Environmental Justice in California." *Policy Studies Journal* 34 (3): 337–62.

Pellow, David (2007) *Resisting Global Toxics: Transnational Movements for Environmental Justice*. Cambridge, MA: MIT Press.

——(2002) *Garbage Wars: The Struggle for Environmental Justice in Chicago*. Cambridge, MA: MIT Press.

Petersen, Dana, Meredith Minkler, Victoria Breckwich Vasquez, and Andrea Baden (2006) "Community-Based Participatory Research as a Tool for Policy Change: A Case Study of the Southern California Environmental Justice Collaborative." *Review of Policy Research* 23(2): 339–54.

Philpott, Tom (2008) "Schlosser: Food Industry Abuses Workers as Matter of Course." *Grist Magazine*, www.grist.org/article/slow-food-nation-farmworkers-at-the-table/ (accessed October 30, 2009).

Pinderhughes, Raquel (2006) "Green Collar Jobs: Work Force Opportunities in the Growing Green Economy." *Journal of Race, Poverty and the Environment* 13(1).

Pinderhughes, Raquel and Joshua Miner. (2002) *Good Farming, Healthy Communities: Strengthening Regional Sustainable Agriculture Sectors and Local Food Systems*. San Francisco, CA: Independent Monograph.

Pollan, Michael (2010) "The Food Movement, Rising." *The New York Review of Books*. www.nybooks.com/articles/archives/2010/jun/10/food-movement-rising/ (accessed June 1, 2011).

Princen, Thomas, Michael Manites, and Kenneth Conca (2002) *Confronting Consumption*. Cambridge, MA: MIT Press.

Pulido, Laura (2000) "Rethinking Environmental Racism: White Privilege and Urban Development in Southern California." *Annals of the Association of American Geographers* 90: 12–40.

——(1996) "A Critical Review of the Methodology of Environmental Racism Research." *Antipode* 28(2): 142–59.

Roberts, J. Timmons (2009) *A Climate of Injustice: Global Inequality, North–South Politics, and Climate Policy*. Cambridge, MA: MIT Press.

Romm, Jeff (2001) "The Coincidental Order of Environmental Justice." Katheryn Mutz, Gary Bryner, and Douglas Kenney (eds.) *Justice and Natural Resources: Concepts, Strategies, and Applications*, Washington, DC: Island Press.

Sloan, David C. (2004) "Bad Meat and Brown Bananas: Building a Legacy of Health by Confronting Health Disparities Around Food." *Planners Network* (Winter): 49–50.

Slocum, Rachel (2006) "Anti-racist Practice and the Work of Community Food Organizations." *Antipode* 38(2): 327–49.

Szasz, Andrew (2007) *Shopping Our Way to Safety: How We Changed from Protecting the Environment to Protecting Ourselves*. Minneapolis, MN: University of Minneapolis Press.

Sze, Julie (2006) *Noxious New York: The Racial Politics of Urban Health and Environmental Justice*. Cambridge, MA: MIT Press.

Trauger, A. (2004) "Because They Can Do the Work: Women Farmers in Sustainable Agriculture in Pennsylvania, USA." *Gender, Place, and Culture* 11: 289–307.

Tuchman, Gail and Harry Gene Levine (1993) "New York Jews and Chinese Food: The Social Construction of an Ethnic Pattern." *Journal of Contemporary Ethnography* 22(3): 382–407.

United Church of Christ. (2007) *Toxic Waste and Race at Twenty*. New York: United Church of Christ.

——(1987) *Toxic Wastes and Race in the United States: A National Report on the Racial and Socio-Economic Characteristics Associated with Hazardous Waste Sites*. New York: United Church of Christ.

Watson, James L. (1997) *Golden Arches East: McDonald's in East Asia*. Palo Alto, CA: Stanford University Press.

White, Monica Marie (2010) "Shouldering Responsibility for the Delivery of Human Rights: A Case Study of the D-Town Farmers of Detroit." *Race/Ethnicity: Multidisciplinary Global Perspectives* 3(2): 189–211.

Williams, Amy Bennett (2008) "Five Plead Guilty in Immokalee Slavery Case." www.democraticunderground. com (accessed October 30, 2009).

Williams-Forson, Psyche (2006) *Building Houses out of Chicken Legs: Black Women, Food and Power*. Chapel Hill: University of North Carolina Press.

Witt, Doris (1999) *Black Hunger: Soul Food and America*. Mineapolis: University of Minnesota Press.

Zenk, Shannon N., Amy J. Schultz, Barbara A. Israel, Sherman A. James, Shuming Bao, and Mark L. Wilson (2005) "Neighborhood Racial Composition, Neighborhood Poverty, and the Spatial Accessibility of Supermarkets in Metropolitan Detroit." *American Journal of Public Health* 95: 660–67.

28

Food studies and animal rights

Carol Helstosky

This article evaluates the impact that the animal rights and animal welfare movements have had on contemporary food habits. After tracing the history of vegetarianism, the article argues that food studies scholars should take more seriously animal rights and animal welfare movements, not only for their philosophical and moral underpinnings, but also in terms of their very real and measurable impact on meat eating. Although seemingly opposed in viewpoints, animal rights advocates and food studies scholars have much to learn from each other. After decades of publication on vegetarianism and the costs of meat consumption, the time is right for a new generation of food studies scholars to evaluate the relationship between humans and non-humans in terms of food consumption and to bring the field of food studies squarely into current debates about the social and environmental costs of food choice, the malleability of food habits, and the ethics of certain food traditions.

Introduction

It would seem that food studies scholars and animal rights advocates are on opposite ends of the table when it comes to thinking about food choice. A pure animal rights advocate believes that animals are not "ours" to do with as we please and, therefore, we should not eat them, nor should we extract any products (milk, eggs) from them; thus a fully committed animal rights advocate is a vegan. Veganism is about limiting one's diet and while a vegan may eat food that tastes good, morality, not taste, is the primary motivator for food choices. Abstaining from all animal products involves a radical change, not only in one's diet but also in one's attitudes towards food traditions, rituals, and trends, many of which involve the consumption of animals. Given the abundance of meat and animal products in the American diet, a choice to reject this norm can meet with hostility or ridicule from those who enjoy the taste of meat or do not care to think about where their meat comes from. Thus, for many ethical vegans, food choice can become a point of tension or discord with the broader community. Food studies scholars understand food quite differently. They enjoy chronicling the expansion, not the restriction, of diet, through improvements in agriculture, refinements in food preparation, and the development of a food market. They write about food traditions and rituals with a seriousness of purpose, if not reverence, because food traditions and rituals, scholars argue, make us who we are. Moreover, rediscovering or preserving (not radically altering) food traditions reassures food studies scholars and their audiences that food still means something in a fast-food world. Lastly, food studies scholars write more about how taste, not ethics, motivates food choices and they tend to see food as a unifying, not dividing, element in society.

Despite these differences, the history and impact of the animal rights movement are significant for understanding many key concepts and ideas relevant to the discipline of food studies (the intersection between politics and diet; environmental consequences of consumption; health and diet; food reform movements). This essay will chart the history of how the animal rights and animal welfare movements have shaped attitudes towards using animals as food sources. Although there are key differences between the animal rights and the animal welfare philosophies, this essay will assesses their impact as social movements and as political forces and thus, they must be viewed together, as both have had measurable effects on how consumers think about the consumption of animals and animal products. Observers and critics of animal rights often focus on the philosophy behind the movement, which many see as unrealistic, overly rigid, or preposterous (what will happen to all the animals if we do not eat them?). However, to measure the impact of animal rights exclusively by philosophical writings is to tell only part of the story. Animal rights is much more than a philosophy; local and national organizations have had to make strategic decisions about how, when, and where to help animals, decisions that have had very real impact on how people think about eating animals. As much as animal rights advocates may desire a world in which no animal is used or exploited, they have chosen to expose and combat some of the worst abuses of animals first (though not exclusively), in an effort to promote public awareness about the extent of animal abuse. Some of the worst cases of abuse have been uncovered in the meat production industries; therefore, animal rights and animal welfare advocates have pushed some critical issues out into the public realm regarding our consumption of animals and animal products. The public campaigns of both animal rights and animal welfare advocates are as significant as their philosophies in shaping debates about food choices.

Historical background and major theoretical approaches

Before the rise of the animal rights social movement in the 1970s and 1980s, there has been a lengthy history of individuals refusing to eat or sacrifice animals on ethical grounds. Humans may have practiced vegetarianism for moral or health reasons, or economic concerns may have limited individual meat consumption levels, but the word vegetarian was not coined until the mid-nineteenth century, around the time of the founding of the first secular vegetarian society in England in the 1840s. Although some vegetarians abstained from meat for health or religious reasons, a growing number of people who supported the anti-cruelty and anti-vivisection movements of the late nineteenth century also abstained from meat because of their concern for all animals, not just working animals or animals used for scientific experimentation. Ethical vegetarians were viewed with much skepticism, as Howard Williams complained in *The Ethics of Diet* (1883); despite a continuous tradition of individuals refusing to eat meat, vegetarianism was frequently dismissed as a "fad." Unintentional vegetarianism, born of poor economic circumstances, was widely practiced until the mid-twentieth century. In the late nineteenth century, physiologists advocated high levels of protein in order to furnish more labor power. Meat was considered by experts to be an optimal protein source, but for many, meat was still a scarce commodity, consumed on special occasions or when one was sick. During both World Wars, consumers were urged to reduce their meat consumption in order to conserve scarce proteins and fats; vegetarian and vegan dishes became patriotic. As Donna Gabaccia has argued, the wars brought ethnic cuisines that utilized little or no meat into the American mainstream. After the Second World War, improved economic circumstances led to a steady increase in meat consumption in the United States and throughout Europe; vegetarianism once again was regarded as an odd or "bohemian" fad.

In the 1970s, Francis Moore Lappé's *Diet for a Small Planet* (1971) and Peter Singer's *Animal Liberation* (1975) moved ethical vegetarianism out from the fringes of culinary practice and into the mainstream of thinking about the consequences of one's diet. Lappé was motivated to conserve the world's resources, while Singer proposed an entirely new system of evaluating nonhuman life. Yet the two authors reached the same conclusion: One does not have to, nor should one, eat meat. Additionally, Singer and Lappé advocated vegetarianism within a larger ethical and environmental framework: one should abstain from meat and animal products not merely because one liked animals, but because to do so fitted into a broader vision of how to transform the world.

Lappé's book emerged out of the international debate over how to use the world's resources in order to produce enough food for everybody. Using the American example, Lappé described the relationship between the overconsumption of meat and the misallocation of agricultural resources to meet rising demand. At the time, Americans consumed more meat than any other country in the world. In particular, Americans loved steak, considered a definitive marker of social prestige (of "making it") and the most demanding to produce in terms of food, water, and land use. Eschewing meat in favor of vegetable protein was a significant step toward solving problems like world hunger and also a step toward responsible environmental stewardship. For Lappé, humans had a choice about what to eat and, if they ate conscientiously, they did not have to make meat their main source of protein. Lappé concludes her social and environmental critique with lessons and recipes in how to combine proteins so as to achieve maximum nutritional benefit from a vegetarian diet. For today's reader, Lappé's concerns about protein consumption may seem excessive and her hope that agricultural concerns would shift production seems idealistic. Still, the book and its subsequent revisions (today, Frances and her daughter Anna are active in maintaining the Small Planet Institute) comprised an important first step in questioning the allocation of agricultural resources and challenging scientific theories about protein consumption in the decades after 1945.

A few years later, philosopher Peter Singer published *Animal Liberation*, which he researched and wrote after a conversation with a vegetarian. Singer popularized the concept of *speciesism*, to subjugate nonhuman animals for human purposes, including eating, as wrong and akin to other forms of prejudicial behavior. Because they have the capacity to suffer (not think or express emotions or act like humans), animals have an interest in *not suffering* and, therefore, they have the right to exist without exploitation or abuse from humans. Providing animals with these rights, then, would furnish the greatest good for the greatest number of all living creatures. According to Singer's reasoning, humans might consume animals if they could find a way to do so without causing the animal to suffer. Yet Singer argued that the conditions of industrial meat production and the fact that alternatives to meat exist meant that vegetarianism is the only ethically acceptable diet. Gustatory pleasure cannot outweigh the rights of the animals not to suffer. *Animal Liberation* deeply offended many readers and others who did not read it (but certainly had opinions about it) because of Singer's suggestion that animals deserve equal consideration.

Although quite different in focus and intent, Lappé's and Singer's books are worth examining together, not only because they were published around the same time, but also because they interrogated the moral consequences of food choices. Neither book was intended to make readers particularly comfortable with eating meat, and both books sought to persuade readers by urging them to move beyond matters of individual preference or taste and to think about their diet within larger political, environmental, and ethical frameworks.

In the wake of the natural foods and health food trends in America, more cookbooks and recipe collections included vegetarian and vegan recipes. Among these books, the *Moosewood Cookbook* (1978) by Mollie Katzen and *Laurel's Kitchen* (1975) by Laurel Robertson were the most popular vegetarian cookbooks, adapting ethnic recipes for vegetarians and refining protein combinations in order to make vegetarian food more attractive to curious readers. A few years later, Dudley Giehl's *Vegetarianism* (1979) and Mark Braunstein's *Radical Vegetarianism* (1981) explained and defended vegetarianism while also encouraging vegetarian readers to maintain and extend their ethical considerations (especially in the case of Braunstein, who advocated a vegan diet). Both works combined history, nutritional advice, information about factory farming, and even economic and legal analyses of the costs of meat consumption. This multi-disciplinary approach to discussing vegetarianism never lost sight of the main ethical reasons for rejecting meat, but their approach highlighted how modern systems of meat production affected so many aspects of daily life in the United States.

As the animal rights movements grew in popularity and impact throughout the 1980s, the initial "targets" for change were those considered egregious in terms of cruelty: Fur coats, fox hunting, cosmetics testing, and certain types of vivisection (i.e. surgical staple demonstrations using live dogs). High-profile investigations, coupled with animal "liberations" at research facilities, focused attention on the use of animals for scientific purposes and later animals used for entertainment, although a few organizations, like FARM and Farm Sanctuary, were dedicated to raising awareness about the use of animals for food. Yet, high-profile campaigns against the use of animals for food were rare, given that levels of public sympathy for animals did not yet extend to farm animals and the public was not fully aware of the potential threats posed by industrial agricultural systems.

Increased public attention to the plight of animals in factory farms resulted from a constellation of events in the late 1980s and early 1990s. In the United Kingdom, the first fatalities from cases of Bovine Spongiform Encephalopathy (BSE or mad cow disease) happened in 1986; subsequently, humans acquired and died of a new variant of Creutzfeldt-Jacob disease, which had similar neurological symptoms. The epidemic and public health threat invited public scrutiny of factory farm practices such as feeding cattle rendered animal parts in commercial feed. Activists and journalists also described the use of antibiotics, hormones, pesticides, and fertilizers in commercial feeds and medical treatments for livestock. John Robbins' book, *Diet for a New America* (1987), boldly referred to "America the Poisoned" in one chapter on factory farming. Robbins urged readers to adopt veganism for health, environmental, and humane reasons. Throughout the 1980s, a growing number of individuals and organizations protested the rapid expansion of McDonald's restaurants in Europe. Activists opposed to the "McDonaldization" of Europe came from all ideological viewpoints, but the animal rights perspective was well represented, especially in the United Kingdom, home to the "McLibel" case of 20 years against a pair of London activists. Once again, the public was made aware of the conditions inside factory farms and the scale of such practices in the wake of the massive global expansion of McDonald's and other fast food restaurants. Mad cow disease and the McDonald's protests raised awareness among European and later American consumers, regarding food choice, health, and morality in a fast-paced global economy.

In the United States, journalist Eric Schlosser expanded an article he wrote for *Rolling Stone* in 1999 into a book-length study of human and animal exploitation by McDonald's, *Fast Food Nation* (2001). The book is frequently compared to Upton Sinclair's *The Jungle* but, in addition to dredging up some rather unpleasant truths about the McDonald's food system, *Fast Food Nation* described the history of America's evolving relationship with meat production, chronicling how embedded the factory farm system became after the Second World War and forecasting the global consequences of sustained growth of this system. The graphic details about animal exploitation were underemphasized in ensuing analyses of the "McDonaldization" phenomenon, yet under pressure from animal rights and animal welfare advocates, McDonald's adopted new standards for procuring meat and the rest of the fast food world followed suit. Initially, the fast food industry adopted partial measures for reform in order to assure the public that the meat they ate was safe. Schlosser's book returned readers to the issue of food safety with regard to factory farming, a topic which seems to gain only irregular scholarly attention (Marion Nestle's *Food Politics* in 2002 was an early example). Certainly, food safety scares encompass more than just animal products, but the public health and public safety dimensions of meat eating are yet to be explored thoroughly. One of the gravest concerns about food safety stems directly from animal cruelty in meat-processing plants: The treatment and use of injured or sick animals or "downers." Undercover investigations and graphic video footage documented the brutal treatment of injured animals in meat-processing plants, evidence not only of a lack of concern or care, but also the economic stakes involved in pushing as many animals as quickly as possible through the slaughterhouse. The USDA recently (2010) banned the use of downed cattle for food, but other downed animals may still be slaughtered and consumed. And, despite more official assurances that meat is safe, meat and poultry recalls indicate that the current regulatory system is not 100 percent effective.

Animal rights and animal welfare organizations were not alone in bringing public attention to the high stakes of agribusiness; the organic food movement gained strength in the 1990s and 2000s from greater public awareness of pesticide and GMO use on large farms. Although united in opposition to factory farming, animal rights and organic/local food advocates do not necessarily agree on the issue of meat consumption, especially when it comes to non-factory-farmed meat. Michael Pollan, for example, wrote *The Omnivore's Dilemma*, not *The Vegetarian's Travail*, and while the book is a tour de force of careful research and insightful observations, Pollan's chapter on vegetarianism is perhaps the weakest in the book, lacking focus and offering nothing new in defense of meat eating. Pollan and others have written on the prospects for ethical meat consumption, i.e. meat raised on small family farms where the suffering of animals would be kept to a minimum. Proponents of ethical meat consumption sidestep the issue of whether small farms could sustainably or realistically satisfy all Americans' (and not just those who can afford it) desire for meat and inexpensive meat at that. While ethical consumption advocates focus public attention on the wrongs of the food factory system, they tend to avoid any deep or sustained engagement with the ethics of eating meat, opting to leave the choice up to the individual consumer.

Though much of the news about CAFOs (concentrated animal feeding operations) and slaughterhouse cruelty shocked the public, it failed to dramatically change eating habits, and ultimately, it had little impact on industrial meat production. Between 1970 and 2008, worldwide beef production almost doubled, pork production nearly tripled, and poultry production increased six times over. In that same time period, milk production has doubled and egg production has tripled. However, in the last two years (2010–11), beef production has leveled off and decreased very slightly (most likely because industrial hog production has now flooded the market with inexpensive pork). Increases on this scale were only possible through intensive factory farm methods. In the face of such daunting figures, animal rights advocates have expanded their work beyond exposing cruelty in the animal production business. Organizations like PETA have presented a more upbeat vision of veganism for consumers, one that highlights vegan celebrities, publicity stunts (that some have found offensive), and a social network of health tips, recipes, and lifestyle advice. Despite the positive attributes of such campaigns, the popular media continue to characterize vegetarians and vegans in a negative light, as fanatics or hypocrites or worse. Such characterizations constitute "vegaphobia" and are found even in the liberal mainstream press, according to a recent British study (Cole 2011). Certain vegetarian campaigns have been more successful than others; the public may be sympathetic to downed cows and pigs locked in gestation crates, but less willing to give up eating chicken, fish, and lobster (David Foster Wallace's brilliant essay, "Consider the Lobster," notwithstanding). Recent studies of fishing (*The End of the Line* and *An Unnatural History of the Sea*) highlight the dire environmental consequences of overfishing while animal rights advocates have made the public aware that fish do indeed feel pain when they are hooked.

Despite greater public knowledge of the environmental and health consequences of consuming meat, few are committed vegetarians and far fewer are vegans.[1] The question of why so few people are vegetarian is usually answered by conspiracy theories about the meat lobby or justifications rooted in our genetic predisposition to eat bacon double cheeseburgers. Yet it seems worthwhile to at least attempt to answer this question more systematically, because the stakes for our current meat production system are high, and an increase in meat production, experts predict, would create the conditions for an environmental disaster. It seems valid to explore why humans continue to eat meat – out of habit, force, tradition, or preference? Although we smirk at the phrase "you are what you eat," some very intriguing studies in the field of psychology suggest that one's food choices may directly affect one's behavior, at least with regard to respect for animals. Studies published in the journal *Appetite* explore the psychology of food consumption, with suggestive, yet tentative, results. A 2010 study by psychologists on meat eating, for example, posits that consuming animals can, in the short term, make the individual consumer less concerned about issues of animal cruelty. Their conclusion is worth quoting at length:

> We started this paper with a paradox: that people both like animals and like eating animals. The current study suggests one way in which people may resolve these conflicting beliefs. When eating meat, people appear to suppress their moral concern, and this leads to a reduction in the perceived capacity of meat animals to suffer. It appears that when faced with the dilemma of participating in the potentially immoral treatment of an animal people shift the animal's moral status.
>
> (*Loughnan* et al., *2010: 159*)

Studies like this raise some very intriguing and perhaps troubling questions about how food choice may shape our behaviors and attitudes towards animals … as opposed to the other way around.

Research methodologies

As both a philosophy and a political movement, animal rights embrace a variety of disciplinary influences. Moreover, as concerns mount over the health and environmental consequences of industrial farming, new voices have entered the debate from the fields of nutrition, the environmental sciences, and journalism. It is not surprising, then, that research methodology in this field varies tremendously, depending on context, audience, and one's personal views on animals. Because animal rights advocates speak for others, not for themselves, their findings and arguments are consistently challenged or rejected because they are, in the words of their critics, untrue, sentimental, or misguided. The contentiousness of these debates frequently obscures important questions like how do we find out about the use of animals for food and how do we evaluate this information? Those who attempt to answer these questions adopt a range of methodological strategies, some more convincing than others.

The most successful methodological approaches are those that offer extensive *and* critical evaluation of sources. Multi-authored works like *The CAFO Reader* are extremely useful to academics because they approach a substantial issue from a variety of viewpoints, in this case, examining the history and consequences of the corporate animal-feeding operation in the United States, while evaluating alternative models for food production and considering multiple perspectives (from farmers, animal rights advocates, environmentalists, and others) on the issue. Single-authored studies that combine careful research, material from published works, and personal observations are also useful, although it must be pointed out that reliable statistics on meat consumption, vegetarianism, and the treatment of animals (particularly the abuse of animals) are difficult to obtain or verify. And, given the highly partisan nature of the debate about meat eating, available statistics tend to come from either animal rights groups or the meat industries. There is clearly a need for more reliable statistical studies in this area, given that there has been increased public awareness of, and interest in, the industrial production of meat and animal products.

Perhaps some of the most influential books in this field are those that combine ethical or moral reflection and argument with data on the scope and consequences of animal exploitation. Matthew Scully's *Dominion* and Peter Singer's *Animal Liberation* are diametrically opposed in terms of their philosophical underpinnings, but they arrive at the same conclusion: That society should condemn and reject the widespread use and abuse of animals as a food source. Their methodology combines a philosophical/moral argument with a literature review and personal observations of animal and human behavior.

Less known or publicized works on the history of vegetarianism trace the intellectual roots and history of vegetarian thought. Given that vegetarians from the past had so many diverse reasons for rejecting meat consumption, it is difficult to establish a coherent or unified history of vegetarianism, and more reasonable, it seems, to write a history of vegetarians. However, Tristram Stuart's erudite work, *The Bloodless Revolution*, approaches the topic provocatively, as the history of exchange between "Western" and "Eastern" ideas about animals-as-food. It is perhaps now possible to write a history of modern vegetarianism (post-*Animal Liberation*) as a cultural or social movement. Historical interpretations of the rise of animal food industries (ranching, factory farming, fishing) tend to deal more with the social and environmental consequences of these systems of production, and less with the popular attitudes toward the consumption of animals and animal products.

More recently, highly personal studies of animal farming seek to bring the issue of lived experience to the debate on the use of animals for food. Gene Baur, who founded the organization Animal Sanctuary, and Nicolette Hahn Niman, who shifted from animal welfare lawyer to livestock farmer, both offer interpretations of how their experience determines whether or not they consume animals and animal products. This personal engagement with the issue is convincing as a methodology only when it is backed up by more general information from secondary sources, or details from the authors' work in the field of animal welfare/animal rights.

Although many authors attempt to connect to their audiences through their personal experiences with animals and/or animal consumption, their arguments rather obviously become more suspect when they are rooted in emotions and/or desire. Paradoxically, perhaps, this highly personalized or subjective approach (the overuse of the "I") proves to be the most popular among reading audiences. Although Michael Pollan's *The Omnivore's Dilemma* is thoroughly researched, some of the central arguments dealing with meat consumption rely on Pollan's subjective interpretation of the relationship between evolution and meat eating and his explanations of how he feels when hunting and/or consuming animals. Similarly, Jonathan

Safran Foer's *Eating Animals* is full of useful information, but his argument against meat consumption sometimes rests on his own experiences, such as gazing into the eyes of a dying turkey. Whether one is appalled by or grateful for the death of an animal, descriptions of such experiences offer little in the way of a critical perspective on one of the most significant issues facing communities and societies today: That our current system of meat production hurts our health, the environment, and our sense of morality. As the next section details, the time is ripe for a new generation of scholars to move beyond the highly personalized frame of reference, to re-evaluate the relationship between humans and non-humans in terms of food consumption, and to bring the field of food studies squarely into contemporary debates on vegetarianism and veganism.

Avenues for future research

One of the most significant food-related developments of the twentieth century was the increase in global meat consumption, facilitated by the industrial production of meats and by the cultural association of meat eating with wealth and status. In the United States, where this system of intensive meat production originated, meat consumption reached an all-time high in 2007 of 222 pounds per person of meat and poultry. Pizzas are piled high with three or four different types of meat; bacon tops most sandwiches in fast food outlets and restaurants alike; even salads are routinely tossed with chicken or steak. The meat-centered diet, popular in the United States, is now rising in popularity throughout the world. The ubiquity of meat should strike food historians as significant. Whereas for centuries in most countries, meat was consumed rarely by the majority of that country's population, it is now available everywhere at relative low cost. The consequences of the spread of the "American" meat-focused diet are significant, not just for moral concerns about the numbers of animals slaughtered in the United States each year (estimates vary, but roughly three billion animals were slaughtered for meat in 1975, now the number fluctuates between nine and ten billion), but also for the aforementioned environmental and health consequences of eating inexpensive meat.

Although works like Eric Schlosser's *Fast Food Nation*, Erik Marcus' *Meat Market*, and Daniel Imhoff's *The CAFO Reader* have traced the history of industrial meat production in broader terms, much of the recent discussion about meat consumption has stalled into an unproductive debate about "happy meat" or ethical meat consumption. Proponents of "happy meat" think mostly about themselves, recounting how they as individuals "feel" about the experience of consuming animals. Thus, meat consumption is not understood or interpreted in a scholarly way, as a societal or global phenomenon, but as a matter of individual choice, a choice that is not practical for many other consumers. Defending "happy meat" rather neatly assuages one's individual conscience, but it does little to situate food choice within larger consequences and developments. It also does little to stem the tide of industrial meat production, as it views meat consumption as an individual preference. Similarly, animal rights advocates, by narrowing their focus to the viability of "happy meat," have lost track of the larger issues that deserve scholarly attention. Individual or personal choices do indeed matter, but they must be evaluated within the broader context of political, economic, social, and environmental responsibility.

Scholars interested in both food studies and animal rights could potentially focus public attention back to the broader contexts of, and consequences for, the consumption of animals and animal products. Scholars have traced the history of factory farming in the United States, though much more could be said about the political dimensions of these developments, especially the ways in which meat-producing interests have influenced American consumer habits through federal agencies like the USDA or the National School Lunch Program. Marion Nestle (*Food Politics*) first described the role of agricultural interest groups in influencing nutritional recommendations, through the creation of the food pyramid, for example. More recently, Erik Marcus has questioned the control of the USDA (as opposed to the National Institutes of Health) over nutritional recommendations. Future work might continue to examine the history of how agricultural interests influence our consumption habits not only through the foods they produce, but also through the political influence they wield. Americans' current addiction to "cheap meat" is a direct result of a vast system of agricultural subsidies; more studies and a history of this subsidy system would shed light on how much of our "cheap meat" habit is publicly financed. The political and economic dimensions of meat consumption are as significant as the environmental and health-related ones.

It is worth emphasizing that the meat-centered diet[2] is a relatively recent historical development, born in the United States after the Depression and the Second World War. A recent controversial article by B. R. Myers on "foodie" writing argues that some authors in the field of food studies have manipulated human history and the history of evolution, concluding that centuries of meat eating have somehow made humans into hard-wired carnivores and meat has shaped (and therefore should continue to shape) our very souls. Such peculiar assertions fly in the face of historical reality. Perhaps our evolutionary ancestors hunted and ate a great deal of meat, but there were many centuries of scarcity in between then and now. Food studies scholars need to be more attentive to the actual history of meat eating in terms of the practical realities of dietary constrictions and shortages: What did people eat? What could they afford to eat? What types of animals were consumed when and why? Histories of meat consumption should offer a scholarly corrective to assertions about the evolution of our souls as meat eaters (given that popular arguments against vegetarianism are that humans were "made" to eat meat or that humans have always eaten meat). Similarly, histories of eating little or no meat, as opposed to histories of vegetarianism, would correct the ethnocentric assumption that "our" souls have been shaped by centuries of meat eating. Meat consumption may define the twentieth-century American culture, but what about other cultures? It seems worth noting, for example, that some of the most popular, and complex, cuisines developed in cultures where meat was rarely consumed, and if it was consumed it was used sparingly (India and Italy are the two most obvious examples). This preoccupation with meat, as a central foundation of diet and therefore human identity, is worth interrogating further for what it reveals about the politics of meat consumption and cultural attitudes towards vegetarianism.

Another venue of future research pertains to cultural attitudes towards vegetarianism and veganism, particularly the latent and overt hostility toward consumers who choose not to eat meat. The previously mentioned study of "vegaphobia" in the British press revealed the extent to which vegetarians and vegans are still depicted as inconsistent or hypocritical fanatics, motivated by ideology rather than a culinary or ethical choice. And, despite a greater public awareness of animal rights and animal welfare issues, vegetarian and vegan cooking remain on the margins of the vast food media network in the United States. Although many chefs on the Food Network prepare dishes without meat or animal products, there have only been a handful of shows that deal explicitly with vegetarianism. Rather, the opposite trend toward excessive or unusual meat consumption seems to have captured the public imagination. Thus, hosts of Food Network programs consume vast amounts of barbecued meat in a single sitting while the food faddist group the "Gastronauts" consume unusual meats (like live octopus, horse, and guinea pig) and post the videos on YouTube. Food studies scholars interested in contemporary social trends should explore this seeming paradox more thoroughly. Despite greater awareness of the suffering of animals used for food, why does latent and overt hostility toward more ethical eating habits still persist? How have recent trends in excessive, unusual, or extreme meat consumption influenced popular eating habits? Although food manufacturers have made meat alternatives and vegetarian options more readily available, why is the American food media industry so slow to acknowledge vegetarian and/or vegan cooking? Our simultaneous cultural unease with killing animals for food and our cultural distaste for vegetarian/veganism deserves more rigorous scholarly treatment than it has received thus far.

Lastly, it seems fair to say that in recent years, much of the debate about animals in food production has focused on the humane treatment of animals in factory farms and, to a lesser extent, the morality of consuming any animals or animal products. Participants in these debates have justified their positions by relying on a large body of scientific studies regarding animal consciousness, or the animals' ability to think, feel pain, suffer, and demonstrate something that humans would recognize as emotions. Still other participants have focused on the social, environmental, and public health consequences of industrialized meat production. The range of opinions in these debates clearly demonstrates the impact of the animal rights/animal welfare movements in moving such questions and concerns out into the public domain, as well as the growing number of individuals and communities who have something to contribute to these debates. It is curious, then, that the field of food studies is relatively quiet on such debates, save for a few books on the history of vegetarianism. Given that so much of the contemporary debates about eating animals focus on traditions and habits ("we have always eaten meat, therefore we are supposed to eat meat and will continue to eat meat"), food studies scholars could offer much in the way of evaluating and interrogating culinary habits and traditions. Are all food habits and traditions "okay" and therefore should they be preserved without question or resistance or can a substantial number of people change the way they eat if they decide to do so? Have there been past cases of dietary or culinary change, when populations chose to adopt new habits or does change only come through coercion or necessity? Should tradition be subject to moral or ethical interrogation?

Practical considerations for getting started

There is no lack of sources about vegetarianism and veganism. There are many websites and blogs dealing with health and nutritional information, practical tips for becoming a vegetarian or vegan, recipes, information about new products, and, in some cases, information about animal rights activism. The website of the Vegetarian Resource Group contains a great deal of information, recipes, announcements, and articles about vegetarian and vegan foods (www.vrg.org). The magazine and website *Vegetarian Times* contains recipes and articles about vegetarianism and veganism (www.vegetariantimes.com). In the United Kingdom, the Vegetarian Society (www.vegsoc.org) maintains a very detailed and extensive website. As for vegetarian and vegan blogs, there are too many to review here. A useful website for browsing the blog offerings is the Vegan and Vegetarian Blog Tracker, www.vegblogs.com, which lists some of the highlights from a variety of blogs.

Moreover, the major animal rights and animal welfare organizations have devoted substantial attention to vegetarianism and veganism. People for the Ethical Treatment of Animals (www.peta.org) and the Humane Society of the United States (www.hsus.org) offer the most comprehensive coverage, with PETA espousing a more radical line on dietary change. Organizations specifically dedicated to farm animal issues include Farm Animal Rights or FARM (www.farmusa.org), the Humane Farming Association (www.hfa.org), and Farm Sanctuary (www.farmsanctuary.org), which maintains a website about both of its sanctuaries in New York and California. All of the farm animal websites contain information about legislation regarding animals and agriculture.

One can find much statistical information about meat production and consumption from the meat industries themselves. The American Meat Institute (www.meatami.com) is the oldest and largest trade association for the meat and poultry industries. Other organizations include the National Meat Association (www.nmaonline.org); the American Association of Meat Processors (www.aamp.com); the American Meat Science Association (www.meatscience.org); the US Poultry and Egg Association (www.poultryegg.org); the American Poultry Association (www. amerpoultryassn.com); and the National Pork Producers Council (www.nppc.org). In addition, there are numerous state councils and associations, as well as many non-US organizations.

However, to think about this issue as animal rights organizations versus the meat industry representatives is to think in overly narrow terms. Scholars interested in how these issues relate to broader contexts may want to look into research in the emerging field of animal studies. An internet clearing house for animal studies is H–Animal, an H–Net discussion group (www.h-net. org\~animal). H–Animal sponsors an email list-serve as well as discussion boards, calls for papers and submissions, a syllabus exchange, reviews of conferences, and thoughtful essays. H–Animal is dedicated to understanding animals in human culture; therefore, the use of animals as food figures prominently in this list-serve's content. H–Animal also lists university programs and academic centers where scholars and students can go to study the human–animal bond with experts in the field. Centers for studying human–animal relations are becoming popular at veterinary schools (there are centers at the University of Pennsylvania, Tuskegee University, Washington State University, Purdue University, and the University of California at Davis). Animal studies programs are located at Michigan State University (animal studies, graduate specialization), Colorado State University (animality studies, animalitystudies.colostate.edu, accessed April 9, 2011), and Eastern Kentucky University (www.psychology.eku.edu/animalstu dy.php, accessed April 9, 2011). In addition, the Humane Society of the United States (www. hsus.org) has a Humane Society University. Outside the United States, there are animal study groups in New Zealand (the New Zealand Centre for Human–Animal Studies, www.nzchas. canterbury.ac.nz, accessed on April 9, 2012) and Australia (the Australian Animal Studies Group www.aasg.org.au, accessed on April 9, 2012).

Scholars looking for archival material related to the history of the animal rights and animal welfare movements may wish to consult the Tom Regan Animal Rights Archive at North Carolina State University, which contains an animal rights manuscript collection (www.lib.ncsu. edu/animalrights, accessed on April 9, 2012). Another interesting source of archival material is the Guither Papers, housed at the University of Illinois (www.library.illinois.edu/archives, accessed on April 9, 2012). Harold D. Guither, formerly a professor of agricultural economics at the University of Illinois, chronicled the history of the animal rights and animal welfare movements between 1977 and 2001.

Most of the funding available for projects in the areas of animal rights and vegetarianism relates to activism and support for organizations; there are few grants given out to individuals who want to do independent research. Similarly, grants in the field of animal studies focus more on human–domestic pet interactions. Scholars would be well advised to apply for funding in their respective disciplines (sociology, history, psychology, etc.) or in the field of food studies.

Notes

1 Estimates vary according to polls and studies. According to a 2008 *Vegetarian Times* poll, in the United States, less than 1 percent of the population follows a vegan diet. An estimated 3–5 percent of the population is vegetarian (no meat, poultry, or fish) and around 10 percent of the population follows a "vegetarian-inclined" diet.

2 By "meat-centered" I mean a diet where meat and animal products assume a central role in most, if not all, meals. I am not arguing that societies in the past were vegetarian or ate few animal products because they were concerned about animal welfare. Rather, societies in the past did not consume nearly as much meat as we do today for many reasons, chief among them being economic ones.

Key reading

Adams, Carol J. (2001) *Living Among Meat Eaters. The Vegetarian's Survival Handbook*. New York: Three Rivers.

——(2000) *The Sexual Politics of Meat: A Feminist-Vegetarian Critical Theory. Tenth Anniversary Edition*. New York: Continuum.

Baur, Gene (2008) *Farm Sanctuary: Changing Hearts and Minds About Animals and Food*. New York: Touchstone.

Brauntein, Mark Matthew (1993) *Radical Vegetarianism: A Dialectic of Diet and Ethic*. Revised Edition. Quaker Hill, CT: Panacea Press.

Clover, Charles (2006) *The End of the Line. How Overfishing is Changing the World and What We Eat*. New York: The New Press.

Cole, Matthew and Karen Morgan (2011) "Vegaphobia: Derogatory Discourses of Veganism and the Reproduction of Speciesism in UK National Newspapers." *British Journal of Sociology* 62, 1: 134–53.

Foer, Jonathan Safran (2009) *Eating Animals*. New York: Little Brown and Company.

Fox, Michael Allen (1999) *Deep Vegetarianism*. Philadelphia, PA: Temple University Press.

Friend, Catherine (2005) *The Compassionate Carnivore: Or, How to Keep Animals Happy, Save Old MacDonald's Farm, Reduce Your Hoofprint, and Still Eat Meat*. Cambridge, MA: Da Capo Press.

Giehl, Dudley (1979) *Vegetarianism. A Way of Life*. New York: Harper and Row.

Imhoff, Daniel, ed. (2010) *The CAFO Reader. The Tragedy of Industrial Animal Factories*. Healdsburg, CA: Watershed Media.

Lappé, Frances Moore (1971) *Diet for a Small Planet*. New York: Ballantine Books.

Loughan, Steve, Haslam, Nick, and Bastian, Brock (2010) "The Role of Meat Consumption and the Denial of Moral Status and Mind to Meat Animals." *Appetite* 55: 156–59.

Marcus, Erik (2005) *Meat Market: Animals, Ethics, and Morality*. Cupertino, CA: Brio Press.

Myers, B. R. "The Moral Crusade Against Foodies." *The Atlantic*. March 2011. www.theatlantic.com/magazine/archive/2011/03/the-moral-crusade-against-foodies/8370/ (accessed May 1, 2012).

Niman, Nicolette Hahn (2009) *Righteous Porkchop: Finding a Life and Good Food Beyond Factory Farms*. New York: Harper Collins.

Preece, Rod (2008) *Sins of the Flesh: A History of Ethical Vegetarian Thought*. Vancouver: UBC Press.

Robbins, John (1987) *Diet for a New America*. Walpole, NH: Stillpoint.

Roberts, Callum (2007) *The Unnatural History of the Sea*. Washington, DC: Island Press.

Schlosser, Eric (2001) *Fast Food Nation. The Dark Side of the All-American Meal*. New York: Perennial.

Scully, Matthew (2002) *Dominion. The Power of Man, the Suffering of Animals, and the Call to Mercy*. New York: St Martin's Press.

Singer, Peter (1975) *Animal Liberation: A New Ethics for Our Treatment of Animals*. New York: Avon Books.

Singer, Peter and Mason, Jim (2006) *The Ethics of What We Eat. Why Our Food Choices Matter*. Emmaus, PA: Rodale Press.

Spencer, Colin (2002) *Vegetarianism. A History*. London: Four Walls, Eight Windows, (originally published as *The Heretic's Feast* in 1993).

Stuart, Tristram (2006) *The Bloodless Revolution. A Cultural History of Vegetarianism from 1600 to Modern Times*. New York: W.W. Norton.

Wallace, David Foster (2004) "Consider the Lobster." *Gourmet* August.

Williams, Howard (2003) *The Ethics of Diet: A Catena of Authorities Deprecatory of the Practice of Flesh-Eating*. Carol J. Adams. ed. Chicago, IL: University of Illinois Press, first published 1882.

29

Qualitative and mixed methods approaches to explore social dimensions of food and nutrition security

Stefanie Lemke and Anne C. Bellows

Social dimensions of food and nutrition security form one aspect of the growing field of food studies. We introduce qualitative and mixed methods research designs that embrace the disconnect between diverse disciplines, and that further bridge the academic/non-academic divide, towards collaborative efforts between universities and civil society organizations, in order to inform and influence public policy. Theoretical approaches outlined are household-level indicators to assess food and nutrition security; sustainable livelihood approaches; community food security; food sovereignty; and rights-based approaches. Emphasis is being laid on ethical considerations and criteria for demonstrating rigor and trustworthiness of qualitative research.

Introduction

The social dimensions of food and nutrition security form one aspect of the growing field of food studies. We argue that qualitative and mixed methods approaches are relevant for the growing spectrum of subjects in this field. We have found it useful to tailor our discussion here to qualitative methods in the context of food and nutrition security, specifically.

Quantitative surveys and nutritional assessments incompletely capture underlying causes of food and nutrition insecurity at the household and community level. These underlying causes are often crucial for the food situation and well-being of household members. While acknowledging global challenges such as the world food crisis, we argue for the need to take into account the micro-level perspective, in addition to or as an alternative to standardized surveys, as only local realities can provide in-depth case studies that reveal underlying location-specific social and structural conditions. Researchers might find themselves being part of heterogenous research teams, from diverse disciplines that apply different theoretical concepts and scientific language, i.e., nutrition, public health, economics, agriculture, development, geography, sociology, anthropology, education, psychology. Qualitative and mixed methods approaches can provide strategies to embrace disconnects between disciplines and paradigms, with the argument being made here for qualitatively driven approaches to mixing methods. This is in line with Creswell (2009), who calls for holistic approaches towards participatory and pragmatic methodologies, taking into account issues of social justice and embracing different perspectives, assumptions, and forms of data collection in order to provide the best under-standing of a research problem. This article aims to encourage researchers and students engaging in food and nutrition research who want to apply interdisciplinary approaches and qualitative and mixed methods research designs, placing specific emphasis on ethical considerations and criteria for rigor and trustworthiness of qualitative research.

Historical background of food and nutrition security scholarship and major theoretical approaches in use

Something is wrong with the way research on food and nutrition security is conducted and used. The International Assessment of Agricultural Science, Knowledge and Technology for Devel-opment (IAASTD, 2009: 3–4) revealed that despite significant scientific and technological achievements to increase agricultural productivity, hunger has increased, and there has been too little attention on social and environmental consequences, neglecting vulnerable groups. It is important therefore to understand how concepts around food and nutrition security developed and how this was linked to research methods that supported data-driven policy directions. Government and donor organizations often still require quantitative information such as data on food production and nutritional status, and are seldom willing or able to spend time and resources to obtain information on local indicators. This information is required to design appropriate and sustainable strategies for improved food and nutrition security.

The concept of food security emerged as a result of the challenge to provide sufficient food at national and global levels. It was propelled forward in the 1948 Universal Declaration of Human Rights (UDHR, 1948: Art. 25[1]. "Everyone has the right to a standard of living adequate for the health and well-being of himself and of his family, including food"). In the 1960s, food security evolved in largely economic delivery terms, referring to food supply rela-tive to production, trade, marketing, stocks, and reserves at global, regional, and national levels. This macro-level approach was gradually replaced in the 1970s and 1980s, with three main shifts since the first World Food Conference in 1974: From the global and national level to the household and individual, from a food first perspective to a livelihood perspective, and from objective indicators to subjective perceptions (Maxwell, 1996: 155).

The Food and Agriculture Organization (FAO) (2002) defines food security as: "[A] situation that exists if all people, at all times, have physical, social and economic access to adequate, safe and nutritious food that meets their dietary needs and food preferences for an active and healthy life." While food insecurity is often, but not always, characterized by hunger, its principal meaning refers to the *risk* of people being hungry (Kracht 1999: 55). The concept has been criticized for its narrow focus on food and disregard of nutrition- and health-related aspects, as food security is not identical with nutritional well-being. Decisive factors for adequate nutritional status are access to and avail-ability of health services, a healthy environment, and care for women and children (United Nations Children's Fund, 1990). Attempts to reflect the complexity of nutrition problems have led to recommended terms like "nutrition security" or "food and nutrition security" (Kracht, 1999: 55–56; Klennert *et al.*, 2009: 25). The following section outlines holistic and integrated theoretical approaches that address the multi-dimensional topic of food and nutrition security, originating from diverse backgrounds and geographies and suited to complement each other.

Key indicators for assessing household-level food and nutrition security

Maxwell and Frankenberger (1992) introduced key indicators for assessing the multi-dimensional phenomenon of household-level food and nutrition security. This approach derives from the realization that sufficient national food supplies can have absolutely nothing to do with individual, group, or community food access. Household and household–community scale indicators identify locations and triggers of food access inequalities. Key indicators are: Household demographics; socio-economic characteristics, including access to various resources, and expenditure on food in percent of total expenditure; infrastructure, including clean drinking water, sanitation, housing, energy sources, health services, education; access to and availability of food, including household dietary diversity; gender and other intra-household dynamics impacting on decision making regarding resources; experience of hunger, food shortage and worries about food; and coping strategies.

Sustainable livelihoods approaches

The Sustainable Livelihoods Framework (Department for International Development, 1999) can serve as a theoretical framework and analytical tool to explore structural and underlying causes of food security. The initial concept "sustainable livelihoods approaches" (SLA) was largely developed and applied in a Southern context and became increasingly central to the international debate about development, poverty reduction, and environmental management in the 1990s (Scoones, 2009). A livelihood "comprises the capabilities, assets (including both material and social resources) and activities required for a means of living. A livelihood is sustainable when it can cope with and recover from stresses and shocks, maintains or enhances its capabilities and assets, while not undermining the natural resource base" (Scoones, 1998: 5). At the micro and meso level, livelihood assets (physical, natural, financial, social, and human capital) play an essential role for households to pursue livelihood strategies and desired livelihood outcomes, largely influenced by institutional and policy structures at the national and provincial level, that to a great extent determine the vulnerability context of people. SLA can and should integrate its approach with rights-based research methods that foreground individual and local interpretation of realities and causes of food and nutrition insecurity, as well as needed changes for sustainable food systems, in the context of human rights claims (Eide and Kracht, 2007).

Community food security

Community food security was introduced by Hamm and Bellows (2003: 37) and is defined as "a condition in which all community residents obtain a safe, culturally acceptable, nutritionally adequate diet through a sustainable food system that maximizes community self-reliance and social justice." Community food security was developed and is largely applied in a Northern context, rooted in civil society, civic agriculture (Lyson, 2004) and cross-sectoral partnerships (public, private, and private non-profit) that leverage a "community voice" into traditional power structures to redefine food and nutrition needs, security, and local-based strategies. It developed in part from theories of food and economic democracy (Koc *et al.*, 1999) as well as the international human right to food (Bellows and Hamm, 2003). Communities are understood as integrated into social fabric, not as isolated units, and community food assessments serve as a strategy to enumerate diverse resources and challenges faced by local populations. The goal of community food security is self-determination, not economic dependency or even self-sufficiency. In some contexts, social protection remains necessary because not everyone can afford adequate food for a healthy life.

Food sovereignty, local governance, and rights-based approaches

Food sovereignty was introduced at the World Food Summit 1996 placing emphasis on human rights and specific needs of smallholder farmers and addressing core problems of hunger and poverty (Windfuhr and Jonsén, 2005). The concept developed in the South, but is increasingly adopted in Northern contexts. Based on the initiative of civil society organizations, the FAO of the United Nations developed the *Voluntary Guidelines on the progressive realisation of the right to adequate food in the context of national food security* (FAO, 2005; cf. Eide and Kracht, 2007) to encourage national states to develop a systematic evaluation approach through the development and inclusion of benchmarks and indicators to monitor progress towards achieving the right to adequate food. The *Voluntary Guidelines* serve the additional purpose of providing civil society organizations the same tools for developing shadow reports that can contest or complement those of national states. Additional support for the development of rights-based research methods for academic and non-academic publics alike is available from the FAO (FAO Right to Food Unit, 2009).

Research methodologies

This anthropological orientation, deeply humanistic, concerned with meanings rather than formal abstractions, remains valuable and even urgent in a world increasingly dominated by technocracy.

(Keesing 1981: 4)

Students and researchers who were trained in the natural or social quantitative sciences are at first usually irritated when being introduced to qualitative approaches. However, they might already have experienced the frustrations that quantitative surveys do not accommodate the "real" or day-to-day issues people are concerned about; or they might find themselves sitting in front of large datasets that do not provide the answers they were looking for. Qualitative research often has been and still is criticized for being inferior, subjective, non-scientific, representing "soft sciences," compared to "hard sciences" that are still perceived by some as being objective, value and bias free. In 2004 an editorial in *The Lancet* on "The soft science of medicine" called for integrating social aspects of medicine into the training of doctors, as nearly half of all causes of morbidity and mortality in the US were known to be linked to behavioral and social factors. The following statement at the time seemed somewhat groundbreaking, but it also distinguished between hard and soft sciences:

Medical training emphasises hard sciences […] yet when young doctors go out into practice they find that much of their day is spent involved in the untidy business of dealing with patients – trying to understand them, their histories, their personalities […] this "softer" side of medicine can be a messy, bewildering process for which the hard sciences provide little help.

(The Lancet, 2004: 1247)

Although the necessity for holistic approaches and in-depth research on food and nutrition security and related issues is increasingly acknowledged, in nutrition sciences so-called evidence-based and bio-medical models of research seem to have become the desired approach in recent years. According to Denzin, Lincoln, and Smith (2008: 4): "[T]he very act of labeling some research as 'evidence-based' implies that some research fails to mount evidence – a strongly political and decidedly nonobjective stance." In support of this view, Cassel (2002: 182) states that "the definition of 'science' is contestable and 'rigor' is not inevitably yoked to value-free – or soporific – social sciences." Research, whether qualitative or quantitative, will always be influenced by the researcher's personality, what s/he intends to investigate and how s/he is doing it, not to mention how funding sources might drive the research question. While most indicators of validity and reliability do not fit qualitative research, extensive criteria for demonstrating rigor, legitimacy, and trustworthiness of qualitative research are available, as will be illustrated later.

Before entering the field: gaining access and ethical considerations

Gaining access to research communities requires sensitive and flexible measures that have to be adapted to the specific research setting. Introductory visits and consultations with communities are crucial for establishing trust and relationships. Ethical conduct must receive exacting scrutiny, especially among vulnerable communities. This not only implies obtaining ethical approval by ethics committees or informed consent from research participants, but also implies awareness that ethical relations extend beyond these formal contracts. This is especially important as researchers might not have full control over how the material will be used when a research project has ended (Ross, 2005; Association Anthropology Southern Africa, 2005). Further, codes of ethics cannot dictate the forms of interaction: For example, when is it appropriate to ask follow-up questions and to continue an interview, when is it advisable to retreat? According to Henderson (2005), this responsibility in interactions with research participants has to be the subject of ongoing attention and reflexive engagement. This includes ethical questions such as: What is the value to research participants? What is the relationship between researcher and research participant; how will it change? This has similarly been argued by Denzin, Lincoln, and Smith (2008: 9–10).

Mixed methods approaches

> [I]t is ultimately more helpful to think in terms of multi-dimensional research strategies that transcend or even subvert the so-called qualitative–quantitative divide. Mixing methods helps us to think creatively and "outside the box".
>
> *(Mason, 2006: 9)*

Mixed methods research combines or associates qualitative and quantitative research designs (including spatial, anthropometric, and others), utilizing the strengths of both approaches and enabling more insights than by employing either form by itself (Creswell, 2009: 203). When applying mixed methods research it should be stated clearly why certain methods are used, and this should correspond with their application in research activities. In mixed methods research, qualitative and quantitative data can be collected following various strategies. The following designs are outlined by Creswell (2009: 209–10):

Sequential designs: qualitative and quantitative data are collected in clearly separated stages, with the following distinctions:
- first, collect quantitative data and analyze, followed by a second phase of collecting and analysing qualitative data (*sequential explanatory strategy*)
- conduct two distinct data collection phases as above, drawing on a theoretical perspective to guide the study (*sequential transformative design*)

Concurrent designs: qualitative and quantitative data are collected during one phase of data collection simultaneously, with the following designs:
- collect qualitative and quantitative data concurrently, then compare (*concurrent triangulation strategy*)
- collect qualitative and quantitative data concurrently, with a primary method (quantitative or qualitative) guiding the research and a secondary database (quantitative or

qualitative) providing a supporting role, with the latter having less priority (*concurrent embedded strategy*)

- in addition to collecting quantitative and qualitative data concurrently, guide approach with a theoretical perspective (*concurrent transformative design*)

Research methods

The following descriptions are based on Cassel (2002), Rubin and Rubin (2005), Denzin and Lincoln (2008), and Creswell (2009), as well as on field research carried out in various contexts and settings. Some of the methods, such as interviews and observations, can either be qualitative or quantitative, depending on how open (qualitative) or closed (quantitative) the response options or checklists for observations are (Creswell, 2009: 217).

Structured interviews

Structured interviews consist of a set of well-thought-out questions that are designed in line with research objectives. In a qualitative approach, mostly open-ended questions should be asked, to allow research participants to elaborate on the underlying reasons for their answer. However, the interview can also entail a section with closed questions, if the issues researched are largely known in a specific context, for example quantitative information relating to infra-structure. Structured interviews are especially advised if the language of research participants is not understood and a translator is needed. Besides adequate wording and culturally sensitive formulation of questions, major attention should be given to the order of topics in an interview. Socio-demographic and socio-economic information are in many populations perceived as highly sensitive and should be shifted to the end of an interview. Other sensitive issues, such as intra-household dynamics and resource allocation, or experiences of hunger and food shortage, should also be placed towards later sections. Such topics can be approached by framing a series of non-threatening questions, to explore them from various angles and to avoid direct and confrontational questions. Depth is obtained by probing and asking follow-up questions whenever this seems appropriate and helpful, signalling to the interviewee the expected level of depth. With research participants' consent interviews can be tape recorded, in addition to written notes, so as not to lose any important information. If interviews are conducted in a language foreign to the interviewer transcripts should be translated, with some interviews being back translated to ensure that the translation adequately reflects the contents. Answers to open-ended questions are then coded, to establish emerging categories and sub-categories, and analyzed and interpreted. Depending on sample size and sampling procedures, simple descriptive statistics such as frequencies, means, cross-correlations might be performed, using the Statistical Package for the Social Sciences (SPSS).

Semi-structured interviews

Semi-structured interviews are designed as interview guides or interview schedules, consisting of key questions. This allows the interviewer more flexibility in conducting the interview, and participants more freedom to elaborate and to be less influenced. Conducting semi-structured interviews requires interviewing skills and experience. Given that consent is obtained, tape recordings can bolster written notes. Recordings should be transcribed and answers are coded to establish categories and sub-categories, to enable analysis and interpretation, using programs for qualitative data analysis (e.g. NVivo). Semi-structured interviews usually provide more depth than structured interviews, for example to illustrate a specific case or event, or to explore perceptions in more depth, as illustrated in research on infant-feeding decision making and practices among HIV-positive women in South Africa (Doherty *et al.* 2006).

Observations

Observations provide valuable additional information to other research methods and should be encouraged in all research activities. The value of observations is often too little appreciated.

Non-participant observation

In non-participant observation, the researcher records human activities and the physical settings in which such activities take place, enabling direct information to be obtained about research settings and behavior of individuals or groups. Observations can be obtained by means of an observation schedule, recording, e.g. the type and material of the house, number of rooms, household appliances, food-storage facilities (quantitative), and/or taking notes of the general surroundings, social atmosphere, and interpersonal dynamics or other events before, during, and after the interview (qualitative). These notes can be coded and categorized, adding understanding and insights to information obtained through interviews. Even though labeled "non-participant," the researcher enters a social sphere and influences the research setting: "[I]f you are there for some time, as a living, reacting fellow human being, rather than a human pretending to be a disembodied fly-on-the-wall, the people you are studying create a space, a role for you" (Cassel, 2002: 180).

Participant observations

In participant observation, the researcher actively participates in daily activities of the people studied. One aim can be to enhance acceptance when investigating sensitive topics. Another aim is to gain insights into social dynamics and situations, e.g. in certain environments (communities, hospitals, schools) or within certain social groups (support or self-help groups, associations, institutions). If possible, the researcher takes brief notes that are written up at the end of the same day. Besides recording all events observed the researcher should also record personal feelings, so as to reveal possible bias. Notes are coded to establish categories, e.g. using SPSS or NVivo. Coding places distance between the researcher, the occurrences, and personal feelings; writing and reflecting on findings creates additional distance, with interpretations possibly being reinterpreted. Drawing back to these records later enables one to perceive how one might have been manipulated in specific situations.

Focus groups

Focus groups are discussions around a specific topic of interest and are usually carried out with six to 12 participants, following specific guidelines. They can be applied before designing an interview for a qualitative or quantitative study, or to explore general perceptions on sensitive issues. If consent has been obtained, discussions can be tape recorded in addition to written notes. As with interviews, answers are coded to establish categories and sub-categories and analyzed. Focus groups can further enable participants to learn more about their own situation and provide possibilities for future networking.

Kitchen audits/household food inventories

Kitchen audits or household food inventories allow the enumeration and evaluation of food stored in individual homes. Researchers have to look into cupboards, closets, storerooms, refrigerators, and freezers, thus entering private spaces. This requires a high level of trust and absolute respect, tolerance, and discretion on the part of the researcher. The level of precision employed in a household food inventory depends on the research objectives. However, a consistent structure of analysis and establishing what is relevant to count is important. In some studies, it might be appropriate to take photographs (Counihan, 2011) or list the different foods and approximate quantities. However, if for example the nutrient potential of a household is being evaluated, scales to weigh foods and calculators to assess percentage weights of partially opened packages are needed. Data analysis might employ Universal Product Codes (UPC) necessitating packing in a computer with barcode scanner, or software systems for identifying and linking food items without barcodes to their nutrient characteristics (Byrd-Bredbenner and Mauer Abbot, 2009; Schefske et al., 2010).

Validation of qualitative research

To avoid the criticism of "subjectivity" often directed at qualitative research, continuous reflection, critical review, and solid documentation are absolutely necessary. The following frameworks enable the critical assessment of processes of qualitative research.

Rubin and Rubin (2005) present the following guidelines:

- *Transparency:* Providing insight into data collection processes, including strengths, weaknesses, biases, comments, and interpretations.
- *Consistency-coherence:* Credibility is increased when core concepts occur in a variety of cases and different settings, acknowledging that people make contradictory statements.
- *Communicability:* Research should be well documented, vivid, and transparent.

According to Creswell (1994), "internal validity" can be achieved by applying:

- triangulation (employing various data sources, methods, researchers, data types);
- member checking (ensuring that an accurate account of the interviewees' perception has been obtained);
- peer examination/review and supervision within the research team and other peers;
- feedback from key informants to reflect on findings and emerging concepts (also called critical reference group);
- translation and back translation of selected interviews if the language of participants is foreign to the researcher.

"External validity" is provided by describing all steps of the research process and the methodology, making it possible that the procedure might be replicated in another setting, while the uniqueness of each study mitigates against replicating it in exactly the same way.

Guba and Lincoln (1985) provide a useful framework and systematic checklist for documenting credibility, transferability, dependability, and conformability, as is especially useful when engaging in qualitative research for the first time.

Lastly, Pyett (2003) provides a useful and critical discussion on the challenges of validation of qualitative research.

Avenues for future research

Along with working interdisciplinarily and creatively engaging mixed methods approaches, we encourage researchers to apply their rich capacity in the context of bridging the academic/non-academic divide and to engage in collaborative efforts between universities, non-governmental organizations, and other civil society groups, in order to inform and influence public policy. Our approach is in line with Denzin, Lincoln, and Smith (2008: 15) who lay out a visionary scenario of a collaborative social sciences research model. With an emphasis on qualitative methodological approaches, they call for making researchers responsible to those being studied; stressing personal accountability, caring, the value of individual expressiveness, the capacity for empathy, and the sharing of emotionality; forcefully aligning the ethics of research with a politics of the oppressed; directing scholars to take up moral projects that respect and reclaim indigenous cultural practices. Such work, these authors argue, produces spiritual, social, and psychological healing; leads to multiple forms of transformation at the personal and social levels; shapes processes of mobilization and collective action; and helps people realize a radical performative politics of possibility. While part of the above is being said in the context of indigenous methodologies, it seems obvious that this also holds true for the broader population, North and South, facing diverse challenges including under-nutrition, food and nutrition insecurity, but also over- and malnutrition in the context of changing lifestyles and nutrition transition, both in Northern and Southern contexts.

Practical considerations for getting started

Food and nutrition security and related topics, whether at the global or national level, are increasingly at the centre of attention, due to the global rising demand for food supplies – as is reflected in the recent food crises and rising food and energy prices – the scarcity and increasing competition for natural resources, the negative impact of the food system on the environment as well as negative effects of over and undernutrition on health. Approaches as outlined here can bridge disciplines and sectors. More than anything else, time and depth are needed if taking this type of research on. This includes developing trust and personal relationships with local actors and organizations and establishing networks that will last when the immediate research phase has ended. It further necessitates access to funding that allows for independent research. Lastly, we have to realize the limitations of what can be achieved. We believe, however, that combining the strengths of diverse and interdisciplinary approaches and engaging both the academy and non-academic local actors can make important and meaningful contributions to guide future research as well as programs towards more holistic, sustainable, and just approaches.

Key reading

Bryman, A. (2006) "Integrating quantitative and qualitative research: how is it done?" *Qualitative Research* 6 (1): 97–113.

Cassel, J. (2002) "Perturbing the system: 'hard science', 'soft science', and social science, the anxiety and madness of method." *Human Organisation* 61 (2): 177–85.

Creswell, J. W. (2009) *Research Design. Qualitative, Quantitative and Mixed Methods Approaches.* 3rd ed. Thousand Oaks, CA: SAGE.

Denzin, N. K. and Y. S. Lincoln, eds. (2008) *Collecting and interpreting qualitative materials.* 3rd ed. Thousand Oaks, CA: SAGE.

Guba, E. G. and Y. S. Lincoln (1985) *Effective evaluation: Improving the usefulness of evaluation results through responses and naturalistic approaches.* San Francisco: Pub Jossey Bass.

Pyett, P. M. (2003) "Validation of qualitative research in the 'real world'." *Qualitative Health Research* 13 (8): 1170–79.

Rubin, H. J. and I. S. Rubin, (2005) *Qualitative Interviewing. The Art of Hearing Data.* 2nd ed. Thousand Oaks, CA: SAGE.

Silvermann, S. (2010) *Doing qualitative research. A practical handbook.* 3rd ed. Thousand Oaks, CA: SAGE.

Bibliography

Association Anthropology Southern Africa (AASA) (2005) "Ethical guidelines and principles of conduct for anthropologists." *Anthropology Southern Africa* 28 (3&4): 142–43.

Bellows, A. C. and Hamm, M. W. (2003) "International Origins of Community Food Security Policies and Practices in the U.S." *Critical Public Health,* Special Issue: Food Policy 13 (2): 107–23.

Byrd-Bredbenner, C, Mauer Abbot, J. (2009) "Differences in food supplies of U.S. households with and without overweight individuals." *Appetite* 52: 479–84.

Cassel, J. (2002) "Perturbing the system: 'hard science', 'soft science', and social science, the anxiety and madness of method." *Human Organisation* 61 (2): 177–85.

Counihan, C. (2011) "Mexicanas taking food public: the power of the kitchen in the San Luis Valley." In Williams-Forson, P. and Counihan, C. (eds.) *Taking Food Public: Redefining Foodways in a Changing World.* New York: Routledge.

Creswell, J. W. (1994) *Research Design. Qualitative and Quantitative Methods.* Thousand Oaks, CA: SAGE.

——(2009) *Research Design. Qualitative, Quantitative and Mixed Methods Approaches.* 3rd ed. Thousand Oaks, CA: SAGE.

Denzin, N. K., Y. S. Lincoln, eds. (2008) *Collecting and interpreting qualitative materials.* 3rd ed. Thousand Oaks, CA: SAGE.

Denzin, N. K., Y. S. Lincoln, and L. T. Smith, eds. (2008) *Handbook of Critical and Indigenous Methodologies.* Thousand Oaks, CA: SAGE.

Department for International Development (DFID) (1999) *Sustainable Livelihoods Guidance Sheets.* London: DFID, www.eldis.org/vfile/upload/1/document/0901/section2.pdf (accessed March 10, 2011).

Doherty, T., M. Chopra, L. Nkonki, D. Jackson, and L. A. Persson, (2006) "A longitudinal qualitative study of infant-feeding decision making and practices among HIV-positive women in South Africa." *The Journal of Nutrition* 136: 2421–26.

Eide, W. B. and U. Kracht, (eds) (2007) *Food and Human Rights in Development. Evolving issues and emerging applications.* Vol. II. Antwerpen–Oxford: Intersentia.

Food and Agriculture Organization (FAO) (2002) *The State of Food Insecurity in the World 2001.* Rome, www.fao.org/docrep/003/y1500e/y1500e00.htm (accessed March 10, 2011).

——(2005) *Voluntary Guidelines to support the progressive realization of the right to adequate food in the context of national food security.* www.fao.org/righttofood/publi_01_en.htm (accessed March 10, 2011).

Food and Agriculture Organization (FAO) Right to Food Unit. (2009) *Right to Food Methodological Toolbox.* Rome: FAO, www.fao.org/righttofood/publi_02_en.htm (accessed November 3, 2011).

Guba, E. G. and Y. S. Lincoln (1985) *Effective evaluation: Improving the usefulness of evaluation results through responses and naturalistic approaches.* San Francisco, CA: Pub Jossey Bass.

Hamm, M. W. and A. C. Bellows (2003) "Community Food Security and Nutrition Educators." *Journal of Nutrition Education and Behavior* 35 (1): 37–43.

Henderson, P. C. (2005) "Mortality and the ethics of qualitative research in a context of HIV/AIDS." *Anthropology Southern Africa* 28 (3&4): 78–90.

IAASTD (International Assessment of Agricultural Knowledge, Science and Technology for Development). (2009) *Agriculture at a crossroads. Synthesis report.* Washington, DC: Island Press, www.agassessment.org/docs/SR_Exec_Sum_280508_English.pdf (accessed February 16, 2011).

Keesing, R. M. (1981) *Cultural Anthropology: A Contemporary Perspective.* New York: Holt, Rinehart & Winston.

Klennert, K. (ed.) (2009) *Achieving Food and Nutrition Security. Actions to Meet the Global Challenge.* In Went, www.inwent.org/imperia/md/content/a-internet2008/portaliz/umweltundernaehrung/achieving_food_and_nutrition_security_2010.pdf (accessed February 16, 2011).

Koc, M., MacRae, R., Mougeot, L. J. A., and Walsh, J. eds. (1999) *For Hunger-Proof Cities: Sustainable Urban Food Systems.* International Development Research Centre (IDRC) and The Centre for Studies in Food Security. Toronto: Ryerson Polytechnic University.

Kracht, U. (1999) "Hunger, Malnutrition and Poverty: Trends and Prospects Towards the 21st Century." In *Food Security and Nutrition. The Global Challenge.* U. Kracht, and M. Schulz, eds. New York: St Martin's.

The Lancet (2004) "Editorial." 363 (9417): 1247.

Lyson, T. A. (2004) *Civic Agriculture: Reconnecting Farm, Food and Community*. Boston, MA: Tufts University Press.

Mason, J. (2006) "Mixing methods in a qualitatively driven way." *Qualitative Research* 6(1): 9–25.

Maxwell, S. (1996) "Food Security: A Post-Modern Perspective." *Food Policy* 21 (2): 155–70.

Maxwell, S. and Frankenberger, T. R. (eds.) (1992) *Household Food Security: Concepts, Indicators, Measurements. A Technical Review*. New York: UNICEF.

Pyett, P. M. (2003) "Validation of qualitative research in the 'real world'." *Qualitative Health Research* 13 (8): 1170–79.

Ross, F. C. (2005) "Codes and Dignity: Thinking about ethics in relation to research on violence." *Anthropology Southern Africa* 28 (3&4): 99–107.

Rubin, H. J. and I. S. Rubin, (2005) *Qualitative Interviewing. The Art of Hearing Data*. 2nd ed. Thousand Oaks, CA: SAGE.

Schefske, S. D., C. L. Cuite, A. C. Bellows, C. Byrd-Bredbenner, T. Vivar, H. Rapport, and W. K. Hallman, (2010) "Nutrient Analysis of Varying Socioeconomic Status Home Food Environments in New Jersey State." *Appetite* 54 (2): 384–89.

Scoones, I. (1998) *Sustainable rural livelihoods: A framework for analysis*. IDS Working Paper, 72. Sussex: Institute for Development Studies.

——(2009) "Livelihoods perspectives and rural development." *Journal of Peasant Studies*, 36 (1), www.tandf.co.uk/journals/pdf/papers/FJPS_36_1_2009.pdf (accessed March 16, 2011).

United Nations Children's Fund (UNICEF). (1990) *Strategy for Improved Nutrition of Children and Women in Developing Countries*. A UNICEF Policy Review. New York: UNICEF.

The Universal Declaration of Human Rights, 25 (1). www.un.org/en/documents/udhr/index.shtml. (accessed October 31, 2010).

Windfuhr, M. and Jonsén, J. (2005) *Food Sovereignty: Towards Democracy in Localized Food Systems*. London: ITDG Publishing, The Schumacher Centre for Technology and Development.

30

School food

Janet Poppendieck

"School Food" covers the National School Lunch Program and the School Breakfast Program in the United States, along with other foods sold or consumed at school. A social constructionist framework looks at cycles in which claims become problems, generating action in the form of policies, which in turn become the basis for new claims and new problems. Basic themes include hunger among school children, the nutritional quality of school food, health outcomes, program access and participation, program integrity and payment accuracy, innovations, and the environmental and economic impact of school food.

In the United States, more than 31 million children eat federally subsidized, nutritionally regulated school lunches each school day; thus about three-fifths of the nation's school-aged children participate in the National School Lunch Program (NSLP). Just over two-thirds of these meals are served free or at sharply reduced prices to children from low-income families. Families with incomes above the cut-off for reduced price meals (185 percent of the poverty line or currently $34,281 annually for a family of three) pay a price set locally. Most schools also offer a school breakfast program, and on a typical day in the most recent school year, some 11.3 million children participated in the School Breakfast Program (SBP), 83 percent of them on a free or reduced-price basis.

Most of the scholarship on school food in the US is concerned with these "official" school meals, but children eat other food at school as well, and in recent years, school food scholarship has come to embrace so-called "competitive foods"—foods sold in competition with the publicly subsidized meals such as foods dispensed by vending machines, sold in fundraisers or school stores, or sold à la carte in the cafeteria—and the foods that parents send to school in backpacks and lunch boxes, food brought from home.

Research on school food follows the classic cycle identified in the social constructionist literature on social problems. (See, for example, Blumer, 1971; Best, 2008; Spector and Kitsue, 1987.) First there are claims that a problem exists—that school children are going hungry, or that they are eating unsafe or unhealthy foods. Such claims are seldom uncontested, and researchers are drawn in, collecting data to support or disprove or measure the accuracy of the claims. If enough people are convinced that the problem is real and merits attention, demands for response accumulate and pass a crucial threshold; a problem achieves legitimacy. At this point, there are prescriptions and proposals for action. In school food, this phase has generated a substantial "how-to" literature—how to design a cafeteria, how to prepare nutritious, safe, and palatable meals, how to get children to eat them—and an extensive array of studies of innovations and pilot programs. Once a course of action is chosen and implemented, typically in the form of a policy or program, there are assessments and evaluations and the cycle begins again as the program's shortcomings become the new "problem," about which claims are made. In terms of public policy in the United States, such cycles take place at the local, state, and federal levels.

Historical background of scholarship on school food and major theoretical approaches

It is really impossible to disentangle the history of school food scholarship from the history of school feeding itself. The early development of school food in the US is intimately linked to the spread of compulsory public education. As new school attendance laws took effect, they brought into the schools many of the nation's poorest children. With family income reduced by the loss of children's wages, substantial numbers of families had little or no food to send to school with their offspring. Hunger in the classroom began attracting the attention of reformers. As Robert Hunter declared in his classic 1904 volume *Poverty*: "It is utter folly, from the point of view of learning, to have a compulsory school law which compels children, in that weak physical and mental state which results from poverty, to sit at their desks, day in and day out, for several years, learning little or nothing" (Hunter, 1904: 217). True to the constructionist model, Hunter's allegations were followed by efforts to document the extent of child hunger, most notably John Spargo's *The Bitter Cry of the Children*) published in 1906, and then a whole series of studies using income calculations and another series using height and weight measurements, leading to what Harvey Levenstein (2003: 109–20) has called "The Great Malnutrition Scare" of 1907–21. Both the *Journal of Home Economics* and more popular vehicles such as *Parents Magazine* regularly published studies of childhood malnutrition throughout the early 1910s and 1920s.

In keeping with the general American preference for private charity and the conviction that education was a local responsibility, the first responses to reports of child hunger were local and voluntary in nature. Women's organizations, especially, undertook a wide variety of school food projects: Penny meals, free milk, even hot lunches. Once such programs were started, the initiating organizations often turned their attention to persuading local Boards of Education to take them over (Gunderson, 1971; Reese, 1980). They received considerable support in these efforts from another group of reformers known collectively as the School Hygiene Movement. Their concern was not so much hunger as food safety and nutrition; they were distressed by the unhealthy foods that students were purchasing from pushcarts and school janitors, and they proposed school lunchrooms under the supervision of a dietician as a way to instruct students in the fundamentals of healthy eating (Boughton, 1914, 1916; Levine, 2008). Some, following the example and urging of John Dewey (1899), saw a role for students themselves in the preparation and serving of school food that would teach them not only nutrition and food safety but also arithmetic, biology, geography, and many other elements of the curriculum. Together, the advocates of better sanitation and nutrition, the proponents of occupation-based education, and those concerned about the hunger of the poorest students achieved considerable success. By 1918, a study conducted by the Municipal Research Bureau in New York City, of school feeding operations in cities with populations of 50,000 or more, found that three-quarters offered meals in their high schools, though only a quarter did so in their elementary schools (Southworth and Klayman, 1941: 13).

Following the predictable lifecycle of the social problem, the social service and home economics publications of the day offered many descriptions of programs: The "how-to" literature mentioned earlier. Especially noteworthy were the papers prepared for the International Congresses on School Hygiene, some of which were reprinted in the *Journal of Home Economics,* and a remarkable chapter entitled "Household Arts and School Lunches" prepared for the Cleveland Survey (Boughton, 1916).

School lunch programs proliferated in the 1920s, and as they did so, they also became professionalized. More and more were under the direction of trained dieticians or home economics teachers. According to historian Susan Levine (2008: 34, 35) the Bureau of Home Economics in the United States Department of Agriculture (USDA), the largest employer of women scientists in the nation, provided both an ongoing research base and substantial programmatic guidance for the rapidly professionalizing field of school food service. It took the Great Depression of the 1930s, however, to get the higher levels of government involved in providing material support to school food. As the suffering attendant upon unemployment became obvious, claims of widespread malnutrition among children surfaced once again, and again researchers undertook to investigate them. Meanwhile, more and more communities started school lunch programs or expanded those that already existed. Charitable contributions of money and food, and especially donations from teachers, helped to fund these, but as the Depression wore on, several states got involved, passing legislation authorizing local school boards to operate lunch rooms, and in a few cases, appropriating funds to assist (Southworth and Klayman, 1941). Consistent with the model above, "how to" documents and descriptive reports abounded in the social work, education, and home economics literature of the depression. The era saw the publication of two major works on child nutrition: Mary Bryan's *The School Cafeteria,* which ran to 726 pages, and an update of Lydia Roberts *Nutrition Work with Children*, which weighed in at 639, were published in the mid–1930s.

Ironically, it was agricultural abundance, not food deprivation, that brought the federal government into the picture. Programs to control farm surpluses in order to stabilize prices left the USDA and its affiliated agencies with enormous supplies of both storable and perishable crops, and in the mid-1930s the USDA began donating surplus farm products to school lunch programs (Poppendieck, 1986). The newly organized Works Progress Administration (WPA), perceiving that school lunchrooms provided an ideal setting for work relief assignments for unemployed women, contributed labor, and the second half of the 1930s saw a major expansion of school food. True to the constructionist paradigm, with the "problem" variously defined as agricultural surpluses and female unemployment, new research assessed the impact of school lunch programs on surplus disposal and farm prices (Southworth and Klayman, 1941) and work relief opportunities for women (Woodward, 1936). The rules and regulations established to govern federal donations of food and labor laid the foundation for a permanent federal program forged in the wartime crucible of "defense nutrition."

The Second World War focused the nation's attention on nutrition as never before. As surpluses gave way to scarcity, the Federal Security Agency asked the National Research Council to establish nutrition standards that could serve as a basis for rationing (Roberts, 1958). The resulting RDAs became the basis for generations of studies assessing the diets of Americans, including those of school children, and food programs, including school meals. Meanwhile, widespread publicity for a public health service study linking failure of Selective Service physicals with malnutrition in childhood forged a clear link between adequate diet and national defense (Ciocco, Klein, and Palmer, 1941). With surpluses a receding memory, food prices rising, and the WPA facing termination, a new "problem" surfaced in school meals: without federal donations of food and labor, schools could not afford to continue their programs (Flanagan, 1969). Anticipating huge surpluses at the end of the war, agricultural economists seeking stable markets for farm products, and nutritionists seeking to improve American diets joined forces to persuade

Congress to appropriate funds to reimburse schools for money spent on food. It was crucial, they argued, to keep the school lunch program operating so that it would be there to absorb the surpluses that would surely accumulate once European nations resumed agricultural production, and to make sure that the children of mothers working in war industries got a nutritious meal at school. By the end of the war, the elements of what became the National School Lunch Program (NSLP) were all in place: Cash indemnities and commodity donations to subsidize meals and keep the prices low, rules requiring schools to provide free meals for children too poor to pay for them, and federal regulations governing the nutrition profile of meals served with federal assistance. The National School Lunch Act was passed in 1946 "as a matter of national security, to safeguard the health and well-being of the nation's children and to encourage the domestic consumption of nutritious agricultural commodities and other foods" (Levine, 2008; Poppendieck, 2010).

The program grew and expanded, but generated little controversy, and little research, until the nation discovered poverty in the midst of plenty in the 1960s. When the civil rights movement and the war on poverty called attention to the needs of hungry school children, a new cycle of claims, research, proposals for action, and programmatic changes was launched. Responding to arguments that school lunch came too late in the day for the hungriest school children, a pilot school breakfast program was established in 1966. Shortly thereafter, a national coalition of women's organizations, called the Committee on School Lunch Participation, undertook an extensive study that revealed major shortcomings in the National School Lunch Program. The Committee found that the previous generation's solution had itself become the problem; the NSLP was not serving most of the nation's poorest children—they were too poor to purchase the lunch even at the subsidized price, and their schools and communities did not have the resources to serve the meals without charge (Fairfax, 1968). The Committee's findings, reinforced by the work of other high-profile investigations of hunger (Citizens Board of Inquiry into Hunger and Malnutrition in the United States, 1968) resulted in a dramatic overhaul of the NSLP. New national standards specified which children were eligible for free meals, and the federal government undertook to reimburse local communities for meals served free in addition to continuing the general subsidy for all meals (Maney, 1989; Martin, 1999).

The renewed focus on hunger, and the success of the research and advocacy work of the ad hoc projects led to the establishment of a set of permanent anti-hunger organizations: The Food Research and Action Center (FRAC), Bread for the World, and World Hunger Year (now WhyHunger?) were all established in the 1970s with research, public education, and lobbying as core parts of their mission, giving rise to a national anti-hunger network that has grown in the ensuing decades (Eisinger, 1998).

One result of the school lunch reform legislation of the early 1970s was a dramatic rise in participation, and with it a steep escalation in costs. As program expenditures rose, so did Congressional interest, and in 1979, the Senate asked the USDA to conduct an evaluation of the School Lunch, School Breakfast, and Special Milk Programs. In research terms, this might be regarded as the dawn of the era of evaluation. The first major national assessment of the nutrient quality and impact of, and participation in, school meals began in October, 1979, and issued a final report in 1983 (Wellisch et al., 1983), producing data that were mined for school food research for a decade.

The election of Ronald Reagan in 1980 signaled the start of a new era in domestic social programs with cutbacks in funding and increased demands for accountability. In the school lunch program, the Reagan-era cuts had dramatic impact. Faced with reductions in commodity donations and sharply curtailed subsidies for both reduced-price and full-price meals, local school food authorities raised prices abruptly, and participation by "full price" customers dropped precipitously. The NSLP lost a quarter of its full price customers in the several years after the cuts were implemented. The consequences were nutritional as well as fiscal. Food service directors across the nation tried to lure student customers back into the school cafeteria by offering more and more of youngsters' favorite foods, expanding their à la carte offerings and installing vending machines in the cafeteria in an attempt to balance the budget (Martin, 1999; Poppendieck, 2010). The how-to literature again proliferated—this time focused on techniques for controlling costs and ways of attracting customers.

The expansion of à la carte with its emphasis on fries, pizza, burgers, and nuggets was soon reflected in the regular, subsidized meal as well, as schools sought cost savings by replacing expensive dishwashing systems with disposables and cutlery with hand-held foods. A glut of high-fat federal commodities fueled a conversion of the school food menu to fast food clones. In the ongoing cycle of problem identification, yesterday's solution once again became today's problem as the fat content of school meals elicited sharp criticism from an emerging group of health-oriented activists. In annual "report cards," Public Voice for Food and Health Policy (1988–90) called attention to the high fat content of school meals and called on the USDA to bring its meals into compliance with the *Dietary Guidelines for Americans* that it helped to formulate (Sims, 1998). The Center for Science in the Public Interest (CSPI) convened a Citizens Committee reminiscent of the ad hoc organizations of the hunger exposés two decades earlier, and issued a white paper calling for limits on fat, sugar, and sodium in school meals. Health began to trump hunger in the national conversation about school food.

In the early 1990s, then Secretary of Agriculture Edwin Madigan launched the contemporary era of school food research by initiating the School Nutrition Dietary Assessment or SNDA, and asking the contractor, Mathematic Policy Research Inc., to measure school meals against the standards of the *Dietary Guidelines for Americans*. When the results were in, the meals proved to be so far from the recommended standards that Congress passed a law requiring the meals to meet the guidelines, and the Department of Agriculture launched a major reform effort, the School Meals Initiative for Healthy Children or SMI for short. SMI generated its own set of literature, both the "how-to" proposals and case studies (c.f. FNS *et al.*, 2005) and a raft of program evaluations. Meanwhile, the SNDA series has become a recurrent phenomenon, and each of these studies has generated significant publications in such journals as *Pediatrics* and the *Journal of the American Dietetic Association*.

The rising concern about the health impacts of school food was fueled in the new millennium by the Surgeon General's Call to Action on Childhood Obesity, and by the publication of several works aimed at popular audiences. Eric Schlosser's *Fast Food Nation* (2001) raised the alarm about the marketing of soft drinks and fast food through schools, while Morgan Spurlock's film *Supersize Me* provided a graphic portrayal of the use of branded items and fast food clones in school lunchrooms. Marion Nestle's *Food Politics* (2002) investigated marketing food to children in greater depth. Both the Campaign for a Commercial Free Childhood and the Alliance for Children took up the issue of food marketing to children through schools. Meanwhile, several high-profile incidents of food-borne illness and growing attention to food allergies expanded the health frame. Additional federal agencies joined the research effort, notably the Centers for Disease Control and Prevention (CDC) with the School Health Policies and Programs Study (SHPPS) (2000) (Wechsler *et al.*, 2001) and 2010, and the Government Accountability Office (GAO) with two studies of outbreaks of food-borne illnesses in schools (2002, 2003), and others of nutritional quality of school meals (2003), and the role of competitive foods in both diet and revenue (2005).

Solutions became problems yet again as efforts to provide healthier foods increased costs and reduced revenues, placing food service operators in a bind. In short, schools feared losing revenues from competitive food sales, and food service directors feared lower participation if healthier menus proved less appealing to children. Recognition of the "School Food Tri-lemma" of trade-offs among nutritional quality, costs, and student participation sparked addi-tional research, notably an extensive assessment of School Lunch and Breakfast costs (Bartlett, Glantz, and Logan, 2008), and a study by The School Nutrition Association of the growing tendency of Local Educational Authorities to charge foodservice operations "indirect costs" for services that they had once contributed (SNA, 2006). Among school food professionals, rising costs are particularly troublesome when they induce school districts to contract out the provision of meals to food service management companies.

Participation may be seen as the intersection of the various concerns and problem definitions in school food research for several reasons. First, school meals can neither promote health nor relieve hunger for children who do not eat them. Second, as participation declines, the unit cost of producing each meal rises; maintaining participation is essential to the fiscal health of school food programs. And third, students from impoverished families typically cannot participate unless they are certified to receive free or reduced-price meals, and the certification process itself is fraught with problems and suffers from high levels of inaccuracy. Thus, the USDA has undertaken substantial research over the years to identify the characteristics of participants and those of eligible non-participants (Glantz, 1994; Ralston et al., 2008; and all of the SNDA series), and to devise and test alternatives to the family application for certification. Anti-hunger advocates also use participation as a benchmark, and the annual School Breakfast Scorecard issued by the Food Research and Action Center tracks the extent to which children who eat free and reduced-price lunches are also receiving breakfast (FRAC, 1991–2010).

Approximately every five years, the school food programs along with other child nutrition programs are subject to a Congressional review and "reauthorization." In the run-up to the 2004 Child Nutrition Reauthorization (CNR), participation data were subject to new scrutiny when officials within the Bush administration claimed that more children were certified to receive free or reduced-price meals than were eligible to receive them. The "over-certification" issue generated a host of new research on income volatility and related issues, research that resulted in significant improvements to program design in the 2004 reauthorization (Newman, 2006; Neuberger and Greenstein, 2003).

While the "overcertification" challenge receded in the face of the data, the underlying con-cern about fraud, abuse, and error did not. The terms "erroneous payments" and "program integrity" gained prominence, and the USDA undertook a series of studies to explore aspects of the application, certification, and verification process (Hulsey, Gleason and Ohls, 2004; Burghardt, Silva and Hulsey, 2004; Burghardt, Devancy and Gordon, 2004; Gleason, 1995; and USDA, FNS, 2005), culminating in a nationally representative study of erroneous payments made in the 2005–06 school year, entitled "National School Lunch Program/School Breakfast Program Access, Participation, Eligibility, and Certification Study" (Ponza et al., 2007), commonly referred to as APEC.

While hunger, health, costs, participation, and program integrity or payment accuracy reflect the primary concerns of the USDA, they do not exhaust the problem frames used to study the program. A new set of concerns has arisen from the environmental movement about the carbon footprint of school food operations, and a very old set of concerns about the impact of school meals on farmers has resurfaced as an emphasis on local and regional procurement: Farm to school or farm to cafeteria.

The latter are intimately connected to the issue of what children are learning from the food they eat at school, and a new round of "how-to" and program evaluation literature has sprung up in conjunction with farm to cafeteria, cooking in school, school garden, and agriculture in the classroom curricula (Gottlieb and Joshi, 2010; Joshi, Kalb and Beery, 2006; Valianatos, Gottlieb, and Haase, 2004; USDA Farm to School Team, 2011; and the publications listed on the website of the National Farm to School Network: www.farmtoschool.org).

Innovations and school food reform have themselves become topics for research, with another round of both popular, "how-to," and scholarly literature, including Anne Cooper and Lisa Holmes's *Lunch Lessons: Changing the Way We Feed Our Children* (2006), historian Susan Levine's *School Lunch Politics* (2008), Kevin Morgan and Roberta Sonnino's *The School Food Revolution: Public Food and the Challenge of Sustainable Development* (2008), Janet Poppendieck's *Free For All: Fixing School Lunch in America* (2010), Sarah Robert and Marcus Weaver-Hightower's *School Food Politics: The Complex Ecology of Hunger and Feeding in Schools Around the World* (2011), Amy Kalafas's *Lunch Wars: How to Start a School Food Revolution and Win the Battle for Our Children's Health* (2011), Sarah Wu (Mrs Q)'s *Fed Up With Lunch: How One Anonymous Teacher Revealed the Truth About School Lunches—and How We Can Change Them* (2011), and Kate Adamick's forthcoming *Lunch Money: Serving Healthy School Food in a Sick Economy.*

Research methodologies

It is difficult to identify a methodology that has *not* been used in school food research. Studies range from the intimate—a single school or even a single classroom—to the massive—nationally representative samples as in the SNDA series. They involve survey data, menu analysis, analysis of production records, 24-hour food recalls, cafeteria observations, interviews in person and by phone with participants, non-participants, their parents, food service personnel, and other key informants. Photo documentation has been used to study students' food choices and actual food consumption. The public health and dietetics literature, predictably, tends to use nutrient analysis, the economics literature uses cost and revenue data, the political science and historical literature uses Congressional documents such as the Congressional Record and committee hearings and the policy instruments of the USDA. Anti-hunger advocates analyze access and participation data. *The Journal of Child Nutrition and Management* publishes many case studies of innovations. Because so many households are touched by the school food programs, so many of us have eaten school meals at some point in life, so many people have opinions about how school food ought to be, there is room for a wide variety of methods and approaches.

The one approach that is severely limited at the macro scale is any variant of the experimental method. Researchers trying to assess the impact of programs on outcomes such as nutrition and health status face special challenges in regard to the NSLP. In general, impact research seeks to compare outcomes with the program in place to those that would have taken place in its absence, the so-called "counterfactual." Researchers usually seek to "establish the counterfactual," that is, to estimate what would have happened in the absence of a given program, by examining a population that has not been exposed to it. In the case of the NSLP, is difficult because the program is so widely available—in more than 90 percent of public schools. Within any school with the program, it is possible to compare participants and non-participants, but these groups tend to differ based on other factors that are highly relevant to the outcomes being studied. For example, if one wants to measure the impact of school lunch on body mass index (BMI), a comparison would need to take into account that lower income children are far more likely to participate than upper income children, and that poverty is correlated with BMI, even in the absence of school food. Such "selection bias" has posed enormous challenges for school food research; in order to "control for" such biases, samples often need to be very large (Fox, Hamilton and Lin, 2004: 13–19).

Most researchers will not have the resources to undertake research with samples large enough to allow such controls, but fortunately, the Department of Agriculture does fund such very large studies through the SNDA series. These studies are normally awarded to large-scale research contractors such as Mathematica Policy Research and Abt Associates. Researchers with questions that need such large-scale samples for answers are advised to contact the Economic Research Service of the US Department of Agriculture to explore the possibility of including their issues in the next round of SNDA.

Avenues for future research

Alternatives and innovations

Because there is currently a great deal of energy and effort directed to efforts to improve school food, one of the most promising avenues of research is the assessment of innovations and alternatives, both here in the US and in other societies from which we might learn. Case studies of innovations offer a rich opportunity. Two very different types of work are needed here. First, with so much experimentation going on, there is an almost insatiable need for evaluations of pilot programs and new approaches, and these might be conducted at a variety of levels including the individual school or classroom, the school system, the state, the federal, and the global. Multiple case research designs can offer the benefits of comparative studies and illuminate the barriers to achieving desired outcomes. Where program innovations reflect policy change, there is also a need for historical and contextual assessments: How did it happen? What explains the adoption of stricter standards for competitive foods in some state legislatures and their failure to secure passage in others, for example. As the provisions of the most recent Child Nutrition Reauthorization Act, the Healthy and Hunger Free Kids Act of 2010, are gradually implemented, there will be a great need for close observation of the way reforms in nutrient standards for competitive foods, revised nutrition standards for school meals, and changes in access to school food play out "on the ground" in varied community settings. Finally, case studies of school food in other nations can provide insights into their food cultures and a reservoir of policy ideas for the US.

The business of school food

A second area of needed study is that of the business of school food, particularly the roles of suppliers, vendors, brokers, food manufacturers, and food service management companies. Studies need to focus on procurement decisions—how they are made—and on supply chains. Again, case studies are needed—of both standard practices and of innovations in supply like farm to cafeteria programs. Most school districts in the US still operate their own programs (called self-operated or "self-ops"), but a growing number have entered into contracts with food service management companies such as Aramark, Sodexo, or Chartwells, generally referred to as FSMCs. Case studies of transitions from one approach to the other would be particularly useful, as would comparative evaluations of food quality, participation, and health outcomes. Recent attention to the violation of federal rules requiring FSMCs to pass along to their public sector clients the value of the rebates offered by food manufacturers should raise interest in the whole process of marketing to schools. Content analysis of the advertising directed at food service procurement decision makers is an opportunity ripe for excavation.

The work and the workforce

The current public interest in food quality has directed attention to the actual work of preparing and serving school food. As parents began to ask why there was so little preparation of fresh food going on in the school kitchen, they were often surprised to learn that defrost-and-reheat technologies had long ago replaced stoves and cooking skills. Again, case studies of efforts to retrain foodservice workers and to upgrade culinary skills and knowledge seem promising. The work of Cook for America, Food Systems Solutions LLC, the Orfalea Foundation in Santa Barbara, CA and Wellness in the Schools in New York City, are examples of culinary training initiatives that could be studied. Because school food jobs are on the school calendar, they are particularly desirable for parents, especially single parents. More study of the role of school food employment in local economies would be welcome. Comparisons of work life, salaries, benefits, and human capital development in FSMC and self-op systems would be particularly useful.

The social relations of the cafeteria

There is a real gap in the existing literature when it comes to what actually happens in the school cafeteria. Murray Milner's *Freaks, Geeks and Cool Kids* shows just how much we can learn from careful observation in school lunchrooms. We need more ethnographic study of the social relations that arise, both among consumers (and non-consumers) of school meals, between students and staff, and among staff. Given the importance of shared meals to human social interaction, it seems odd that there is so little literature about what students experience in the school food setting.

School food reform as social movement

There is ample room for studies of school food reform efforts from a social movements perspective. Again, case studies, multiple case studies, and international comparisons would all be helpful.

Practical considerations for getting started

Because the National School Lunch Program and the School Breakfast Program are federal programs, and the federal research investment is both deep and extensive, almost any school food research project should begin by consulting the relevant federal research, and the USDA does a good job of making the research accessible through its websites. For a listing of available studies, go to: www.fns.usda.gov/ora/MENU/Published/CNP/cnp.htm (accessed on April 10, 2012). In addition, in 2008 the Economic Research Service, the branch of USDA that oversees most large-scale research studies, published a useful overview of recent research entitled "The National School Lunch Program: Background, Trends and Issues," by Katherine Ralston, Constance Newman, Annettte Clauson, Joanne Guthrie, and Jean Buzby (Ralston *et al.*, 2008). It is an essential starting point.

Within the corpus of USDA-sponsored research, the SNDA series continues to be a treasure trove. The original SNDA was completed by Mathematica Policy Research using data collected in 1991–92 and released in 1993. SNDA-II was conducted by Abt Associates, Inc., using data collected during the 1998–99 school year and released in 2001. SNDA-III was done by Mathematica, collecting data in 2004–05 and released late in 2007. And SNDA-IV, again conducted by Mathematica, is currently in progress with data collected at the time of writing, January–June, 2010.

Another important starting point is also a result of federal investment in research. In 2004, Abt Associates prepared for the USDA a major report on the *Effects of Food Assistance and Nutrition Programs on Nutrition and Health* (Fox, Hamilton, and Lin, 2004). This very useful document included a volume of literature review, with a chapter on the NSLP and another on the SBP. It is available on the web at www.ers.usda.gov/publications/fanrr19–3/fanrr19-3.pdf (accessed on April 10, 2012).

A different federal resource for studying school food is the USDA system for publicizing policy, rules, and guidance to regional offices and school food authorities.

Note that all policy memos are available online at www.fns.usda.gov/cnd/Governance/regulations. htm (accessed on April 10, 2012), as are guidance letters issued by the USDA for states and school food authorities at www.fns.usda.gov/cnd/guidance/default.htm (accessed on April 10, 2012).

For scholars interested in the history of school food, there are several collections of particular interest. The National School Food Management Institute (NSFMI) located at the University of Mississippi has a wonderful collection of papers and oral histories in its "Child Nutrition Archive," substantial portions of which can be accessed online. These papers include those of Thelma Flanagan, long the Director of Food and Nutrition Services for the State of Florida, who gathered material for a history of school food that she wrote in the 1960s, an excellent starting point for any historical venture (Flanagan, 1969). Similarly, the papers of Dr Josephine Martin, the first director of the NSFMI and the editor of a major textbook on food service management, contain a great deal of material helpful for historical study. Over the years the Congressional Research Service has done a number of historical summaries for Congressional committees, and some of these are also available through the Child Nutrition Archive. One of these summaries was incorporated into a document released in 1989 by the House Committee on Education and Labor, and then reprinted in full in the *School Food Service Research Review*, Vol. 13, No. 1, under the title "Child Nutrition Programs: Issues for the 101st Congress." The HEARTH (Home Economics Archive: Research Tradition and History) prepared by the Mann Library at Cornell University is a fabulous collection of books and journals in home economics and related disciplines from 1850 until 1950; the entire collection is available electronically.

The NSFMI also conducts studies of its own and collects literature on school food operations; students interested in the inner workings of the menu planning and food preparation process or in the finances and management of school food would do well to search the NSFMI databases. The *Journal of Child Nutrition and Management* began publishing in 1977 as the *School Foodservice Research Review*. Thus it serves as an essential source for both historical scholarship and contemporary studies of innovations and practices. The *Journal of the American Dietetic Association*, the *Journal of the American Public Health Association*, *Pediatrics*, and the *Journal of Nutrition Education and Behavior* (*Journal of the Society for Nutrition Education and Behavior*) are also important sources for school food research.

The School Nutrition Association (SNA) (formerly the American School Foodservice Association) is the professional association of school food service workers; its membership embraces both frontline workers (aka "lunch ladies") and food service directors and school business officials. Its monthly magazine, currently called *School Nutrition*, is another essential for scholars looking to understand the realties of school food in the United States. A monthly publication aimed at a broader range of food service managers including hospital, correctional, and other institutional settings, corporate dining services and employee cafeterias of all sorts, and college campuses as well as K–12 school meals is *Food Management*, available in both print and online editions. School business managers have their own association, ASBO, the Association of School Business Officials International (see www.asbointl.org) and their own monthly magazine, *School Business Affairs*. Similarly, the National School Boards Association has a website (www.nsba.org) and a monthly publication, *American School Board Journal*.

A number of the advocacy groups active in the school food arena maintain active websites and conduct and publicize research. The School Nutrition Association is a major resource at the national level, and every state has a state association of school food service workers, usually called the [name of state] School Nutrition Association. The Center for Ecoliteracy maintains a web-based resource called Rethinking School Lunch (www.ecoliteracy.org/downloads/rethinking-school-lunch-guide, accessed on April 10, 2012).

Essential resources for the study of school food and school food activism can be found on the websites—and in the libraries—of national organizations including Action for Healthy Kids (www.actionforhealthykids.org), the Center for Science in the Public Interest (www.cspinet.org), the Center on Budget and Policy Priorities (cbpp.org), the Food Research and Action Center (www.frac.org), Bread For the World (www.bread.org), Mazon: a Jewish Response to Hunger (www.mazon.org), Kids Can Make a Difference (www.kidscanmakeadifference.org), WhyHunger? (www.whyhunger.org), the Community Food Security Coalition (www.foodsecurity.org), the National Farm to School Network (www.farmtoschool.org), the Physicians Committee for Responsible Medicine (www.pcrm.org), the Alliance to End Hunger (www.allinacetoendhunger.org), Share Our Strength (www.strength.org), the Congressional Hunger Center (www.hungercenter.org), Feeding America (www.feedingamerica.org), Slow Food USA (www.slowfoodusa.org), the Children's Defense Fund (www.childrensdefense.org), School Food Focus (www.schoolfoodfocus.org), and an alliance of many of these organizations called NAHO, the National Anti Hunger Organizations (www.wecanendhunger.org). In addition, links to resources are provided on the website of Let's Move, the First Lady's initiative to end childhood obesity (www.letsmove.gov).

Within each state, there is a branch of Action for Healthy Kids, and most states have at least one statewide anti-hunger organization. Some states have an organization that specializes in child nutrition. In some states, statewide organizations of PTAs or of school boards have useful websites. Typically, the state Action for Healthy Kids site will have links to other relevant voluntary associations within the states.

Several philanthropic foundations have taken an interest in school food. The Alliance for a Healthier Generation is composed of the American Heart Association and the William J. Clinton Foundation. The W. K. Kellogg Foundation has made significant investments in better school food as has the Robert Wood Johnson Foundation. The Pew Charitable Trusts, the Chez Panisse Foundation, the Whole Kids Foundation, and the Food Family Farming Foundation all consider grants in this arena, though the federal government remains by far the largest funder of research on school food.

Bibliography

Bartlett, Susan, Frederic Glantz, and Christopher Logan (2008) "School Lunch and Breakfast Cost Study II." United States Department of Agriculture, Special Nutrition Programs Report No. CN-08-MCII.

Best, Joel (2008) *Social Problems*. New York: W. W. Norton & Company.

Blumer, Herbert (1971) "Social Problems as Collective Behavior." *Social Problems* 18: 298–306.

Boughton, Alice (1914) "The Administration of School Lunches in Cities." *Journal of Home Economics* 6: 3 (June): 213–18.

——(1916) "Household Arts and School Lunches." In *Cleveland Educational Survey*. Cleveland, OH: The Survey Committeee of the Cleveland Foundation.

Burghardt, John A., Barbara Devaney, and Anne R. Gordon (2004) "School Nutrition Dietary Assessment Study: Summary and Discussion." *The American Journal of Clinical Nutrition*, 61 (suppl.): S252-57.

Burghardt, John, Tim Silva, and Lara Hulsey (2004) "Case Study of National School Lunch Program Verification Outcomes in Large Metropolitan School Districts." USDA Food and Nutrition Service, Special Nutrition Programs Report No. CN-04-AV3.

Ciocco, A., H. Klein, and C. Palmer (1941) "Child health and the selective service physical standards." *Pub Health Rep* 56: 2365–75.

Eisinger, Peter (1998) *Toward an End to Hunger in America*. Washington, DC: The Brookings Institution.

Fairfax, Jean. (1968) *Their Daily Bread*, Committee on School Lunch Participation. Atlanta, GA: McNelley-Rudd Printing Service, Inc.

Flanagan, Thelma. (1969) "School Food Services," in *Education in the States: Nationwide Development since 1900*, eds. Edgar Fuller and Jim B. Pearson. Washington, DC: National Education Association.

Food and Nutrition Service (FNS), (2005) US Department of Agriculture, Centers for Disease Control and Prevention, and US Department of Education. *Make it Happen! School Nutrition Success Stories*. FN p.3.S-374. Alexandria, VA, January.

Food Research Action Center (FRAC). (1991–2010) *An Advocate's Guide to School Nutrition Programs*. Washington, DC: FRAC.

Fox, Mary Kay, William Hamilton, and Biing-Hwan Lin. (2004) *Effects of Food Assistance and Nutrition Programs on Nutrition and Health*, Volume 4, Executive Summary of the Literature Review, www.ers.usda.gov/publications/fanrr19-4/fanrr19-4a.pdf (accessed on May 1, 2012).

Glantz, Frederic B. (1994) *School Lunch Eligible Non-Participants*, Final Report. Cambridge, MA: Abt Associates.

Gleason, Philip M. (1995) "Participation in the National School Lunch Program and the School Breakfast Program," *American Journal of Clinical Nutrition*, 611 (suppl.): S213-20.

Gottlieb, Robert and Anupama Joshi (2010) *Food Justice (Food, Health and Environment)*. Cambridge, MA: MIT Press.

Gunderson, Gordon (1971) *The National School Lunch Program: Background and Development*, FNS 63. Washington, DC: US Government Printing Office, 14–15.

Hulsey, Lara, Philip Gleason, and James Ohls. (2004) "Evaluation of the National School Lunch Program Application/Verification Pilot Projects." USDA Food and Nutrition Service, Special Nutrition Programs Report No. CN-04-AV4.

Hunter, Robert (1904) *Poverty*. New York: MacMillan.

Institute of Medicine. Committee on Nutrition Standards for National School Lunch and Breakfast Programs. (2010) *School Meals: Building Blocks for Healthy Children*. Edited by Virginia A. Stallings, Carol West Suitor, and Christine L. Taylor. Washington, DC: The National Academies Press.

Joshi, Anupama, Marion Kalb, and Moira Beery. (2006) *Going Local: Paths to Success for Farm to School Programs*. agmarketing.extension.psu.edu/Wholesale/PDFs/goinglocal.pdf (accessed May 1, 2012).

Levenstein, Harvey (2003) *Paradox of Plenty*. Berkeley: University of California Press.

Levine, Susan (2008) *School Lunch Politics: The Surprising History of America's Favorite Welfare Program*. Princeton, NJ: Princeton University Press.

Maney, Ardith (1989) *Still Hungry after All These Years: Food Assistance from Kennedy to Reagan*. Westport, CT: Greenwood Press.

Martin, Josephine (1999) "History of Child Nutrition Programs." In *Managing Child Nutrition Programs: Leadership for the Twenty First Century*, Josephine Martin and Martha T. Conklin, eds. Gaithersburg, MD: Aspen Publishers, Inc., 29–85.

Morgan, Kevin and Roberta Sonnino (2008) *The School Food Revolution: Public Food and the Challenge of Sustainable Development*. London: Earthscan.

Nestle, Marion (2002) *Food Politics: How the Food Industry Influences Nutrition and Health*. Berkeley, CA: University of California Press.

Neuberger, Zoe and Robert Greenstein (2003) "'What Have We Learned from the FNS' New Research Findings about Overcertification in the School Meals Programs." Center on Budget and Policy Priorities, November 13.

Newman, Constance (2006) *The Income Volatility See-Saw: Implications for School Lunch*. US Department of Agriculture, Economic Research Service ERR-23, August.

Ponza, Michael, Philip Gleason, Lara Hulsey, and Quinn Moore (2007) *NSLP/SBP Access, Participation, Eligibility, and Certification Study: Erroneous Payments in the NSLP and SBP. Volume 1: Study Findings*. Special Nutrition programs Report No. CN-07-APEC. US Department of Agriculture, Food and Nutrition Service, Office of Research and Analysis.

Poppendieck, Janet (1986) *Breadlines Knee Deep in Wheat. Food Assistance in the Great Depression*. New Brunswick, NJ: Rutgers University Press.

——(2010) *Free for All: Fixing School Food in America*. Berkeley, CA: University of California Press.

Ralston, Katherine, Constance Newman, Annette Clauson, Joanne Guthrie, and Jean Buzby (2008) *The National School Lunch Program, Background, Trends and Issues*. Washington, DC: USDA, Economic Research Service, ERR-61.

Reese, William (1980) "After Bread, Education: Nutrition and Urban School Children, 1890–1920," *Teacher's College Record* 18:4 (Summer): 496–525.

Robert, Sarah A. and Marcus B. Weaver-Hightower, eds. (2011) *School Food Politics: The Complex Ecology of Hunger and Feeding in Schools Around the World.* New York: Peter Lang.

Roberts, Lydia (1958) "Beginnings of the Recommended Daily Allowances." *Journal of American Dietetic Association* 34 (September): 903–08.

Sims, Laura S. (1998) *The Politics of Fat: Food and Nutrition Policy in America.* Armonk, NY: M. E. Sharpe.

Southworth, H. M. and M. I. Klayman (1941) *The School Lunch Program and Agricultural Surplus Disposal.* Washington, DC: United States Department of Agriculture, Bureau of Agricultural Economics, Miscellaneous publication 467. US Government Printing Office.

Spector, Malcolm and John I. Kitsue (1987) *Constructing Social Problems.* Piscataway, NJ: Aldine Transaction.

United States Congress. House Committee on Education and Labor (1989) "Child Nutrition Programs: Issues for the 101st Congress." Reprinted in full as Kathleen Stitt, Mary Klatko, Mary Nix (on behalf of the American School Food Service Association), and Jean Yavis-Jones (Congressional Research Service) "Child Nutrition Programs, Issues for the 101st Congress," *School Food Service Research Review* 13 (1).

US Department of Agriculture, Food and Nutrition Service, Office of Research, Nutrition and Analysis. (2007) *School Nutrition Dietary Assessment-III, Volume I: School Foodservice, School Food Environment, and Meals Offered and Served.* Alexandria, VA: USDA, by Anne Gordon, Mary Kay Crepinsek, Renee Nogales, and Elizabeth Condon. Project Officer: Patricia McKinney.

——(2007) *School Nutrition Dietary Assessment-III: Volume II: Student Participation and Dietary Intakes.* Alexandria, VA: USDA, by Anne Gordon, Mary K. Fox, Melissa Clark, Renee Nogales, Elizabeth Condon, Philip Gleason, Ankur Sarin. Project Officer: Patricia McKinney.

Wechsler, H. *et al.* (2001) "Food Service and Foods and Beverages Available at School: Results from the School Health Policies and Program Study 2000." *Journal of School Health* 71:7 (2001).

Wellisch, Jean B. *et al.* (1983) *The National Evaluation of School Nutrition Programs, Final Report.* Santa Monica, CA: Systems Development Corporation.

31

Food in tourism studies

Lucy M. Long

Food has always been a part of hospitality services required by tourism, but it has only been recognized within tourism studies as a tourist attraction or destination since the late 1990s. Much of this work has focused on how to develop distinctive and memorable dining experiences ("culinary tourism" or "food tourism"). Scholars in New Zealand, Australia, Canada, and England have led the field, and some explore the potential impacts of tourist activities on local food cultures and cuisines. Also, scholars and businesses working with wine, agritourism, eco-tourism, and sustainable tourism are particularly interested in food.

Introduction

Tourism studies is an interdisciplinary field, oftentimes professionally oriented in training students to work within the industry, but increasingly drawing upon both social sciences and the humanities to explore the practices, the impacts, and the meanings of tourism. As an academic field at educational institutions it is usually aligned with hospitality management or recreation and leisure, and frequently has a strong marketing component, although classes examining it as a cultural, economic, and political phenomen might be offered within other departments.

Food surprisingly played an insignificant role in tourism studies until the late 1990s, and is still frequently treated as simply another hospitality service that accompanies tourism. Starting in 2002, publications brought attention to food as a potential attraction and destination in its own right. The tourism industry also "discovered" food in the middle of the first decade of 2000, leading to "culinary tourism" becoming a fast-growing niche within the industry and a popular subject for research. It is also treated as part of agritourism, sustainable tourism, and cultural tourism.

Historical background

People have always traveled, but historically it was out of necessity rather than pleasure and was full of hardship and danger. Food could be an object of travel in that travelers sought new food sources, trade routes for carrying food, and new foods that could be traded as a commodities. Food was central to the survival of travelers, but, unless the traveler was of a high status, it was usually treated as fuel rather than a pleasurable culinary experience. For example, the hard tack, or "ship's biscuits," given to British sailors in the 1700 and 1800s would barely qualify as food for most culinary tourists today.

Debates abound among tourism scholars as to when tourism started as an actual industry. Food is part of the debate since it is an integral part of the hospitality services supporting travelers. The issues around food tended to be not on food itself but on how to ensure adequate and safe supplies to fortify/nourish tourists traveling to and at their destination. Pilgrimages during the European Middle Ages, for example, encouraged the growth of inns, convent and monastery gardens and food specialties (such as cheeses, candies, breads, beer, and wine). Mass tourism is seen as beginning in the 1700s in Great Britain as a way to help the working classes escape the unhealthy industrial centers. Emphasis here was on healthy and hearty food as a necessary part of the experience rather than the focus of attention. Similarly, travel for health reasons to a climate or environment better suited for human habitation or to cure specific ailments (tuberculosis) usually included food that would be healthier, but was not the destination itself. The European Grand Tour of the seventeenth and eighteenth centuries took well-to-do upper-class youth to the great sights of Europe, but travelers oftentimes ate the foods they were accustomed to rather than try new foods. In fact, eating local foods was frequently out of necessity rather than choice since there tended to be among most cultures a fear of what others eat.

It should be mentioned that a certain amount of "domestic tourism" (tourism within one's own .country) has always occurred around food, especially in places known for regional specialties. In Spain, for example, towns in the north were famous for their distinctive varieties of beans. Aficionados would travel to restaurants in season specializing in dishes made with those beans. Cheeses, meats, vegetables, and fruits with strong place associations tended to attract consumers, even though they frequently were not seen as tourism attractions per se. Even now, individuals travel to a favorite restaurant or to a region where they can obtain a particular specialty without thinking of themselves as tourists. Similarly certain countries have reputations for their cuisines, and individuals knowledgeable in those cuisines enjoy traveling there, not as tourists but as well-informed connoisseurs. France has a long history of attracting gourmands for its excellent and distinctive foods, as do Spain, Italy, Mexico, parts of China, and numerous other countries and geographic regions.

Recognition within the tourism industry that food could be an attraction in itself began in the 1990s with wine, in which connoisseurs would travel to the source of excellent wines in order to experience for themselves the origin of a wine and to taste it in its natural setting. Such tours involved not only tasting wines, but also learning about the varieties and nuances of tastes. All of this usually was directed at heightening the aesthetic pleasure of the visit and tended to lend itself to tourism as status marker. Similarly, the tourism industry had always recognized gourmet dining experiences as an "added value" to a tour, but in the early 2000s, businesses began thinking of food as a potential attraction and even destination. The focus tended to be on famous restaurants, famous chefs, and exceptional and unique fine-dining experiences, and these were marketed to tourists usually with some prior knowledge of the culinary world and characterized as having extra money that could be spent on extravagant services. Numerous organizations specializing in culinary tourism have since been established.

Meanwhile, scholars from a variety of fields were exploring the concepts of eating and otherness in tourism and suggested several terms for such tourism focused on food: "Tasting tourism" (Boniface), "food tourism" (Hall), "gastronomic tourism" (Zelinski), and "culinary tourism" (Long, 1998, 2004) and "food pilgrimages" (Long, 2006). Each term represented a slightly different approach to the subject, but the industry now most commonly uses "culinary tourism," changing the scholarly meaning of the phrase from the original "voluntary, exploratory participation in the foodways of an Other" (Long, 2004) to "the pursuit of unique and memorable eating and drinking experiences" (Wolf, 2006).

Major theoretical approaches

Tourism is both an industry and a human activity. Correspondingly, tourism studies is both a professional and academic field. Theory, therefore, falls into two large categories of operation: how best to run tourism operations; and anthropological, cultural and philosophical theories exploring the meanings of the tourism experience. Both sets of scholarship deal with the motivations behind tourism as well as its impacts, but they tend to differ in that the first is concerned primarily with applied knowledge, and the second with interpretation of the activities of tourism. Also, the two approaches define tourism very differently, and those definitions then drive theory.

The tourism industry tends to define it as an activity involving travel that then requires hospitality services away from home: "[T]ourism comprises the activities of persons traveling to and staying in places outside their usual environment for not more than one consecutive year for leisure, business, and other purposes" (United Nations World Tourism Organization, 1993), and a tourist is "[one] who travels away from home for a distance of at least 50 miles (one way) for business, pleasure, personal affairs, or any other purpose except to commute to work, whether he stay overnight or returns the same day" (the National Tourism Resources Review Commission, 1973). These definitions focus on the potential money spent on services needed by an individual in a new place or on services that would normally occur at home, such as eating, laundering one's clothes, sleeping. Most tourism scholars now add that tourism is a complex phenomenon involving multiple activities and multiple players: "[T]ourism may be defined as the processes, activities, and outcomes arising from the relationships and the interactions among tourist, tourism suppliers, host governments, host communities, and surrounding environments that are involved in the attracting and hosting of visitors" (Goeldner and Ritchie, 2009: 6). Food is included as one of the activities involved in such interactions and is a physical need and therefore a service, and potentially an attraction for tourists.

Operational theories are closely aligned with business, hospitality management, marketing, travel, lodging, and food services. These theories provide models for best practices and making predictions within tourism and hospitality providers, usually with the aim of improving efficiency and profitability. There is a tendency within tourism scholarship to focus primarily on the businesses providing services, but there is a push to take into account all the players, including the tourist, tourist services, governments of host and guest cultures, and host community. Established tourism scholars and textbook writers, Charles Goeldner and Brent Ritchie, encourage a systems approach, defining a system as "a set of interrelated groups coordinated to form a unified whole and organized to accomplish a set of goals. It integrates the other approaches into a comprehensive method dealing with both micro and macro issues" (2009: 25).

Within operational theories, until the early 2000s, food was generally approached as a hospitality service with little attention paid to the cultural or symbolic meanings of that food. Seminal work was done by European, Australian, and New Zealand tourism scholars who began researching and theorizing food as an attraction and destination. Much of this work addresses the planning, implementation, and management of tourism operations around food and wine, but it also recognizes food as a cultural phenomenon.

Mitchell and Hall define food tourism as "visitation to primary and secondary food producers, food festivals, restaurants, and specific locations for which food tasting and/or experiencing the attributes of specialist food production regions are the primary motivating factor for travel"

(2001: 308). They propose that one of the unique features of this type of tourism is the association between specific foods and locales, so marketing needs to pay special attention to images attached to place.

In 2000 Hall, Sharples, Cambourne, and Macionis edited *Wine Tourism Around the World: Development, Management and Markets*, giving cross-displinary perspectives from business, the social sciences, and policy studies. Hall, Sharples, *et al.* edited *Food Tourism Around the World: Development, Management and Markets* in 2003, exploring motivations for food tourism, models for developing and managing it, strategies for connecting it to regional economic development, and the implications of tourism for culinary identity. Similar to earlier tourism scholarship, they attempt to develop typologies – of culinary tourists, of attractions, of dining experiences. Although some of the authors in this volume address cultural issues and questions of authenticity and identity, most of the articles offer models for applying the research to developing and managing tourism. In the introductory chapter, for example, Hall and Sharples state that food is significant in tourism because it represents a large percentage of expenditures, it is useful for marketing, and it "can be used as a means of differentiation for a destination in an increasingly competitive global marketplace" (2003: 5). Hall and Sharples later edited a third volume, *Food and Wine Festivals and Events Around the World*, in 2008, which continues their earlier work but brings in a new emphasis on ecological concerns surrounding tourism events. Consistent with trends within tourism studies and the tourism industry towards sustainability, the authors promote models that are collaborative, community based, environmentally friendly, and encouraging of local economic development.

Another significant volume was edited by Anne-Mette Hjalager and Greg Richards in 2002. *Gastronomy and Tourism* is also directed towards the application of theory, but it brings in a more cultural perspective, examining both tourism and gastronomy as impacted by globalization. They point out that both fields have always been dynamic, and that a holistic understanding of them together will enable tourism policy makers and operators to develop programs that will allow for creative change while simultaneously encouraging regional cuisines. The authors also offer an epistemological framework for gastronomic tourism, and outline the types of knowledge that are needed to further develop the field. This volume includes articles going beyond impact studies to discuss food as intellectual property, as representing regional and national identities, and as a force in globalization and localization as well as a major tool in economic development.

The anthropology of tourism explores the meanings of the tourism. It emerged as a field in the mid-1970s when anthropologists recognized that tourism was both culturally shaped and an activity involving cultural implications. Definitions were introduced that focused on tourism as a type of mind-set or attitude of the tourist rather than just physical movement away from home. Valene Smith defined a tourist as "a temporarily leisured person who voluntarily visits a place away from home for the purpose of experiencing a change" (1997: 1) and developed typologies of types of tourists as well as forms of tourism. Another seminal scholar, Dean MacCannell, stated that "touristic consciousness is motivated by its desire for authentic experience" (1999: 277). Tourists accordingly were fleeing modernity and seeking a feeling of connection with nature, other people, and even themselves that was thought to exist outside the industrialized world. He explored how sites became "sacralized" into a tourist attraction, and how authenticity was "staged" so that tourists had the illusion of experiencing another culture. Similarly, Nelson Graburn defined the tourist experience as a journey from the profane to the sacred in that tourism is a way in which people "embellish and add meaning to their lives" (1989: 22). John Urry took these notions further in his concept of the "tourist gaze" as essentially different from "everyday looking" (2002): "[T]he potential objects of the tourist gaze must be different in some way or other. They must be out of the ordinary. People must experience particularly distinct pleasures which involve different senses or are on a different scale from those typically encountered in everyday life" (Urry, 2002: 45).

These anthropological definitions and theories did not address food per se, but they called for more nuanced understandings of culture in general, laying the foundation for food to be recognized as part of the experience of tourism—and tourism as a way of experiencing the world. Several tourism scholars recognized the potential of food as a subject for understanding tourism as a cultural experience. Priscilla Boniface takes this approach in her *Tasting Tourism: Travelling for Food and Drink* (2003). She recognizes that culture defines and shapes tourism and the forms it takes. What one group of people see as tourism may then be perceived differently by another group. She then suggests that food and drink have recently become tourist attractions in their own right because tourism itself has changed. Tourism now overlaps with everyday life, and difference is no longer important in defining an experience as a touristic one. Instead, tourism acts as a medium through which society works out issues and concerns. Tourism offers "liminal" spaces, in which individuals feel out of the ordinary. This then frees them to experiment and explore not only another culture, but their own identities, beliefs, and practices.

Folklorist Lucy Long (1998, 2004, 2006) also drew from this literature in developing her culinary tourism model, which has been adopted by much of the tourism industry. She applied Urry's concept of "tourist gaze" to food and eating, emphasizing tourism as a type of experience based on curiosity and perception of otherness in food. Otherness can be more than another culture; it can be a time, age, region, religion, socioeconomic class, or any other category that is perceived as being out of the norm for an individual. This means that tourism can occur in a number of venues without a person actually traveling away from home—cookbooks, films, fiction, etc. The definition also expands the range of activities that are involved in culinary tourism, moving from food to foodways, the total system of activities and conceptualizations surrounding eating (procurement, preservation, preparation, product, consumption, disposal, performance). This connects culinary tourism to other varieties of tourism—agri-, heritage, eco-, sustainable—and also to a food culture as a whole.

Tourism scholarship is continuing to incorporate more interdisciplinary perspectives on food and tourism. It is refining operational models, developing criteria for successful implementation, conducting case studies, and exploring the potential for channeling culinary tourism for sustainability. A perusal through tourism and hospitality journals demonstrates that food is now a serious subject in scholarship. Two major questions drive much of this work: The motivations of tourists and the impacts of tourism.

The anthropological theories that tourism is actually a search for authenticity have also been applied to culinary tourism. Accordingly, tourists go to other places to consume the food of that place because it offers an authentic experience of food connected to place. This then gives the tourist a sense of connection, of being whole and integrated. It also gives an "added value" to the food in that it is unique to that place, requires physical travel, and therefore an out-of-ordinary experience. Others theorize that the motivation is a desire for memorable dining experiences or unique ones that give the tourist a higher status. Long (2004) posits that curiosity is the basic motivation, and that the curiosity can be about the food or the culture behind the food. Boniface (2003) identified five "driving motivations: anxiety over food safety, the need for comradeship in uncertain times and the need for comfort and escape; a need to show distinction, affluence and individualism; curiosity and the wish for knowledge and discovery; the need to feel grounded amid globalization; and the need for sensory and tactile pleasure." Sharples offers a typology of culinary tourists based on the depth of interest in food. Most scholars recognize that motivations can be mixed, and that individual tourists may change motivations at any time.

A second general trend of theory in tourism scholarship explores the impacts of tourism on host communities. This can be done from a social science perspective, measuring economic, health, safety, and social "costs and benefits" arising from tourism. Costs are the negative results of tourism, while benefits are the positive ones, and ideally benefits would outweigh the costs of any tourist activity. Problems arise in the interpretation of what is a cost and to whom.

Erik Cohen and Nir Avieli claimed that food could actually be an obstacle to tourism. Unpleasant food experiences could lead to cultural misunderstandings, and treating food as an attraction could have harmful effects on the host culture (2004). Many tourism scholars, however, see food in tourism as beneficial by affirming culinary identities and providing a market base for the continuation of culinary traditions. Priscilla Boniface, in *Tasting Tourism: Travelling for Food and Drink* (2003) sees food tourism as actually stimulating local cuisine rather than stifling it, since such tourists are seeking authentic experiences through food. A number of articles in *Food Tourism Around the World* suggest similar conclusions; food tourism is partially responsible for the development of regional cuisines.

Another theory interpreting the impacts of tourism tends to see it as an inherently colonialist enterprise. Coming primarily from Marxist-influenced cultural studies, these scholars see tourism as representing an unequal power structure in which hosts must cater to guests for their approval and financial "gifts." In economic terms, this creates dependency on the tourism industry, which is often controlled by players outside the actual tourism destinations. In cultural terms, it creates shame and embarrassment within the tourist culture and, rather than encouraging cultural understanding, perpetuates stereotypes of both the host and guest cultures. Food plays a role by representing culture, so that eating the food of an Other can symbolically be a domination, even annihilation of that other. While that interpretation may seem extreme, tourism does put cultures on display for the entertainment or edification of tourists, as anthropologist-folklorist Barbara Kirshenblatt-Gimblett points out in *Destination Culture: Tourism, Museums, and Heritage* (1998). In such displays, the host culture performs itself self-consciously to the audience, shaping itself according to the perceived expectations of that audience. Restaurants catering to tourists similarly design their menus and recipes with tourist tastes in mind. Whether that is colonialism or simply good marketing on their part depends on the amount of agency and choice they feel they have in making their decisions.

Tourism scholarship and policy has attempted to address the issues of costs and benefits and inequalities by developing the concept of sustainable tourism, tourism that wisely uses environmental, economic, social, and cultural resources so that they will be available in the future. Food can play a significant role in sustainability since it easily links the various tourism components and has obvious ties to the environment and culture. Furthermore, Rosario Scarpato argues that tourism should be able to support a "sustainable gastronomy" by providing economic and social support for local foods (in Hall and Sharples *et al.*, 2003: 132–53).

Methods

Tourism studies emphasizes social science and quantitative methods of research. Data are collected through surveys, questionnaires, observation, and brief interviews, and are interpreted using statistics and methods. Case studies are a common tool for examining the implementation of theories.

These methods are then applied to the specific approach and concerns of the researcher. Applied researchers focusing on improving tourism as an industry utilize models for efficiency and profitability, including the economics of tourism – amounts of money spent and on what services, multiplier effects (other businesses benefiting from tourism dollars), and distribution of profits. A productive method is to "follow the money" to see who actually benefits financially from tourism. Consumer behavior is studied in order to determine who responds to what marketing efforts, as well as to identify clientele for specific tourism activities. Environmental impacts of tourism are easily measured, and the affects of tourism on social institutions, demographics, crime, and public cultural practices and expressive forms are also quantifiable subjects. These measurements are crucial to the assessment of "costs" and "benefits" in tourism to all the "stakeholders" (tourist, host community, host government, host environment, and tourism businesses).

Interpretation of data frequently involves developing typologies addressing the spectrum of tourism components: Tourists (motivations, primary interests, place of origin, socioeconomic characteristics), tourist activities (shopping, eating, sleeping, visiting sites, etc.), destinations and attractions (types of sites, popularity, length of time spent there), and impacts (particularly economic and environmental). Typologies can then be utilized in marketing, planning of tourism programs and in making public policy decisions concerning tourism. They also allow for the application of models with different variables and for objective evaluation of the efficacy of models. Relevant to food in tourism is a typology of food tourists based on their depth of interest in food (Hall and Sharples *et al.*, 2003). Similarly, Boniface offers five motivations for food tourism, and Long suggests typologies of "otherness," venues for tourism, and strategies for negotiating exoticness and familiarity in the culinary tourism experience.

Qualitative research methods tend to be used by those tourism scholars coming from anthropological and humanities perspectives. They approach tourism as a cultural and social construction, reflecting and shaping cultural beliefs and worldviews as well as social values and identity. These intangible aspects of tourism require research methods that help to identify perceptions of individuals as well as collective understandings. This type of ethnography allows individuals to speak for themselves, recognizing that behavior stems from perception, but places those individuals within the larger historical, economic, political, social, and cultural context. It frequently addresses the experience of tourism and how that affects the ways in which that individual might see the world.

By 2010, much tourism scholarship recognized the need to integrate quantitative and qualitative methods, and to recognize the cultural and experiential aspects of tourism. The sub-field of sustainable tourism, although frequently focused on economic and ecological sustainability, encourages collaborative and integrative research and assessments.

It recognizes that tourism is both an economic enterprise and a cultural one and attempts to develop approaches that allow for a holistic understanding of how all components work together.

Avenues for future research

As one of the largest industries in the world, tourism offers numerous directions for further research. Tourism studies is becoming increasingly multi- and interdisciplinary, and the cultural aspects of the field are more recognized among both professionals and scholars. It now makes room for more input from scholars from a variety of humanities and social science disciplines.

Culinary tourism is currently seen as a positive force in economic development. Initiatives have developed throughout the world that use food to attract tourist dollars. The best of these create networks between food producers (farmers), processors (chefs, artisinal preservation and preparation), and distributors (shops, restaurants), so that tourists gain a broader perspective on where their food comes from and who is involved. They also tend to feature local production, strengthening local food businesses and creating stable markets for small-scale farmers. Some culinary tourism initiatives also promote local foodways and food cultures, such as preparation methods, everyday foods, or eating styles and contexts (think of Amish suppers). More research is needed in order to identify foodways, but the local and everyday does not always fit the criteria of gourmet, unique, or exotic.

Research on the impacts of food tourism is crucial. Tourism oftentimes introduces new ingredients, dishes, and cuisines to both hosts and tourists. In what ways might that shape individual experiences and perceptions of the other? Can food be an entrée into understanding another culture, or is it simply entertainment or fuel? Also, tourism may cause some established food traditions to be overshadowed, even obliterated, by the new foods. How do such changes affect the local food culture (the beliefs and practices surrounding food) and food system (system of production, distribution, and consumption)? Tourism may actually bring seemingly beneficial changes, encouraging healthier eating habits, more environmentally friendly production methods with local foods, and a stronger sense of pride in food traditions. What is the long-term effect of these benefits, however? They may shift cultural values and perceptions in ways that affect other aspects of that culture in unforeseen ways.

Another area of research concerns issues surrounding intangible heritage and intellectual property in tourism. Food studies can contribute to a better understanding of these concepts, partly because food's ubiquitousness and materiality make it productive to "think with." Everyone can participate in discussions about food, and everyone can participate in the consumption of it. Also, specific cuisines and dishes are now being designated as UNESCO world heritage items, turning them into official tourism attractions. What are the implications?

Sustainable tourism is a growing trend within the tourism industry, and food can play a part in encouraging sustainability. Research can help push the role of food beyond its obvious connections to economies and environments to help promote social and cultural sustainability as well. Culture is not fully understood in much sustainable tourism and tends to be perceived as simply artistic forms or everyday practices of a group of people. An understanding of the complexity of culture as a worldview and ethos as well as practices can be developed through the study of food as a cultural phenomenon.

Similarly, scholars and professionals are recognizing that tourism can shape perceptions of others and interactions between cultures and even nations. Anthropological and folkloristic approaches to culinary tourism tend to emphasize ways in which it can be channeled towards education, cultural understanding, and peaceful relations between diverse groups of people. Much more work is needed in this area.

Tourism involving food also offers employment opportunities for individuals trained in food studies or culinary arts. Along with working in food services, such backgrounds are an "added value" in planning, developing, and executing tourism programs.

Practical considerations for getting started

Tourism degrees are offered at both the undergraduate and graduate level at universities throughout the world. Frequently connected with travel, hospitality, leisure or recreation, the degree is a professional one preparing students for work in the tourism industry. Depending on the program, students can specialize in tourism administration, programming, management, and policy. Some programs offer an emphasis in sustainable or "responsible" tourism. The PhD in tourism tends to emphasize research that can be applied to the profession. Tourism programs in the US and China tend to emphasize the business and marketing aspects of the field, while

Canadian, European, and Australian/New Zealand ones recognize its interdisciplinarity and require courses in anthropology, sociology, and psychology.

Tourism classes are also offered in other disciplines, particularly anthropology, folklore, and cultural studies. Many food studies programs frequently include a class or lectures on culinary tourism.

There are numerous tourism organizations, both professional and scholarly. At the global level, there are two primary organizations: The United Nations World Tourism Organization, which aims to insure that tourism contributes to economic development, international understanding, and peace, and the World Travel and Tourism Council, made up of industry leaders and highlighting the positive benefits of tourism. This division between promotion of the tourism industry and oversight of tourism activities is then seen at the national, regional, and even town level. Many of these are connected to the travel and tourism industry, and frequently every country, region, and even town has its own organization to promote and oversee tourism within its boundaries. A number of organizations specialize in culinary tourism, and these tend towards promotion of the tourism industry: The International Culinary Tourism Association (based in the US), the Ontario Culinary Tourism Alliance and BC Culinary Tourism Society (Canada), and Australia on a Silver Platter. There also are numerous scholarly organizations for tourism study, and culinary tourism is included as a subject within those.

There are no journals dealing specifically with culinary tourism, but articles about the subject appear in peer-reviewed academic journals, including the *Journal of Travel Research*, *Tourism Management*, *Tourism Economics*, *Journal of Leisure Research*, *Tourism Geographies*, and *Annals of Tourism Research*. A journal that addresses tourism from an interdisciplinary perspective, including cultural studies, as part of a larger treatment of strangers and newcomers, was established in 2011, *Hospitality & Society*.

Key reading

Boniface, Priscilla (2003) *Tasting Tourism: Travelling for Food Drink*. Aldershot: Ashgate.

Chambers, Erve (2010) *Native Tours: The Anthropology of Travel and Tourism*. Long Grove, IL: Waveland Press Inc.

Cohen, Erik and Nir Avieli (2004) "Food in Tourism: Attraction and Impediment." *Annals of Tourism Research* 31, no. 4: 755–78.

Gmelch, Sharon Bohn, ed. (2010) *Tourists and Tourism: Reader*. Long Grove, IL: Waveland Press, Inc.

Goeldner, Charles R. and J. R. Brent Ritchie (2009) *Tourism: Principles, Practices, Philosophies*. Hoboken, NJ: John Wiley & Sons Inc.

Graburn, Nelson (1989) "'Tourism' the Sacred Journey." In *Hosts and Guests: The Anthropology of Tourism*, V. Smith, ed., 2nd edn, pp. 21–3. Philadelphia: University of Pennsylvania Press6.

Hall, C. Michael and Liz Sharples, eds. (2008) *Food and Wine Festivals and Events around the World: Development, Managment and Markets*. Burlington, VT: Butterworth-Heinemann.

Hall, C. Michael, Liz Sharples, Richard Mitchell, Niki Macionis, and Brock Cambourne, eds. (2003) *Food Tourism Around the World: Development, Management and Markets*. London: Butterworth-Heinemann.

Hall, C. Michael, Liz Sharples, B. Cambourne and N. Macionis (2000) *Wine Tourism Around the World: Development, Management and Markets*. Oxford: Butterworth Heinemann.

Harris, Rob, Tony Griffin, and Peter Williams (2002) *Sustainable Tourism: A Global Perspective*. Jordan Hill: Butterworth-Heinemann.

Hjalager, Ane-Mette and Greg Richards, eds. (2002) *Tourism and Gastronomy*. London: Routledge.

Kirshenblatt-Gimblett, Barbara (1998) *Destination Culture: Tourism, Museums, and Heritage*. Berkeley and Los Angeles: University of California Press.

Long, Lucy M. (1998) "Culinary Tourism: A Folkloristic Perspective on Eating and Otherness." *Southern Folklore* 55: 181–204.

——(2004) *Culinary Tourism*. Lexington: University of Kentucky Press.

——"Food pilgrimages: seeking the sacred and the authentic in food." *Appetite* 47, no. 3 (November 2006).

MacCannell, Dean (1999) *The Tourist: A New Theory of the Leisure Class*. Berkeley and Los Angeles: University of California Press.

Mill, Robert Christie and Alastair M. Morrison (2009) *The Tourism System*. Dubuque, IA: Kendall Hunt Publishing Company.

Mitchell, R. and C. M. Hall (2001) "The Winery Consumer: a New Zealand Perspective." *Tourism Recreation Research* 25(2): 63–75.

Smith, Valene L., ed. (1997) *Hosts and Guests: The Anthropology of Tourism*. Philadelphia: University of Pennsylvania Press.

Urry, John (2002) *The Tourist Gaze*. Thousand Oaks, CA: SAGE Publications Ltd.

Weaver, David (2006) *Sustainable Tourism: Theory and Practice*. Kidlington: Butterworth-Heinemann.

Williams, Stephen (2009) *Tourism Geography: A New Synthesis*. New York: Routledge.

Wolf, Eric (2006) *Culinary Tourism: The Hidden Harvest*. Dubuque, IA: Kendall Hunt Publishing.

32

Food and the senses

Beth M. Forrest and Deirdre Murphy

The interdisciplinary field of sensory studies has bloomed in the last three decades and, more recently, has converged with food studies. Given that one's encounters with food are both ephemeral and individual, food as a subject of sensory studies scholarship provides a way to think about the shifting encounters between subjective individual experience, and the social and cultural construction of reality. The charge of sensory studies of food and taste is to trace out this cycle that creates and is created by physical, individual, and communal experiences; and that does so in ways that are both immediate and historic.

Introduction

An assessment of the scholarship on food and the senses might well begin by looking back to the fictional experiences of a miserable miser who neither ate much, nor was sensitive to the pleasures of food, nor valued the community of the table at all. When Charles Dickens' now-famous Scrooge first encountered the wildly bombastic Spirit of Christmas Present in his chill, dark, sparse apartments in the middle of a frigid night in 1843, it was a moment of gastronomic overload for his curmudgeonly senses. For one used to subsisting on thin gruels rather than real meals, the shock was profound:

> Heaped up upon the floor, to form a kind of throne, were turkeys, geese, game, poultry, brawn, great joints of meat, sucking-pigs, long wreaths of sausages, mince-pies, plum puddings, barrels of oysters, red-hot chestnuts, cherry-cheeked apples, juicy oranges, luscious pears, immense twelfth-cakes, and seething bowls of punch, that made the chamber dim with their delicious steam. In easy estate upon this couch, there sat a jolly giant, glorious to see; who bore a glowing torch, in shape not unlike Plenty's horn, and held it up, high up, to shed its light on Scrooge, as he came peeping round the door.
>
> *(Dickens, 1989: 109–10)*

Overwhelmed by this ghostly presence, the anti-social Scrooge peers from a distance. Given the multi-sensory offerings at hand, he holds himself apart and cannot at first make sense of the manner in which the spirit reveals himself, nor of the images the spectre goes on to conjure for him on the state of society. The experience is a whirlwind of contrasts as the Spirit shows him examples of abundance and pleasure in society, mixed with those of poverty and suffering. Finally, as the visit draws to a close, we have the introduction of a "Yellow, meagre, ragged, scowling, wolfish" boy and girl. They are "Ignorance" and "Want," and they grovel pathetically though threateningly at the skirts of the ghost of Christmas of 1843. "Beware them both and all their degree," warns the Spirit, for upon their forms "I see that written which is Doom" (ibid.: 141–42).

As Dickens (the social critic) knew nearly two centuries ago, and as scholars within sensory studies continue to examine it today, food is the nexus of the "sensing" self and the "sensible" society, the meeting point of the individual and the communal. Through the experience of tasting, smelling, touching, seeing, and even hearing food, the individual encounters culture, and becomes a part of society. Thus, the problem with Scrooge and the skeletally starved and anthropomorphized social problems, "Ignorance" and "Want," is that, with respect to food, they do not sense anything at all. These characters either do not or cannot partake of gustatory pleasures, and this is the basis of their characterization as various incarnations of social dysfunction. Conversely, Scrooge at the moment of his social and spiritual rehabilitation becomes a more sensing and sensitive individual. He celebrates his moment of rebirth at the end of the tale by reclaiming his physical appetite: First, he sends a goose to the family of his much-abused assistant, Bob Cratchit, and then he rushes off to reknit the social fabric of his world even further by joining his own previously alienated family for a feast.

What Dickens's famous redemption story demonstrates for scholars, is that paying attention to food from the perspective of the senses allows us to place individual experience within cultural and social context, and to examine how social and cultural context shapes individual sensory experience. Sensory studies of food are positioned to do both because food is such a relentlessly material subject, even as tasting it is also a richly abstract field for the cultural imagination. As Mikhail Bakhtin has characterized the role of "table talks," and feasting in the work of sixteenth-century satirist Rabelais, the act of eating food, as well as the representation of such, expresses a complex and multi-layered "conception of truth": "The merry, triumphant encounter with the world in the act of eating and drinking, in which man partakes of the world instead of being devoured by it," constitutes a "victory over the world." For Bakhtin, "the act of eating [i]s concrete, tangible, bodily." Simultaneously, feasting "gave the very taste of the defeated world, which had fed and would feed mankind" (Bakhtin, 1989: 285). Given that our encounters with food are both ephemeral and individual, food as a subject of sensory studies scholarship provides, as Bakhtin's comments reveal, a way to think about the shifting encounters between subjective individual experience, and the social and cultural construction of reality.

Historical background of scholarship and major theoretical approaches

Within sensory studies scholarship, Karl Marx's daunting assertion in 1844 that "The forming of the five senses is a labour of the entire history of the world down to the present" is rightly and frequently pressed into service (Marx, 2011). It is repeated not nearly so much nor with such evident fondness as a certain memory about a certain madeleine, but its recurrence is still notable, and not only for the way in which it succinctly outlines the enormity of the task set for the serious sensory studies scholar. What Marx was insisting upon was an awareness that it is our ability to engage our sensory perceptions, to be cognizant of them, that makes us fully human, and embedded in this declaration was a warning against alienation from sensory experience (Howes, 2005). We might consider then, the way in which Marx's comment (as well as Scrooge's rehabilitation) usefully characterizes a broadly developed sensory studies approach to the subject of food as cyclical: Over time and repeatedly, people and societies produce food, which is then consumed by individuals who, through the act of eating it, express their participation in culture, and thus reaffirm their place in society. Through our encounters with food, in other words, we sustain the body and express the individual self, even as we also create culture and submit to society. The charge of sensory studies of food and taste is to trace out this cycle that creates and is created by physical, individual, and communal experiences; and that does so in ways that are both immediate and historic.

Ironically enough, the first scholars to take up the "labor" of examining the senses as a subject of academic research were anthropologists and sociologists who left the sense of taste far in the background of their scholarship. The work of nineteenth-century anthropologists was an ethnographic calculation and categorization of the sensory experiences of "primitives," and part of the way they accomplished this task was through the maintenance of a long-established "hierarchy of the senses" (Classen, 1997; Howes, 2003; Jütte, 2005; Ferguson, 2011). For these scholars, vision, followed by hearing, was regarded as the most "elevated" of all forms of perception.

For early researchers, hearing and seeing were the senses most closely associated with the thinking, rational brain as it observed phenomena. These senses extended out farthest from the body, visual and aural experiences could be most easily shared with others, and they were assumed to allow their possessors to encounter the world more objectively than other senses could. As historian Mark Smith has described it, they were imbued with the ability to promote "perspective, distance, balance, coolness, detachment, and a growing sense of self" (Smith, 2008: 10). Taste, meanwhile, historically often ranked between the senses of smell and touch, was both dependent upon these other "lower order" senses, and far less objective: Not only did it require touching the sense object (food), it changed it through mastication, which led to swallowing, and then digesting (Ferguson, 2011). Tasting food then, was understood to be a deeply subjective, and even brute sense because it altered the object it encountered: Taste, base sense that it was, simply could not leave an object alone.

By the time sociologist George Simmel published his seminal "Sociology of the Senses" in 1907, the scholarly predilection for the visual and the aural was firmly in place. So much so that taste, as one of "the lower senses [which are] of secondary importance," according to Simmel, received no direct mention at all in this work, which is among the very earliest to outline the possibilities for sensory research (Simmel, 1998: 117). As the study of the senses moved forward through the middle decades of the twentieth century, largely in anthropology and sociology, taste remained for most scholars a footnote or an overlooked realm of experience. The reasons for this are two-fold. The first of these was the continued privileging of seeing and hearing over smelling, tasting, and touching, and this was abetted starting in the early decades of the twentieth century by the invention of technologies of reproduction that recorded only sights and sounds (Howes, 2003).

In fact, this preference for the visual and the aural remained intact for decades, and in many respects it is still in place. Emphasis on visual and aural forms of experience was a principal characteristic of some of the early theoretical work that influenced what would formally become recognized as sensory studies, that of Marshall McLuhan and his student, Walter Ong. What McLuhan attempted, in works like *The Gutenberg Galaxy: The Making of Typographic Man* (1962) and *Understanding Media: The Extensions of Man* (1965) was nothing less than "to explain all of human history, as well as social organization between the West and the 'tribal' societies of Africa and the Orient, in terms of transformations in the 'ratio of senses' brought on by changes in the technology of communications" (Howes, 1991). McLuhan's scholarship extended the framework of sensory studies by examining as varying and variable the "ratios" of sensory organization through which different cultures perceived the world. However, as far-reaching as his research remains, its emphasis on technologies like writing and movable type as extensions of the senses also meant that near-exclusive attention to the visual and the aural remained intact.

While McLuhan's work offered concepts for sensory research that were also more nuanced than a "great divide" between the visual and aural on the one hand, and scent, taste, and touch on the other, his scholarship also functioned to keep this binary in place, and compelling to a range of sensory scholars for years. Furthermore, the dominance of the ocular was supported through the 1970s in the work of other theorists whose scholarship shaped thought across multiple fields. Alongside McLuhan's work we might also think, for instance, of the long shadow cast by Michel Foucault in his studies of surveillance and observation, particularly in works like *The Birth of the Clinic* (1966), *The Order of Things* (1970), and *Discipline and Punish* (1975).

In terms of the trajectory of sensory studies through the mid-point of the twentieth century, then, it was shaped first by a tight focus on which senses were most worthy of research, and next by a wrangling over theoretical approaches that would determine how sensory experience would be studied. And herein we arrive at a second reason for a relative "tastelessness" to the field up through the later decades of the twentieth century. As anthropologist David Howes summarizes, theoretical approaches that emphasized the study of "culture as text" remained at the forefront of scholarship, and necessarily imparted "both a visual and a verbal bias to any analysis" (Howes, 2003: 19). What this meant for scholarly investigations into sensory experiences, was that they ran the risk of fitting their subjects into textual analysis, or "reading" them, as any written or envisioned object might be read. The result of this is a theoretical framing that replicates visual and aural experiences while continuing to veer away from other forms of sensory experience. Considered as text, certainly culture could be engaged from multiple theoretical positions: One could "dialogue" with it, one could "interpret" it, or, one could "negotiate" with it. Even so, what all of these verbs demonstrate profoundly, is the continued entrenchment of the visual/aural bias.

By the 1980s this dynamic was set to shift, and the question of how to take the senses "on their own terms," how to treat them more fully sensually, has since come to the forefront of a wide-ranging sensory scholarship. One result of this is that research on the senses across disciplinary fields has become far more aware of taste and food; in other words, it has become more fully "tasteful" as scholars have begun to engage the sensual subject of food.

In considering how this came about, it is worth noting that, while a visual/aural privileging of analysis may have been dominant through the 1970s, these had never been the only theoretical frameworks for examining the senses. Sensory studies may be a newly identified field; nonetheless, its slender roots go deep. For instance, David Howes points to a thread of anthropological research which he refers to as the work of the early "sensualists," that goes back to the work of scholars like Margaret Mead and Rhoda Metraux in the 1930s (Howes, 2003). Scholars such as these, known (though not always necessarily celebrated by dominant trends in their field) as participant observers, took sensory experience on its own, varied, and individual terms. This was a crucial aspect of their research: "For sensualists (as they could be called) were committed to using all their senses," and at the same time, "they also set great store in achieving empathy, or sensing along with their informants" (Howes, 2003: 13). Further, scholarly interest in the senses beyond anthropology also has significant depth. There is no better example of this than sociologist Norbert Elias's *The Civilizing Process* (1939). Although it did not receive the scholarly attention it deserved until nearly three decades after it was first published, Elias's work was groundbreaking in its examination of "habitus," meaning the psychological frameworks or habits formed out of exposure to social structures. Interestingly, for the scholar wishing to study the link between food and the senses, Elias's work paid close attention to the formation of table manners in European history. More broadly, we might also think back, for instance, to early work on sensory subjects within the French Annales school of historians, and particularly the work of Lucien Febvre in *The Problem of Unbelief in the Sixteenth Century* (1942).

For so many scholars in the humanities and social sciences then, we might conceive of the 1980s and 1990s as a watershed moment in which major older theoretical positions were dismantled, and areas of research that emphasized the particular, the individual, the contingent, and even the intimate gained attention. The flowering of post-modern theory in so many academic circles meant the abandonment of a coolly detached pursuit of objective knowledge. If objective knowledge was dead, then the subjective experiences of groups and individuals was worth exploring. For anthropologists, this meant the formulation of an "anthropology of the senses," led by scholars such as Howes, Constance Classen, Paul Stoller, David Sutton, and Nadia Seremetakis. And as this area of research evolved, it merged with a sensory turn in other disciplines. This included, very significantly, history, and also sociology, literary studies, and philosophy. For scholars who wanted to study culture and power "from the bottom up," and analyze the intimate aspects of "everyday life," making room for a serious contemplation of the senses was the sensible thing to do. At the same time, for food studies as a whole, it could take advantage of this theoretically creative moment, and emerge as a self-conscious, formally acknowledged field of research.

Thus, the opportunity for realizing a synchronized study of food and the senses was realized. Within major works to treat sensory research on food, we can identify at least two major and consistent trends: Those that treat the taste of food as commodity, and those that treat the taste of food as aesthetic.

Among the first profound studies to examine specifically the role of food and the senses are those that understand taste as a driving force in transforming food into commodities, which then had the power to shape national economies, develop global markets, shift (often through force or coercion) labor pools from one place to another, and alter the ways in which whole classes of people self-identified (Smith, 2008: 151). Among the earliest of such works are Wolfgang Schivelbusch's *Tastes of Paradise: A Social History of Spices, Stimulants, and Intoxicants*, (1980, trans. English 1992), Sidney Mintz's *Sweetness and Power: The Place of Sugar in Modern History* (1986), and Warren Belasco's *Appetite for Change: How the Counter Culture Took on the Food Industry, 1966–1988* (1986). More recently, important works such as Andrew Dalby's *Dangerous Tastes: The History of Spices* (2000) and Marcy Norton's, *Sacred Gifts, Profane Pleasures: A History of Tobacco and Chocolate in the Atlantic World* (2010) have continued in this vein.

And just as food and the sense of taste matters on the broadest levels of human experience, scholarship has also demonstrated their place as actors on more intimate scales of interaction. Here, the growing body of scholarship on the sense of taste and the construction of social "Taste," continues to demonstrate the marked interdisciplinarity of sensory studies in general. Sociologist Stephen Mennell's *All Manners of Food: Eating and Taste in England and France from the Middle Ages to the Present* may have opened the floodgates on the aesthetic study of food (1985). However, this area of research has been carried on in the work of such diverse researchers as philosopher, Carolyn Korsmeyer in *Making Sense of Taste* (1999), historian Rebecca Spang with *The Invention of the Restaurant: Paris and Modern Gastronomic Culture* (2001), anthropologist David Sutton in *Remembrance of Repasts: An Anthropology of Food and Memory* (2001), historian Woodruff Smith in *Consumption and the Making of Respectability: 1600–1800* (2002), sociologist Priscilla Parkhust Ferguson in *Accounting for Taste: The Triumph of French Cuisine* (2004), and literary studies scholar, Denise Gigante with *Taste: a Literary History* (2005).

Happily, the above-mentioned texts hardly constitute an exhaustive list of important works on food and the senses. Instead, we might think of them as an entering wedge of research on issues of sensory perception as they concern our bodies and minds and the consumption of food. This interrelationship has recently been defined by political and cultural theorist Davide Panagia, who notes that the mouth is a "complex organ," and one that society often (and problematically) considers through a "normative partition: the mouth can not eat and speak at the same time." It is either "the conduit for the mind's ideas," or it "must be the avenue for the consumption of food, the origins of sustenance, and a gustatory medium of bodily restorations" (Panagia, 2009: 123). While this divide might have served the purposes of different arenas of scholarship, it does not do full justice to our experience of and thoughtful engagement with food. When sensory studies scholarship pays close attention to food, and when food studies scholarship returns to the senses, we come closer to bridging this gap, and considering human experience from a more fully complex position.

Research methodologies

Much like food interacts with all of the senses, so too does sensory studies, when focused on food, often interweave methods of scholarship from traditional disciplines to form rich interdisciplinary research. At the core, however, the base method of food and sensory studies is to keep the senses at the forefront of the investigation. Likewise, across disciplines, the central questions remain the same: How can we attempt to understand the place and meaning of the senses for an individual and for a culture, for it encompasses both physical action and experience that falls within and reflects cognitive knowledge? Sensations accompany an idea, become a form of communication, have meaning, and are embedded as part of a system of awareness (Panagia, 2009; Bourdieu, 1984; Ferguson, 2011). What then, is the location of food and taste within this constellation of making meaning through the senses? How does one's taste of food and one's taste for food shape – and reflect – people's world?

These broad considerations must be pondered on multiple levels: For an individual, as part of a distinct culture, and in a particular context. For example, how might one's unique relationship with food influence the sensorium? On a biological and physiological level, a shared experience is never quite the same and can differ from person to person – and thus the complete understanding, memory, and future expectation of a food or meal might also change. A "non-taster," whose perception of taste is limited, and a "super-taster," who perceives taste much more intensely, might have a different knowledge of the meal. Along these lines, a personal or cultural memory, closely linked to aroma neurologically, will affect the action, meaning, and attitude of eating or eating particular foods (Sutton, 2001; Wolfe, 2005). Even place matters, as eating a familiar food in an exotic setting (or vice versa), will change the sensorial experience (Long, 2003; Trubek, 2008).

Within a culture, having particular roles in society (for example: Hunters, farmers, chefs, mothers, doctors) whose specified tasks intersect with foodstuffs might alter one's sensorium. On a broader scale the difference between an agricultural, rural society and an urban, industrial society, divorced from much of the food chain, will have a different relationship to food and eating resulting in divergent realities. Regarding class distinctions, food is a necessity when populations are faced with scarcity; when overflowing from a cornucopia, it is a luxury (Bourdieu, 1984). With technology and broad-based consumerism, the growth of mass media and post-modern marketing, with the rampant exposure to "food porn," and "virtual food," the context of expectation, satisfaction, and thus eating experience has complicated (Haden, 2005; Korsmeyer, 1999). From these considerations, as well as countless others, a scholar can seek greater understanding and patterns of constructed knowledge including how and why knowledge of food, and the sensory awareness of it, shifts and evolves.

Ethnographic research, the descriptive branch of anthropology, gives perhaps the most complete entry into sensory studies of food. For although the researcher brings her/his own biases to the table, there is still the possibility to have access to multi-sensorial experiences surrounding food when at a site. To do so successfully, however, one should have a thorough context of the meaning of food in a particular culture by understanding how each food and all of the senses are embodied as well as how moralities are attached to them (Stoller, 1989; Mennell, 1996; Rasmussen, 1999; Spang, 2000; Pink, 2009). Prior to research, a self-reflexive analysis of one's own sensorial sensitivity will encourage awareness of prejudice of sensorial subjectivity, or biases, and will enable a scholar to experience a heightened understanding of the senses when conducting participant–observation fieldwork, in terms of both hierarchy and intensity (Pink, 2009).

Historians have borrowed heavily from the methodology of anthropologists when considering how to try to understand the senses in culture. This approach has led to the call for historians to follow anthropologists literally "into the field" (in terms of both the area of sensory studies, as well as becoming participant-observers). This, obviously, is problematic when studying the past, but some scholars suggest that a historian might overcome this time-travel hurdle by visiting museums and living history heritage centers that "bring the past alive" (Hoffer, 2003). The vast array of eras and places that can be visited at open air museums range significantly, but similarly suggest that visitors will "experience the authentic sights, sounds, smells and tastes from the past" (www.bclm.co.uk, Black Country Living Museum).

More radically, might scholars frame their lives to replicate those that they are studying, as many ethnographers do? During Lent, 2007 historian Ken Albala fasted while researching the Reformation in Wolfenbüttel, Germany. On his blog, he wrote of an internalized sense of control over what food he consumed, followed by the "swoon" of joy from his first bite of meat after abstinence. This realization led him to wonder if he better understood the Reformation intellectually because of this viseral experience (Albala, 2007). Albala, like a number of other scholars, has recreated historic meals, in an attempt to better understand food of the past and all of the tangible and intangible qualities of it (Albala, 2006; Bottero, 2006; Braund and Wilkins, 2000). As a method, however, trying to (re)experience or (re)live the past is controversial in that one's own experiences have changed the context from the past (Smith, 2007). The ephemeral nature of food (and one might argue of the context of the senses) prohibits reliability of authenticity or of a shared experience and understanding, yet it remains the burden of the scholar to try to understand.

Luckily, for those scholars who cannot experience a particular culture first hand, understanding might still be gleaned remotely (Métraux and Mead, 2001). Howes and Classen suggest that for sensory studies, a scholar look at a range of sources, including existing ethnographies, text-based literature, and visually based sources (art and film). From these, there is a four-step process: Extract all references to the sensorium; analyze data for each sense individually; consider the consociation among each modality, or sense, and how they help construct the meaning of experience; conclude with an organization of the senses for a culture (Howes, 1991). It becomes, then, an epistemological exercise by which to understand how culture internalizes the senses (Stoller, 1997).

Within the aforementioned process, or any analysis, the key becomes paying particular attention to references regarding the senses in the sources. Within a text-based narrative, closely considering the characteristic nature of gustatory passages serves to further the understanding of a person or culture and/through their food. The "thick description" that surrounds food and the senses becomes the informative medium and message for scholars to embrace (Camporesi, 1989, 1994). The narrative, then, frequently based on repetition and memory, becomes the collective norm, percolating as metaphor and metonymy throughout a culture (Sutton, 2001).

The same idea holds true when examining non-text-based sources, including oral histories, artwork, archaeological sites and evidence, photography, films, and material culture, which can not only reveal visual aspects of food and aesthetics, but a better understanding of all senses (Schama, 1987; Métraux, 1951; Pennell, 1998). But, as is the case whenever doing research, it is the task of the scholar to closely consider who has produced the source as well as their motivation for doing so.

Even with a range of cultural "goods" pointing us toward understanding sensibility, however, Braudel reminds us that when researching a "totality" a scholar should limit the locus by geography and time, paying particular attention to a culture's (or an individual's for that matter) frontiers, borrowings, and refusals (Braudel, 1980). These boundary lines offer awareness of a deeper understanding of an individual or a culture precisely because the actions involving food, the body, and knowledge are bound together. Food and the senses intimately embody aesthetic taste and regurgitate philosophies and desires, and one makes distinctions because eating and experiencing the sensorial is part of being alive (a necessity) but is also part of an intellectual pursuit (a luxury) (Bourdieu, 1984; Rozin and Siegal, 2003; Fleissner, 2008). Thus action, or the process of sensing, reveals ontology, knowledge, and greater understanding of the intellectual, reuniting the body and the mind. Pierre Bourdieu perhaps explains this cycle best: "[T]he philosophical sense of distinction is another form of the visceral disgust at vulgarity which defines pure taste as an internalized social relationship, a social relationship made flesh" (Bourdieu, 1984: 499–500). While Bourdieu is referring specifically to class relations, it serves to remind us that visceral disgust is both biologically and culturally formed and frequently surfaces when the "us" is faced with the "them" and food choice (Rozin et al., 2000).

Ultimately, food choice and the senses intersects the material and intellect, becomes the point of the cognitive and the aesthetic, inextricably tied to the sensorium. For medieval Norman-Anglo, for example, taste was thought to be transmitted through the tongue's pores, where it would be considered by the "judgement of the soul" (Woolgar, 2007), while it is the sensorial modes of the Japanese tea ceremony that provides "symbolic efficacy and power" in an attempt to reach transcendence (Kondo, 1985). As such, looking at food studies and sensorial studies can help to understand other cultural questions including, but not limited to, religion, philosophy, and ethics. Perhaps this will lead us to the most complete understanding of the individual and the cultural, the tangible and the intellectual, in an attempt to reach a "conception of truth."

Future research

The relatively nascent fields of food studies and sensory studies are ripe with possible areas to consider and investigate. Certainly, recent studies strive to give greater consideration of cultural relativity toward the senses, but Western scholarship historically has investigated the five senses with which we are familiar. This widely accepted truism, however, is more recently being contested as neither a static nor a universal understanding. Additional senses that have been argued that need attention include speech, hunger, thirst, pain, kinesthetic, and even, as scholars of medieval history have revealed, holiness, or, as Brillat-Savarin himself suggested, desire (Howes, 2007; Bynum 1987; Woolgar, 2007). The role of emotions needs also to be considered when researching the senses as influencing and reflecting personal experience. Certainly, scholars who look at food choice, nutrition, marketing, and consumer behavior find it integral, but rarely is it explored in tandem with food studies and the senses (Pink, 2009).

Scholars also need to ruminate on what one tastes when tasting. For much of Western history, the culture identified four "tastes": sweet, salty, sour, and bitter. Included with these, Aristotle incorporated the tastes of pungent and astringent, while current ideology (especially if one listens to marketing) embraces umami, long identified in Japanese culture, and even calcium. Cross culturally, the number of tastes that are categorized also varies. In Indonesia, the Weyéwa categorize sweet, sour, salty, bitter, pungent, and bland, while the Sereer Ndut of Senegal only recognize three (Kuipers, 1991).

Physiologically, taste is rarely experienced in isolation, but rather as an intimate joining with flavor. Food molecules, dissolved in saliva, are noted by taste receptors (found in the taste buds) and travel to the brain. Simultaneously, additional molecules are released both through our nose (orthonasal) and at the back of our mouths through the nasal cavity (retronasal). These aroma molecules stimulate the olfactory system and alert us to flavor (for example the difference between strawberry and cherry). The third sense that happens in the mouth is the somatosensory, which includes pain (for example, capsaicin) and pleasure, but also mouthfeel, which can often change with textures of food, but also components such as fat. When studying the senses, rarely do scholars consider all of these aspects, culturally, when in fact there is a diplomacy of the mouth. This becomes an extremely difficult task to consider as the general population are rarely cognizant of the nuances of these components. Thus, it remains an exciting frontier for scholars of the humanities and social sciences, to work across the hallway with hard scientists, to strengthen the understanding between biologically driven food sensation and experiences and those constructed via culture (Korsmeyer, 1999; Rozin, 1999; Peynaud, 2005; Wolfe, 2005).

Finally, to take up the mantle suggested by David Howes, it remains somewhat ironic that sensorial studies (along with food) is often presented through one sense, the visual. In this way, scholars perpetuate the continuation of the dominance of the visual and of written communication devoid of the other senses. How, instead, might we change this? Certainly, within the halls of academia, more scholars incorporate experiential teaching and learning in the classroom, but as a group this also needs to be considered on a larger scale of dissemination. We don't have the answer to this, but we sense future scholars might (Howes, 2007).

Getting started

For one wishing to embark on the sensory study of food, the range of options is expanding as the field matures. The sensory analysis of food is one that can be undertaken throughout the humanities and social sciences, particularly in anthropology, sociology, and history departments. However, a more compelling approach to the scholar interested in the sensorial approach to food might consider interdisciplinary programs in food studies, cultural studies, and American studies.

While not specifically focused on food and the senses, there are a number of research institutes, doing compelling work on sensorial studies that include "The Sense Lab" at Concordia University, New York Institute of Philosophy, and Sensory Stories at the University of York. A comprehensive list of programs is listed at the website www.senorialstudies.org, which also has additional resources including a research directory, events, syllabi and curricula, and information on the excellent journal, *The Senses and Society*, which was founded in 2006.

Key reading

Howes, David ed. (2005) *The Empire of the Senses: The Sensual Culture Reader*. New York: Berg.
——(2007) *Sensual Relations: Engaging the Senses in Culture and Social Theory*. Ann Arbor, MI: University of Michigan Press.
Jütte Robert (2005) *A History of the Senses: From Antiquity to Cyberspace*. Malden, MA: Polity Press.
Korsmeyer Carolyn, ed. (2005) *The Taste Culture Reader: Experiencing Food and Drink*. New York: Berg.
——(1999) *Making Sense of Taste: Food and Philosophy*. Ithaca, NY: Cornell University Press.
Mintz Sydney (1985) *Sweetness and Power: The Place of Sugar in Modern History*. New York: Viking Adult.

Rozin, Paul Jonathan, Haidt and McCauley, R. Clark (2000) "Disgust." In *Handbook of Emotions*, 2nd Edition. M. Lewis, ed. New York: The Guildford Press.

Mark M. Smith (2007) *Sensing the Past: Seeing, Hearing, Smelling, Tasting, and Touching in History*. Berkeley: University of California Press.

Paul Stoller (1989) *A Taste of Ethnographic Things: The Senses in Anthropology*. Philadelphia: University of Pennsylvania Press.

David Sutton (2001) *Remembrance of Repasts: An Anthropology of Food and Memory*. New York: Berg.

Jeremy M. Wolfe, Kluender, Keith R., and Levi, Dennis M. (2005) *Sensations & Perception*. Sunderland, MA: Sinauer Associates, Inc.

Bibliography

Ken Albala (2006) *Cooking in Europe, 1250–1650* (The Greenwood Press Daily Life Through History Series). Westport, CT: Greenwood.

——(2007) *Ken Albala's Food Rant: Fasting in Schlarrafenland*. kenalbala.blogspot.com/2007/06/fasting-in-schlarrafenland.html (accessed on April 10, 2012).

Mikhail Bakhtin (1989) *Rabelais and His World*. Bloomington: Indiana University Press.

Linda Bartoshuk (1997) *Tasting and Smelling*. Waltham, MA: Academic Press.

Warren J. Belasco (2006) *Appetite for Change: How the Counterculture Took on the Food Industry*, 2nd ed. Ithaca, NY: Cornell University Press.

Jean Bottero (2006) *The Oldest Cuisine in the World: Cooking in Mesopotamia*. Chicago, IL: University of Chicago Press.

Pierre Bourdieu (1984) *Distinction: A Social Critique of the Judgement of Taste*. Cambridge, MA: Harvard University Press.

Fernand Braudel (1980) *On History*. London: Weidenfeld and Nicolson.

David Braund and John Wilkins (2000) *Athenaeus and his World: Reading Greek Culture in the Roman Empire*. Exeter: University of Exeter Press.

Jean Anthelme Brillat-Savarin and M. F. K. Fisher (2009) *The Physiology of Taste: or Meditations on Transcendental Gastronomy*. New York: Random House Digital, Inc.

Caroline Walker Bynum (1987) *Holy Feast and Holy Fast: The Religious Significance of Food to Medieval Women*. Berkeley: University of California Press.

Piero Camporesi, (1989) *Bread of Dreams: Food and Fantasy in Early Modern Europe*. Chicago, IL: University of Chicago Press.

——(1994) *Exotic Brew: The Art of Living in the Age of Enlightenment*. Cambridge: Polity.

Constance Classen, (1997) "Foundations for an anthropology of the senses," *International Social Science Journal* 49, 153 (September 1): 401–12.

Francis J. Coleman, (1965) "Can a Smell or a Taste or a Touch Be Beautiful?," *American Philosophical Quarterly* 2, 4 (October 1): 319–24.

Alexander Cowan and Jill Steward (2007) *The City and the Senses: Urban Culture Since 1500*. Farnham: Ashgate Publishing, Ltd.

Patricia Curran (1989) *Grace before Meals: Food Ritual and Body Discipline in Convent Culture*. Chicago, IL: University of Illinois Press.

Andrew Dalby (2000) *Dangerous Tastes: The Story of Spices*. Berkeley: University of California Press.

Charles Dickens (1989) *Annotated Christmas Carol, Deluxe*. New York: Random House Value Publishing.

Norbert Elias (2000) *The Civilizing Process: Sociogenetic and Psychogenetic Investigations*. Oxford: Wiley-Blackwell.

Lucien Febvre and Beatrice Gottlieb (1985) *The Problem of Unbelief in the Sixteenth Century, the Religion of Rabelais*. Cambridge, MA: Harvard University Press.

Priscilla Parkhurst Ferguson (2004) *Accounting for Taste: The Triumph of French Cuisine.*. Chicago, IL: University of Chicago Press.

——(2011) "The Senses of Taste," *The American Historical Review* 16: 371–84.

Jennifer L. Fleissner (2008) "Henry James's Art of Eating," *ELH* 75, 1: 27–62.

Michel Foucault (1975) *The Birth of the Clinic: An Archaeology of Medical Perception*. New York: Vintage Books.

——(1970) *The Order of Things: An Archaeology of the Human Sciences*. New York: Vintage Books.

——(1977) *Discipline & Punish*. New York: Random House Digital, Inc.

Denise Gigante (2005) *Taste: A Literary History*. New Haven, CT: Yale University Press.

Jack Goody (2010) *Food and Love: A Cultural History of East and West*. London: Verso.

Jukka Gronow (1997) *The Sociology of Taste*. London: Taylor & Francis.

Roger Haden (2005) "Taste in an Age of Convenience: From Frozen Food to Meals in 'the Matrix'," in *The Taste Culture Reader: Experiencing Food and Drink*. Oxford: Berg.

Peter Charles Hoffer (2003) *Sensory Worlds in Early America*. Baltimore, MD: The Johns Hopkins University Press.

David Howes (1991a) *The Varieties of Sensory Experience: a Sourcebook in the Anthropology of the Senses*. Toronto: University of Toronto Press.

——(1991b) "Sensorial Anthropology," in *The Varieties of Sensory Experience: A Sourcebook in the Anthropology of the Senses* Toronto: University of Toronto Press.

——2003) *Sensual Relations: Engaging the Senses in Culture and Social Theory*. Anne Arbor, MI: University of Michigan Press.

——(2005) "Hyperesthesia, or The Sensual Logic of Late Capitalism." *Empire of the Senses: the Sensual Culture Reader*. Oxford: Berg.

David Hume (1952) *An Enquiry Concerning Human Understanding*. Charleston, SC: Forgotten Books.

Robert Jütte (2004) *A History of the Senses: From Antiquity to Cyberspace*. Cambridge: Polity.

Dorinne Kondo, (1985) "The Way of Tea: A Symbolic Analysis," *Man* 20, 2, New Series (June 1): 287–306.

Carolyn Korsmeyer (1999) *Making Sense of Taste: Food and Philosophy*. Ithaca, NY: Cornell University Press.

Carolyn Korsmeyer and David Sutton, "The Sensory Experience of Food," *Food, Culture & Society* Vol. 14, No. 4 (Dec. 2001): 461–75.

Joel C. Kuipers (1991) "Matters of Taste in Weyéwa," in *The Varieties of Sensory Experience: a Sourcebook in the Anthropology of the Senses*. David Howes, ed. Toronto: University of Toronto Press.

Lucy Long (2003) *Culinary Tourism*. Lexington: University Press of Kentucky.

Karl Marx (2011) *Economic and Philosophic Manuscripts of 1844*. Eastford, CT: Martino Publishing.

Marshall McLuhan (1962) *The Gutenberg Galaxy: The Making of Typographic Man*. Toronto: University of Toronto Press.

——(1964) *Understanding Media: The Extensions of Man*. Cambridge, MA: MIT Press.

Stephen Mennell (1996) *All Manners of Food: Eating and Taste in England and France from the Middle Ages to the Present*. Chicago: University of Illinois Press.

Rhoda Métraux and Margaret Mead (2001) *Themes in French Culture: A Preface to a Study of French Community*. Oxford: Berghahn Books.

Sidney W. Mintz (1985) *Sweetness and Power: The Place of Sugar in Modern History*, New York: Viking Adult.

Marcy Norton (2008) *Sacred Gifts, Profane Pleasures: A History of Tobacco and Chocolate in the Atlantic World*. Ithaca, NY: Cornell University Press.

Davide Panagia (2009) *The Political Life of Sensation*. Durham, NC: Duke University Press Books.

Carolyn de la Peña (2010) *Empty Pleasures: The Story of Artificial Sweeteners from Saccharin to Splenda*. Chapel Hill: The University of North Carolina Press.

Sara Pennell, "'Pots and Pans History': The Material Culture of the Kitchen in Early Modern England," *Journal of Design History* Vol. 11, No. 3 (January 1, 1998): 201–16.

Émile Peynaud (2005) "Tasting Problems and Errors of Perception," in *The Taste Culture Reader: Experiencing Food and Drink*. Carolyn Korsmeyer, ed. Oxford: Berg.

Sarah Pink (2009) *Doing Sensory Ethnography*. Thousand Oaks, CA: Sage.

Susan Rasmussen, (1999) "Making Better 'Scents' in Anthropology: Aroma in Tuareg Sociocultural Systems and the Shaping of Ethnography," *Anthropological Quarterly* 72, 2 (April 1): 55–73.

Antonius C. G. M. Robben and Jeffrey A. Sluka (2007) *Ethnographic Fieldwork: An Anthropological Reader*. Hoboken, NJ: Wiley-Blackwell.

Paul Rozin and Michael Siegal "Vegemite as a Marker of National Identity," *Gastronomica: The Journal of Food and Culture* Vol. 3, No. 4 (November 1, 2003): 63–67.

Paul Rozin, Jonathan Haidt, and Clark McCauley (2000) "Disgust," in *Handbook of Emotions*, 2nd edn, Michael Lewis, ed. New York: The Guilford Press.

Simon Schama (1987) *The Embarrassment of Riches: An Interpretation of Dutch Culture in the Golden Age*. New York: Knopf.

Lawrence R. Schehr and Allen S. Weiss (2001) *French Food: On the Table, On the Page, and in French Culture*. London: Routledge.

Wolfgang Schivelbusch (1993) *Tastes of Paradise: A Social History of Spices, Stimulants, and Intoxicants*. New York: Vintage Books.

Nadia Seremetakis (1994) *The Senses Still: Perception and Memory as Material Culture in Modernity*. Boulder, CO: Westview Press.

Georg Simmel (1998) *Simmel on Culture: Selected Writings*, Thousand Oaks, CA: Sage Publications Ltd.

Mark M. Smith (2007) "Producing Sense, Consuming Sense, Making Sense: Perils and Prospects for Sensory History," *Journal of Social History* 40, 4: 841–58.

——(2008) *Sensing the Past: Seeing, Hearing, Smelling, Tasting, and Touching in History*. Berkeley: University of California Press.

Woodruff Smith (2002) *Consumption and the Making of Respectability, 1600–1800*. London: Routledge.

Rebecca L. Spang (2000) *The Invention of the Restaurant: Paris and Modern Gastronomic Culture*. Cambridge, MA: Harvard University Press.

Stephane Spoiden (2001) "The Betrayal of Moules-frites: This is (Not) Belgium," in *French Food: On the Table, On the Page, and in French Culture*, Lawrence. R. Scherr and Allen S. Weiss, eds., pp. 157–69. Oxford: Routledge.

Paul Stoller (1989) *Taste of Ethnographic Things: The Senses in Anthropology*, illustrated edition Philadelphia, University of Pennsylvania Press.

——(1997) *Sensuous Scholarship*. Philadelphia: University of Pennsylvania Press.

David E. Sutton (2001) *Remembrance of Repasts: An Anthropology of Food and Memory*. Oxford: Berg.

Susan J. Terrio (2000) *Crafting the Culture and History of French Chocolate*. Berkeley: University of California Press.

Laurel Thatcher Ulrich (1990) *A Midwife's Tale: The Life of Martha Ballard, Based on Her Diary, 1785–1812.*, New York: Knopf.

Maguelonne Toussaint-Samat (2008) *A History of Food*. Oxford: Wiley-Blackwell.

Amy B. Trubek (2008) *The Taste of Place: A Cultural Journey into Terroir*. Berkeley: University of California Press.

Jeremy M. Wolfe *et al.* (2008) *Sensation and Perception*. Sunderland, MA: Sinauer Associates Inc.

C. M. Woolgar (2007) *The Senses in Late Medieval England*. New Haven, CT: Yale University Press.

33

Anticipating a new agricultural research agenda for the twenty-first century[1]

Frederick L. Kirschenmann

The food system we have created during the past half century is designed to achieve a singular goal: Maximum efficient production for short-term economic return. To achieve that goal we have created farming systems that feature specialization, management simplification and economies of scale. Furthermore, our public policies for agriculture have been designed to further that singular goal. But there is nothing in that goal, or the policies created to support it, that is designed to achieve sustainability—a resilient food and agriculture system. It is now imperative that we explore alternative food and agriculture systems, and foster public policies and research agendas, that produce resilient food systems that can maintain productivity in the face of future challenges—the end of cheap energy, depleting minerals, fresh water, and biodiversity, and more unstable climates.

> The real problem of food production occurs within a complex, mutually influential relationship of soil, plants, animals, and people. A real solution to that problem will therefore be ecologically, agriculturally, and culturally healthful … a bad solution solves for a single purpose or goal, such as increased production. And it is typical of such solutions that they achieve stupendous increases in production at exorbitant biological and social costs.
>
> (Wendell Berry)

The challenges facing agriculture at the turn of the century clearly will play a role in shaping our food and agriculture future. Population growth, persistent poverty, the end of cheap energy, food security, erosion of ecological capital and unstable climates, will all be integral parts of the challenges facing our agricultural and food system and therefore the agriculture research agenda for most of this century.

The question we face as we develop a research agenda to meet these challenges is *not* whether we will use technology to shape the new future. Clearly we will. Nor is the pertinent question what *kind* of technology we will use. We likely will use all of the available technologies that hold any promise for developing an agriculture capable of meeting these challenges. The more important question is *how* we will use the technologies available to us.

Through most of the industrial era we have tended to use technologies almost exclusively to perform one-dimensional, single-tactic functions. We developed and applied pesticides to control a target pest. We manufactured and applied fertilizers to replace soil nutrients. We produced and injected antibiotics to fight disease. It is a methodology that Joe Lewis, pest

364

management specialist with the USDA's Agricultural Research Service, calls "therapeutic intervention."[2] This approach uses technology to intervene in a system to solve a specific problem. Based on field experience Lewis argues that this approach has failed. He suggests that we now need to use technology to better understand how systems function and to redesign systems to reduce the sources of the problem.

The single-tactic approach can, however, certainly lay claim to many successes. We dramatically reduced the labor required to produce essential crops. We increased the yields of those crops beyond anyone's expectations. And we made it possible for citizens of the United States to spend less of their disposable income on food than any other nation in the world—only 10 percent in 2001 according to USDA/ERS estimates.[3] Although what we pay *per calorie of food* consumed is more than what 95 percent of the rest of humanity pays.

Ecological failure

This one-dimensional approach, despite its successes, has, however, led to unanticipated consequences. Manufacturing and applying nutrients to overcome nutrient deficiencies allowed us to ignore the larger issues of deteriorating soil health and soil erosion. Healthy soil, in turn, can provide a range of benefits to healthy, resilient production systems while making major contributions to water quality.[4] Soil erosion not only seriously depletes our ecological capital but, together with excess nutrient application and highly specialized production systems, fosters nutrient pollution in rivers and streams that eventually contributes to the hypoxic zones in major bodies of water, such as the Gulf of Mexico. Poor-quality soils also require increased irrigation, which depletes aquifers, rivers, and lakes, and adds to soil salinity. Land degradation has reached epic proportions. By some estimates, 36 percent of the world's cropland is "losing topsoil at a rate that is undermining its productivity."[5] This does not bode well for meeting the twin challenges of feeding a growing population while reversing environmental degradation.

Similarly, use of a broad-spectrum pesticide to control a target pest (another single-tactic approach) failed to acknowledge the ecological connections within the system in which the pesticide is applied. The results, once again, yielded unintended side effects. The pesticide not only kills the target pest, it also harms many beneficial organisms that previously kept other pests in check, creating new pest problems. Since a pesticide never kills all the target pests, those that survive become resistant to the pesticide and create a new population of hardier pests. In the process, the biological evenness of a system is undermined, encouraging pest resurgence. Meanwhile, the correlations among soil quality, nutrition, and plant protection remain largely unexplored, and agriculturalists too often resist exploring the potential human and wildlife health effects of the pesticides being used.

A further complication arises from the fact that the one-dimensional agriculture of the past century achieved its success because of two resources that had been readily available: (1) ample natural resources (especially cheap fossil fuels and mined minerals, such as rock phosphate) to supply the inputs, and (2) adequate sinks in nature to absorb the wastes. Today both of these resources are increasingly in short supply. Some agriculturalists argue that this altered situation will be enough to force the agriculture of the future to change from a one-dimensional input-dependent system to a more complex, symbiotic ecologically driven system.

> The present system of agriculture, which depends on consumption of tremendous quantities of fossil fuel energy, is now being forced to change to a system where the interactions between organisms and the environment are properly used. There are two reasons for this transformation. The first is the depletion of readily available fossil fuel resources. The

second is that consumption of fossil fuels has induced deterioration of the environment ... Is it possible to replace current technologies based on fossil energy with proper interactions operating between crops/livestock and other organisms to enhance agricultural production? If the answer is yes, then modern agriculture, which uses only the simplest biotic responses, can be transformed into an alternative system of agriculture, in which the use of complex biotic interactions becomes the key technology.[6]

Lester Brown argues that even if we could stretch available fossil fuel resources several decades into the future, the need to develop "clean, climate-benign fuels" will drive a global transition to alternative systems.[7] In other words, the depletion of fossil fuels and the need to reduce environmental degradation are tightly coupled.

Despite these signals for the need for change the culture of one-dimensional, input-dependent functions continues to pervade most of the agricultural sciences. The new generation of technologies being introduced into agricultural research follows the same paradigm as the chemical technologies of the past half century. Most applications of transgenic technologies, for example, are still intended as single-tactic approaches to problems – designing corn plants to resist the corn borer; designing soybean plants to resist a broad spectrum herbicide to control weeds; designing pharmaceutical crops to produce specific properties as therapeutic intervention in disease. Lewis argues that since the new technologies follow a similar blueprint as yesterday's chemical technologies, they are likely to meet with similar constraints. And in the process, he argues, they will hamper our progress toward developing more ecologically sound strategies.

> As spectacular and exciting as biotechnology is, its breakthroughs have tended to delay our shift to long-term, ecologically based pest management because the rapid array of new products provide a sense of security just as did synthetic pesticides at the time of their discovery in the 1940s ... the crops engineered to express toxins of pathogens are simply targeted as replacements for synthetic pesticides and will become ineffective in the same way that pesticides have.[8]

Lewis's observation is now being corroborated, not only by the appearance of pest resistance to transgenic technologies in the field, but also by a growing awareness among scientists that genetic mechanisms are much more complex than biological determinists had previously assumed. Richard Strohman, molecular biologist at the University of California, described the matter succinctly.

> Molecular biologists have rediscovered the profound complexity of the genotype–phenotype relationship, but are unable to explain it: Something is missing. The missing element was described 35 years ago by Michael Polanyi, who characterized live mechanisms and information in DNA as "boundary conditions with a sequence of boundaries above them."[9]

Harold Morowitz, professor of Biology and Natural Philosophy at George Mason University, also acknowledges this complexity and the paradigm shift it portends.

> [There] is a startling change in the paradigm of genetics following from the dogma of molecular biology. It suggests bionic laws at the level of phenotype and a somewhat noisier background of genes that are required to reify these laws in a not overly precise way. It tends to turn the present paradigm rather on its head ... All of this suggests the possibility

of a substantive change in the paradigm of biology and a reconsideration of how we are spending our research funds.[10]

These scientific findings will, as Evelyn Fox Keller has observed, "necessitate the introduction of … other ways of thinking about biological organization, thereby loosening the grip that genes have had on the imagination of life sciences these many decades." She also suggests that this "success" will finally teach us the necessary "humility" that will lead us to appreciate, and perhaps honor, the complexity and interdependence of the living systems of which we are a part.[11] In other words, we might begin to take ecology seriously in all of our human endeavors, and these new discoveries in the functions of biology and ecology may impose a significant paradigm shift on agricultural research. It would seem prudent, therefore, on countless ecological fronts, to begin the shift from a one-dimensional, single-tactic strategy to a systems–restructuring strategy as the guiding principle of our agricultural research agenda. This shift would lead to the development of systems that focus on "harnessing inherent strengths within ecosystems" rather than continuing to invent single-tactic, therapeutic intervention solutions.[12]

Socio-economic adversity

Biological and ecological constraints are not the only reasons we need to explore alternatives for the future of agriculture. In addition to the *ecological* failures, one-dimensional approaches to agriculture also have failed to provide *economic* sustainability—at least for farmers.

Perhaps it goes without saying that an agricultural system must be economically viable in order to be sustainable. But there is an assumption, deeply rooted in current economic philosophy, which contends that economic viability is largely limited to economic *efficiency*. Amartya Sen, Nobel Prize-winning economist, calls this the "engineering-based" approach to economics. It is an approach that concerns itself only with the "logistic and engineering problems within economics" instead of the economic wealth and well-being of society. While the engineering-based approach "predicts" that such societal well-being will automatically be served, that assumption, according to Sen, rests more on theory than on empirical verification.[13]

Classical economists such as Adam Smith insisted that economic *freedom* and economic *power* were as important to a healthy economy as economic *efficiency*. As our food and agriculture systems become increasingly consolidated, there is little freedom to move in and out of most segments of the agricultural economy. Currently, economic power in our food and agriculture enterprises is so heavily concentrated that neither free market competition nor efficiency is evident. Such concentration ultimately fails to serve the best interests of either producers or consumers. Farmers increasingly must sell bulk commodities at prices below their cost of production, and the potential benefits of market efficiencies are no longer passed on to consumers. This scenario hardly lends itself to an agricultural future that is economically viable or sustainable.

Our current economic philosophy also has made it difficult for us to address the third component of the sustainability formula—social responsiveness. Our laissez-faire economic ideology regards any interference in the free market to achieve social goals as "social engineering" and therefore suspect. But it has long been recognized that it is impossible to achieve either the economic or environmental goals of agriculture in any community without the "proper functioning of those social institutions which are essential to satisfactory farm life."[14] To insure a durable, economically healthy culture, civil society and the state must be equal partners with free markets. As Aldo Leopold reminded us, the "economic parts of the biotic clock" will not function well without the "uneconomic parts."[15]

The economic, ecological, and community components of agricultural sustainability are therefore interdependent. If we focus only on the economic viability of the farm while ignoring the ecology, soil quality soon will become degraded, requiring larger infusions of fertilizer and thereby affecting the economic viability of the farm. Likewise, if we ignore the welfare of the community in which the farm exists, the public services the community provides that support the farm's economy—such as public roads, quality education, and local research—begin to deteriorate and eventually affect the economic viability of the farm. Similarly, if we only attend to the ecology and the community and ignore the farm's economic viability, then the deteriorating economy of the farm will make it impossible for the farmer to be active in supporting the community or to properly care for the ecology. These three components are simply inextricably linked, and one cannot imagine a sustainable agriculture without acknowledging their interdependence.

The fact that one-dimensional approaches to agricultural productivity have failed to allow farmers to become economically sustainable is now evident. Richard Levins, Department of Applied Economics at the University of Minnesota, and Michael Duffy, Extension Economist at Iowa State University, demonstrated this with unusual clarity some time ago. Levins pointed out that "the one consistent part" of the farm economy story of the past 40 years is that "farmers, as a group, have been left out of the enormous growth in the value of what they sell."[16] Levins pointed out that while gross farm income grew dramatically since 1960, net farm income remained essentially flat. Average national gross farm income rose from less than $50,000 to $250,000 while average net income remained below $50,000.

Duffy demonstrated similar findings regarding Iowa farmers. His research demonstrated that while Iowa farmers had succeeded in increasing their gross income dramatically between 1950 and 2001 (albeit with the help of government subsidies), their net income remained essentially flat through most of that period. Nearly all of the farmers' yearly gross income was used for the expenses required to produce the income!

This, of course, puts Iowa's farmers under constant pressure to add more units (animals and/ or acres) to their farms each year to generate more gross income just to pay the bills. In the process, Iowa's net farm income as a percentage of total expenses dropped from more than 80 percent in 1950 to 13 percent in 2001.

Under such dire economic conditions, farmers cannot reasonably be expected to contribute to the ecological and community services necessary to a healthy, sustainable future.

How can we make agriculture more sustainable?

If the previous observations are valid, we cannot reduce our goal of making agriculture more sustainable to some kind of universal prescription using one-dimensional tactics for changing our farming practices—switching from chemical to biological inputs, for example. Nor can we condense it to a simple formula for increasing the yields of a few commodities to "feed the world." What we *can* do, and perhaps *must* do, is to redesign our food and agriculture system so that its functions are more consistent with our best understanding of how the biotic community, in which the farm exists, works. We can seek to provide adequate amounts of food by nurturing the potential for increased productivity inherent in redesigned multi-species systems. It seems imperative to pursue at least three objectives to that end.

First, we should begin to *refocus* our public research agenda. We should focus on research that helps us better understand the synergies and synchronies of the diverse species in each agricultural watershed, and determine how they can be employed to increase our agricultural productivity while simultaneously reducing farmers' costs, and enhancing the capacity of the land to renew itself. This would mean, among other things, that we would begin using ecological screens to determine what technologies to employ and how to use them to achieve these larger objectives.

Second, we should begin to *expand* our research agendas to include new market designs. We can map out new food marketing relationships that would enable farmers to produce more value on their farms and *retain a larger share of that value on their farms and in local economies*. There can be no sustainable future for farmers when they produce only undifferentiated raw materials as cheaply as possible, with all of the value of that production accruing to distant shareholders. The federal Sustainable Agriculture Research and Education (SARE) program might well be expanded to include such total food systems research.

Third, we should *explore policy options* at both federal and local levels that give these new production and marketing systems a competitive advantage so that farmers can begin to transition to them. If a healthy economy, ecology and community must be achieved in concert, then our public policies must be redesigned to embrace that larger, integrated goal. In the face of declining fossil fuel resources, resources that have been used to mask ecological deterioration, ecological restoration must be a centerpiece of the new policies. Such policies should be geared to encourage micro enterprises and local solutions rather than consolidation and regulation. The new policies must also be designed to attract a new generation of farmers to the land. Sound ecological management can be achieved only by farmers living in local ecologies long enough and intimately enough to learn how to manage them well. This means we need *more* farmers, not fewer.

This broadening of the research agenda is consistent with recommendations in an earlier National Academy of Sciences (NAS) report, *Frontiers in Agricultural Research: Food, Health, Environment and Communities*. The report recommended that the USDA refocus its two billion-dollar annual research budget, shifting its emphasis from increased food and fiber production to environmentally sound farming alternatives, quality of life in rural communities, diet and health, food safety, and the impact of globalization on US farming.

The NAS report writers were well aware that these new demands on agricultural researchers would tax the ability of the land grant system in many dimensions. In a coda to the report, they warned: "To meet new demands, established processes and partnerships in agricultural research must evolve without losing their unique value. Those tensions in the research agenda can be managed only through sustained vision, leadership, and political will."

It may well be that Wendell Berry had it right all along. In an essay on "Solving for Pattern," published in 1980, he suggested:

> A good solution acts within the larger pattern the way a healthy organ acts with the body. But it must at once be understood that a healthy organ does not – as the mechanistic or industrial mind would like to say – "give" health to the body, is not exploited for the body's health, but is *a part* of its health. The health of organ and organism is the same, just as the health of organism and ecosystem is the same.[17]

Or as Morowitz put it, in more scientific, but less poetic language: "The primary metabolic chart of every species maps onto the universal metabolic chart ... The metabolic chart is part of the phenotype of every organism. The phenotype ... has a robustness in spite of the constant buzz of noise in the underlying genomes."[18]

Notes

1 An earlier version of this paper was presented at the Iowa State University Department of Agronomy Baker Council annual meeting, March 25, 2003. Portions of this paper were presented earlier at the

Tri-Societies plenary meeting in Charlotte, NC, October 22, 2001. Other parts were published previously in *Renewable Resources Journal*, "Why American Agriculture is Not Sustainable." Autumn, 2002.

2 W. J. Lewis, J. C. van Lenteren, S. C. Phatak, and J. H. Tumlinson, III (1997) "A Total System Approach to Sustainable Pest Management." *Proceedings of the National Academy of Sciences* 94: 12243–8.

3 One should be cautious about translating the percentage of disposable income spent on food into a "cheap food" claim, however. What Americans pay per calorie of food consumed is more than what 95 percent of the rest of humanity pays according to some estimates. See Charles Benbrook, "Principles Governing the Long-Run Risks, Benefits, and Costs of Agricultural Biotechnology." Unpublished manuscript, available from the author.

4 National Research Council (1993) *Soil and Water Quality: An Agenda for Agriculture*. Washington, DC: National Academy Press.

5 L. R. Brown (2001) *Eco-Economy: Building an Economy for the Earth*. New York: W. W. Norton & Company, 63.

6 M. Shiyomi and H. Koizumi, eds. (2001) *Structure and Function in Agroecosystem Design and Management*. New York: CRC Press.

7 Brown, *Eco-Economy*, 98.

8 Lewis *et al.*, "A Total System Approach."

9 R. Strohman (2002) "Maneuvering in the Complex Path from Genotype to Phenotype." *Science* 296, 26 April 701–3.

10 H. Morowitz (2003) "Phenetics, A Born Again Science." *Complexity* 8, 1, 12–13.

11 E. F. Keller (2001) *The Century of the Gene*. Cambridge, MA: Harvard University Press, 7, 147.

12 Lewis *et al.*, "A Total System Approach."

13 A. Sen (1989) *On Ethics and Economics*. Oxford: Blackwell.

14 H. C. Hanson (1939) "Ecology in Agriculture." *Ecology*, 20, 2, April: 111–17.

15 A. Leopold (1949) *A Sand County Almanac*. New York: Oxford University Press.

16 R. A. Levins (2001) "An Essay on Farm Income." Staff Paper Series, Department of Applied Economics, College of Agricultural, Food, and Environmental Sciences. University of Minnesota. April.

17 W. Berry (1983) *The Gift of Good Land*. San Francisco, CA: North Point Press.

18 Morowitz, "Phenetics."

34

Food and ethics

Julia Abramson

Addressing goodness, right action, and moral responsibility, ethics considered with food is universal in its applications. Since all people eat, issues of food and ethics should interest everyone, whether consumers, producers, or both. Food is, moreover, natural in origin, as well as cultural, and it is indispensable to life. Just as food mirrors our relationships to community and society, it similarly reflects our interactions with nature. In our technological, industrial, and interconnected global society, food and ethics addresses humans and human cultures, but also other forms of life and the environment, and the future as well as the present.

Overview

Issues of food and ethics are universal in their interest and applications. Since all people eat, food and ethics should interest all people, whether as consumers or producers or both. Food is, moreover, natural in origin, as well as cultural, and it is indispensable to life. Just as food mirrors our relationships to community and society, it also reflects our interactions with nature. Correspondingly, food and ethics addresses humans and human cultures, but also other forms of life and the environment. Contemporary research in food and ethics shares concerns with related applied ethical fields, including environmental ethics, agricultural ethics, bioethics, medical ethics, business ethics, corporate ethics, and ethics and economics, as well as with the scientific, social, and cultural questions such as those of ecology and with social movements and activism such as for food justice.

Historical background and major theoretical approaches

An anthropocentric, local, and presentist purview long shaped most ethics of food. Western ethics, or moral science, addresses goodness and right action, with implications for moral responsibility. To what ends should we apply ourselves? What moral principles should govern our choices and pursuits (Deigh, 1999)? In Aristotelian terms, ethics theorizes about the good life, but also conceptualizes practical steps for its realization. For most of human history, subsistence diets meant that the primary concern was simply to acquire sufficient food to sustain life, while social groups were relatively atomized. Agricultural systems, and associated forms of provisioning such as hunting, were diverse and adapted to local conditions. Ancient Greek dietetics, which emphasized temperance, morality, and rationality, and which focused on consumption by the individual, exemplifies the approach. Foods themselves are neutral from a moral perspective, as Zwart (2001) observes, while their use by the individual carries moral valence, as judged by the effect of the foods on the constitution, health, and behavior of the individual. By contrast, Hebraic testamentary laws transferred morality to foods themselves, whether clean or unclean, allowed or forbidden. Here, expression of the social values begins with the foods themselves. In both examples, however, it is the immediate human experience, understood as unique, that informs value. To be sure, some early moral philosophies began to widen the sphere of food ethics, notably to consider the animal experience. Forms of vegetarianism, understood as a positive choice to subsist on a vegetable diet while deliberately avoiding animal flesh or all animal foods, constitute a long history not only of religious, medical, scientific, and economic thought pertaining to diet, but also of moral considerations (Walters and Portmess, 1999; Stuart, 2007; Preece, 2009; Puskar-Pasewicz, 2010). Yet historical vegetarian philosophies have inconsistently invested the animal experience with dignity and importance or questioned the dominant position assigned to the human. Rather, they have been as likely ultimately to formalize human concerns, such as for personal health and moral purity.

Material, political, and economic changes traceable to the early modern era frame modern debates about food and ethics. In the West, in the account of Thompson (1998), as rural, feudal, and agricultural societies transformed to become predominantly urban, commercial, and industrial, the explicitation of relationships in contracts emphasized the universal aspects of human existence and reimagined human dependencies in terms of legal obligations rather than personal loyalty. At the same time, the decline of manorial society in favor of manufacturing and trade changed the relationship of people to the land required for agriculture, thus to food. Rewards diminished for attachment to and cultivation of a particular place and plot. Instead, the new paradigm privileged mobility, distance from the land and from the primary source of food production, the abstraction of other humans who become substitutable contracting parties, and accountability to universal expectations and obligations. Motivation for personal loyalty to others engaged in the agricultural enterprise on which the common livelihood depended—that is, the impetus for intimate bonds among food producers, food consumers, and the land that sustains them—declined in the face of the different demands of industrialization, specialization, and urbanization. Following the decline of the manorial system, landowners increasingly produced for profit and on a contractual basis, but without, as Thompson (1998) notes, further political obligations. Rhetorics of social and civil engagement have regularly accompanied forms of economic expansion and conquest, such as calls for increased agricultural yield to feed the hungry. In the modern context, structural motivation to adopt innovations designed to increase agricultural yield and profit is strong. Innovation and profit as such now rival, if they do not actually supplant, modernist democratic socio-political ideals such as equality and justice, as well as considerations such as cultural continuity and personal loyalty, now viewed as traditionalist.

At present, food and ethics come into relation within the contexts of the global industrial food system, a transformed scientific landscape, and intensified conditions of higher global population and greater exploitation than ever before of natural resources for agricultural and other purposes. Once again, it is useful to recall the structures in which contemporary ethics as related to food is practiced. Norberg-Hodge, Goering, and Page (2001) point to the importance of the post-Depression Bretton Woods conference of 1944, where Western leaders sought to design a new financial underpinning for post-Second World War society, and which resulted in the articulation of imperatives of global economic growth and international trade cooperation. Thereafter the United States as well as European nations, such as France, which are food producing powerhouses but also massive consumers, further promulgated expansionist but also protectionist agricultural policies. The Bretton Woods framework established the International Monetary Fund, the World Bank, and the General Agreement on Tariffs and Trade, whose member nations would in 1994 create the World Trade Organization. In the name of development and free trade, the Bretton Woods agreements have served to promote exploitative and asymmetrical systems and structures. A result has been the funneling of resources from the global and post-colonial South to the global North, the channeling of wealth toward an ever-smaller number of increasingly powerful producers intent on financial gain, and the impoverishment and descent into hunger notably of the many small producers and others on whose backs the superstructures are built in neo-colonial arrangement. The spectacles of hunger and poverty have provoked responses in the form of political and charitable aid, yet debates about "lifeboat ethics," as well as documentation about impoverished communities in a variety of circumstances, raise doubts about the ultimate effectiveness of assistance that does not address the root causes of poverty and hunger (Lucas and Ogletree, 1976; Patel, 2007; Winne, 2008). Debate about food and ethics and about values now takes place within dominant structures that privilege commodification and consumerism as outcomes, but that also, within the global theatre, promotes unequal access to food products, the natural resources necessary for agriculture, and other goods.

Concurrently following the Second World War, both government policies and subventions for selected forms of farming, and new technological and scientific agricultural practices developed and supported in both university and corporate settings, served to increase food production by some measure, but at costs that are still being calculated. The "Green Revolution" multiplied yields of selected food crops through heavy inputs of chemical fertilizers, pesticides, and herbicides. The industrial agricultural practices depend upon natural cycles, yet do not complete them. The model of production is linear rather than cyclical, and it depends upon chemical inputs and monocultures. Early critics began to observe that industrial agricultural practices lead ultimately to the degradation of soils, pollution of the ecosystem, and a variety of human, plant, and animal ills (Carson, 1962; Lappé, 1978; Hardin, 1972; Berry, 1977). The subsequent generation of agricultural innovations based on genetic engineering has intensified ancient natural and human processes of hybridization and selection, moved genetic material among species that do not exchange genes in nature, and changed characteristics of species through genetic manipulation, in view of promoting or creating selected characteristics of plants and animals in agriculture and for food production, but also to further economic goals of producers. Problematic aspects and results associated with the "Genetic Engineering Agricultural Revolution" include the monopolization of seeds and other natural products and entities as property by corporations, loss of genetic diversity in nature, punitive measures pursued by powerful corporations that directly or indirectly target practitioners of alternative forms of agriculture, and the psychological and cultural unease as well as the dangers of a Faustian bargain with nature (Fowler and Mooney, 1990; Thompson, 1997; Ho, 1998; Shiva, 2000).

In the corporate industrial agricultural and food system, the scope of food ethics changes relative to older conceptions. Food-related activities and food choices of the individual and communities as well as of governments and corporations now always impinge consequentially—if often imperceptibly in the immediate term and local arena—on those of other people and other regions and on the environment. Today, considerations of food and ethics necessarily focus not only on the regulation of the self per se. They must further examine how the self co-exists with the Other, given different if not disparate interests, and within structures and conditions in which issues of responsibility and consequences are essential. The ethical innovations of Lockean social and political contractarianism interested in ideal terms of social cooperation, of Kantian universalism and deontology concerned with obligation to duty and rules, of

Rousseauist principles of justice and equality of process, and of the utilitarian consequentialism developed by Bentham and elaborated by Mill that takes as its business the "greatest happiness" as judged by outcomes, frame debates about food and ethics in modernity. At the same time, the notion of the autonomous or independent self, if a necessary fiction for forms of political democracy, becomes increasingly problematic in the real conditions of late modern society, in which nearly any action of an individual exerts effects, whether intended or not, upon others. Recent philosophies have, correspondingly, shown a particular preoccupation with relational issues. Lévinas (1969) "name[s] this calling into question of my spontaneity by the presence of the Other ethics," while Ricoeur, influenced by phenomenology and existentialism, argues for the active choice to "live well with and for others" (1992) and for the ethical intersubjective or mutual social "recognition" of others (2004). Yet who, and what, is the Other?

Within the peculiar context of industrialized, technical, and global society, ethics further expands its sphere beyond the human to include other species and the natural world, beyond the present time to consider future generations and future existence, and beyond local geographies to consider remote effects in far-flung places. This is not to suggest that issues of human goods and right actions have found their resolutions, but rather to state that it has additionally become necessary to consider, if only for the good of humans themselves, non-human entities such as soil, trees, and water as possible participants in ethics (Stone, 1974; Ferry, 1995; Shiva, 2002). These views broaden from more familiar ethical debates about non-humans, including whether animals should serve as food sources for humans and how animals should be treated in agriculture (Singer, 1975, 1999; Schlosser, 2001; Singer and Mason, 2006). The lasting and severe qualities of the effects of human interventions in the age of science and technology and within a populous industrial global society adds the issue of responsibility to the claims of posterity as well as of present-day actors to contemporary ethical research (Jonas, 1984). Moving away from the older, presentist, individualistic, anthropocentric mode, a variety of ideas and practices currently converges around the search for ways to redress natural balances; respect natural and cyclical processes and natural limits; conserve and nurture rather than exploit; and encourage cooperation, fairness, diversity, and community, rather than widely destructive forms of competition and totalitarian simplification (Beatley, 1994; Beatley and Manning, 1997; Nabhan, 2002, 2008a, 2008b; Lyson, 2004; Patel, 2008; Cobb, 2011). Food and ethics must now take as its business human goods, but also competing claims of other species besides the human and of the environment; future as well as present concerns; and sustainable interactions among economic, ecological, and cultural systems, and their relation to political institutions and social justice. Consideration of food and ethics in the broadest sense must encompass as its object or objects goodness, right action, and the good life relative to all spheres, phases, aspects, and circumstances of food, its production and its consumption.

Like other forms of ethics, food and ethics provides a basis for people, whether specialists or not, and whether acting alone or in community or corporative settings, to consider from the perspective of food how to conduct their lives and affairs. Within the complex circumstances of late modern society, it is clear that any possibility of rigorous and penetrating ethical reflection, much less of ethical action, reposes first and foremost upon knowledge, but also upon means and will, and that any inquiry about food and ethics depends on situation and structure. In order for a person to have or to develop an ethical relationship to food, that individual requires knowledge, not only to carry out a right action that has an immediately perceptible consequence, but also, as Coff (2006) writes, to abstract consequences of the choice that may not be immediately or locally perceptible. The conditions of the corporate industrial food system have made knowledge difficult to acquire, for the majority. The system has fostered the radical separation of food producers from consumers, while it has also attained an all-encompassing reach and extraordinary degree of interconnectedness from continent to continent, and shrouded processes of food cultivation, for example, in obscurity. Significant difficulties for food and ethics result. For the consumer, for instance, who knows nothing about noisome production practices and is, furthermore, not aware of his or her ignorance nor perhaps interested in overcoming it, food ethics is, as Coff (2006) observes, irrelevant. Functionally, for that individual, food ethics does not exist, nor is there a need for it. For the producer guided uniquely by a zero-sum vision of profit, on the other hand, ethics is perceived as irrelevant if not actually an obstacle or is perverted to suit claims that do not consider the welfare of the majority of people (Nestle, 2002, 2003; Brownell and Horgen, 2004), of non-human species, and of the environment. Society and the food system foster asymmetrical relationships characterized by unequal access to and control of information and means and goods, and are productive of market-sanctioned forms of censorship and other constraints that counter the pursuit of justice and liberty. In these conditions, the need for research, teaching, and public debate about food and ethics is clear.

Research methodologies

Scholarship in food and ethics is eclectic. One approach is to begin, at least rhetorically, with a grounding in a traditional philosophical or ethical school of thought, and then apply the concepts to the analysis of a practical question or situation whose parameters must also be thoroughly researched. The responses of Singer (1975, 1999), for example, to the question, "Should people eat meat?" pursue a teleological, utilitarian line of analysis, drawing conclusions that form a moral code that can be universally applied, in view of realizing what is considered to be the greatest good for the greatest number. It is by no means clear that such an approach is dominant. The move to reflection and research about food and ethics may stem from a far more general sense or from a particular experience of injustice, or from a broad interest in pursuing some course of action perceived as more virtuous than a present, unsatisfactory one. It is also the case that local conditions in which research and debate about food and ethics are pursued vary widely by location and among groups and themselves evolve constantly. While most countries across the globe do not legislate for the ethical treatment of animals used as food sources, for instance, the European Union does so, changing the terms and possibly the outcome of any debate. Like other forms of applied ethics, food and ethics must consider structure and circumstance as a part of analysis. Finally, work in food and ethics may emerge from a background in an area such as the law, or agriculture, or nutrition, which provides the deep knowledge of a specific field in which food and ethical issues can eventually be pursued. The scholarship of Stone (1973) about granting legal standing to natural objects has attracted the interest of environmentalists, but inasmuch as foods such as water and edible plants are natural objects, such work has implications for food and ethics.

Avenues for future research

The range of food topics and questions that deserve ethical analysis or continued research through ethics is nearly limitless. The list includes conditions of food production in its impact on workers and the environment, the issue of good food and its availability to people, analysis of food-related behavior and responsibility as connected with the science and politics of moral agency, the marketplace for food, food distribution, climate change and food, responsibility for feeding others, the science and culture of taste, genetically modified foods, food and biodiversity, and issues of transparency and traceability. Given the universal need for food, but also the contingent nature of available food choices for any person, and the inevitability of those choices having consequences for others and for the environment, the question of access to debate and knowledge about food and ethics will need to be addressed. Should food and ethics be taught in schools? If research in food and ethics can be situationist, occasional, and reactive, having an interest in ameliorative but also preventive consequences or outcomes, its utility for activism, social justice, and social change, is clear. An area that is ripe for development is the bridging of gaps between theoretical work, and the implementation of its recommendations and conclusions in the real world. Law and regulation, as well as culture more broadly, are venues to which findings in food and ethics could usefully be applied, although an array of forces oppose structural change.

Practical considerations for getting started

Researchers and students interested in food and ethics arrive at the subject from a variety of perspectives and approaches. The study of ethics as such traditionally takes place within departments of philosophy; however, applied ethics courses feature in a range of academic programs in the humanities, social sciences, hard sciences, and professions. Specific courses on food and ethics have historically not featured in universities, but have begun to proliferate recently with the gradual maturation and institutionalization of food studies more generally and as both public and scholarly interest in the topic increases. New undergraduate courses are currently being added in a variety of departments and faculties on topics in food and ethics and in the philosophy of food. Such classes provide a useful starting point for students to analyze the implications of their own eating patterns, for example, but also to draw connections between traditional works of philosophy and ethics and research in all aspects of food, agriculture, and the environment. The content and inflection of these courses varies widely, from, say, a focus on cultural and social aspects of food, to issues in nutrition, to the science and technology of food, and so on, and may not at all depend on familiarity with any literature that has been traditional to the study of Western ethics but that is not about food specifically. Applied ethical issues in different fields—legal, medical, environmental, and so on—occupy common ground with food and ethics, and debate about food can and should enter into these realms. Within the context of departments or institutes devoted to philosophy or ethics, recent years have seen an increase in conferences and colloquia specifically devoted to food ethical themes, while scholarly journals as well as the popular media, now interested in issues of food justice, expand the space devoted to food and ethics. Food and ethics is relevant in many traditional and newer fields, such as public policy, public health, political science, government, urban studies, rural studies, gender studies, anthropology, ecology, agriculture, sustainability studies, nutrition, molecular biology, genetics, and economics. Students and researchers can benefit from a variety of funding sources, from foundations, academic agencies, and institutes that address a similarly wide range of issues and disciplines.

Key reading

Aristotle (1995) *Nicomachean Ethics*, translator W. D. Ross and J. O. Urmson. In *The Complete Works of Aristotle: The Revised Oxford Translation*, vol. 2. Jonathan Barnes, ed. Princeton, NJ: Princeton University Press, pp. 1729–1867.

Beatley, Timothy (1994) *Ethical Land Use: Principles of Policy and Planning*. Baltimore, MD: The Johns Hopkins University Press.

Beatley, Timothy and Kristy Manning (1997) *The Ecology of Place: Planning for Environment, Economy, and Community*. Washington, DC: Island Press.

Bentham, Jeremy (1970 [1789]) *An Introduction to the Principles of Morals and Legislation*. Editors James Henderson Burns and Herbert Lionel Adolphus Hart. London: Athlone Press.

Berry, Wendell (1977) *The Unsettling of America: Culture and Agriculture*. San Francisco, CA: Sierra Club Books.

Brownell, Kelly D. and Katherine Battle Horgen (2004) *Food Fight: The Inside Story of the Food Industry, America's Obesity Crisis, and What We Can Do About It*. New York: Contemporary Books.

Carson, Rachel (1962) *Silent Spring*. Cambridge, MA: Riverside Press.

Cobb, Tanya Denckla (2011) *Reclaiming Our Food: How the Grassroots Food Movement Is Changing the Way We Eat*. Foreword by Gary Paul Nabhan. North Adams, MA: Storey.

Coff, Christian (2006) *The Taste for Ethics: An Ethic of Food Consumption*. Translator Edward Broadbridge. Dordrecht: Springer Verlag.

Crocker, David and Toby Linden, eds. (1998) *Ethics of Consumption: The Good Life, Justice and Global Stewardship*. Boston, MA: Rowman and Littlefield.

Deigh, John (1999) "Ethics." In *The Cambridge Dictionary of Philosophy*. Second edition. Robert Audi, ed. New York: Cambridge University Press, pp. 284–89.

Ferry, Luc. (1995 [1992]) *The New Ecological Order*. Chicago, IL: The University of Chicago Press.

Fowler, Cary and Pat Mooney (1990) *Shattering: Food, Politics, and the Loss of Genetic Diversity*. Tucson: University of Arizona Press.

Gottwald, Franz-Theo, Hans Werner Ingensiep, and Marc Meinhardt, eds. (2010) *Food Ethics*. Dordrecht: Springer Verlag.

Hardin, Garrett James (1972) *Exploring New Ethics for Survival: The Voyage of the Spaceship Beagle*. New York: Viking.

Ho, Mae-Wan (1998) *Genetic Engineering—Dream or Nightmare?: The Brave New World of Bad Science and Big Business*. Bath: Gateway Books.

Jonas, Hans (1984 [1979]) *The Imperative of Responsibility: In Search of an Ethics for a Technological Age*. Translator Hans Jonas with David Herr. Chicago, IL: University of Chicago Press.

Kant, Immanuel (1998 [1785]) *Groundwork of the Metaphysics of Morals*. Mary J. Gregor, ed. New York: Cambridge University Press.

Kemp, Peter (1997) *L'Irremplaçable: Une éthique de la technologie*. Paris: Les Éditions du Cerf.

Korthals, Michiel (2004) *Before Dinner: Philosophy and Ethics of Food*. Translator Frans Kooymans. Dordrecht: Springer Verlag.

Lappé, Frances Moore (1978 [1971]) *Diet for a Small Planet*. Revised edition. New York: Ballantine Books.

Lévinas, Emmanuel (1969 [1961]) *Totality and Infinity: An Essay on Exteriority*. Pittsburgh, PA: Duquesne University Press.

Locke, John (1988 [1690]) *Two Treatises of Government*. Peter Laslett, ed. New York: Cambridge University Press.

Lucas, George R. and Thomas W. Ogletree (1976) *Lifeboat Ethics: The Moral Dilemmas of World Hunger*. New York: Harper and Row.

Lyson, Thomas A. (2004) *Civic Agriculture: Reconnecting Farm, Food, and Community*. Medford, MA: Tufts University Press.

MacIntyre, Alasdair (1981) *After Virtue*. London: Duckworth.

Marino, Gordon, ed. (2010) *Ethics: The Essential Writings*. New York: Modern Library.

Mepham, Ben, ed. (1996) *Food Ethics*. New York: Routledge.

Mill, John Stuart (1998 [1861]) *Utilitarianism*. Editor Roger Crisp. Oxford: Oxford University Press.

Nabhan, Gary Paul (2002) *Coming Home to Eat: The Pleasures and Politics of Local Foods*. New York: W. W. Norton.

——(2008a) *Where Our Food Comes From: Retracing Nikolai Vavilov's Quest to End Famine*. Washington, DC: Shearwater.

——ed. (2008b) *Renewing America's Food Traditions: Saving and Savoring the Continent's Most Endangered Foods*. Foreword by Deborah Madison. White River Junction, VT: Chelsea Green Publishing Company.

Nestle, Marion (2007 [2002]) *Food Politics: How the Food Industry Influences Nutrition and Health*. Revised and expanded edition. Berkeley: University of California Press.

——(2010 [2003]) *Safe Food: The Politics of Food Safety*. Updated and expanded edition. Berkeley: University of California Press.

——(2006) *What to Eat*. New York: North Point Press.

Norberg-Hodge, Helen, Peter Goering, and John Page (2001) *From the Ground Up: Rethinking Industrial Agriculture*. London: Zed Books.

Patel, Raj (2008) *Stuffed and Starved: The Hidden Battle for the World Food System*. New York: Melville House.

Pedrot, Philippe, ed. (2003) *Traçabilité et responsabilité*. Paris: Economica.

Pence, Gregory E., ed. (2002) *The Ethics of Food: A Reader for the Twenty-First Century*. Lanham, MD: Rowman & Littlefield.

Pojman, Paul, ed. (2012) *Food Ethics*. Boston, MA: Wadsworth.

Preece, Rod (2009) *Sins of the Flesh: A History of Ethical Vegetarian Thought*. Vancouver: University of British Columbia Press.

Puskar-Pasewicz, Margaret, ed. (2010) *Cultural Encyclopedia of Vegetarianism*. Santa Barbara, CA: Greenwood Press.

Ricoeur, Paul. (1992 [1990]) *Oneself as Another*. Translator Kathleen Blamey. Chicago, IL: University of Chicago Press.

——(2004) *The Course of Recognition*. Translator David Pellauer. Cambridge, MA: Harvard University Press.

Rousseau, Jean-Jacques (1964 [1750 and 1755]) *The First and Second Discourses*. Translators Roger D. Masters and Judith R. Masters. New York: St Martin's Press.

——(1762 [1978]) *On the Social Contract*. Translators Roger D. Masters and Judith R. Masters. New York: St Martin's Press.

Schlosser, Eric (2001) *Fast Food Nation: The Dark Side of the All-American Meal*. New York: Houghton Mifflin.

Sen, Amartya (1981) *Poverty and Famines: An Essay on Entitlement and Deprivation*. New York: Oxford University Press.

——(1987) *On Ethics and Economics*. New York: Basil Blackwell.

Shiva, Vandana (2000) *Stolen Harvest: The Hijacking of the Global Food Supply*. Cambridge, MA: South End Press.

——(2002) *Water Wars: Privatization, Pollution, and Profit*. Cambridge, MA: South End Press.

Singer, Peter (1975) *Animal Liberation*. New York: Random House.

——(1999 [1979]) *Practical Ethics*. New York: Cambridge University Press.

Singer, Peter and Jim Mason (2006) *The Way We Eat: Why Our Food Choices Matter*. Emmaus, PA: Rodale.

Stone, Christopher D. (1974) *Should Trees Have Standing? Toward Legal Rights for Natural Objects*. Forward by Garrett James Hardin. Los Altos, CA: W. Kaufmann.

Stuart, Tristram (2007 [2006]) *The Bloodless Revolution: A Cultural History of Vegetarianism from 1600 to Modern Times*. New York: W. W. Norton.

Thompson, Paul B. (1998) *Agricultural Ethics: Research, Teaching, and Public Policy*. Ames, IA: Iowa State University Press.

——(1997) *Food Biotechnology in Ethical Perspective*. London: Blackie Academic and Professional.

Walters, Kerry S. and Lisa Portmess, eds. (1999) *Ethical Vegetarianism from Pythagoras to Peter Singer*. Albany, NY: State University of New York Press.

Warde, Alan (1997) *Consumption, Food and Taste: Culinary Antinomies and Commodity Culture*. London: Sage.

Winne, Mark (2008) *Closing the Food Gap: Resetting the Table in the Land of Plenty*. Boston, MA: Beacon Press.

Zwart, Hub (2001) "A Short History of Food Ethics." *Journal of Agricultural and Environmental Ethics* 12: 113–26.

Index

Abarca, Meredith 251, 252, 253, 256, 288
Abrams, H.L. 51
Abramson, Julia viii, 371–78
Academy of Nutrition and Dietetics 71–72
Accounting for Taste: The Triumph of French Cuisine (Ferguson, P.P.) 356
Adamick, Kate 335
Adams, Carol J. 106, 139
Adapon, Joy 277
adaptation, concept of 52–53
Adelman, Janet 123
Adema, Pauline 190, 192, 278
Adler, R.W. 240
administrative law 240
Adolph, Andrea 128
Adrià, Ferran 267
aesthetics: norms of food presentation in Japan 173; philosophy and food 135–36
The Aesthetics of the Greek Banquet (Lissarrague, F.) 171
African American D-Town Farmers 295–96
African American Foodways (Bower, A.) 286
agency theory 15
The Agrarian Roots of Pragmatism (Thompson, P. and Hilde, T., eds.) 139
agribusiness: food justice and system of 295–96; high stakes of 310
agricultural law 240
agricultural research, anticipating a new agenda for 364–70; biological organization, thinking about 367; clean, climate-benign fuels 366; ecological failure 365–67; economic sustainability 367–68; food production, real problem of 364; *Frontiers in Agricultural Research: Food, Health, Environment and Communities* (NAS) 369;

genetics 366–67; Iowa, farming incomes in 368; laissez-faire economic ideology 367; molecular biology 366–67; natural resources 365; pesticides 365; pharmaceutical crops 366; single-tactic approach 364–65; sinks in nature to absorb wastes 365; socio-economic adversity 367–68; summary of themes 364; sustainability 368–70; Sustainable Agriculture Research and Education (SARE) 369; symbiotic ecologically driven system 365–66; USDA Agricultural Research Service 365
Agriculture, Food and Human Values Society (AFHVS) 143, 271, 272
Agyeman, Julian 287, 291n14
Aiello, L. and Key, C. 51
Aiello, L. and Wells, J. 51
Aiello, L. and Wheeler, P. 51
Aiken, William 139
Albala, C. *et al.* 72n2
Albala, Ken viii, xv–xvi, 105, 114–21, 298, 358
Alimentum (LeMay, E.) 89
Alkon, A.H. and Norgaard, K.M. 297
Alkon, Alison Hope viii, 287, 291n12, 291n14, 295–305
All Manners of Food (Mennell, S.): culinary history 115; cultural history of food 104–5; senses, food and the 356
Allen, Barbara L. 296, 297
Allen, P. and Sachs, C. 251, 255, 256–57
Allhoff, Fritz 136
Allison, Dorothy 254
Allison, Margaret Randall 253
Altman, Donald 164
Amberg, S.M. and Hall, T.E. 29, 33
American Culinary Federation 271–72

health outcomes 49, 52–53
Heath, D. and Meneley, A. 8
Hebraic testamentary laws 372
Hegel, Georg W.F. 125
Heiatt, Constance 115
Heinz, B. and Lee, R. 29, 33
Heldke, Lisa x, 135–45, 251, 256, 298
Heller, T. and Moran, P. 123, 253
Helstosky, Carol x, 306–17
Henderson, J.S. et al. 77
Henderson, M.C. 31
Henderson, P.C. 322
Hendley, Joyce 278
Henisch, Bridget Ann 161
Henry, A.G. et al. 76
Herbert, George 123
Herring, E.P. 240
Hershey, Milton 232
Hershey Foods Technical Center 81
Heseltine, Marjorie G. 66
Hess, Karen 115, 153–54, 284
Hesse, B. and Wapnish, P. 79
Hesser, Amanda x, 89–100
Hilde, Thomas 139
Himmelgreen, D. 50
Himmelgreen, D. and Kedia, S. 53
Himmelgreen, D. and Romero-Diaz, N. 54
Hinduism 159–60
Hinrichs, C.C. 18
Hippocrates 104
historic cookbooks 116, 117, 118–19
historical perspectives: American studies, food and 209–10; animal rights and food studies 307–11; anthropology of food 3–5; archaeology of food 74–76; art, food and 170–71; communication, food and 27–28; culinary arts, foodservice management and 265–66; culinary history 114–16; cultural history of food 102–4; cultural studies, food and 275–77; ethics, food and 371–75; film, food in 177–78; folklore 221–23; food justice 296–97; food museums 229–32; food studies programs 201–2; gender and food studies, intersection of 251–54; journalism 90–91; law, food and 239; linguistics and food studies 147–48; literature, food and 123–28; nutritional anthropology 49–50; philosophy and food 136–37; public health nutrition 65–67; race, food and 282–83; school food 330–33; senses, food and the 353–54; social dimensions of food and nutrition security, exploration of 319–21; sociology of food 14; television, food and 188–89; theology, food and 160–61; tourism studies, food in 342–44
historical writing 94
Hitchcock, Alfred 182
Hjalager, A.-M. and Richards, G. 345
Ho, Mae-Wan 373

Hobsbawm, Eric 103
Hock, H.H. and Joseph, B.D. 149, 154
Hockett, B. and Haws, J. 52
Hoecherl-Alden, G. and Lindenfeld, L. 32, 33
Hoefkens, C. et al. 243
Hoffer, Peter Charles 358
Hoffer, T.B. and Welch, Jr., V 215
Hog and Hominy (Opie, F.D.) 283–84
Hoggart, Richard 276
Holden, T.J.M. 190
holistic perspectives 5–6
Holland, Peter 124
Hollington, Michael 127, 128
Hollows, Joanne 32, 33, 189, 190, 192
holocultural studies 7
Holtzman, Jon D. 5, 9, 279
Holy Feast and Holy Fast (Bynum, C.W.): gender and food studies, intersection of 252; literature, food and 124
hominid foods, interpretation of 75–76
honey, archaeology of 77
hooks, bell 257
Horowitz, Irving Louis 16
Horrell, David 162
Hosking, Richard 156
hospitality education 270
household food inventories 325
Houston, Walter 161
Howes, David 354, 355, 356, 358, 359, 360
Howlett, Caroline J. 252
Huey, T.A. 33
Hughes, R. 72n8
Hulsey, L., Gleason, P. and Ohls, J. 334
human diet see nutritional anthropology
Human Food Uses: A Cross-Cultural, Comprehensive Annotated Bibliography (Freedman, R.) 10
Human Relations Area Files (HRAF) 10
human subsistence, ecological impact of 78
Humane Farming Association 315
Hume, David 135, 136
Humphrey, T.C. and Humphrey, L.T. 6, 222
Hunger Overcome: Food and Resistance in Twentieth-Century African American Literature (Warnes, A.) 285
Hunter, Gina x–xi, 3–13
Hunter, Robert 330
Huntington, Helen 126–27
Hurston, Zora Neale 285
Hutt, P.B. 238, 240
Hyman, Gwen 122, 126, 127, 128

identity: expression through 220–21; food and 282–83; identity-value conferred by commodities 104; role of food in creation of 32; theme of 5
imagery, interpretation of 169–70
Imhoff, Daniel 313

and getting started 69–72; professional
associations 72; programs recognized by
Academy of Nutrition and Dietetics 71–72;
reading, key resources 73; research
methodologies 67–68; state health departments
66; sugar-sweetened beverages (SSBs),
consumption of 68; summary of themes 65;
training, education and 70–72; White House
Conference on Aging (1971) 66; World Public
Health Nutrition Association (WPHNA) 72;
Youth Risk Behavior Surveillance System
(YRBSS) 68
Pulido, Laura 299
Puskar-Pasewicz, Margaret 162, 372
Putnam, Robert 17
Pyett, P.M. 325

Qin, W. and Brown, J.L. 29, 33
qualitative research methods: communication,
food and 33; gender and food studies,
intersection of 256; sociology of food 21;
tourism studies, food in 348
Quandt, S. 55
quantitative research methods: communication,
food and 33; social dimensions of food and
nutrition security 318–19; sociology of food 21
queer theories 284–85

Rabelais 353
race, food and 282–91; *African American Foodways*
(Bower, A.) 286; American society, race and
ethnic relations in 283; Asian diaspora 284;
barbecuing 285; *Black Hunger: Food and the
Politics of U.S. Identity* (Witt, D.) 286; black
women, agency of 286; *Cooking in Other
Women's Kitchens* (Sharpless, R.) 284; *Cultivating
Food Justice: Race, Class, and Sustainability*
(Alkon, A. and Agyeman, J.) 287; *Eating
Identities: Reading Food in Asian American
Literature* (Xu, W.) 284; ethnic food and
foodways 288; ethnic relations in American
society 283; food insecurity, roots of 288–89;
food justice 287; foodways, complexities and
differences of 283; future research directions
288–90; historical perspective 282–83; *Hog and
Hominy* (Opie, F.D.) 283–84; *Hunger Overcome:
Food and Resistance in Twentieth-Century African
American Literature* (Warnes, A.) 285; identity,
food and 282–83; literature, food-related
themes in 284; *The Migrant's Table: Meals and
Memories in Bengali-American Households*
(Krishnendu, R.) 288; nativism, nationalism,
and race privilege 285; practical considerations
and getting started 290; queer theories 284–85;
race and food, intersection of 282; racial
formation theory 283; *Regional and Ethnic
Foodways: Performance of Group Identity* (Mussell,

K.) 288; research methodologies 283–87;
Restaurant Opportunities Center United 290;
social market for food 287; structural
inequalities and imbalances in power with
regard to food 290n1; summary of themes 282;
sustainable agriculture 287; theoretical
approaches 283–87; UN Educational, Scientific
and Cultural Organization (UNESCO) 283
Radical Vegetarianism (Braunstein, M.) 309
Ragas, M.W. and Roberts, M.S. 29, 34
Rahn, Millie 223
Raizman, D.J. *et al.* 270
Raja, S. *et al.* 299
Ralston, K. *et al.* 334, 337
Randall, Margaret 253
Rappaport, R. 4
Rasmussen, Susan 358
rational observation 354
Ray, Krishnendu 16, 48, 189, 190, 191, 277, 288
Ray, Rachael 266
Reader, John 102
reading, key resources: American studies, food and
216–19; animal rights and food studies 317;
anthropology of food 11–13; archaeology of
food 82; art, food and 175–76; communication,
food and 35; culinary arts, foodservice
management and 272–73; culinary history 120;
cultural history of food 110; cultural studies,
food and 280; ethics, food and 376–78; film,
food in 185–86; food justice 302; food
museums 237; food scholarship, historical
background 45–46; food studies programs 208;
gender and food studies, intersection of 258–
61; journalism 100; law, food and 246;
linguistics and food studies 155–56; literature,
food and 131–34; philosophy and food 143–45;
public health nutrition 73; school food 339–41;
senses, food and the 360–61; social dimensions
of food and nutrition security, exploration of
326–27; sociology of food 22; television, food
and 194–95; theology, food and 165–66;
tourism studies, food in 350–51
Reagan, J. and Collins, J. 33
Reagan, Ronald 332–33
Reber, E.A. and Evershed, R.P. 80
recipe and technique writing 92–93
Redfield, Robert 221
Redish, M.H. 240
Reese, William 330
Regan, Tom 136, 137, 139–40
*Regional and Ethnic Foodways: Performance of Group
Identity* (Mussell, K.) 288
Reichl, Ruth 95, 98
Reifschneider, M.J. *et al.* 20
Reinhard, K.J. and Bryant, Jr., V.M. 79
Reinholtz, Eric L. 182
Reitz, E.J. and Wing, E. 76

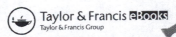